Dieter Beyer Ulrich Mödder

Diagnostic Imaging of the Acute Abdomen

A Clinico-Radiologic Approach

With Contributions by
G. Benz-Bohm W. Gross-Fengels A. E. Horwitz G. P. Krestin
R. Lorenz K. F. R. Neufang P. E. Peters H. Pichlmaier
W. Steinbrich F. E. Zanella

With a Foreword by H. Pichlmaier

With 250 Figures Containing 680 Separate Illustrations

Springer-Verlag Berlin Heidelberg New York
London Paris Tokyo

Professor Dr. Dieter Beyer
Department of Radiology
Krankenhaus Porz am Rhein
Urbacher Weg 19
D-5000 Cologne 90

Professor Dr. Ulrich Mödder
Department of Radiology
University of Düsseldorf Medical School
Moorenstraße 5
D-4000 Düsseldorf 1

Translator:
Terry C. Telger, 6112 Waco Way, Ft. Worth, TX 67133, USA

Title of the German Edition
Diagnostik des akuten Abdomens mit bildgebenden Verfahren
ISBN-13:978-3-642-71886-1

ISBN-13:978-3-642-71886-1 e-ISBN-13:978-3-642-71884-7
DOI: 10.1007/978-3-642-71884-7

Library of Congress Cataloging-in-Publication Data

Diagnostic imaging of the acute abdomen : a clinico-radiologic approach / [edited by] Dieter Beyer, Ulrich Mödder ; with contributions by G. Benz-Bohm ... [et al.] ; with a foreword by H. Pichlmaier.
p. cm.
Includes index.
ISBN-13:978-3-642-71886-1(U.S.)
1. Acute abdomen-Diagnosis. 2. Acute abdomen-Radiography. 3. Abdomen-Imaging. I. Beyer, Dieter, 1946- . II. Mödder, Ulrich, 1945- . III. Benz-Bohm, G. (Gabriele) RD540.D52 1988
617'.550757-dc19 88-28157

Softcover reprint of the hardcover 1st edition 1988

2121/3145-543210 - Printed on acid-free paper

We dedicate this manual with appreciation to
Gerd Friedmann, Cologne, and *Bernhard Swart,* Neuss,
for their inspiration, guidance, and friendship.

Foreword

That radiologists and surgeons work in close cooperation is in the nature of things, as it is the surgeon who is in the best position to verify radiographic findings or reveal errors. At the same time, the surgeon depends more than anyone else on precise diagnosis, accurate preoperative details of topography and pathology, clear description of the relative positions of neighboring organs and structures, and evaluations of function, e.g., by angiography. It was these considerations that gave rise to the idea of this book. The aim is to outline the applications of imaging techniques in examination of the acute abdomen, structured around key words, to give the student and the practising radiologist a conceptual framework for everyday use. This seemed to us all the more necessary in that imaging techniques are in a process of rapid technological development: new ground is broken and new elements are added every year. Appropriate and rational application of these techniques is essential, if only because of the multitude of possibilities available. The correct choice of techniques and the sequence in which they are used is becoming increasingly significant both to the well-being of the patient and to the economics of patient care.

Cologne, June 1988 H. Pichlmaier

Preface

Altes Fundament ehrt man,
darf aber das Recht nicht
aufgeben, irgendwo wieder
einmal von vorn zu gründen.[1]

J. W. von Goethe

The acute abdomen ist one of the most frequent, most dangerous, and most difficult ailments a diagnostic radiologist has to examine and diagnose. It is an everyday, recurring problem for the private practitioner and an interdisciplinary diagnostic and therapeutic challenge for physicians in the hospital setting.

The potential causes range from extra- or intra-abdominal disorders amenable to conservative, nonsurgical treatment to highly acute abdominal conditions after a prompt diagnosis demanding immediate surgical intervention. The outcome of many acute abdominal disorders is decided in a matter of hours, and often diagnosis can be a matter of extreme urgency.

Today the attending physician has to choose from a wide range of diagnostic procedures, because no other field of medicine has changed as dynamically during recent years as diagnostic radiology. An inexperienced physician on call - most patients with acute abdomen are first seen in the evening or at night, even if the symptoms start in the daytime - may find it especially difficult to determine the most suitable sequence of imaging modalities for a given patient ("tailored approach"). Because of their specialized training, it is the radiologists' role to guide the referring physician to the appropriate available examinations, reducing the time needed to establish a diagnosis and decreasing the number of examinations required.

This book, which was designed to serve as a quick reference aid in daily practice, draws on the 1974 publication of Swart and Meyer on plain radiography of the acute abdomen. However, the concept of plain abdominal radiography has undergone marked changes in the last decade, and we wish to show that the newer imaging techniques, most notably ultrasonography and computed tomography, now enable many conditions to be diagnosed earlier, more accurately, and less invasively, with a consequent reduction in the mortality rate. The new imaging modalities and interventional radiology have already greatly changed methods of diagnosis and therapy of a number of acute abdominal conditions and undoubtedly will lead to further changes in the future.

The material and case studies presented are designed to show the current status of diagnostic radiology in the investigation of the acute abdomen. The success of more sophisticated procedures, however, should not make us forget the simpler and less costly method of plain abdominal radiography. It would be unfortunate if this mainstay were to decline due to lack of practice in plain film interpretation, since plain radiographs have not at all been replaced by the newer imaging techniques. This is borne in mind in the staged approach to the diagnostic imaging of the acute abdomen that is presented in this book.

To keep this text within a reasonable length we have followed a pragmatic

[1] One reveres ancient foundations, but must not surrender the right to begin building elsewhere anew

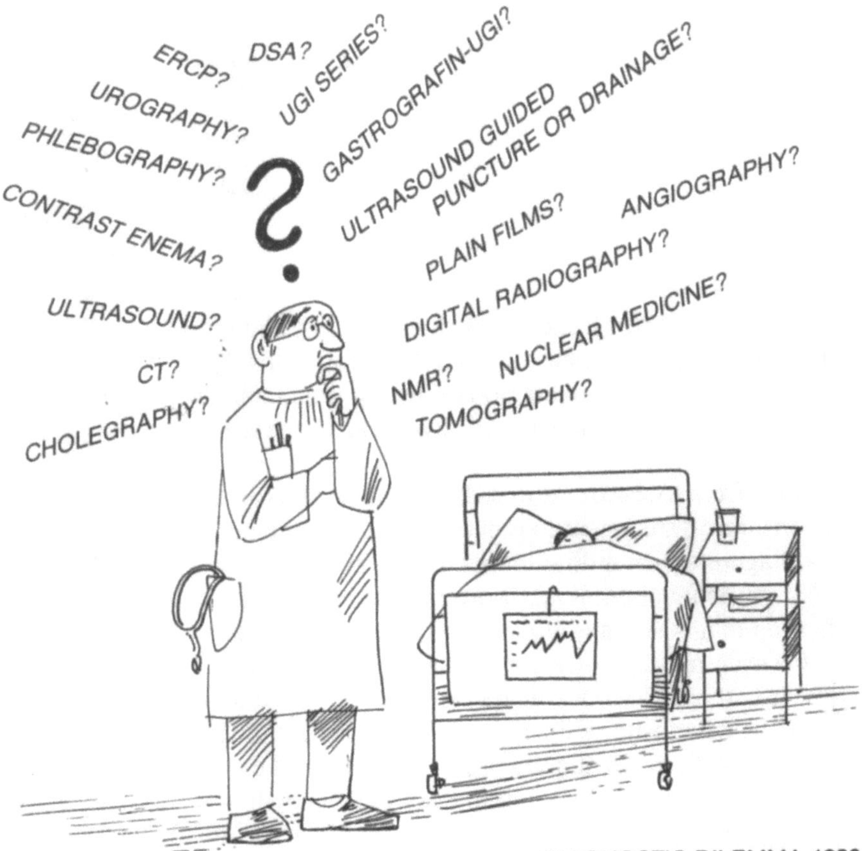

DIAGNOSTIC DILEMMA 1988

approach, giving short and clear presentations and emphasizing the most relevant symptoms and clinical problems. Overlap and repetitions between chapters were, however, necessary so that the various chapters, arranged according to methods, symptoms, and diseases, would each form a complete unit.

The importance of interdisciplinary consultation between the attending physician, the surgeon, and the radiologist is repeatedly emphasized throughout the text. The many years of close cooperation between the Departments of Surgery and Radiology of the University of Cologne Medical School provide an important basis for this. Daily consultations on patient selection and postoperative feedback have produced a continuing follow-up on the results of diagnostic imaging and have provided a mechanism for their improvement. For this we are particularly indebted to Prof. Dr. Dr. H. Pichlmaier and his colleagues.

We wish to express our appreciation to Mr. F. Textoris for his advice on photographic matters and for the processing of illustrations. We are also grateful to Mrs. Schreiber for providing the diagrams, and to Mrs. Milo for typing the manuscripts. Thanks also to the translators, Terry C. Telger, Walter Gross-Fengels and Hans Herlinger. We also thank Springer-Verlag, and especially Mr. B. Lewerich, Dr. U. Heilmann, and Mr. J. Sydor, for their courtesy and personal efforts in the preparation of this book.

We will be grateful if errors and omissions are brought to our attention.

Cologne, June 1988

Dieter Beyer
Ulrich Mödder

Table of Contents

List of Contributors

Professor Dr. med. Dieter Beyer
Department of Radiology,
Krankenhaus Porz am Rhein,
Urbacher Weg 19,
D-5000 Cologne 90, Federal Republic of Germany

Professor Dr. med. Gabriele Benz-Bohm
Dr. med. Walter Gross-Fengels
Dr. med. Gabriel Paul Krestin
Dr. med. René Lorenz
Priv. Doz. Dr. med. Karl Friedrich Rudolf Neufang
Priv. Doz. Dr. med. Wolfgang Steinbrich
Dr. med. Friedhelm E. Zanella

all the above contributors
Department of Radiology,
University of Cologne Medical School,
Joseph-Stelzmann-Str. 9,
D-5000 Cologne 41, Federal Republic of Germany

Dr. med Alfred E. Horwitz
Department of Radiology - Pediatric Clinics,
University of Würzburg Medical School,
Josef-Schneider-Straße 2,
D-8700 Würzburg, Federal Republic of Germany

Professor Dr. med. Ulrich Mödder
Department of Radiology,
University of Düsseldorf Medical School,
Moorenstraße 5,
D-4000 Düsseldorf 1, Federal Republic of Germany

Professor Dr. med. Peter E. Peters
Department of Radiology,
Westfälische Wilhelms University Medical School,
Albert-Schweitzer-Str. 33,
D-4000 Münster, Federal Republic of Germany

Professor Dr. med. Dr. med. dent. Heinz Pichlmaier
Department of Surgery,
University of Cologne Medical School,
Joseph-Stelzmann-Str. 9,
D-5000 Cologne 41, Federal Republic of Germany

1 Clinical Examination and Symptoms

H. PICHLMAIER

The acute abdomen is a syndrome of sudden onset that affects the abdominal and pelvic cavity and is generally accompanied by pain and other abdominal signs and symptoms. Its severity and propensity for rapid progression demand prompt, systematic evaluation and in many cases surgical intervention. Besides history taking, inspection, and clinical examination, imaging procedures are incorporated early into the diagnostic work-up and are of major importance.

Note: To interpret radiographs, sonograms, and CT scans of the acute abdomen correctly, the physician must know the patient's history and clinical symptoms (location and character of pain, rigidity, peristalsis). There fore, the *"clinicoradiologic concept"* is central to the diagnostic evaluation of the acute abdomen.

Equally important is the selection of an imaging procedure and the determination of its place in the sequence of diagnostic studies. Thus, for example, an enema with a water-soluble contrast material as the only radiologic procedure can immediately disclose the need for life-saving surgery in a patient with a perforated sigmoid colon. Overdiagnosis, on the other hand, can be fatal in the acutely ill patient (e.g., ordering CT scans for a ruptured abdominal aortic aneurysm).

Note: The examination ends when the diagnosis is made.

Note: There is no other acute disorder in which evaluation by *eye* (general condition, facial expression, surgical scars, rigid bowel loops, etc.), by *hand* (tenderness, abdominal rigidity, etc.), and by *ear* (hyperperistalsis, silent bowel, pathologic sounds such as vascular murmurs) assume such major importance as in the *acute abdomen*.

Despite the multitude of disorders that must be considered in making a differential diagnosis, there are several *typical cardinal symptoms* which characterize the acute abdomen. These are:

- Pain
- Systemic changes
- Disturbance of bowel function

History
- Family history (vascular disease, carcinoma, gout, diabetes, etc.)
- Prior history (previous operations, ulcer disease, pancreatitis, vascular disease, diabetes, or other metabolic disorders, etc.)
- Current history (description of symptoms - time of onset, type, localization, association with specific events, progression over time)
- Trauma
- Recent history of surgery (postoperative period)

Pain
The presence and characteristics of abdominal pain are of great diagnostic importance: spontaneous pain - provoked pain

Types of Pain
1. Visceral pain (aching, dull, colicky)
   Cause: stretching of a hollow viscus or metabolic acidosis
2. Somatic pain (localized, sharp, burning)
   Cause: inflammation, trauma, embolism of an abdominal organ

Character of Pain: Continous, occuring in waves, stabbing, plateau-forming, colicky, excruciating, etc.

Associated Symptoms
- Muscular rigidity in parietal peritonitis
- Pain aggraveted by respiration with epigastric disorders
- Forward bent posture in retroperitoneal disease
- Radiation to the ipsilateral shoulder with involvement of the diaphragm (phrenic nerve irritation)

Rigidity of the Abdominal Muscles
- No rigidity, compresses easily
- Reflex rigidity
- Induced rigidity
- Local rigidity from irritation of the parietal peritoneum with sustained contraction of the abdominal muscles
- Diffuse rigidity in diffuse parietal peritonitis

Note: Visceral peritonitis of the intestine does *not* produce abdominal rigidity. This occurs only when the *visceral* peritonitis progresses to a *parietal* peritonitis. Even with diffuse peritonitis the patient may show *no muscular rigidity*, e.g., with inflammatory processes in the lesser pelvis, abdominal muscular weakness, drug therapy (opiates?), high-dosage cortisone therapy, certain neurologic disorders, and in patients on respirator therapy (sedatives? muscle relaxants?) or dialysis.

Findings on Auscultation of the Abdomen
- *Normal* sounds associated with peristalsis of the stomach and small bowel
- *Increased* sounds associated with stenotic bowel lesions
  - obstruction of the small bowel
  - colon obstruction and ileocecal valve incompetence
  - enterocolitis
  - incipient mechanical bowel obstruction

- Sounds are *diminished or absent* with small-bowel atony,
  when secondary (e.g., renal colic, myocardial infarction, pancreatitis)
  in metabolic disorders (hypokalemia, metabolic, acidosis, etc.)
  in visceral or parietal peritonitis
  in the atonic recovery phase of mechanical bowel obstruction
  in bowel ischemia progressing to gangrene (stage 3)
  in paralytic ileus

Systemic Signs
- Prostration and shock
- Fever
- Unrest
- Reduced respiratory movements
- Nausea and vomiting
- Diarrhea
- Dehydration

Note: If we wish to translate the information contained in diagnostic images into a *diagnosis*, we can do this with some confidence only if we know the *local clinical findings* and *history* and can correlate the clinical results with the results of the imaging procedures. Otherwise, we may describe the radiologic signs without making a radiologic diagnosis. If the findings are equivocal, an interdisciplinary consultation with the referring physician is advised.

Because imaging studies of the acute abdome are *always* performed immediately after the clinical examination, they generally have to be evaluated without knowledge of laboratory data (white cell count, hemoglobin, hematocrit, blood gases, amylase, lipase, etc.). We will not discuss laboratory findings at this time.
With *abdominal complaints of unknown cause,* consideration should particularly be given to the following disorders:
Diseases of the stomach and duodenum
Diseases of the appendix
Hepatobiliary diseases
Pancreatic disorders
Diseases of the spleen
Diverticulitis
Colon carcinoma
Diseases arising from the genitalia and lesser pelvis
Abdominal pain from poisonings and metabolic disorders
Renal colic and acute inflammatory renal diseases
Peritonitis
Embolism or thrombosis of the abdominal vessels
Referred pain from diseases of the thoracic viscera
Lesions of the abdominal wall
Herpes zoster
Spinal disorders
Tabetic crises, etc.

Note: Pain *cannot* always be definitely localized to the upper abdomen, midabdomen, or lower abdomen, especially since the location of the pain may vary during the course of the illness. Frequently, however, conclusions can be drawn from the location of the pain and its character.

Guidelines for Differential Diagnosis

1. Upper Abdominal Pain

Gastritis
Gastroenteritis
Gastric/duodenal ulcer (penetration or free/confined perforation)
Acute and chronic pancreatitis
Acute appendicitis
Incarcerated umbilical hernia
Gastric volvulus
Reflux esophagitis
Basal pleurisy/pneumonia/pulmonary embolism/pneumothorax
Myocardial infarction
Obstructive lesion of the transverse colon (polyp, carcinoma)

2. Right Upper Quadrant Pain (Fig. 1 a)

Cholelithiasis
Choledocholithiasis
Acute cholecystitis
Gallbladder empyema
Perforation of the gallbladder (pain radiating to right shoulder)
Duodenal ulcer (penetration or confined perforation)
Acute pancreatitis
Secondary pancreatitis (pain radiating to the back)
Nephrolithiasis (pain radiating to the groin/testes)
Right subphrenic abscess
Acute retrocecal appendicitis
Liver abscess
Acute hepatic congestion
Hydatid disease
Right colon flexure lesion (polyp, carcinoma, segmental colitis)
Right basal pleurisy/pneumonia

Fig. 1 a–d. The most common causes of acute abdomen. ▷
a Right upper quadrant: *1,* acute obstruction of the cystic duct; *2,* acute cholecystitis, gallbladder empyema, emphysematous cholecystitis; *3,* cholelithiasis; *4,* duodenal ulcer; *5,* gastric ulcer; *6,* acute pancreatitis; *7,* renal and ureteral calculi; *8,* acute retrocecal appendicitis; *9,* right basal pleurisy/pneumonia; *10,* hepatic abscess, acute hepatic congestion. **b** Left upper quadrant: *1,* gastric perforation; *2,* acute pancreatitis; *3,* left subphrenic abscess; *4,* splenic infarction/rupture; *5,* myocardial infarction; *6,* left basal pleurisy/pneumonia; *7,* incarcerated hiatus hernia; *8,* left-sided renal disease, ureteral stone. **c** Right lower quadrant: *1,* acute appendicitis; *2,* mesenteric lymphadenitis; *3,* Meckel's diverticulitis; *4,* regional enteritis (Crohn's disease); *5,* diverticulitis of elongated sigmoid; *6,* cecal carcinoma; *7,* renal/ureteral calculus; *8,* right-sided acute adnex-

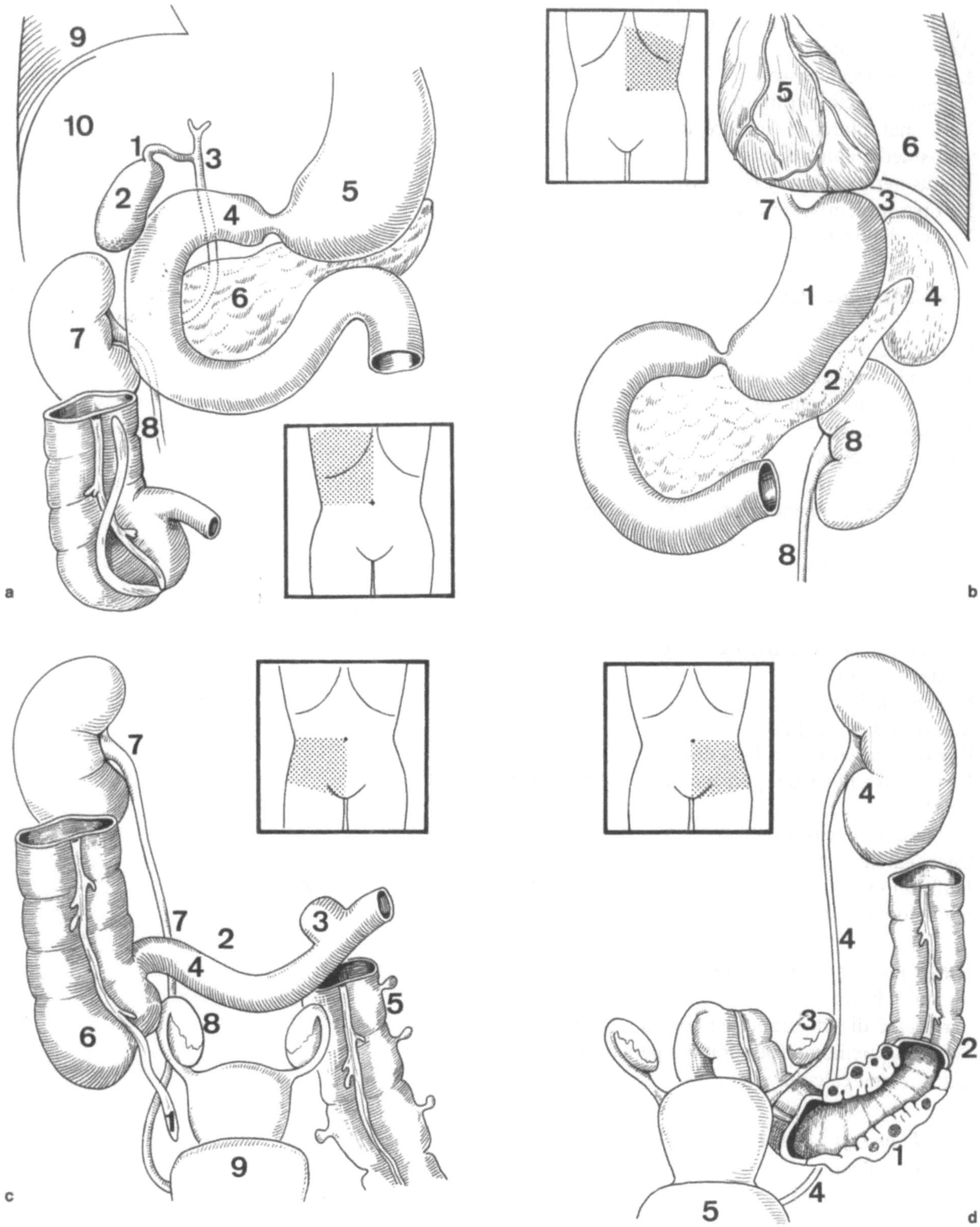

al process, ectopic pregnancy; *9,* acute urinary retention, acute cystitis. **d** Left lower quadrant: *1,* sigmoid diverticulitis, perforated diverticulum, perforation after endoscopic polyp removal; *2,* sigmoid carcinoma; *3,* left-sided acute adnexal process, ectopic pregnancy; *4,* left renal/ureteral calculus; *5,* acute urinary retention, acute cystitis. (Modified from Ungeheuer and Fabian 1984)

3. Left Upper Quadrant Pain (Fig. 1 b)
Gastric perforation (anterior wall)
Acute pancreatitis
Left subphrenic abscess
Splenic infarction/rupture
Left renal infarction/rupture/colic
Left-sided colonic disease
Hiatus hernia (usually painless)
Left basal pleurisy/pneumonia
Myocardial infarction

4. Midabdominal Pain (usually diffuse, poorly localized)
Small-bowel ileus
Colon ileus
Abdominal angina
Mesenteric ischemia and infarction
Nonspecific enterocolitis
Ulcerative colitis
Epigastric hernia
Penetration of an abdominal aortic aneurysm
Porphyria
Diabetic precoma
Lead poisoning

5. Right Lower Quadrant Pain (Fig. 1 c)
Acute appendicitis
Mesenteric lymphadenitis
Meckel's diverticulitis
Regional enteritis (Crohn's disease)
Peridiverticulitis from perforation of sigmoid diverticulum
Amebic colitis
Ileocecal tuberculosis
Cecal carcinoma
Perforation of the stomach or duodenum (which usually occurs more than 6 h before onset of pain)

6. Left Lower Quadrant Pain (Fig. 1 d)
Sigmoid diverticulitis
Perforated diverticulum (pericolic abscess)
Sigmoid carcinoma (perforation/penetration?)
Left ureteral calculus

7. Right or Left Lower Quadrant Pain
Ureteral calculus
Incarcerated hernia
Adnexitis
Tubal rupture
Torsion of ovarian cyst
Ovulation
Pelvic venous thrombosis
Acute urinary retention
Intra-abdominal hemorrhage (e.g., ruptured aneurysm)

Diffuse Peritonitis (Causes)
Gastroduodenal perforation
Perforated appendicitis
Perforated gallbladder (hydrops/empyema)
Hemorrhagic necrotizing pancreatitis
Prior pancreatic injury (rupture)
Perforating tumor in the intestinal tract
Traumatic rupture of the intestinal tract
Perforated small-bowel ulcer (typhus, potassium tablets)
Bowel gangrene (as late complication of ischemia)
Toxic megacolon with perforation
Iatrogenic perforation of the stomach/colon/uterus
Hematogenous peritonitis (children)
Gonorrheal or tuberculous peritonitis

Caution: An acute abdominal disorder can be mimicked by: basal pneumonia, pleurisy, pulmonary embolism, myocardial infarction, periarteritis nodosa, diabetic acidosis, hypoglycemia, uremia, porphyria, hemochromatosis, essential hyperlipidemia, Addison's disease, hemolytic crises, tabes dorsalis, herpes zoster, meningitis, abdominal typhus, lead or thallium poisoning, herniated intervertebral disc, withdrawal symptoms in drug addicts, and in patients on respirator therapy.

Reference

Ungeheuer E, Fabian G (1984) Das akute Abdomen. In: Aus der Sicht der Chirurgen. Dtsch Ärztebl 81: 345-350

2 Imaging Techniques and Systematic Image Analysis (in Adults)

(See Chap. 5 for Special Imaging Techniques in Children)

2.1 Plain Abdominal Radiography

D. BEYER, W. GROSS-FENGELS

A plain abdominal (supine and left lateral films) radiographic examination can be performed in any X-ray department or practice, requires virtually no patient preparation, and can be completed in about 10 min. Patient discomfort is minimal, and radiation exposure is a minor concern in cases of acute abdomen. Male patients can be protected with a gonad shield. Since the procedure is well standardized, the examination can be repeated at any time to allow comparison with previous films. The diagnostic results are influenced by the examination technique, image quality, and other factors.

Note: A standardized radiographic technique in two views is an absolute prerequisite for satisfactory, reproducible diagnostic results.

Radiographic Technique

1. *Supine abdominal film* (Fig. 2a), overhead projection using a low-kV beam (70 kV, 12:1 grid, high-speed screen) to heighten detail of organ contours, soft-tissue structures, and bone. The abdomen has to be imaged from the symphysis to the diaphragm.
2. *Left lateral decubitus film* (L Lat) (Fig. 2b), cross-table projection using a high-kV beam (125 kV, 12:1 grid, high-speed screen, Film-Focus (FF) distance 1 m).
3. Cassettes with a 35 × 43 cm format are recommended for imaging the region from the upper border of the symphysis to the diaphragm.

A 125-kV beam is used for the L Lat film to reduce contrast and avoid motion unsharpness in obese patients who require longer exposure times. This view does *not* produce a highly detailed image. Its purpose is to demonstrate free air, fluid levels inside and outside the bowel, gas bubbles, portal gas, and air in the bile ducts.

We do not advocate erect abdominal films, despite the requests of some surgeons, for the following reasons:

- Seriously ill patients are unable to stand and have to be examined in recumbency.
- Positional inconsistencies lead to diagnostic errors.
- Women and obese patients in particular show considerable lumbar lordosis when standing erect; this increases the abdominal diameter caudally and reduces image quality.

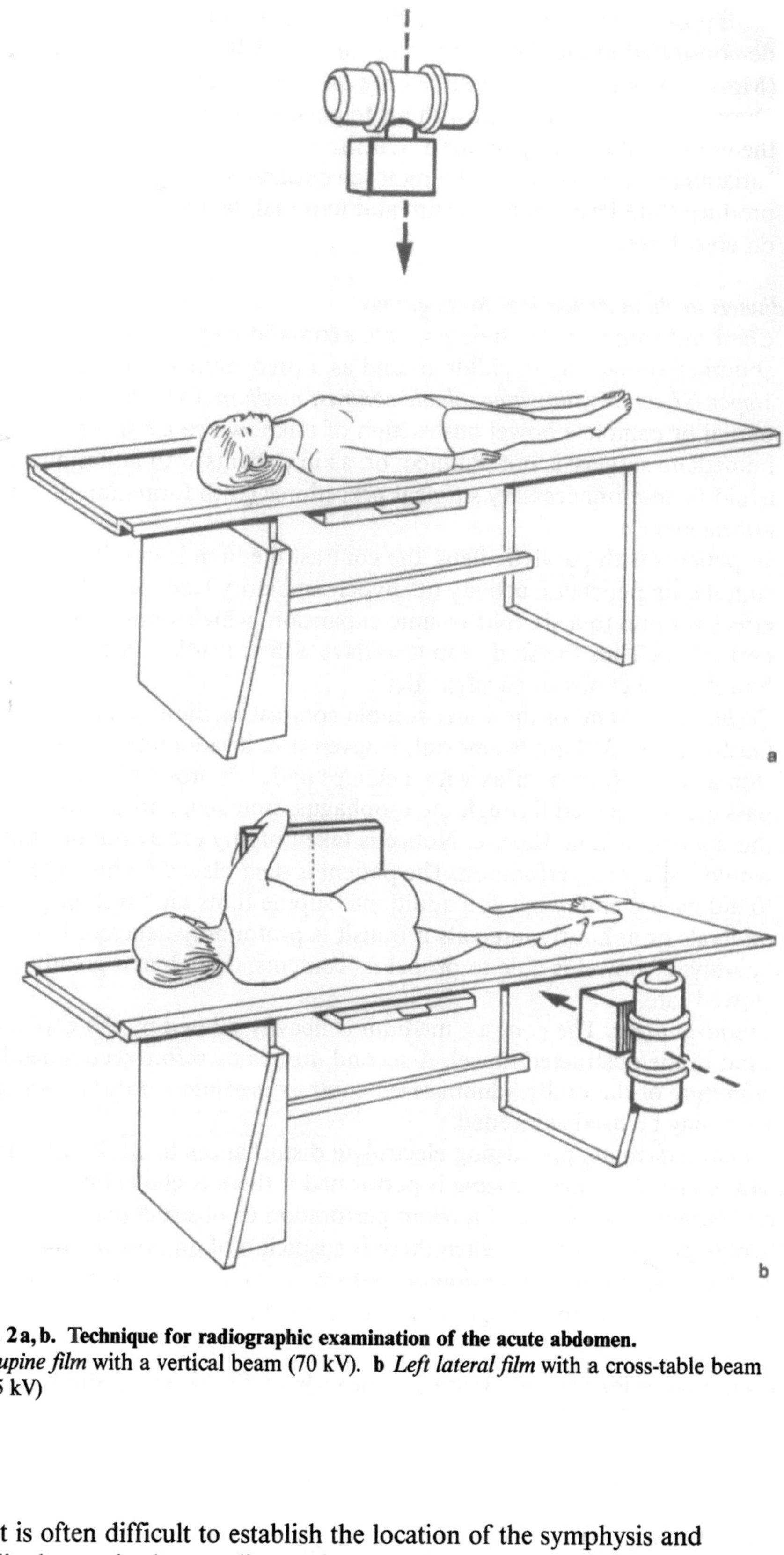

Fig. 2 a, b. Technique for radiographic examination of the acute abdomen.
a *Supine film* with a vertical beam (70 kV). **b** *Left lateral film* with a cross-table beam (125 kV)

- It is often difficult to establish the location of the symphysis and diaphragm in the standing patient, causing a worse projection.
- Free air can be demonstrated only beyond a certain minimum volume, because aerated lung in the anterior and posterior diaphragmatic recesses can obscure small amounts of air.

- With postoperative perihepatic adhesions, free air cannot be demonstrated in the right subphrenic area; it collects beneath the liver (Morison's pouch) and is visible only on supine films.
- Duodenal atony associated with acute pancreatitis is *not* appreciated in the erect position (only on the L Lat film).
- Inflammatory processes in the right lower quadrant (e.g., appendicitis) produce fluid levels in the cecum and terminal ileum that are *not* visible on erect films.

Adjuncts to Plain Abdominal Radiographs

1. *Chest radiograph:* to exclude possible extra-abdominal causes of acute abdomen (especially in children) and as a preoperative study.
2. *Upper GI series with water-soluble contrast medium:* for evaluation of partial or complete bowel obstruction of unknown cause where immediate surgery is not planned, or, as in patients with adhesions, to avoid further unnecessary surgical procedures (with formation of new adhesions).
   In patients with paralytic ileus, the contrast medium is capable of stimulating peristaltic activity (its hyperosmolarity leads to a dilution effect with up to a six fold volume expansion, which stimulates peristalsis). Thus the study can also have a therapeutic value in partial bowel obstructions or paralytic ileus.
   Technique: 100 ml of the water-soluble contrast medium (e.g., Gastrografin; 370 mg Iodine/ml) is given p.o. or administered by stomach tube (avoid reflux with a clamp) under fluoroscopic control. Its passage is observed through the esophagus, stomach, and duodenum to the duodenojejunal flexure. Notice is taken of any extravasations that would indicate a perforation. The patient is then placed on his *right side* to aid gastric emptying, and additional supine films are taken at 30-min intervals or at hourly intervals if transit is profoundly delayed. Even the "paralytic" bowel is able to propel its contents, though at a greatly slowed rate.
   Disadvantages: The contrast medium is heavily diluted by the copious fluid in the obstructed bowel. A second dose is therefore recommended. Vomiting of the orally administered contrast medium is rare; a gastric tube may be used as needed.
   Contraindication: preexisting electrolyte disturbances in adult patients.
3. *Water-soluble contrast enema* is performed if there is clinical or radiographic suspicion of a colon perforation or obstruction.
4. *Urography* is performed when there is suspicion of an obstructing ureteral calculus or a questionable retroperitoneal mass (sonogram may show unilateral renal congestion; see Sect. 4.4).

Recommendations for Systematic Analysis of Plain Abdominal Radiographs (Checklist)

Recommended sequence: "Bones and stones, gas and mass."

1. Supine Film

- Free air? (see Sect. 3.5.1 for radiographic signs)
- Bowel gas pattern? Isolated distension of a gastrointestinal segment? Combined gaseous distension of multiple bowel segments? (see Sect. 3.1 for radiographic signs)

- Evaluation of the bowel wall (see Sect. 3.2)
  Wall thickening?
  Luminal narrowing?
  Altered wall contours?
  Separation of adjacent loops?
- Pathologic exta- or intraperitoneal gas collections (Sect. 3.5)
  Free or fixed gas? (determined from L Lat decubitus film)
- Gas bubbles in organ parenchyma (liver, pancreas, bowel wall, kidney, uterus?)
- Intraluminal gas collections in tubular structures or hollow viscera? (gallbladder, bile ducts, appendix, renal pelvis, ureter, bladder, mesenteric or portal veins)
- Evidence of intraperitoneal fluid collections (Sect. 3.3)?
- Presence or nonvisualization of physiologic soft-tissue structures? (psoas muscle; flank stripe; hepatic, splenic, and renal outlines; structures of lesser pelvis; bladder; perivesical fat; rectal air) (see Sect. 3.6)
- Pathologic soft-tissue structures? (soft-tissue masses, pseudotumors) (see Sect. 3.6)
- Pathologic calcifications or foreign bodies? (see Sects. 3.7 and 3.8)
- Pathologic skeletal changes? (sequelae of trauma, bony metastases, spondylodiscitis) (see Sect. 3.6)
- Pathologic changes in the lung bases (if shown)?

2. Left Lateral Film
- *Free air* between the liver and lateral abdominal wall? In the right flank at the level of the iliac crest?
- Intra- or extraperitoneal *fixed gas?*
  With or without fluid levels?
- Presence of fluid levels?
  In what part of the gastrointestinal tract?
- Constant separation and bowel wall thickening?
  Rigid-loop sign (immobility of edematous bowel loops with position change)?
- Duodenal atony

Note: Systematic evaluation of the plain abdominal radiographs according to the checklist is essential; otherwise important features may be overlooked. Remember, however, that a consideration of radiologic findings together with the history and clinical presentation is necessary before definitive diagnosis is possible.

References

Friedmann G, Wenz W, Ebel KD, Bücheler E (1983) Dringliche Röntgendiagnostik. Traumatologie und akute Erkrankungen. Thieme, Stuttgart
Frimann-Dahl J (1968) The acute abdomen. In: Strnad F (Hrsg) Röntgendiagnostik des Digestionstraktes und des Abdomens. Springer, Berlin Heidelberg New York (Handbuch der medizinischen Radiologie, Bd 11/2)
Greenbaum EJ (1982) Radiology of the emergency patient. Am atlas approach. Wiley, New York Chichester Brisbane Toronto Singapore

Jansen R, Christ F, Schneider B, Engel C (1982) Wertigkeit der oralen Gastrografin-Passage in der Ileus-Diagnostik. Fortschr Röntgenstr 136/6: 641-648
McCort JJ (1981) Abdominal radiology. Williams & Wilkins, Baltimore London
Mindelzun RE, McCort JJ (1983) Acute abdomen. In: Margulis AR, Burhenne HJ (eds) Alimentary tract radiology, vol 1. Mosby, St. Louis Toronto London
Swart B (1984) Bemerkungen zur Untersuchungstechnik bei akutem Abdomen. Deutsche Röntgengesellschaft, Informationen 2: 2-4
Swart B, Meyer G (1974) Die Diagnostik des akuten Abdomens beim Erwachsenen - ein neues klinisch-roentgenologisches Konzept. Radiologe 14: 1-57
Watkins DT, Robertson CL (1985) Water-soluble radiocontrast material in the treatment of postoperative ileus. Am J obstet Gynecol 152: 450-455

2.2 Real-Time Ultrasonography

D. BEYER

Note: Abdominal real-time sonography frequently supplements plain film radiography of the acute abdomen und is therefore recommended as a *second examination*. It is available in most X-ray departments and practices. The ultrasound examination takes a maximum of 15 min, requires no special preparation, causes no discomfort, and avoids radiation exposure; it may be repeated as often as desired.

Caution: One drawback of sonography is that the results of the examination depend strongly on the triad of patient (obesity, overlying bowel gas, cooperation), equipment, and examiner.

Systematic Image Analysis (Checklist), Examination Procedure, Positioning

Note: In real-time sonography the examination of the patient and the systematic analysis of acoustic and dynamic phenomena are performed *simultaneously!* Permanent image records (Polaroid pictures, multiformat documentation) are made chiefly for the benefit of the attending physician rather than for purposes of primary evaluation.

Checklist

Note: All viscera or pathologic structures should be scanned at least in the longitudinal and transverse planes. Supplementary oblique scans often help to establish the diagnosis and can make it easier to assign an abnormality to a particular organ.

1. Hepatobiliary System

Liver: Size, position, and shape
Echo pattern
Contours (protrusions)
Masses (usually present as abnormalities of contour and/or structure
Solid mass: tumor, metastasis, abscess
Liquid mass: cyst, abscess, post-traumatic hematoma, biloma
Gas-containing mass: gas-forming or gas-containing abscess
Vascular system
Hepatic veins visualized? (if not, Budd-Chiari syndrome?)
Caliber of hepatic veins ("right-heart" failure)
Portal vein visualized? (caliber of vessel, thrombosis, collateral vessels)
Parahepatic space
Free fluid (ascites, pus, blood, bile)
Encapsulated fluid (abscess, ascites, hematoma, subcapsular hematoma)
Gas with reverberation echoes (free air, gas-forming abscess)

Gallbladder: Position, shape, and size. Hydrops?
Evaluation of wall:
Thickened (acute/chronic cholecystitis, other causes)
Thickened with hypoechoic fluid margin (acute cholecystitis)
Evaluation of contents:
Calculi, impacted cystic duct stone
Hyerechoic contents (sludge, empyema)
Gas (emphysematous cholecystitis)

Biliary tract:
Caliber of common bile duct larger than 4 mm?
Intrahepatic dilatation?
Outflow obstruction in porta hepatis or pancreatic head region?
Intracanalicular stones (with or without acoustic shadows)?
Intracanalicular gas (biliary-enteric fistula, gas-forming cholangitis?)

2. Spleen

Position, shape, and size (normal dimensions approx. $4 \times 7 \times 11$ cm)
Echo pattern
Focal lesions (solid, liquid, semiliquid?) (infiltrate, tumor, hematoma, abscess, infarction, trauma)
Parasplenic fluid collection (ascites, pus, blood, bile), shifts freely with position change?
Parasplenic gas (free air, gas-forming subphrenic abscess)

3. Pancreas

Can the pancreas be clearly delineated?
Shape and size
Echo pattern
Caliber of pancreatic duct
Calcifications (chronic calcifying pancreatitis)
Focal lesions (liquid or semiliquid, solid?)

Parapancreatic fluid or a spread of necrosis formation to the right or left pararenal space in pancreatitis.

Caution: A cascading, fluid-filled gastric fundus that projects posteriorly can easily be mistaken for a pancreatic pseudocyst or pancreatic hematoma.

4. Gastrointestinal Tract

Isolated fluid-filled stomach with food residue (pyloric stenosis)
"Target lesion" (circumferential tumor growth or other transmural infiltrative process)
Gastric displacement (by tumor, pancreatic pseudocyst, or hematoma)
Fluid-filled, atonic, or dilated duodenum (acute pancreatitis or cholecystitis, high mechanical bowel obstruction)
Paraduodenal liquid mass (pancreatic hematoma, abscess) (differential diagnosis: fluid-filled duodenal diverticulum)
Fluid-filled small bowel (obstruction, ischemia)
Progression of small-bowel contents (mechanical obstruction or paralytic ileus)
Thickening of small-bowel wall (target lesion due to ischemia, intramural hemorrhage, Crohn's disease, amyloidosis, lymphoma, peritoneal carcinomatosis, primary tumor)
Gas in the bowel wall (ischemia, pneumatosis intestinalis)
Fluid-filled colon (obstruction)
Colon target lesion (tumor, Crohn's disease, ulcerative colitis, ischemia, diverticulosis, diverticulitis)
Paraintestinal abnormalities (abscess, appendicitis, hematoma, free fluid - blood, ascites, pus, bile)

5. Peritoneal Cavity

Free fluid: ventral to the liver, in hepatorenal recess, parasplenic, in the paracolic gutters, retrovesical fluid in the lesser pelvis
Encapsulated fluid (position change): blood, abscess, ascites, biloma, lymphocele
Percutaneous aspiration under sonographic guidance?

6. Chest and Pleural Cavity

Pleural effusion, hemorrhage, empyema
Enterothorax from diaphragmatic rupture
Pericardial effusion

7. Retroperitoneum

Kidneys: Position (displacement?), shape (smooth, bulge, focal lesion?), and size (enlargement - acute renal failure?)
Dilatation of collecting system (congestion, cause of congestion - calculi, retroperitoneal masses)

Intrarenal mass (abscess, pyelonephritis with abscess formation, tumor, cyst)
Perirenal abscess (following renal infection) between the kidney surface and fibrous capsule
Pararenal abscess (usually due to extrarenal cause), less displacement with respiration!
Intra-, peri-, or pararenal gas collections in an abscess with acoustic shadowing or reverberations?
Sequelae of trauma - rupture or organ, subcapsular hematoma, pararenal hematoma, urinary stasis from clotted blood in the collecting system, seroma, urinoma?

Major vessels:
aorta - wall contour (arteriosclerosis) Caliber (ectasia, aneurysm)
Double-lumen effect, "third wall" (aortic dissection)
Course (displacement by para-aortic mass?)
Luminal cutoff (thrombus at bifurcation)

Inferior vena cava: Caliber (stasis? "right-heart" failure?)
Luminal contents (thrombus, tumor?)
Extrinsic compression (mass, abscess, hematoma)
Course (displacement by abscess, hematoma, tumor)

8. Lesser Pelvis

Bladder: Shape (indentation by extravesical lesion?)
Fullnes
Paravesical fluid?
Bladder calculi
Bladder tamponade (bladder filled with partly sonodense and partly liquid material)
"Snowstorm" pattern (small, floating blood clots), possibly with sedimentation
Bladder wall tumor with unilateral renal congestion

Uterus and adnexa: Consider ectopic pregnancy, tubal abortion and rupture, and ovulation
Exclude pyosalpinx and tubo-ovarian abscess
Watch for free fluid in the cul-de-sac (blood, ascites, pus, urine)

Prostate: Shape, position, size
Evidence of prostatic abscess?

References

Braun B, Günther R, Schwerk W (1983) Ultraschalldiagnostik. Lehrbuch u. Atlas. Acomed, Landsberg
Bücheler E, Friedmann G, Thelen M (1983) Real-time-Sonographie des Körpers. Thieme, Stuttgart New York

Dinkel E, Grosser G, Beck A, Brambs HJ (1986) Sonographische Diagnostik des Gastrointestinaltraktes. Radiologe 26: 144-153
Hansmann M, Hackelöer BJ, Staudach A (1985) Ultraschalldiagnostik in Geburtshilfe und Gynäkologie. Springer, Berlin Heidelberg New York Tokyo
Simeone JF, Novelline RA, Ferrucci JT Jr et al. (1985) Comparison of sonography and plain films in evaluation of the acute abdomen. AJR 144: 49-52

2.3 Computed Tomography

U. MÖDDER

Capabilities
Computed tomography (CT) allows the *direct* visualization of intra-abdominal parenchymatous organs, muscles, bone, and fatty tissue on cross-sectional whole body images in true scale and with exquisite differentiation of tissue densities. It surpasses other radiologic methods in its ability to depict density changes (due to edema, fatty degeneration, storage disease) and small fluid collections (ascites, abscess, bile) and to assign space-occupying lesions, abnormal air collections, and foreign bodies to specific organs.
Other *advantages* are:
- Minimal patient discomfort
- Acceptable radiation exposure
- Good reproducibility and documentation of results
- Accessibility of images to non-radiologists

Disadvantages are:
- High technical cost
- Need for specially trained personnel

Indications
For making or confirming a diagnosis after plain radiography and sonography in patients with:
- Questionable intra-abdominal masses
- Pathologic gas collections, uncertain soft-tissue structures, calcifications
- Suspected abscess, hemorrhage, traumatic lesion, foreign body

CT also permits a highly accurate topographic localization of lesions (peritoneum, retroperitoneum, abdominal wall, intra- or extrapelvic processes, etc.).

Systematic Image Analysis
The *systematic* analysis of CT images focuses on three aspects:

1. Morphology
Size, contour, shape, and position of the organs and supportive tissue.
- Generalized enlargement affecting the entire organ: Diffuse inflammation? Edema? Isodense neoplastic process?
- Focal enlargement of an organ: Tumor? Abscess? Hemorrhage?
- Abnormalities of contour and shape: Primary or secondary neoplastic process? Inflammatory mass? Hemorrhage? Bleeding into a preexisting lesion? Rupture? Infarction? Scar formation?

- Position of the organs: Displacement in the craniocaudal direction is more difficult to appreciate than in the lateral and anteroposterior (AP) directions.

Caution: Marked position shifts may be noted in the upper abdomen following surgical procedures.

2. Deviations from normal attenuation (density) values, possibly combined with changes in organ shape and contour

- The initial step is anatomic localization: Inside or outside a parenchymatous abdominal organ; in peritoneal or retroperitoneal space; in the back, abdominal wall, flank, or pelvic region?
- Fluid-equivalent attenuation values (5–20 Hounsfield units)
  Interpretation: ascites, lymphocele, urinoma, biloma, seroma, old hematoma, ruptured cyst
  Differentiate from necrotic, liquid tissue at the center of a tumor or abscess
- Focal density increase (60–90 Hn units)
  Interpretation: fresh hematoma or hemorrhage; possibly hemorrage within a neoplas
- Calcifications (>90 Hn units)
  Interpretation: calculus (urolithiasis, cholelithiasis), chronic pancreatitis, older, tuberculotic foci in lymph nodes or adrenals, calcifications in old hematomas, chronic calcifying pancreatitis, phleboliths, prostatic calculi, calcified, myofibromas, peritoneal carcinomatosis, metastatic or tumor-associated calcifications
  Differentiate from foreign bodies such as metallic clips, drains, residual contrast material, and projectiles
- Circumscribed lipomatous changes (negative attenuation values to − 100 Hn units)
  Interpretation: lipoma, liposarcoma
- Circumscribed gas collection
  Interpretation: abscess formation (20%–40% of all abdominal abscess contain visible gas), free intra-abdominal air from perforation, postoperative or post-traumatic collection, result of needle biopsy or embolization, pneumatosis intestinalis, foreign body

Caution: Gas collecting in joints and intervertebral discs may be a manifestation of degenerative disease.

Contrast changes after i.v. administration of contrast medium

- Yields information on the vascularization of a lesion, an organ or organ segment → no perfusion → organ-equivalent perfusion → hypervascularization
- Yields information on perfusion of major abdominal vessels → embolization, thrombosis
  In *abscesses,* two stages can be recognized. *Initial stage:* mass with relatively high attenuation value (30–50 Hn units) but showing no enhancement after injection of contrast medium.
  Mature stage: mass with low-density center (0–20 Hn units) but showing enhancement at its periphery ("rim sign").

Examination Technique

CT Scans Without Contrast Medium

The scans are performed from the pelvic floor to the diaphragm and may be centered on specific organs for selctive inquiries. The table may be moved in continuous steps or in an alternating pattern that bypasses intermediate areas. Details of the scans may be enlarged, as in evaluations for spondylodiscitis or intraspinal bleeding after trauma. The examination may be done in the lateral or prone position if pain is significant.

Contrast Scans

Oral: 500-600 ml Gastrografin, (sodium amidotrizoate, meglumine amidotrizoate) diluted to a 3%-4% solution, given about 20 min before the start of the examination.
Rectal: 100-200 ml Gastrografin in same concentration administered by balloon-tipped catheter.
Intravenous: Infusion of 100 ml Angiografin (meglumine amidotrizoate iodine 306 mg/ml); 200 ml is used for vascular imaging (aortic aneurysm, vena cava thrombosis). A bolus of 40-50 ml is injected for diagnosis of abscesses or organ necrosis (acute pancreatitis).

Note: The general contraindications that limit the use of contrast media - impaired renal function, cardiac failure, severe liver damage, latent hyperthyroidism - apply with equal validity in computed tomography!

Artifacts

With the advent of fourth-generation CT scanners with short scan times, rapid scan rates, and improved image quality, it has become possible to utilize CT for acute diagnosis. The frequency and severity of artifacts have decreased markedly. Most important are potentially disruptive factors associated with the object being examined:

- Movement by the patient (may require sedation or analgesic medication)
- Respiration-dependent artifacts, increased intestinal peristalsis (in obstructions), vascular pulsations
- Residual contrast medium (barium sulfate) or metallic objects (endoprostheses, internal fixation material, surgical clips).

System-related errors no longer play a significant role in modern CT scanners.

Radiation Dose

The "surface dose product" gives us an approximate measure of the absorbed integral dose. For a 30-section abdominal CT examination (230 mA, 8-mm section thickness), the surface dose product would be approximately 3000-4000 R/cm^2 and is comparable to the exposure received from a standard upper GI series or contrast enema.
If the ovaries in pelvic examinations are located within the primory beam, they receive a dose of approximately 15-30 mGy. The dose to the testes on direct exposure is approximately 20-40 mGy. The dose to attendant personnel in the examination room is negligible.

References

Friedmann G, Bücheler E, Thurn P (1981) Ganzkörper-Computertomographie. Thieme, Stuttgart New York
Heller M, Jend HH (1984) Computertomographie in der Traumatologie. Thieme, Stuttgart New York
Lee JKT, Sagel SS, Stanley RJ (1983) Computed body tomography. Raven, New York
Schindler G (1984) Stellenwert der Computertomographie in der radiologischen Diagnostik des akuten Abdomens. Röntgenpraxis 37: 48-57

2.4 Angiography

K. F. R. Neufang, P. E. Peters

Note: Angiography under emergency conditions means:
- A restless, uncooperative patient who is in pain and whose general condition is compromised
- Usually inadequate patient preparation (unclean bowel, gaseous bowel distension)
- Urgency - examination must be available 24 h a day
  Treatment must not be delayed!

Technique
Percutaneous transfemoral catheter angiography is standard. The transaxillary approach is an acceptable alternative only in exceptional cases because of its higher rate of complications and more difficult selective catheter placement.
Size French 7 catheters are preferred because they are easier to handle.
Digital subtraction angiography with selective arterial catheterization (selective IA DSA) has two advantages for emergency angiography:
- The immediate image display saves time. The subtracted image appears immediately on the monitor screen following injection of the contrast medium. In selective or super-selective catheterizations the "road mapping" technique makes it easier to locate the desired vessel.
- The improved contrast resolution makes it easier to detect contrast medium extravasation.

The successful use of IA DSA relies on optimum artifact elimination (pharmacologic immobilization of the bowel) and a DSA system with expaned postprocessing capabilities (mask and image integration, pixel shift).
IA DSA may be unsatisfactory in very restless patients, and conventional angiography may be required. Indirect transvenous DSA (IV DSA) has *no* place in emergency examinations of the abdomen.

Abdominal Aortography

Note: General abdominal aortography in acute abdominal vascular disorders is appropriate only in exceptional cases!

Indications
Suspected aortoenteric fistula
Suspected aorto- or iliacoenteric fistula
Suspected iliac AV fistula
Suspected renal polar artery (differential diagnosis: organ infarction)

Technique
Catheter type: French 7 (6, 5) pigtail
Catheter position: approx. 1st lumbar vertebral body
Contrast medium: iodine content approx. 300 mg/ml, non-ionic, e.g., iohexol (Omnipaque), iopamidol (Solutrast), iopromide (Ultravist), better tolerance, less pain and heat sensation
volume 40-60 ml
injection rate 10-12 ml/s.
Filming rate: 2 films/s for 4 s, followed by 1 film every 3 s for 18 s
Compared with traditional film techniques, IA DSA requires only 50% of the volume of contrast medium, with an iodine content of 300 mg/ml.
IV DSA has indicated only in exceptional cases (40 ml of contrast medium, 370 mg I/ml, 17 ml/s, central venous injection):
- Suspicion of a large fistula between minor vessels
- Calm and cooperative patient
- Minimal bowel gas

Selective Arteriography

Indications
Upper gastrointestinal bleeding (see Sect. 4.4.1)
Lower gastrointestinal bleeding (see Sect. 4.4.2)
Acute bowel ischemia (see Sect. 4.2.4)

Technique
Catheter types: cobra, sidewinder, renal, headhunter
Contrast medium: 300 mg I/ml, as in abdominal aortography
Filming rate (unless otherwise recommended): 2 films/s for 2-4 s, followed by 1 film every 3 s for 18-24 s

Celiac arteriography (nondigital technique)
Contrast medium 40-60 ml
Injection rate 8-10 ml/s

Superior mesenteric arteriography:
Contrast medium 50 (-80) ml
Injection rate 6-10 ml/s

Inferior mesenteric arteriography:
Contrast medium 18–25 ml
Injection rate 3–5 ml/s

Superselective angiography (branches of the celiac axis):
Contrast medium 15–20 ml
Injection rate 3–5 ml/s

Systematic Angiographic Image Analysis in the Acute Abdomen (Checklist)

Arterial vascular occlusion?
Main trunk, side branches: embolism, traumatic intimal rupture, dissection, thrombosis

Arterial vascular dilatation?
Traumatic or degenerative aneurysm

Vascular displacement?
Mass or bleeding into surrounding structures (organs, retroperitoneum)

Early venous filling?
AV fistula, angiodysplasia

Contrast medium extravasation?
Persistent bleeding of at least 0.6–6.0 ml/min, depending on vascular region
Free extravasation of blood: hollow viscus, retroperitoneal space, peritoneum
Extravasation confined to organ parenchyma
Detailed analysis - site of contrast medium extravasation
- Afferent vessel (anatomic variants!)
- Configuration of extravasated material (suggestive only): ragged, wispy; intraparenchymal, retroperitoneal; rounded, circumscribed pools; cavities

Organ displacement?
Hemorrhage: subcapsular, extra-/pericapsular, neighboring organs (like vascular displacement, see above)

Organ fragmentation?
Disruption of normal organ continuity (kidney, spleen, liver), usually interfragmental hemorrhage: most severe form of injury to parenchymatous organs following acute, blunt abdominal trauma

Parenchymal defect?
Traumatic infarction
Intraparenchymatous hematoma
Infarction scar (history? source of embolism? mitral valve disease?)

Slowing of blood flow?
Local:
- Nonhomogeneous parenchymal phase
- Intraparenchymal bleeding sites, edema
- Occlusions of small visceral arteries

Venous:
General slowing of arterial and capillary phase:
- Venous thrombosis
- Venous compression (extrinsic, hemorrhage, mass lesion)

Possible Sources of Error in Angiography of the Acute Abdomen

Incomplete arterial opacification, parenchymal defect
Differential diagnosis: embolism, thrombosis, organ infarction
Check catheter position: *reflux?* (e.g., short segment of celiac trunk) or *occlusion of side branches?* (e.g., catheter advanced too far, or short mainstem segment)
Perform abdominal aortography: exclude *polar vessels* (kidney!), exclude *anatomic variants* (liver!, e.g., right hepatic artery arising from superior mesenteric artery)
Overlying gas simulates parenchymal defect or nonhomogeneous parenchymal phase: perform subtraction or 2nd image plane (oblique, abdominal compression belt)

Increased contrast accumulation/staining
Differential diagnosis: free or intraparenchymatous hemorrhage, AV malformation
In parenchymatous organs: richly *vascularized tumors* (angioma, hemangioma), focal nodular hyperplasia (FNH), hepatic adenoma, highly vascularized metastasis, hypernephroma, angiolipoma)
In hollow viscera: hyperemia after *cleansing enema*
In adrenal region: increased contrast accumulation by *adrenals in* (hypovolemic) *shock;* direct organ damage is very rare.

Irregular organ contour
Differential diagnosis: fresh superficial parenchymal defect, infarction scar, anatomic variant, organ rupture, polar vessel, atypical arterial blood supply

Caution: in DSA, saturation artifacts due to image inhomogeneity may produce "burn outs" and thus simulate defects on an irregular contour of the organ.

References

Alfidi RJ (1974) Angiography in identifiying the source of intestinal bleeding. Dis Colon Rectum 17: 442

Athanasoulis CA, Waltman AC, Novelline RA (1976) Angiography, its contribution to the emergency management of gastrointestinal hemorrhage. Radiol Clin North Am 14: 265

Baum S (1983) Arteriography. In: Margulis AR, Burhenne HJ (eds) Alimentary tract radiology, vol 2. Mosby, St. Louis Toronto London
Bookstein JJ, Greenway GD (1981) Gastrointestinal hemorrhage: Angiography and transcatheter therapy. In: Teplick JG, Haskin ME (eds) Surgical radiology. Saunders, Philadelphia London Toronto
Friedmann G, Wenz W, Ebel KD, Bücheler E (1983) Dringliche Röntgendiagnostik. Traumatologie und akute Erkrankungen. Thieme, Stuttgart New York
Haertel M (1975) Röntgendiagnostik viszeraler Verletzungen nach stumpfem Abdominaltrauma. Thieme, Stuttgart
Lang EK (1979) Current and future applications of angiography in the abdomen. Radiol Clin North Am 17: 55

3 Radiographic, Sonographic, and Computed Tomographic Findings

3.1 Pathologic Gaseous Distension of the Intestinal Tract

Note: The gastrointestinal tract secretes approximately *8 liters of fluid* daily (bowel 3, stomach 2.5, saliva 1.5, pancreas 0.7, bile 0.5 liter). Virtually all of this fluid is reabsorbed.
In addition, approximately *50 liters of gas* accumulate from the swallowing of air (2), the liberation of CO_2 (15–30), bacterial gas production (15), and the diffusion of gas into the bowel lumen (15). About 95% of this gas is reabsorbed.

In all *pathologic gaseous distensions* of the intestinal tract, the accumulation of gas is related to the swallowing of air and to a mechanical or functional *obstruction to the passage of intestinal contents,* with an associated decrease in the reabsorption of gas. In addition there is a *fluid shift* into the bowel lumen, especially with mechanical obstruction, due to diminished fluid absorption by the bowel wall as a result of distension and progressive blood flow impairment. These pathologic collections of gas and fluid cause typical *fluid levels* to appear on the L Lat plain abdominal radiograph (Fig. 3 a, b). Fluid levels are a *nonspecific* sign and may result from mechanical or nonmechanical causes. They have diagnostic value only within the context of the clinical presentation.

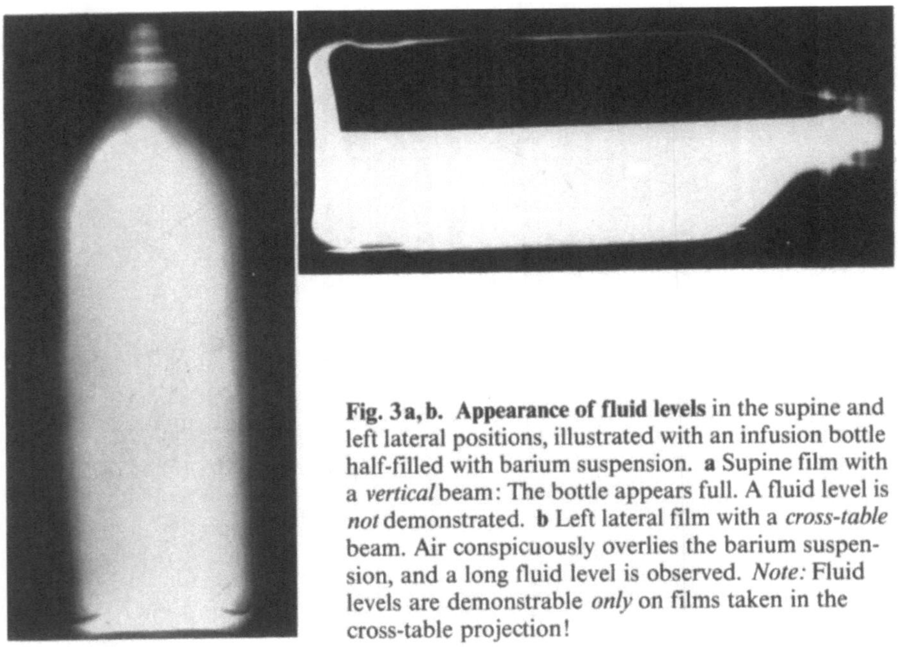

b

a

Fig. 3 a, b. Appearance of fluid levels in the supine and left lateral positions, illustrated with an infusion bottle half-filled with barium suspension. **a** Supine film with a *vertical* beam: The bottle appears full. A fluid level is *not* demonstrated. **b** Left lateral film with a *cross-table* beam. Air conspicuously overlies the barium suspension, and a long fluid level is observed. *Note:* Fluid levels are demonstrable *only* on films taken in the cross-table projection!

Note: A single fluid level may be very important, while multiple fluid levels may be inconsequential, and vice-versa.

3.1.1 Pathologic Gastric Distension

D. Beyer

Causes

Mechanical Causes
Gastric outlet stenosis (Figs. 4–6) → isolated gastric distension with a fluid level.
Peptic ulcer disease, neoplasms, gastric webs, gastric volvulus, tricho- or phytobezoars, narrow surgical anastomosis, and jejunogastric intussusception following a Billroth II resection
In children: congenital hypertrophic pyloric stenosis

Duodenal obstruction → gastric distension and possibly dilatation of the duodenum, depending on the site of the obstruction.
Pancreatic tumor, malignant lymphoma, renal tumor, duodenal carcinoma, foreign body, traumatic or spontaneous duodenal hematoma, superior mesenteric artery syndrome
In children: annular pancreas, duodenal atresia or stenosis, duodenal duplication, preduodenal portal vein

Nonmechanical Causes
Acute gastric distension (Figs. 7, 8) → isolated gastric dilatation with a fluid level.
Acidosis, diabetes, uremia, fasting, vagotomy, heroin abuse, ganglion-blocking drugs, complication of hypotonic duodenography with Pro-Banthine. May relate to a process adjacent to the stomach (gastric ulcer perforating into the omental bursa with abscess formation, acute pancreatitis), or to an intrinsic gastric disorder (acute phlegmonous gastritis, corrosive gastritis from caustic insult, postischemic gastric wall necrosis, vagotomy)

Radiologic Signs

Plain Radiographs
Supine film: The dilated, largely fluid-filled stomach presents as a large, supramesocolic, soft-tissue mass in the upper abdomen that displaces the transverse colon inferiorly → "ground-glass" density of the abdomen (Fig. 8a–c). Gaseous contents may predominate. The greater curvature of the stomach may extend into the lower abdomen (Figs. 4, 8a, c).
With mechanical gastric outlet obstruction, little or no gas is visible in the remainder of the bowel (Fig. 5). The upper abdominal viscera are not displaced, and the renal and psoas muscle contours are not seen. If findings are equivocal, gastric contents may be aspirated with a tube, or a Gastrografin upper GI series may be obtained for selected patients (Fig. 6). In rare cases the inner contour of the stomach is outlined by intraluminal gas ("air luminogram"), allowing visualization of large ulcers, tumors, polyps, or bezoars (Fig. 86a).

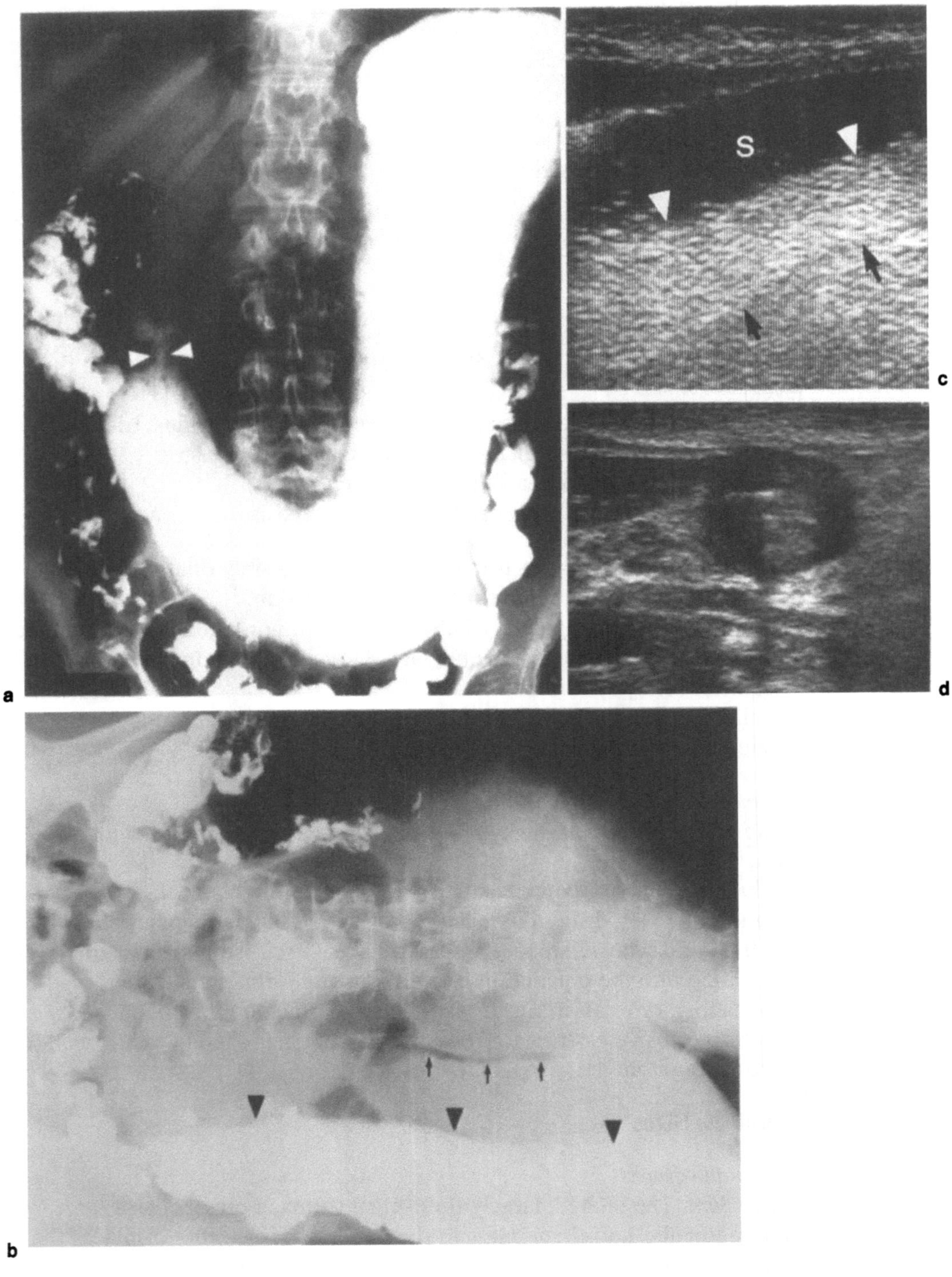

Fig. 4a–d. Pathologic gastric distension secondary to pyloric stenosis in a 72-year-old woman with epigastric pain and recurrent vomiting. A barium upper GI series had been performed 24 h earlier. **a** On *supine film* the dilated, barium-filled stomach sags into the lesser pelvis and exhibits a stenotic area in the presumed position of the pylorus (▶ ◀). **b** *Left lateral film* shows no free air. Double fluid level in the stomach. A long, more posterior fluid level is produced by sedimentation of the barium sulfate (▶). A second air-fluid level is seen under the lesser curvature (→). **c** *Sonogram,* left parasagittal longitudinal scan, shows a markedly dilated stomach *(S)* containing mobile, echogenic material with sedimentation posteriorly (▶). The posterior gastric wall appears as a thin, less echogenic structure (→). **d** Longitudinal right paramedian scan shows a complete target lesion with a small residual lumen. A prepyloric antral carcinoma was found at *operation*

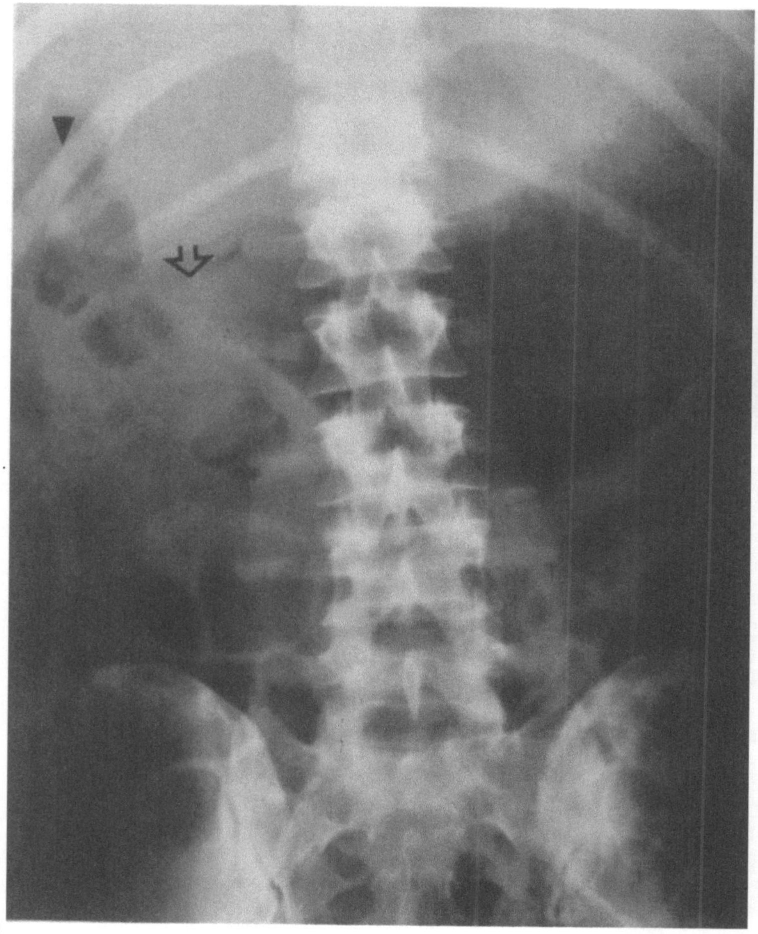

a

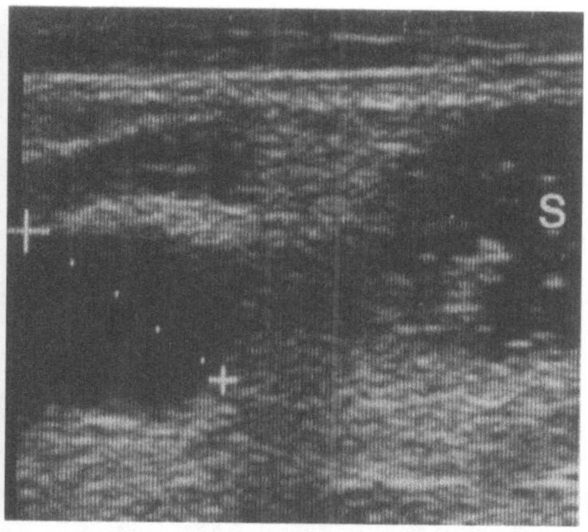

b

Fig. 5 a, b. Pathologic gastric distension of mechanical etiology in a 52-year-old man who had constant postoperative vomiting after a partial hepatic resection for tumor. **a** *Supine film* shows isolated gastric distension with cutoff of the gas column on the right side of the spine (⇨). There is marked elevation of the hepatic flexure following resection of the right lobe of the liver (▶) with otherwise nonspecific gaseous bowel distension. **b** *Sonogram,* transverse scan through the upper abdomen below the left hepatic lobe, shows a markedly fluid- and debris-filled stomach (*S*). A fluid collection 4.5 cm in diameter is visible in the region of the gastric outlet. *Operation* disclosed pyloric stenosis caused by a postoperative biloma

L Lat film: A fluid level in the gastric position outlines the lesser curvature and antrum to the pylorus. Extreme dilatation may produce an elongated fluid level (depending on gas content) projected onto the right iliac fossa and lower flank stripe (Figs. 4, 8).

Sonography

The gas-distended, atonic stomach is usually an *obstacle* to upper abdominal sonography, producing a strong echo front below the abdominal wall with acoustic shadowing and reverberation echoes (Fig. 4 c).

Sonography in the *erect position* displaces the gas upward into the gastric fundus; this may make it easier to identify the stomach and its contents.

In *gastric outlet stenosis* the dilated, fluid-filled stomach has multiple, bright, mobile food particles ("snowstorm" pattern). With a high-grade distension, the gastric wall is not delineated by ultrasound. The cause of the stenosis presents as a complete or incomplete *gastric target lesion* (due to tumor, large ulcer, lymphoma) (Fig. 4 d).

With a *duodenal obstruction* the cause is frequently apparent: pancreatic tumor, lymph node conglomerates, renal tumor, duodenal target lesion caused by transmural process, periduodenal hematoma (Figs. 10, 11).

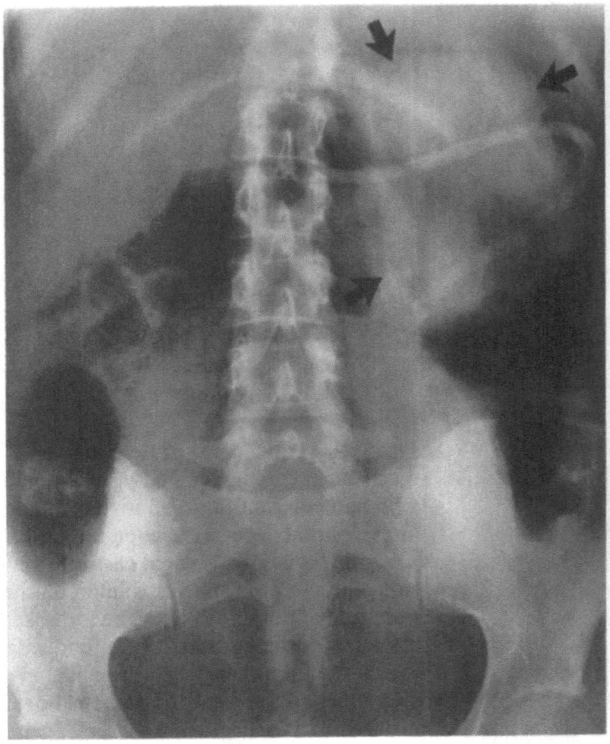
a

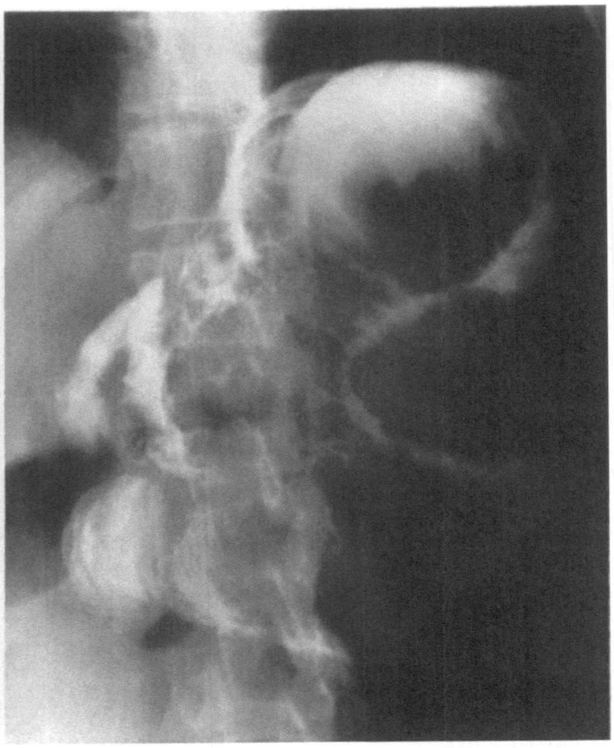
b

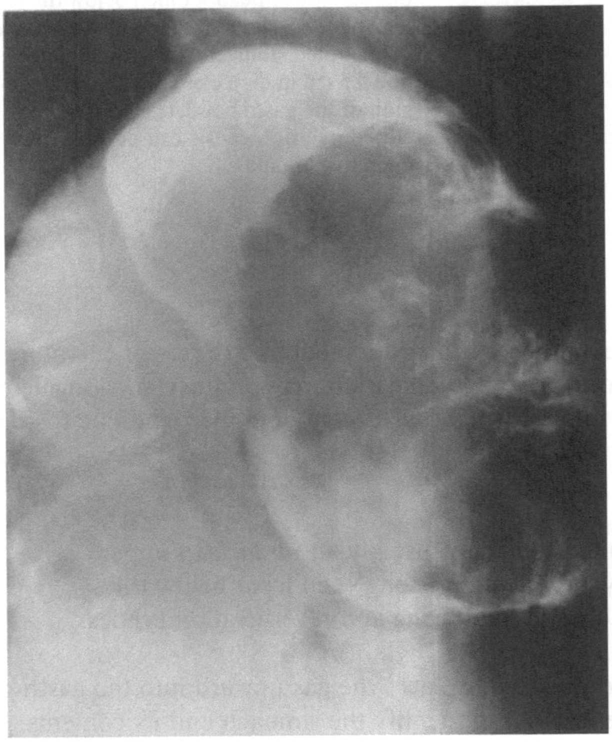
c

Fig. 6a–c. Pathologic gastric distension caused by jejunogastric intussusception in a 55-year-old man who had undergone a Billroth II resection 8 years earlier. Patient presented with increasing blood-stained vomiting of 12-h duration; he was unable to eat. **a** *Supine film* shows nonspecific gaseous bowel distension with a soft-tissue mass in the gastric position (➧), gastric tube. No gas is seen in the gastric region. **b, c** *Gastrografin UGI series,* which provoked continual vomiting, shows cord-like soft-tissue masses with convoluted outlines filling the stomach. Operation confirmed jejunogastric intussusception

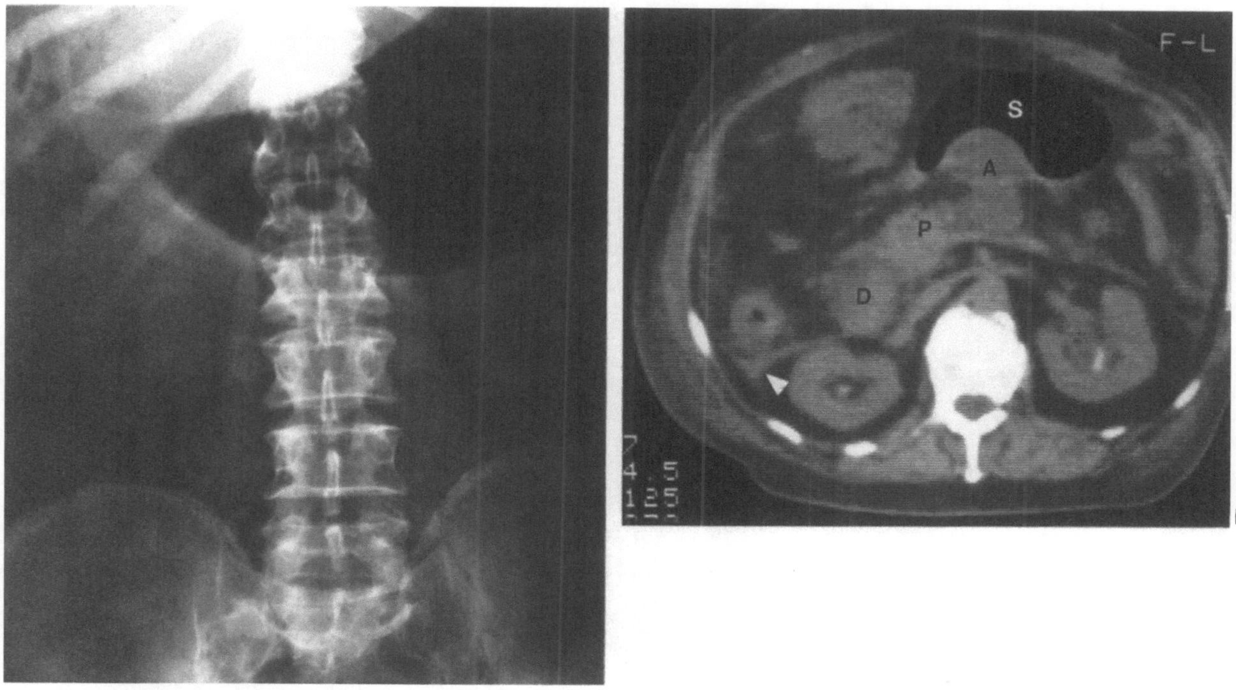

a b

Fig. 7a, b. Pathologic gastric distension of nonmechanical etiology caused by an abscess in the omental bursa. This 67-year-old man had undergone a partial hepatectomy for hepatocellular carcinoma and experienced midabdominal pain 5 days postoperatively. Patient was afebrile. **a** *Supine film* shows an atonic, gas-filled stomach and a gasless abdomen. Sonograms (not shown) demonstrated a fluid-filled mass in the pancreatic region, raising the suspicion of postoperative hematoma. **b** *CT scan* shows a soft-tissue mass *(A)* between the pancreas *(P)* and stomach *(S)* in the omental bursa that impresses upon the posterior gastric wall (*D*, duodenum). There is also an accentuated pattern of striation and reticulation in the right midabdomen and thickening of the retroperitoneal fascia (►) following the partial hepatic resection. *Operation* disclosed a postoperative abscess in the omental bursa

Computed Tomography

CT is *not* a primary study for demonstrating signs of gastric distension, but it can frequently establish the primary cause (Fig. 7b). Scans show a gas-filled cavity in the upper abdomen, occupying the position of the stomach and containing a fluid level (supine position). The distended gastric wall is poorly delineated. Mechanical causes of gastric distension are easily recognized and can be related to a specific organ or disease (e.g., antral carcinoma, pancreatitis, abscess, lymphoma, etc.).

In the hugely distended stomach with predominantly gaseous contents, the "mass" is often difficult to classify. A fluid level is indicative of the stomach. Doubts can be resolved by inserting a gastric tube or by giving diluted, water-soluble contrast medium.

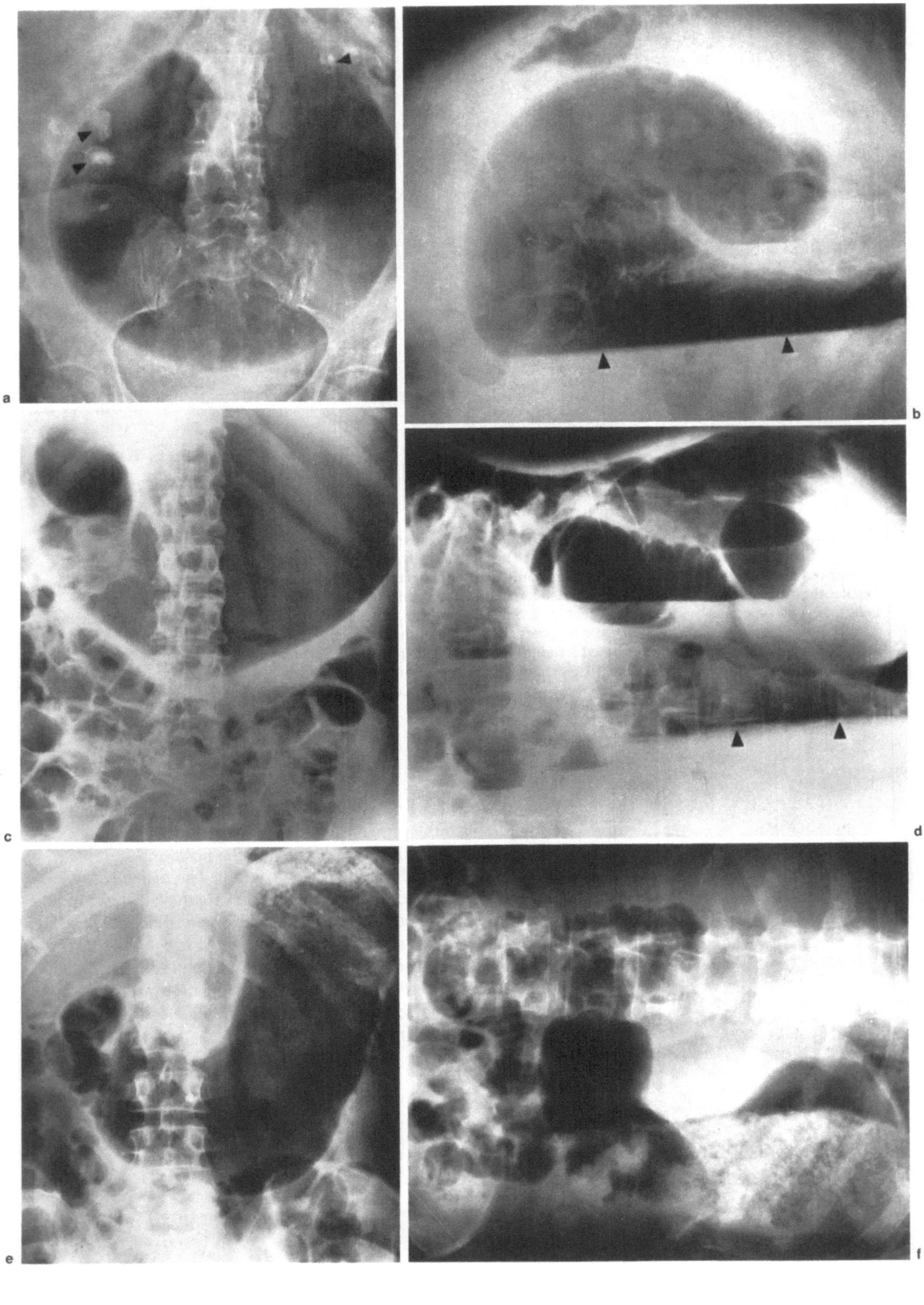
a
b
c
d
e
f

◁ **Fig. 8a–f. Pathologic gastric distension** of nonmechanical etiology. **a** Woman, 72 years of age, with bilateral nephrolithiasis (▶) and uremia, vomiting, and abdominal distension. *Supine film* shows large, oval-shaped, gas-containing mass in the mid- and upper abdomen extending down into the pelvis. **b** *On left lateral* the position and shape of the mass signify an enormously distended stomach with a long fluid level under the lesser curvature (▶). **c, d Pathologic gastric distension** of nonmechanical etiology in diabetic precoma. Man, 52 years of age, with a massively distended, nonrigid abdomen and silent bowel. **c** On *supine film* the massive gastric distension appears as a supramesocolic epigastric mass displacing the distended transverse colon downwards. There is concomitant distension of the small bowel. **d** *Left lateral film* shows a long fluid level in the stomach (▶) without evidence of free air. Additional fluid levels are visible in the duodenum and small bowel. **e, f Pathologic gastric distension** of nonmechanical etiology in a 42-year-old man who had undergone vagotomy 4 weeks earlier. Patient suffered unexplained epigastric and cardiac pain which was most pronounced after meals. **e** *Supine film* shows marked gastric distension with accompanying distension of the colon. **f** *Left lateral film* shows a long fluid level in the stomach produced by fluid and food residue. Free air is not demonstrated. There is moderate small-bowel distension without fluid levels

3.1.2 Duodenal Distension

D. Beyer

Causes

Distension limited to the duodenum

- Acute pancreatitis (see Sect. 4.1.2)
- Acute cholecystitis (see Sect. 4.1.1)
- Regional enteritis of the duodenum
- Scleroderma
- Lupus erythematosus
- Prior radiation to the duodenum
- Abscess in proximity to the duodenum (see Sect. 4.1.5.1)

Combined duodenal and gastric distension

- High mechanical bowel obstruction (involving the jejunum) (Figs. 12, 156, 157) or the same factors which cause isolated duodenal distension

Duodenal distension combined with distension of the ileum and cecum

- Mesenteric lymphadenitis (e.g. *Yersinia* infections) (see Figs. 127c, 134)

Radiologic Signs

Plain Radiographs

Supine film: Duodenal distension is almost never appreciated on the supine film!

L Lat film: With the left side down, air rises from the gastric fundus into the duodenum. Gas transport into the small bowel is absent or delayed because of atony. A gasless abdomen does not exclude duodenal atony: test by administering a gas-forming agent (Fig. 9).
Acute pancreatitis produces a smoothing or a double contour of the medial border of the duodenum with deformity caused by the enlarged head of the pancreas. The lateral aspect of the duodenum appears normal (Fig. 10a).

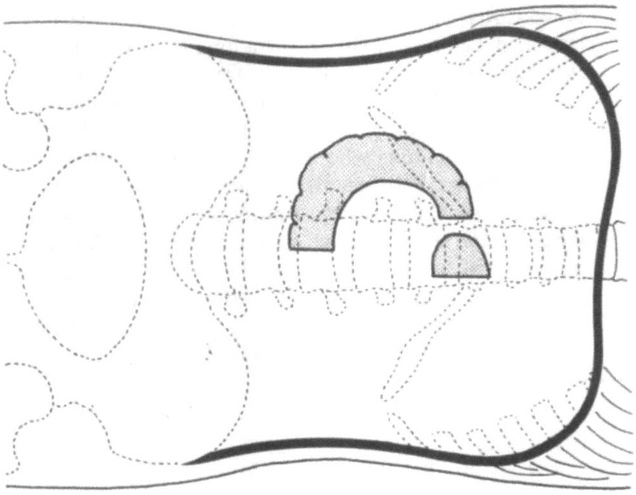

Fig. 9. Schematic representation of **duodenal distension** on the left lateral abdominal radiograph. One must be alert for a flattened or double-contoured appearance of the medial border of the duodenum caused by enlargement and protrusion of the head of the pancreas

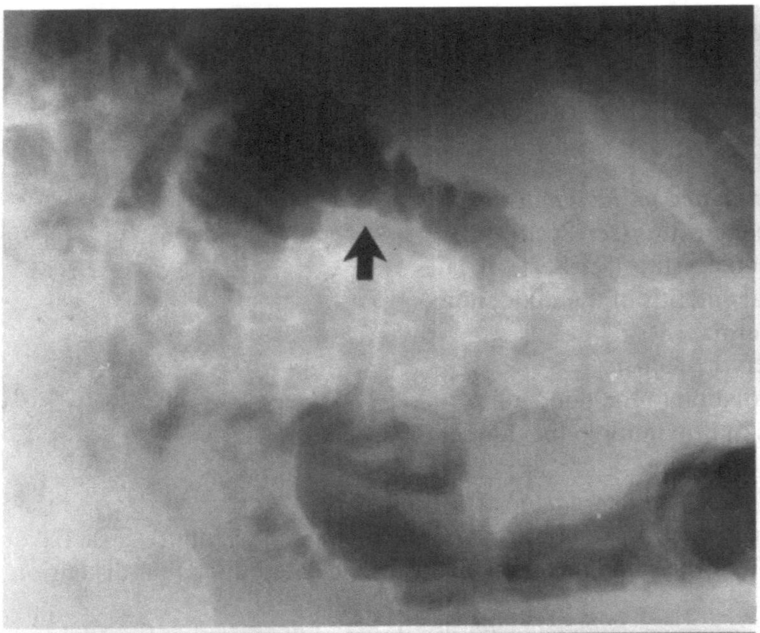

a

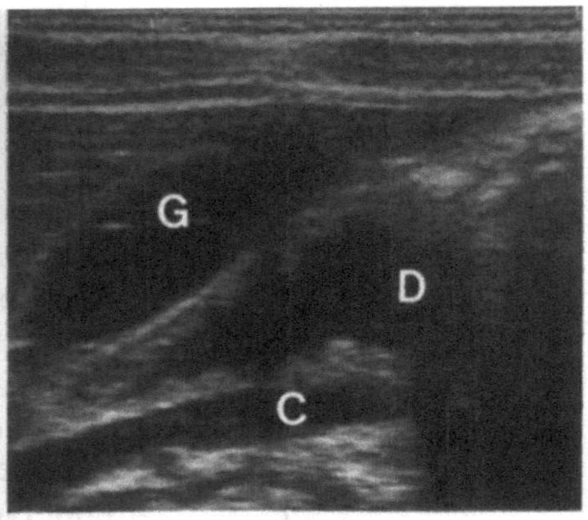

b

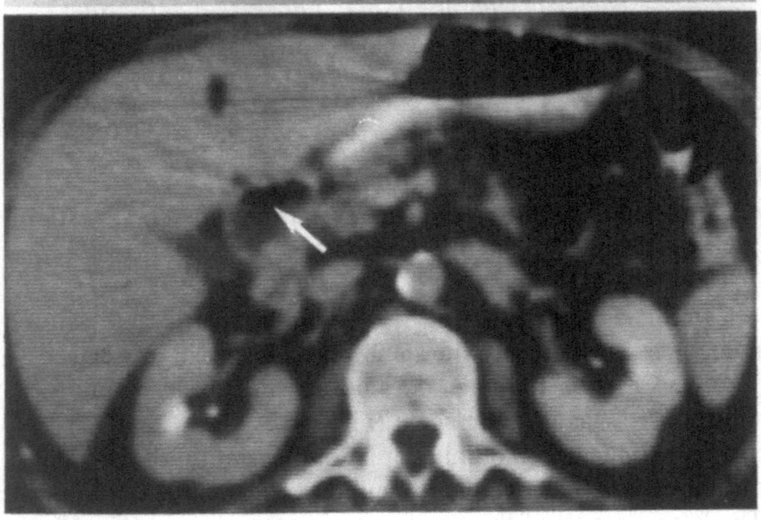

c

Fig. 10a–c. Duodenal distension in acute pancreatitis. **a** *Left lateral film* shows isolated duodenal distension with flattening of the inner border of the duodenum and protrusion of the enlarged pancreatic head (➡). **b** *Sonogram*, longitudinal parasagittal scan through the inferior vena cava *(C)*, shows a markedly dilated, atonic, and fluid-filled duodenum *(D)* as a fluid-filled structure between the gallbladder *(G)* and inferior vena cava. **c** *CT scan* in stage I edematous pancreatitis shows a markedly distended and atonic duodenum with an air-fluid level (→)

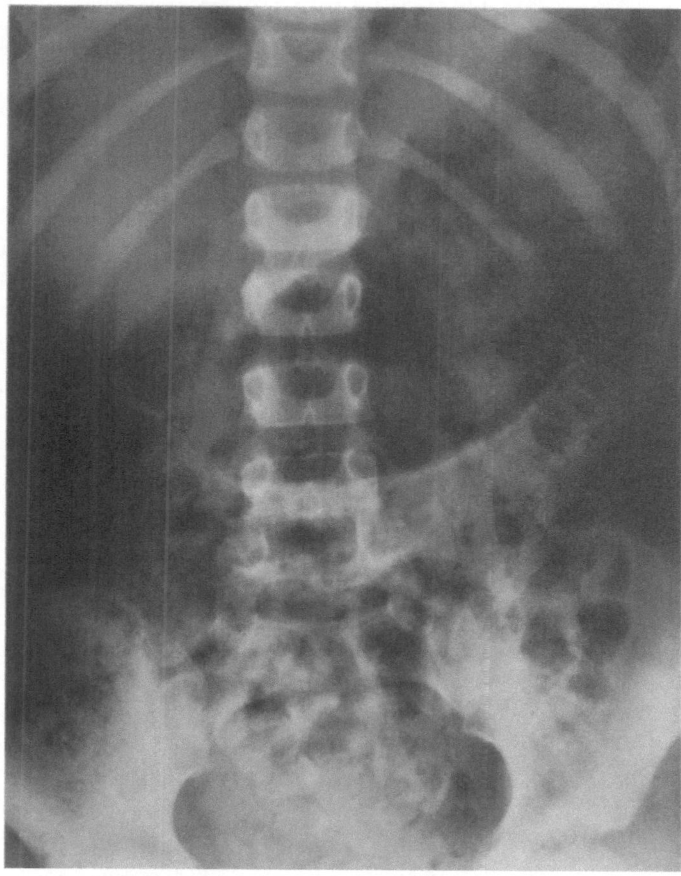

a

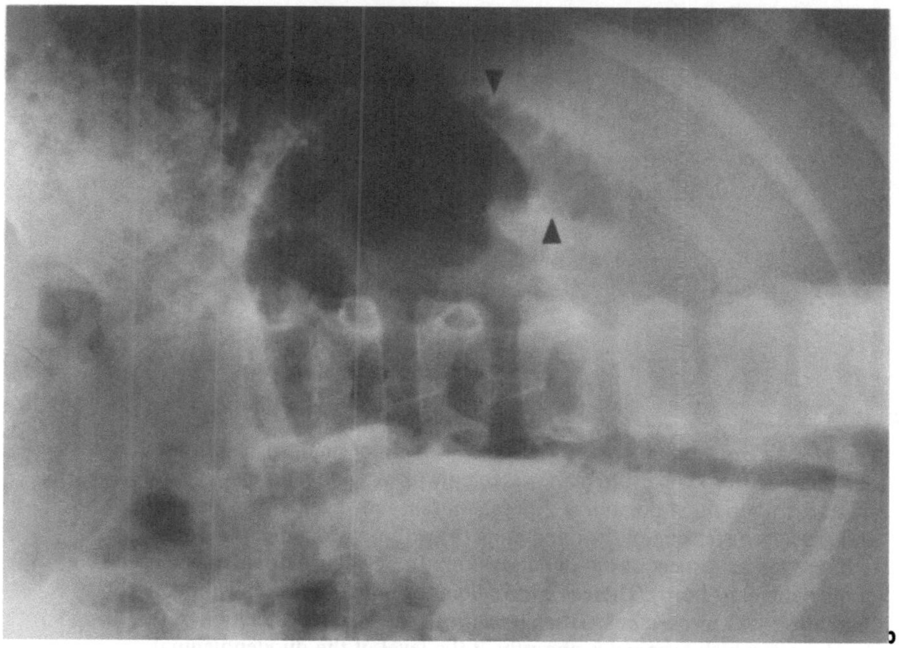

b

Fig. 11 a, b. Gastric and duodenal distension in a 12-year-old boy secondary to posttraumatic pancreatitis from a handlebar injury. **a** *Supine film* shows distension of the stomach, small bowel, and colon. The duodenal distension is *not* apparent on the supine film. **b** *Left lateral film* shows gastric and duodenal distension (▲) with a long fluid level in the stomach

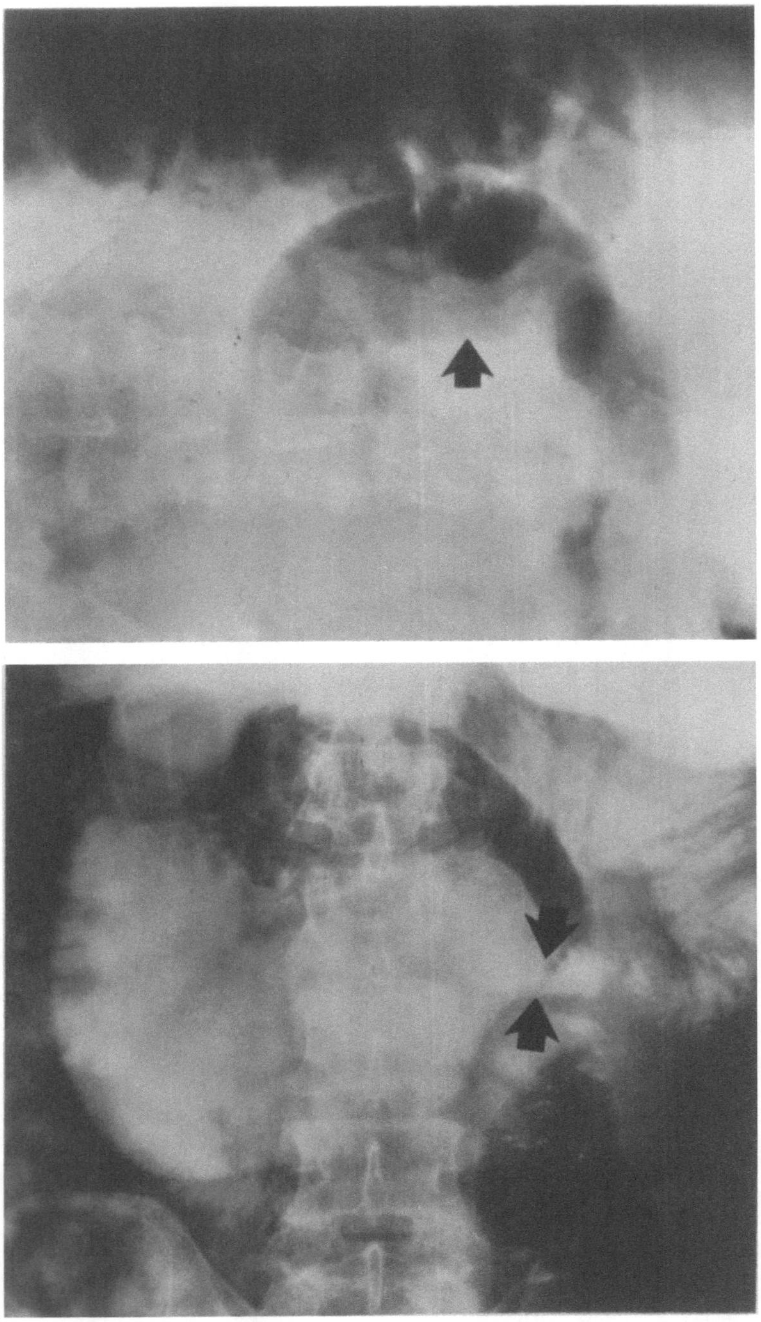

a

b

Fig. 12a, b. Duodenal distension caused by a high mechanical small-bowel obstruction. The 45-year-old man presented with vomiting, normal peristalsis, and a nonrigid abdomen. **a** *Left lateral film* shows massive widening and gaseous distension of the duodenum (➧) without widening or deformity of the medial aspect of the duodenal loop (no evidence of enlargement of the pancreatic head). There is concomitant colonic distension without a fluid level. **b** *Gastrografin UGI series* confirms the massive dilatation of the duodenum, which terminates abruptly at the level of the duodenojejunal flexure (⬆). The filling of the distal small-bowel loops signifies an incomplete obstruction. *Operation* disclosed adhesive bands directly behind the duodenojejunal flexure relating to a previous appendectomy

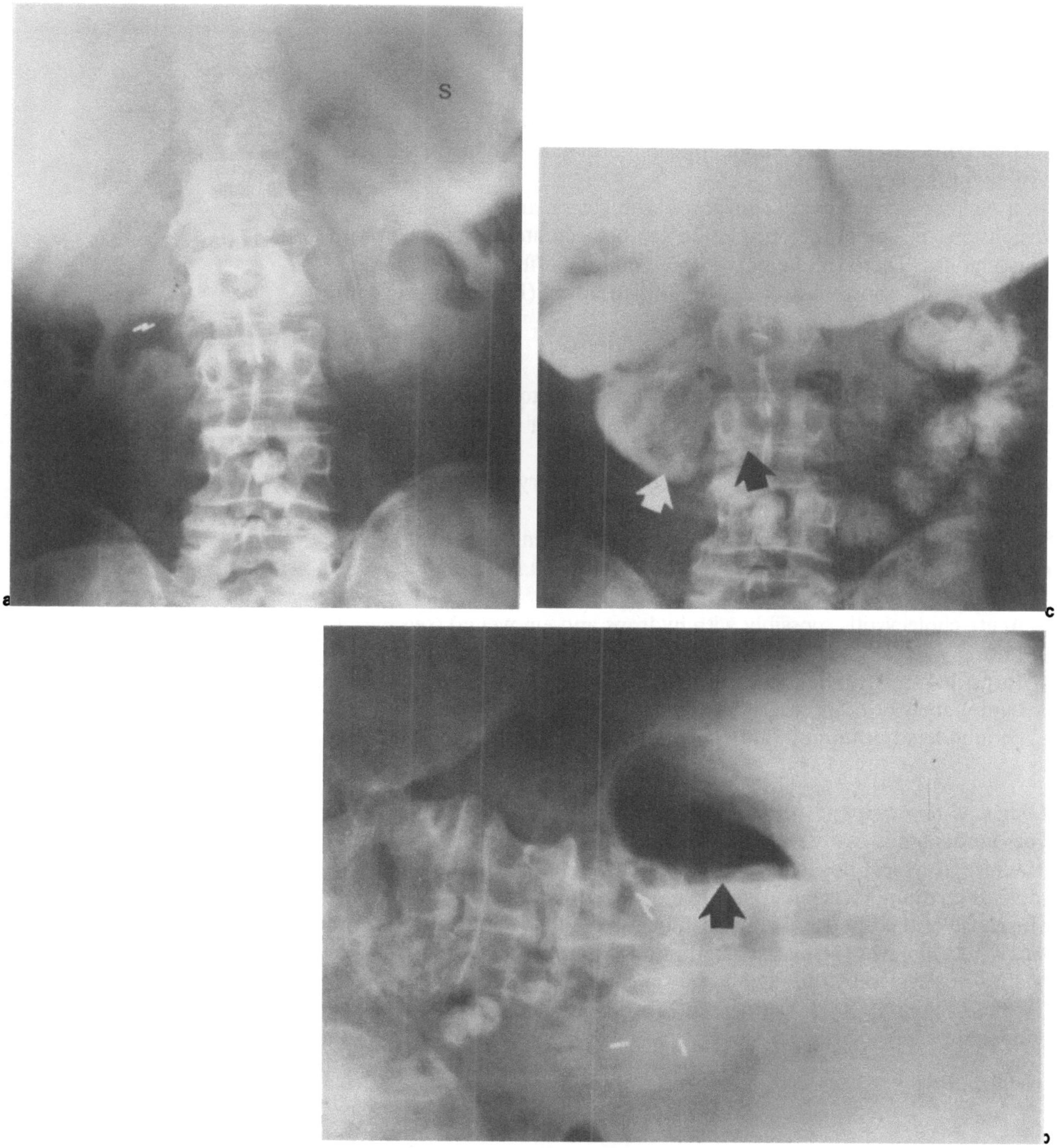

a c b

Fig. 13a–c. Atypical duodenal distension secondary to high mechanical bowel obstruction caused by invasion by a pancreatic carcinoma into the duodenum. The patient, a 61-year-old woman, had previously undergone an exploratory laparotomy for the inoperable tumor. She presented with vomiting, epigastric pain and tenderness, and depressed peristalsis. **a** *Supine film* shows slight gastric distension *(S)* and a nonspecific gas collection projected over the transverse colon. There is a *clip* in the presumed region of the pancreatic head. **b** *Left lateral film* shows atypical distension of the duodenum and an overlying, air-filled, gastric antrum (➡). The remainder of the bowel is gasless. **c** *Gastrografin UGI series* shows dilatation of the stomach and duodenum down to the inferior duodenal flexure. The duodenum is compressed by soft-tissue masses (➡). The Gastrografin examination shows that the obstruction is not yet complete

Note: In 90% of all patients with pancreatitis, duodenal distension is noted on the L Lat radiograph.

With *acute cholecystitis,* possibly with associated hydrops or empyema, the medial border of the duodenum appears normal, and a "pad effect" is visible on the lateral aspect.
In a *high mechanical bowel obstruction* with gastric and duodenal distension, the site of the obstruction can be accurately established with Gastrografin. There will be only a small dilution effect of the contrast medium in the short, obstructed, fluid-filled bowel (Fig. 13, cf. Fig. 156).

Sonography
The gas-distended atonic duodenum is an *obstacle* to upper abdominal sonography, especially in evaluations of the head of the pancreas (e.g., in acute pancreatitis).
A predominantly *fluid-filled* atonic duodenum is very clearly visualized with ultrasound (Fig. 10b).
When there is minimal overlying bowel gas, or when the patient is examined erect, the *cause of duodenal atony may be apparent:*
- Acute pancreatitis (see Figs. 119, 120)
- Acute cholecystitis (possibly with hydrops and empyema) (see Figs. 112, 113)
- Target lesion signifying an obstructing bowel tumor (see Fig. 4d)
- Lymphomas or other space-occupying lesions
- Periduodenal or intramural hematoma

Computed Tomography
The duodenum is easily recognized as an air- and fluid-filled intestinal structure in typical position, especially after a diluted, water-soluble contrast medium has been administered (Fig. 10c).
The cause of the duodenal atony can be assessed (see Sonography). The *major advantage* of CT over sonography is the consistently high image quality, unaffected by obesity and bowel gas.
CT, then, is the *most informative study* for investigations of the duodenal-pancreatic region.

3.1.3 Distension Limited to the Small Bowel

D. BEYER, W. GROSS-FENGELS

Note: The *cause* of limited small-bowel distension with accompanying fluid levels on the L Lat film can be established *only* by correlating radiologic findings with the clinical presentation! Radiologic signs alone cannot reliably differentiate a mechanical bowel obstruction from paralytic ileus.

Causes of limited small-bowel distension with fluid levels
(Differentiation by clinical symptoms)
Nonrigid, nontender abdomen - hyperperistalsis

Mechanical small-bowel obstruction

1. *Strangulation* (early stage of mesenteric vascular torsion or without vascular involvement)
   Incarceration (internal and external hernias)
   Intussusception (ileoileal, ileocecal, colocolic)
   Volvulus (ileocecal)
2. *Obturation* (without vascular involvement)
   Bands and adhesions (postsurgical, inflammatory, congenital), atresia, meconium ileus, duplications of bowel, small-bowel tumor, cecal tumor, strictures (Crohn's disease), gallstone, swallowed foreign body, worm bolus (ascariasis), bezoars and food materials (cherry pits, oranges), impaction of water-insoluble medications (antacids, ion exchangers), stenoses (postoperative, following radiation therapy, periappendicitis)
3. *Mesenteric ischemia and infarction* (in early stage!)
4. *Obstruction of cecum or ascending colon*

Nonrigid abdomen - hyperperistalsis → absence of peristalsis

Long-standing strangling obstruction with ischemic or gangrenous changes
Long-standing mechanical obstruction (transition to paralysis)
Intestinal pseudo-obstruction (see Sect. 4.2.3)

- Mesenteric ischemia and infarction, latent period with wall edema
- Small-bowel intramural hemorrhage (trauma, anticoagulants)
- Acute appendicitis
- Acute pancreatitis
- Mesenteric lymphadenitis
- Drug-related (ganglion-blocking agents)

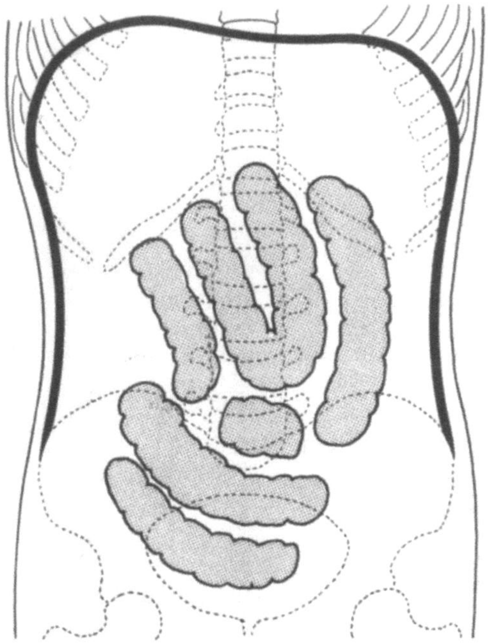

a

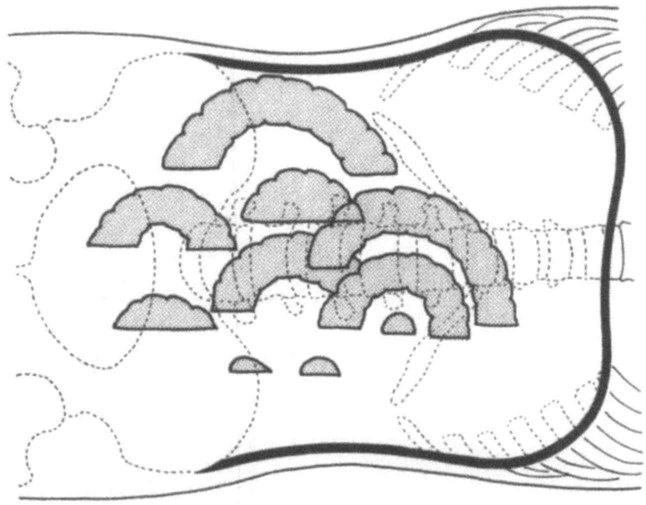

b

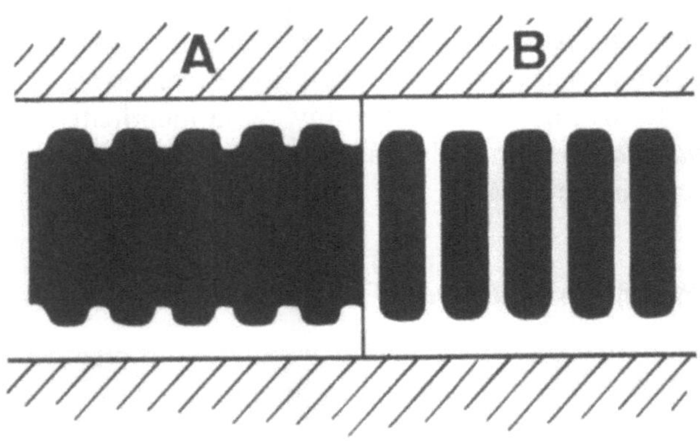

c

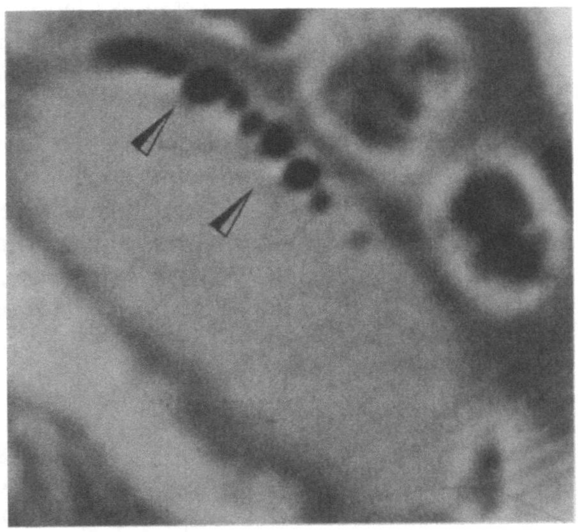

d

Fig. 14 a–d. Schematic illustration of **small-bowel distension** on abdominal plain films and sonograms. **a** *Supine film* of the abdomen shows centralized, distened small-bowel loops with typical Kerckring's folds and an empty colon. **b** *Left lateral film* shows uncoiled, distended small-bowel loops with fluid levels. **c** The "keyboard" sign on sonograms is produced by the characteristic appearance of Kerckring's folds in the dilated, fluid-containing small bowel *(A)*. In an axial scan cutting the bowel wall tangentially, a "stepladder" pattern is created by portions of mucosal folds close to the wall *(B)*. **d** *CT scan* shows a fluid-engorged loop of jejunum with small gas bubbles between Kerckring's folds (▶)

Radiologic Signs

Plain Radiographs (Fig. 14)

- Mild small-bowel distension with a few short fluid levels on the L Lat film:
  Gasless abdomen (supine film) → ground-glass density
  "String-of-beads" sign caused by linear arrangement of small gas bubbles between Kerckring's folds
  → Mechanical small-bowel obstruction with predominantly fluid-filled loops; evaluate by sonography and clinical signs (hyperperistalsis) (see Fig. 156)
  → Early stage of mesenteric arterial embolism with wall edema after evacuation of bowel contens by initial hyperperistalsis (see Fig. 173)

- Marked small-bowel distension with conspicuous fluid levels on L Lat film; supine film shows centralized, distended small-bowel loops with typical Kerckring's folds (stepladder sign) and an "empty" colon (Figs. 15, 16). The *L Lat film* shows uncoiled, hairpinlike, distended small-bowel loops containing fluid levels (Figs. 15b, 16b). The small bowel may be so greatly dilated that it resembles the colon (Fig. 16), but it is identified by the typical spiral arrangement of the Kerckring's folds (Figs. 14, 15, 19).

When combined with *hyperperistalsis*, this constellation is phathognomonic of mechanical bowel obstruction.

Note: The extent of the small-bowel distension on the supine film is *not* an accurate guide to the location of the obstruction, because the distal bowel segments are often filled with fluid before the obstruction.

Caution: The presence of fluid levels at different heights in the same loop on the L Lat film has traditionally been considered a sign of mechanical obstruction; however, the same pattern can occur in paralytic ileus. Differentiation by clinical symptoms (hyperperistalsis) is more dependable.

- Limited small-bowel distension with wall edema (supine) and fluid levels (L Lat): edematous wall thickening, luminal narrowing, wall contour changes, and separation of adjacent loops → strong evidence of *mesenteric ischemia and infarction* (see Sect. 4.2.4) or intramural *bleeding* (see Sect. 4.3.4) (Fig. 18). Rigid loops on the L Lat film that do not move with position changes (rigid loop sign) (Figs. 18c, 174b).
- "Coffee bean" sign signifies a closed loop that is obstructed at both ends by volvulus or incarceration (see Fig. 178a).
- Pseudotumor sign (see Fig. 173a): Because gas cannot escape from the closed loop (volvulus, incarceration), the loop slowly fills with fluid. Wall edema may develop due to accompanying ischemia. There is *no* palpable mass. Diagnosis is established by sonography.
- The cause is visible aboral to the small-bowel distension: intussusceptum, "tumor" (Fig. 17), large calcified gallstone, foreign body.

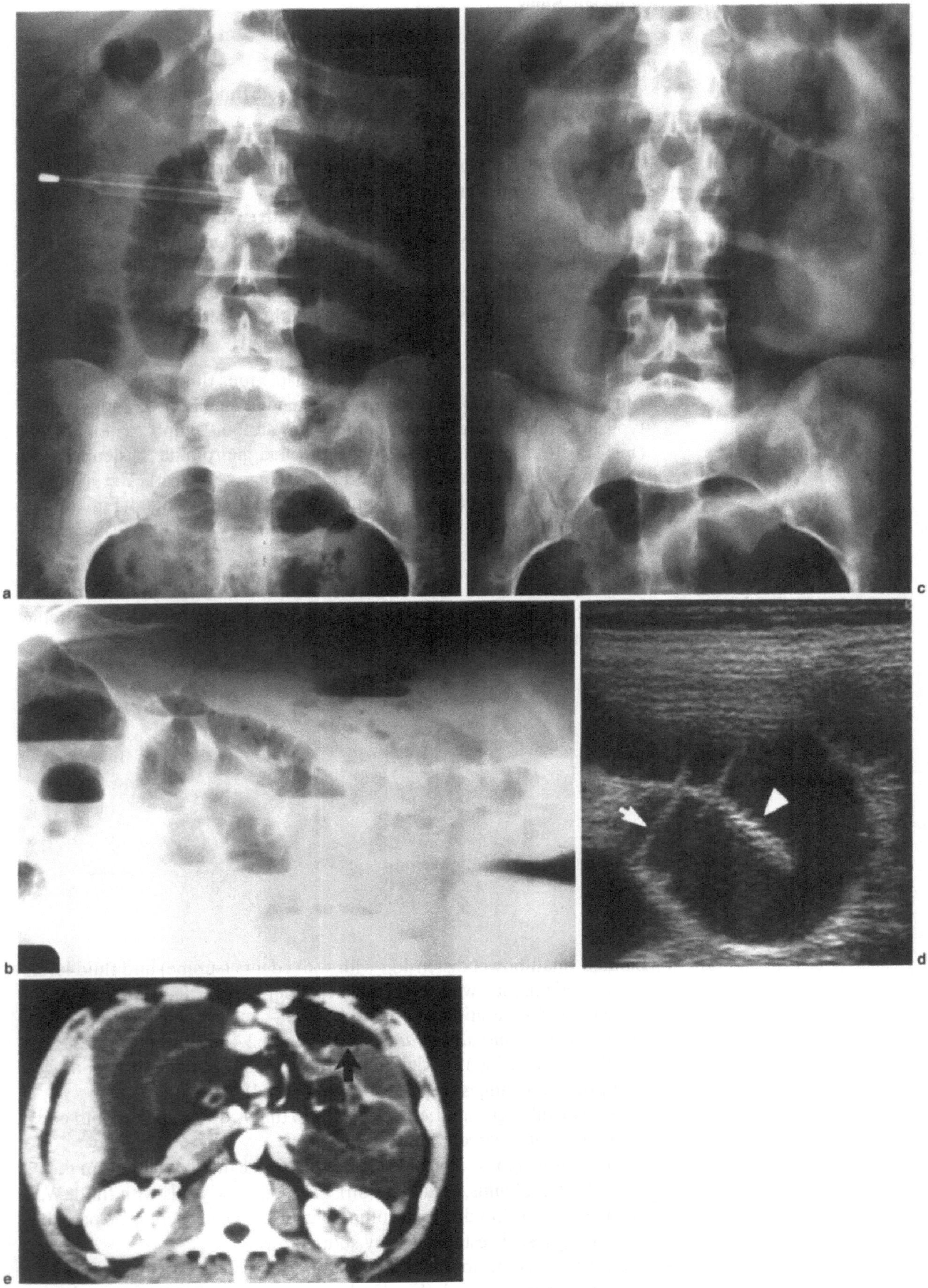
a
c
b
d
e

Contrast Examination (with water-soluble contrast)
This study is indicated for complete or partial bowel obstruction of unknown etiology when the patient's general condition is good and immediate surgery is not planned (Fig. 15 c).
The upper GI series with water-soluble contrast medium (Figs. 155 e, 156 c) can:

- Differentiate mechanical obstruction from paralytic ileus
- Establish the site of the obstruction with reasonable accuracy
- Show whether there is a complete or incomplete obstruction of the small-bowel lumen
- Stimulate peristaltic activity in paralytic ileus owing to hyperosmolarity of the contrast medium (combined diagnostic and therapeutic procedure)

Disadvantage: The water-soluble contrast medium is heavily diluted by the copious secretions in the obstructed bowel.

◁ **Fig. 15 a–e. Small-bowel distension** due to mechanical obstruction. The 35-year-old woman, who had had an appendectomy 16 years earlier, presented with abdominal distension, hyperperistalsis, and diffuse abdominal tenderness; she was afebrile. **a** *Supine film* shows isolated small-bowel distension with centralized, distended, small-bowel loops and typical Kerckring's folds. The colon is empty. The thermometer depicted on the film was *under* the patient! **b** *Left lateral film* shows uncoiled, hairpinlike, distended small-bowel loops with individual fluid levels. Free air is not demonstrated. **c** *Gastrografin UGI series* confirms the plain film findings. The small-bowel loops are markedly distended, and the more anterior loops (which contain more air) are centrally positioned. There is evidence of contrast blockage in the right lower quadrant. The colon still appears empty. **d** *Sonogram* shows dilated, fluid-containing, small-bowel loops with a keyboard sign (►) produced by Kerckring's folds. Bowel wall cut tangentially by the scan shows a stepladder pattern of mucosal folds (➧). **e** (From a different patient) *CT scan* of the abdomen after bolus injection shows predominantly fluid-filled, dilated small-bowel loops with individual fluid levels (➧). There is marked opacification of the small-bowel wall after the bolus injection

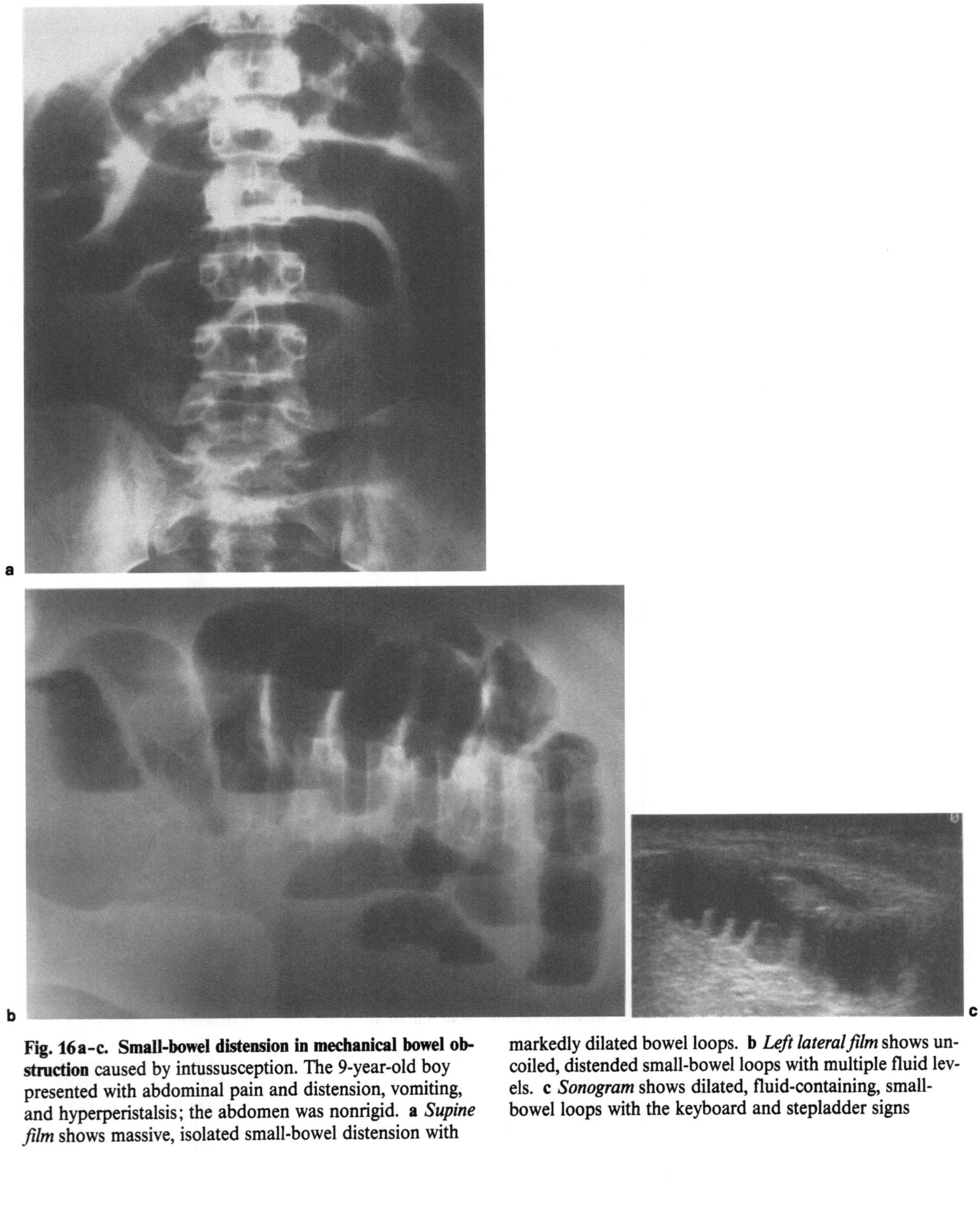

Fig. 16a–c. Small-bowel distension in mechanical bowel obstruction caused by intussusception. The 9-year-old boy presented with abdominal pain and distension, vomiting, and hyperperistalsis; the abdomen was nonrigid. **a** *Supine film* shows massive, isolated small-bowel distension with markedly dilated bowel loops. **b** *Left lateral film* shows uncoiled, distended small-bowel loops with multiple fluid levels. **c** *Sonogram* shows dilated, fluid-containing, small-bowel loops with the keyboard and stepladder signs

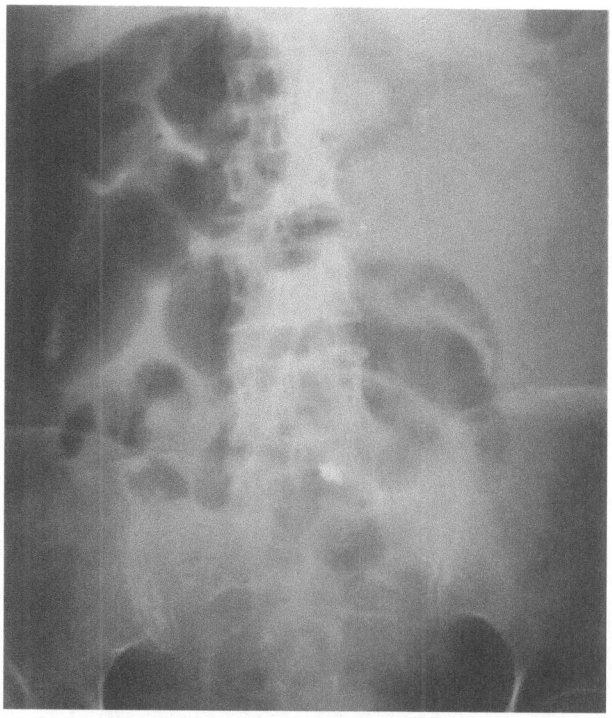
a

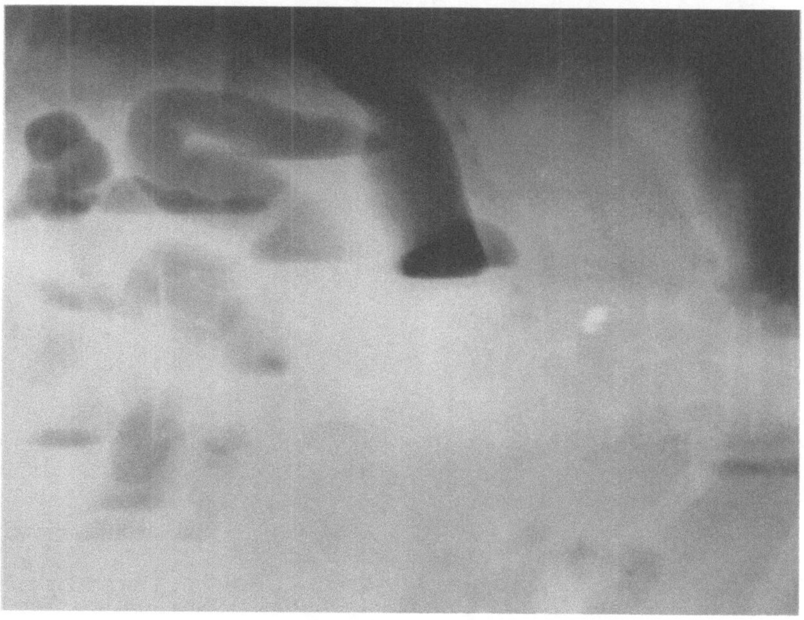
b

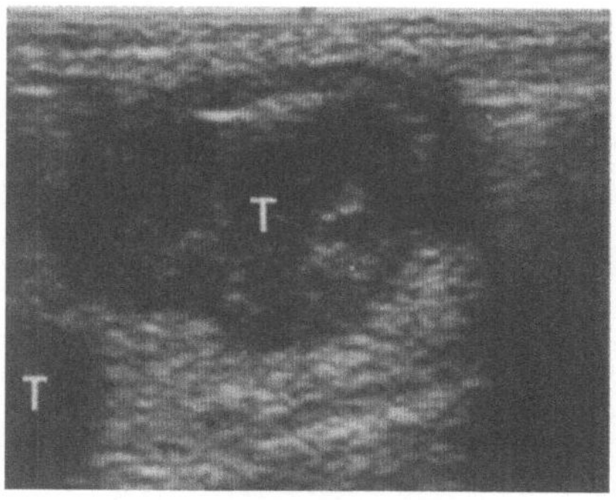

c

Fig. 17 a–c. Atypical small-bowel distension secondary to peritoneal carcinomatosis. The 42-year-old woman had undergone resection of an ovarian carcinoma 2 years earlier and now presented with cramping abdominal pains and weight loss, alternating normal and increased peristalsis, and diffuse tenderness; the abdomen was nonrigid. **a** *Supine film* shows multiple, distended small-bowel loops of variable width in the right upper quadrant and midabdomen. **b** *Left lateral film* shows uncoiled small-bowel loops with fluid levels; the loops appear stiffened and show marked variations in their luminal diameters. **c** *Sonogram* shows marked narrowing and wall thickening of the stiffened small-bowel loops, some of which show asymmetric, hypoechoic areas that represent solid tumor *(T)* deposits of peritoneal carcinomatosis. There is no evidence of ascites

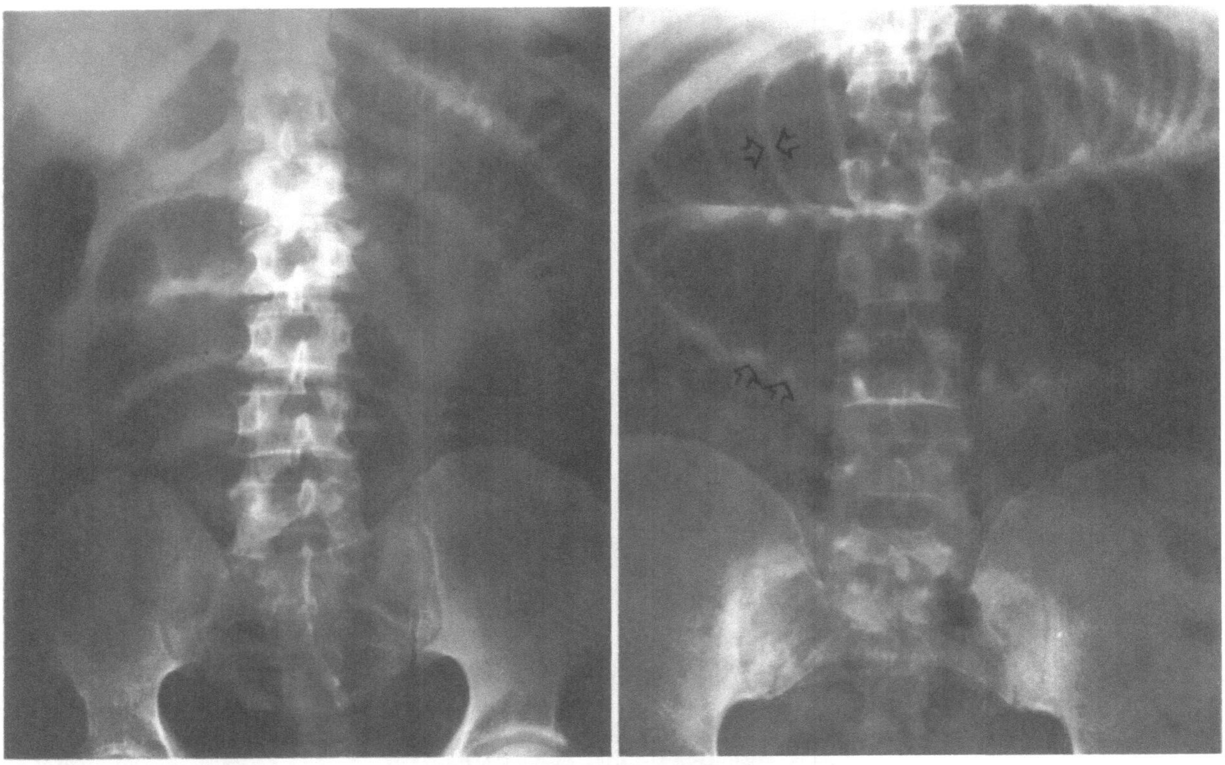

a b

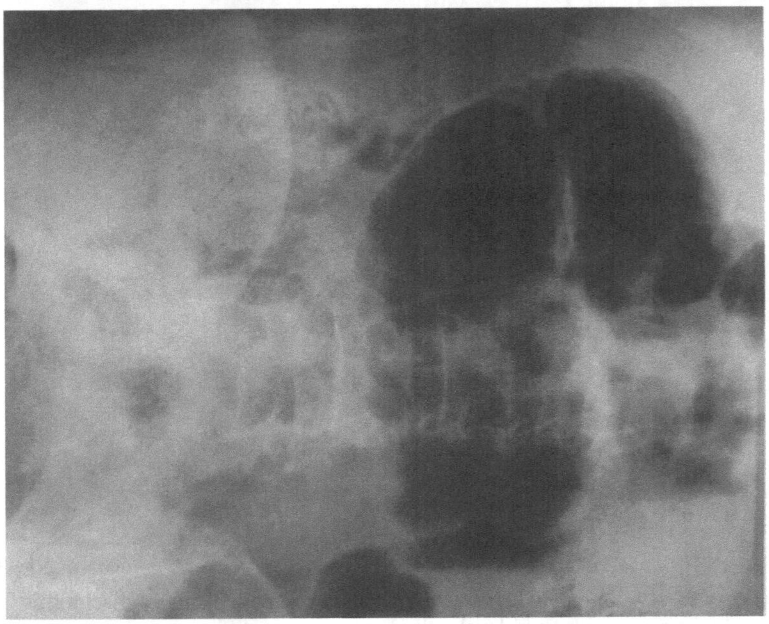

c

Fig. 18 a–c. Small-bowel distension associated with mesenteric ischemia.
a Slow development of mesenteric arterial thrombosis in a 48-year-old man who had had increasing abdominal pain for 2 days and bloody diarrhea for 3 h, prompting hospitalization. Clinical examination showed incipient abdominal rigidity, aperistalsis, and shock. *Supine film* shows isolated distension of the entire small bowel and ascending colon with thickening of the bowel wall from the jejunum to the ileum. There is marked luminal narrowing of the ileum, especially at the flexures. The Kerckring's folds of the jejunum are swollen. The left lateral film (not shown) demonstrated small-bowel distension with fluid levels and accompanying distension of the ascending colon with a fluid level; separation of the small-bowel loops was *not* apparent. *Operation* disclosed hemorrhagic infarction of the entire small bowel and ascending colon to the hepatic flexure due to mesenteric arterial thrombosis, with incipient peritonitis. Surgery entailed total resection of the small bowel and ascending colon. The patient died 4 days postoperatively. **b, c Circumscribed mesenteric venous thrombosis** of a jejunal vein in a 60-year-old woman with increasing abdominal pain and bloody diarrhea. Clinically the entire abdomen was nonrigid and diffusely tender, and peristalsis was diminished. **b** *Supine film,* taken about 10 h after onset of symptoms, shows limited distension of a jejunal loop with wall thickening and pronounced widening of Kerckring's folds (⇨). There is very little gas in the remainder of the bowel. **c** *Left lateral film* shows limited distension of the jejunal loop with a fluid level. Fold edema is apparent. The loop is immobile with position changes (rigid loop sign). Laparotomy disclosed mesenteric thrombosis of a jejunal vein with early hemorrhagic infarction of a 35-cm-long segment of jejunum, which was resected. The patient survived

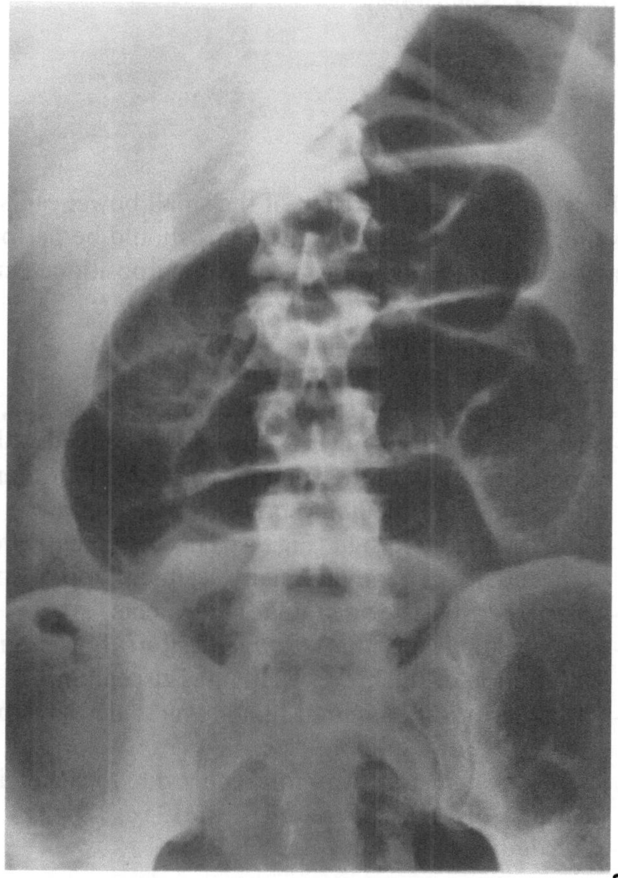

a

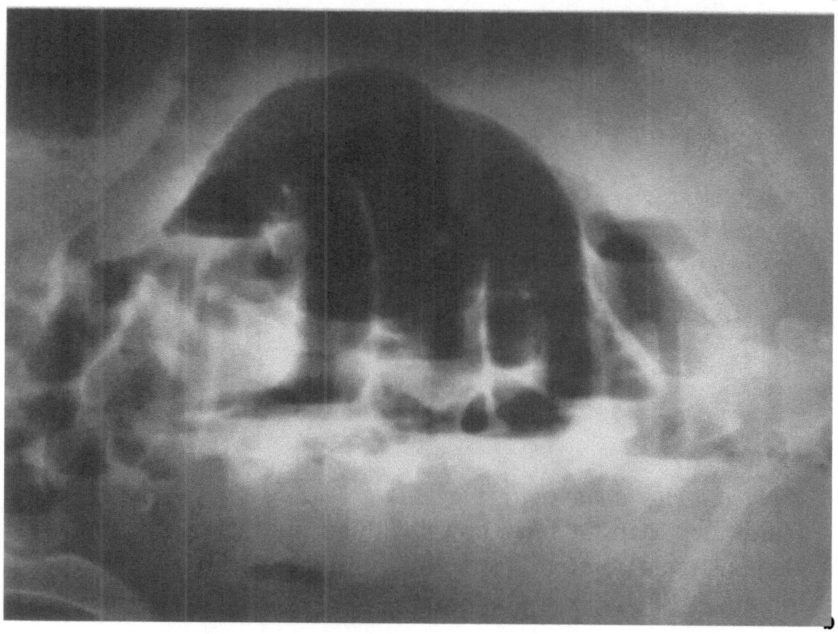

b

Fig. 19 a, b. Small-bowel distension associated with inflammatory bowel disease. **a** Pseudomembranous enteritis in a 42-year-old woman with sepsis who was taking several antibiotics. The patient presented with diarrhea and abdominal distension, hypoperistalsis, and diffuse abdominal tenderness. *Supine film* shows a hugely distended small bowel and stomach and slight, irregular thickening of the mucosal folds in the jejunum. **b** *Left lateral film* shows uncoiled and distended small-bowel loops with fluid levels. Pseudomembranous plaques were identified on the colorectal mucosa, and *Clostridium difficile* was found in the stool

Real-Time Sonography

Note: Today sonography is the *most important* adjunctive study to plain radiography when intestinal obstruction is suspected.

Because gaseous distension of the small bowel can seriously hamper sonographic visualization, the scans should be performed from the lateral aspect (from the flank) with the patient positioned supine.

Real-time sonography can demonstrate:
- Fluid accumulation in the small bowel
- Enlargement of the small-bowel lumen (Figs. 15 d, 16 c)
- The "keyboard" sign (Fig. 14 d): bright, ribbed wall echo patterns, most commonly seen in the jejunum and caused by Kerckring's folds projecting into the liquid bowel contents
- The "stepladder" sign (Fig. 14 d) occurs when Kerckring's folds are cut tangentially in a longitudinally scanned loop of small bowel
- Hyperperistalsis or pendular movements
- An obstructive lesion → "target lesion" (bowel tumor, lymphomatous infiltration of the bowel wall, intussusceptum)
- Mass lesions (extramural tumors, mesenteric lymphomas; Figs. 17 c, 155 d)
- Diffuse edematous wall thickening due to ischemia, amyloidosis, Crohn's disease, etc. (see Figs. 34 b, 35 c, 37)
- Accompanying ascites (see Fig. 37 c)

Note: In any intestinal obstruction of unknown cause, sonography yields information not only on the bowel wall and intraluminal contents but also on *all visible abdominal organs*. Thus, it helps to exclude other causes of acute abdomen with ileus.

Computed Tomography

Note: The purpose of CT is *not* to demonstrate a small-bowel distension with fluid levels but to demonstrate the *cause*. It is indicated only if other imaging procedures fail to give reliable information, and the patient does not have to be examined in a hurry.

Computed tomographic signs (Fig. 157)
- Fluid-filled loops of small bowel with air-fluid levels (see Fig. 15 e)
- Demonstrable point of obstruction (in some cases)

3.1.4 Distension Limited to the Colon

D. BEYER

Note: Approximately 25% of all intestinal obstructions are caused by a colonic process and lead to colonic distension.

Causes
Limited colonic distension with fluid levels in the L Lat position can have various causes. The most frequent one, especially in elderly patients, is colorectal carcinoma (60% incidence).
Other causes can usually be established only by correlating radiologic findings with the history and clinical presentation. A contrast enema may be necessary.

Causes of limited colonic distension with or without fluid levels
(Differentiation by clinical symptoms)

Nonrigid, nontender abdomen – normal peristalsis
Mechanical colon obstruction
1. *Obturation obstruction*
   Colorectal carcinoma
   Tumors of adjacent organs (ovary, uterus, prostate)
   Peritoneal carcinomatosis
   Diverticulitic abscess
   Pelvic abscess of other etiology
   Internal and external hernias
   Lymphogranuloma venereum with rectal stenosis
   Foreign bodies introduced per rectum
   Impaction of water-insoluble medications (antacids, ion exchangers)
   Inspissated barium sulfate after contrast examination
   Inspissated feces in elderly, bedridden, and psychiatric patients (fecal impaction)
2. *Strangulation obstruction*
   Intussusception
   Sigmoid volvulus
   Incarcerated hernia
3. *Enterocolitis* (Fig. 26)
4. *Iatrogenic* (Fig. 22)

Nonrigid abdomen – hypoperistalsis → aperistalsis
1. *Retroperitoneal disorders* (Fig. 25
   Ureteral calculus, acute pyelonephritis
   Retroperitoneal hematoma (postoperative, posttraumatic, after translumbar angiography)
   Trauma with vertebral fracture and/or renal rupture

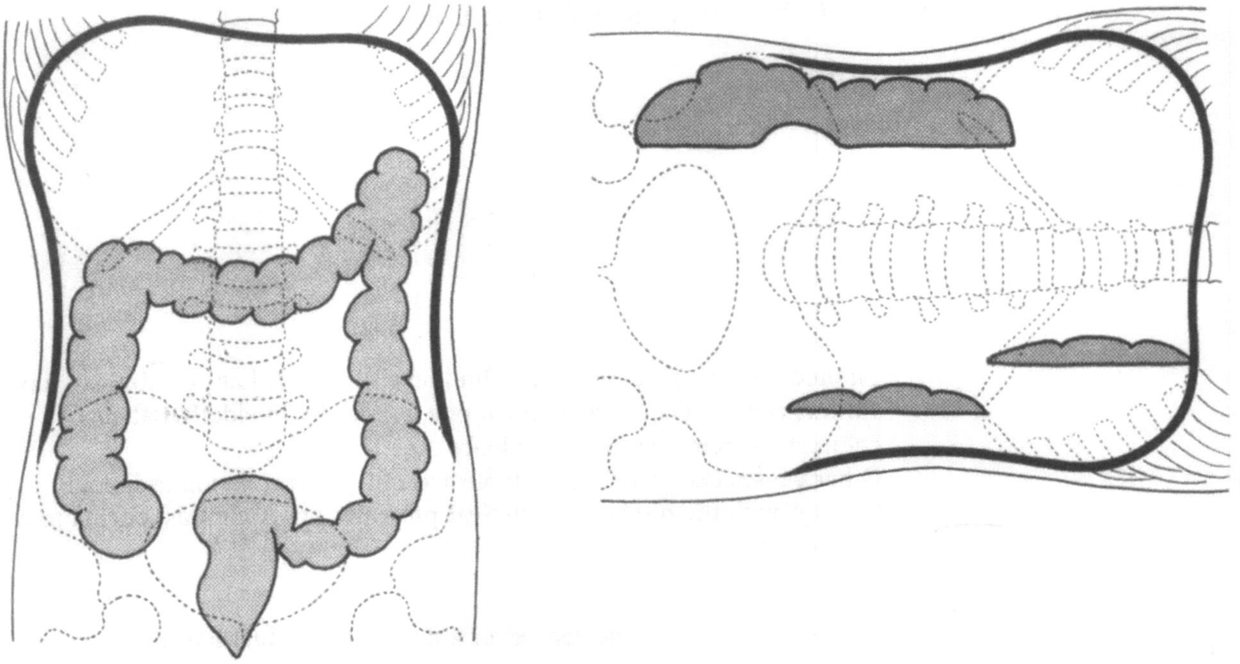

Fig. 20a, b. Schematic illustration of distension limited to the colon. **a** *Supine film* shows distension to be most pronounced in the anterior parts of the colon, especially the transverse colon. Later, distension also affects the ascending colon and cecum. One should watch for cutoff of the gas column proximal to an obstruction. **b** On *left lateral film* the distension is most apparent in the cecum and transverse colon (highest points!). There are extensive fluid levels in the cecum and ascending colon, and individual levels in the transverse colon

2. *Extraperitoneal disorders*
   Basal pneumonia
   Basal pleurisy
   Myocardial infarction, pericarditis
   Hypokalemia - hyperkalemia
   Medications (phenothiazines, tricyclic antidepressants, antiparkinson drugs, morphine, ganglion-blocking drugs)
   Porphyria
   Myxedema, Addison's disease
3. *Colonic ischemia*
   Occlusion of colon-supplying arteries or colon-draining veins
   Acute ulcerative colitis
   Toxic megacolon
   Ischemia in long-standing volvulus of the colon and incarcerated hernia with colonic content

Local abdominal rigidity - normal or diminished peristalsis

Acute cholecystitis
Retrocecal appendicitis
Acute pancreatitis with spread of ezymes to the mesocolon and retroperitoneum
Subhepatic and subphrenic abscess
Sigmoid diverticulitis

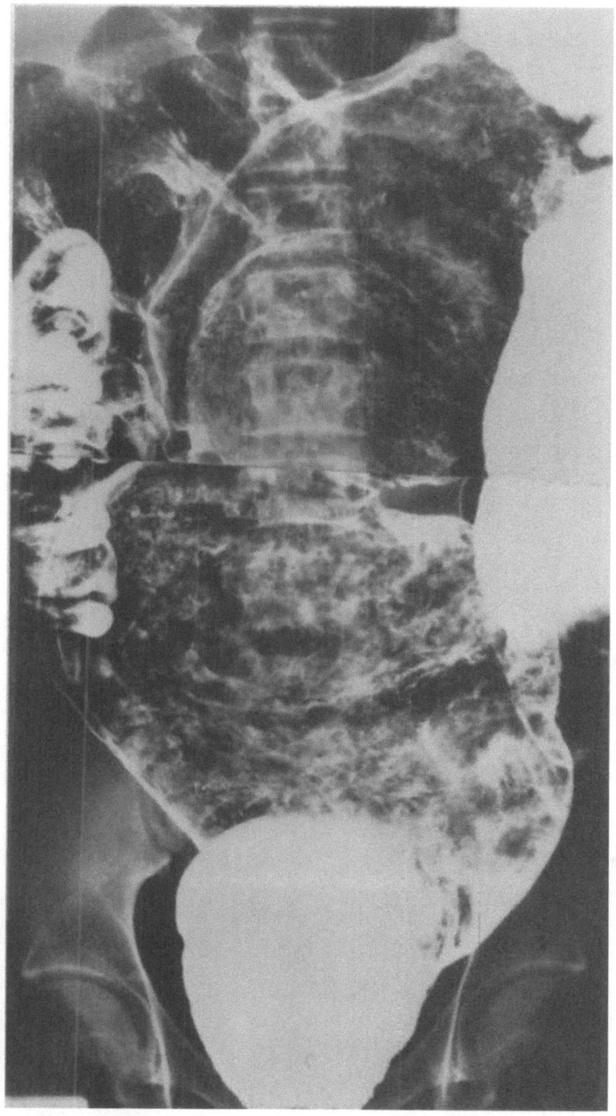

Fig. 21. Distension limited to the colon due to fecal impaction in a bedridden psychiatric patient. The patient ate a strict vegetarian diet and suffered from severe, chronic constipation. He presented with massive abdominal distension, a nonrigid, nontender abdomen, and normal peristalsis. *Contrast enema* in the supine position (composite film) shows massive distension of the rectum and sigmoid colon, which is filled with soft material bathed in contrast medium. The remaining portions of the colon are also dilated. The diaphragm is greatly elevated

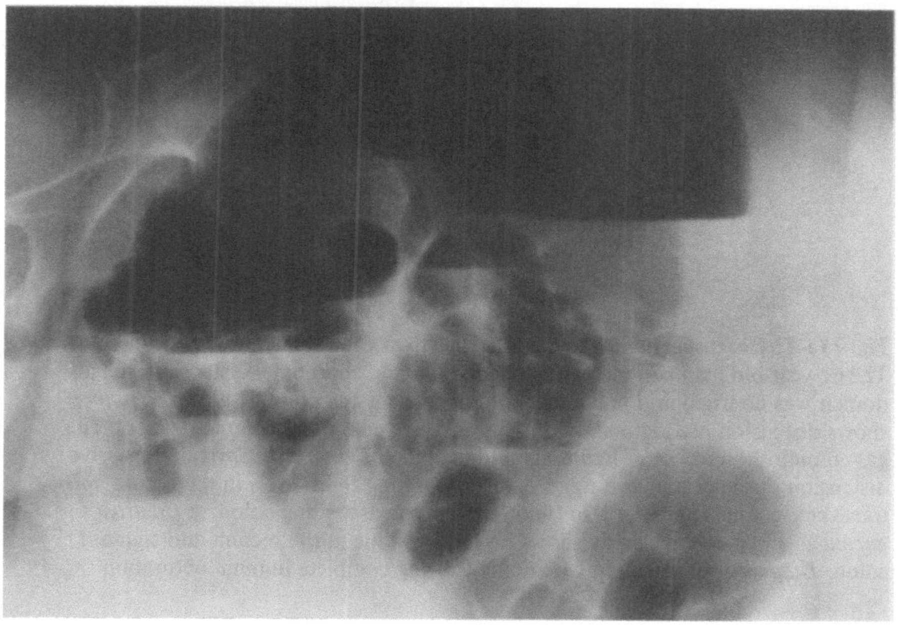

Fig. 22. "Iatrogenic" colonic distension after colonoscopy. The patient complained of abdominal pain following a colonoscopic examination. The abdomen was soft and diffusely tender, and peristalsis was sluggish. *Left lateral film* shows massive colonic distension, especially in the region of the cecum and transverse colon. Some short fluid levels are visible. There is no free air

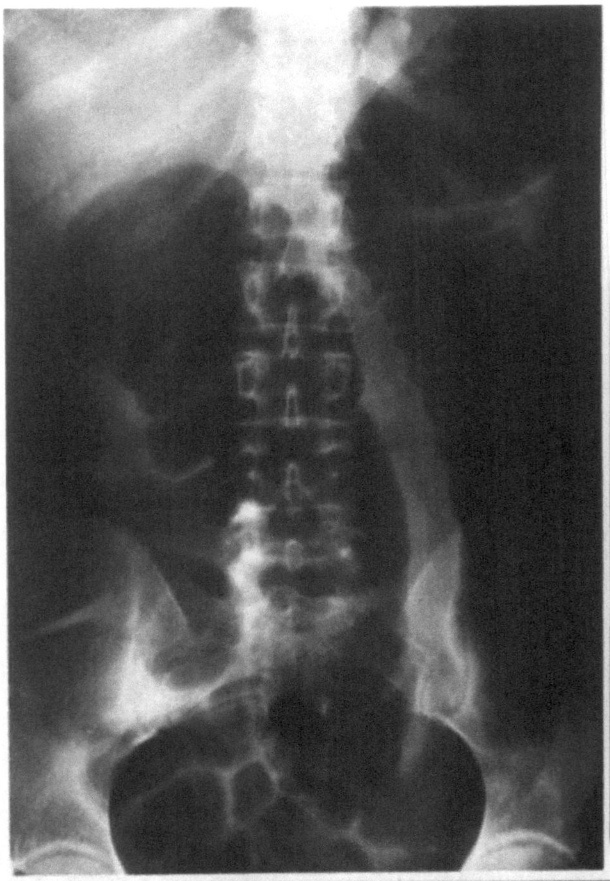

a

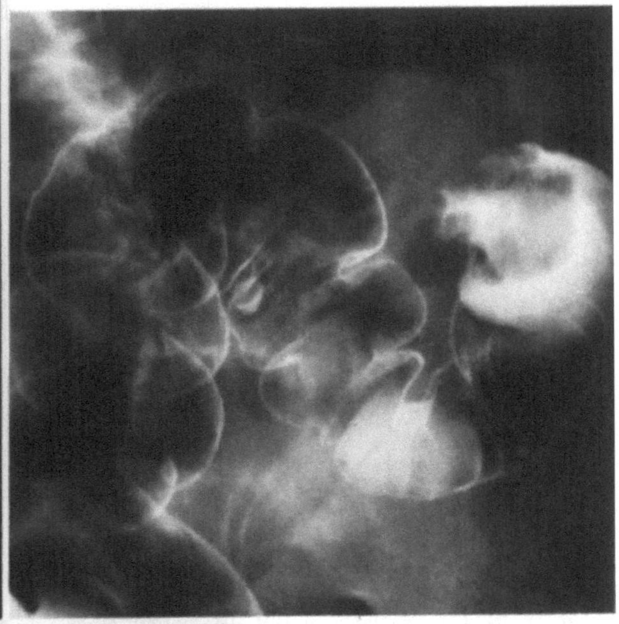

c

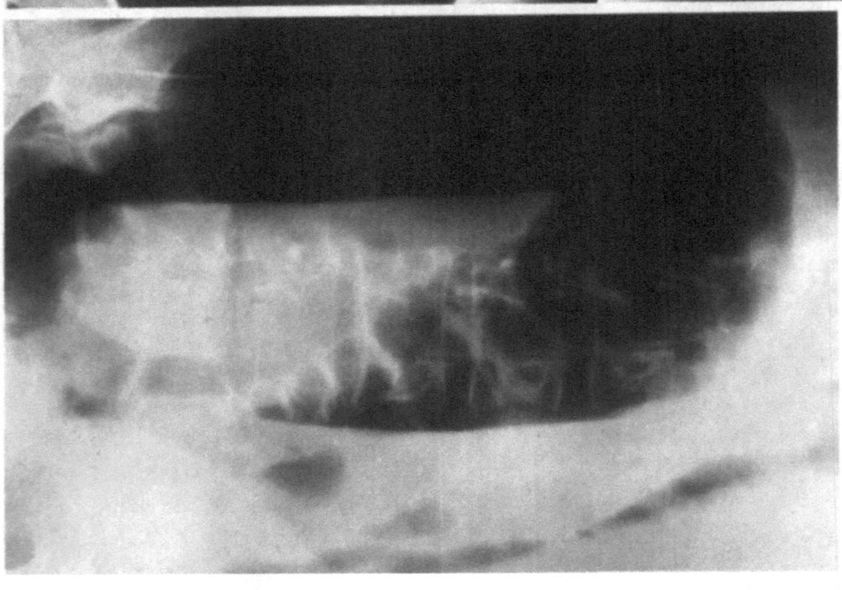

b

Fig. 23 a–f. Distension limited to the colon due to mechanical obturation of the colon. The 62-year-old man had increasing obstipation and abdominal distension; the abdomen was nonrigid and nontender, and peristalsis was normal. **a** *Supine film* shows distension predominantly of the transverse colon and colonic flexures. The gas column shows a cutoff in the sigmoid region. **b** *Left lateral film* shows massive distension of the cecum and right flexure, with long fluid levels in the cecum and transverse colon. There are also fluid levels in the ascending colon. **c** *Contrast enema* as an emergency study shows no fecal residue in the rectum and sigmoid colon. *Diagnosis:* midsigmoid carcinoma causing complete luminal obturation.

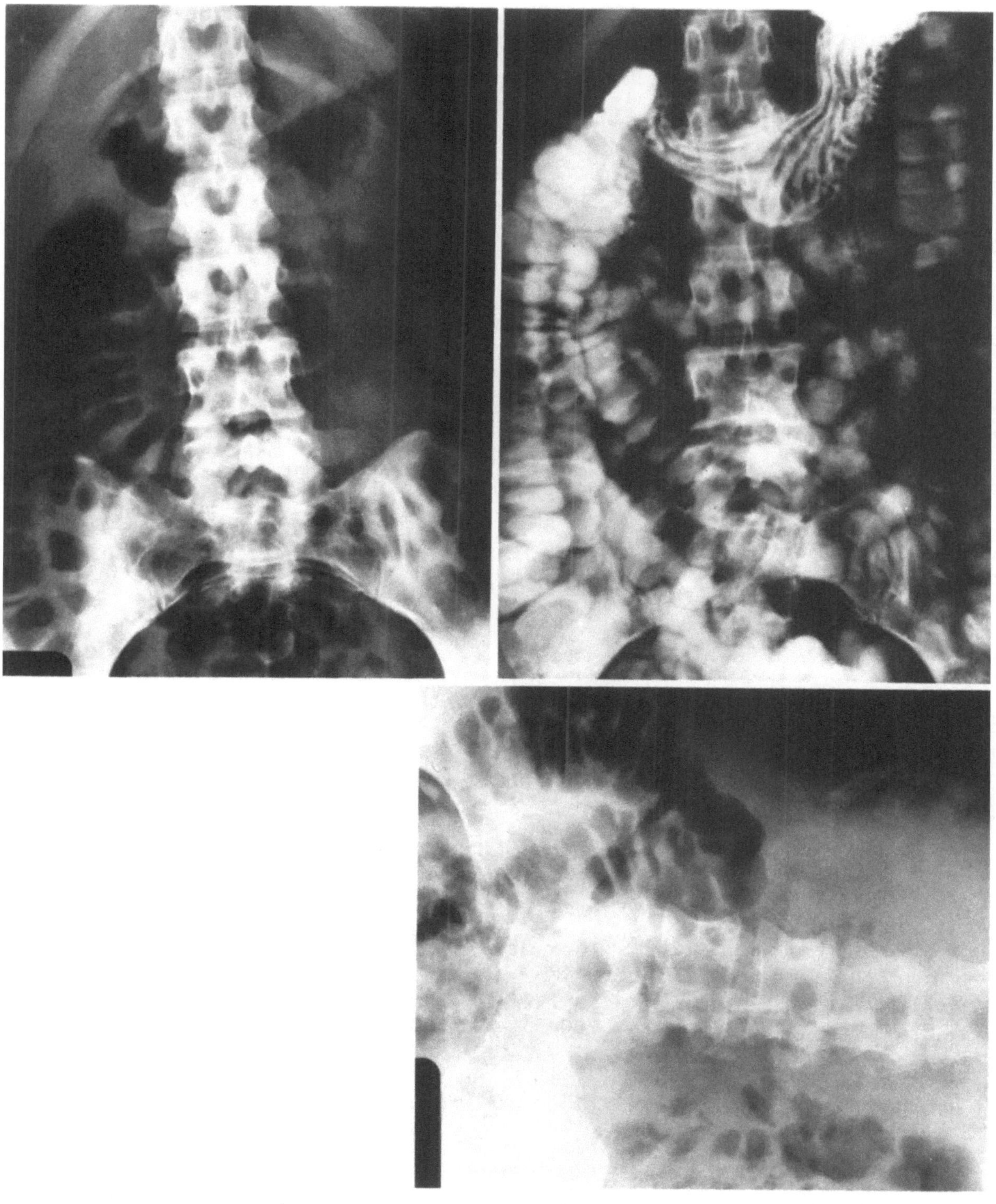

d f e

Fig. 23 (continued)
d–f For comparison: **Colonic distension *without* pathologic significance.** The patient presented with abdominal pain of unknown cause. *Supine film* shows isolated colonic distension with no cutoff of the gas column (**d**). *Left lateral film* shows distension predominantly of the ascending and transverse colon. The cecum is not dilated, and there are no fluid levels (**e**). **f** *UGI series* confirms normal passage of water-soluble contrast medium through the small and large intestines

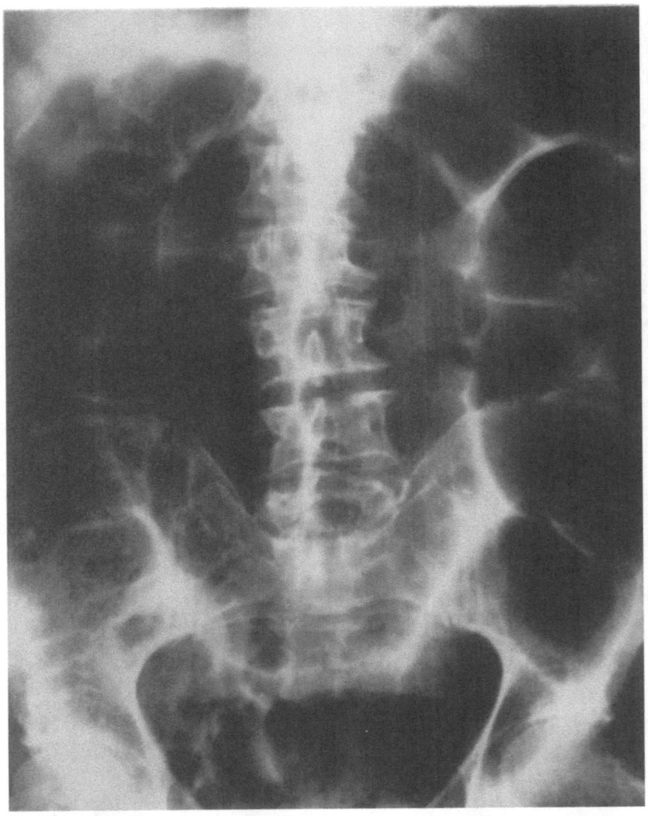

a

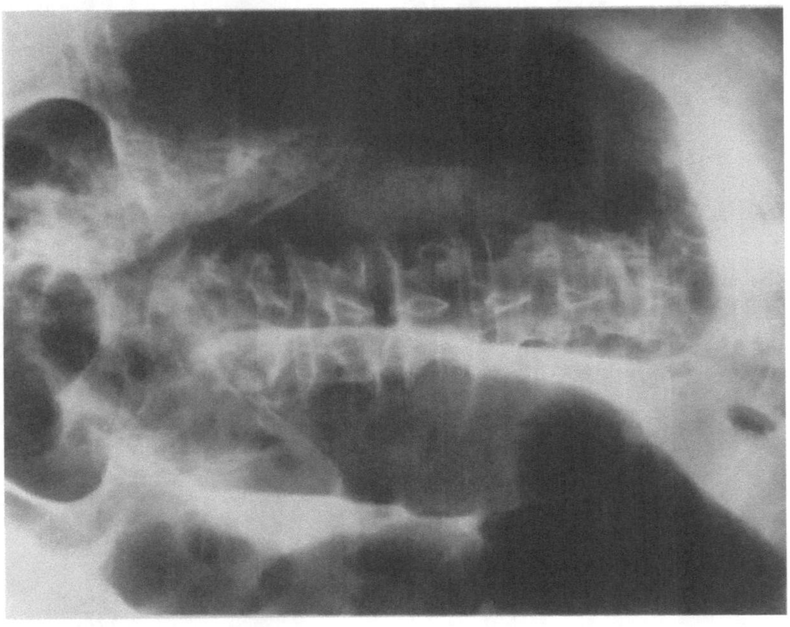

b

Fig. 24 a–d. Colonic distension secondary to extraperitoneal disease. Man, 61 years old, with inferior lobar pleuropneumonia of the right side presented with diffuse abdominal pain of sudden onset with a nonrigid abdomen and aperistalsis. **a** *Supine film* shows massive colonic distension from the cecum to the rectum. **b** On *left lateral film* the absence of marked cecal distension excludes a mechanical obstruction as the cause. Fluid levels are minimal.

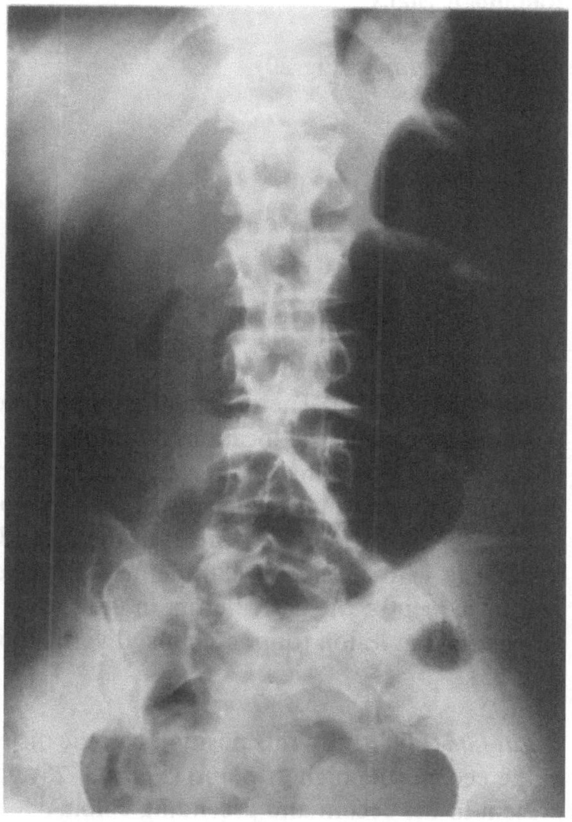

c

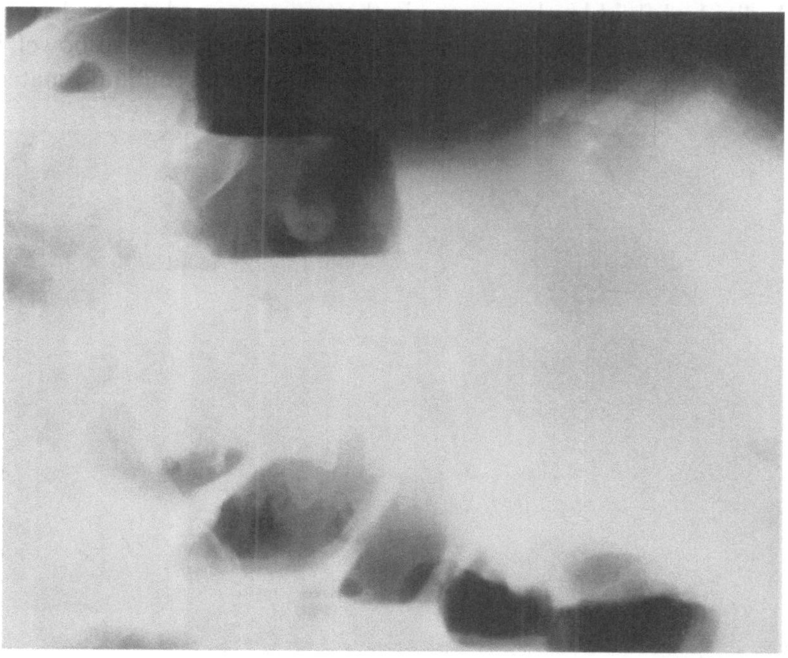

d

Fig. 24 (continued)
c, d Woman, 59 years old, with latent adrenal insufficiency experienced an addisonian crisis with prostration and hypoglycemia. The abdomen was nonrigid, and peristalsis was absent. **c** *Supine film* shows massive distension of the transverse colon to the splenic flexure. The haustrations are preserved. The small bowel is not distended. **d** *Left lateral film* likewise shows nonspecific distension of the cecum and ascending colon. The gas pattern is not characteristic of a mechanical colon obstruction

Radiologic Signs

Plain Radiographs (Fig. 20)

Note: The symptom of limited colonic distension due to mechanical colon obstruction develops much more slowly than a distension limited to the small bowel.
The farther down the intestinal tract the obstruction is located, the longer it takes the colon to become distended (aside from acute volvulus and intussusception).

Supine film (Fig. 20): The degree of colonic distension in the supine position varies with the location, duration, and completeness of the obstruction. Depending on the gas content of the colon, distension may first affect the most anterior parts of the large bowel (especially the transverse colon) and later spread to the ascending colon and cecum (especially with a retro- or extraperitoneal cause) (Figs. 23-25).
Not infrequently, the gas column on the supine film terminates *in front of* an obstructing lesion (tumor, colitis, diverticulitis) → Gastrografin enema (Fig. 23).

L Lat film (Fig. 20): In this position colonic distension is most pronounced in the cecum (the highest point) (Figs. 23-25). Extensive fluid levels are present in the cecum and ascending colon.
Individual fluid levels are seen in the transverse and descending colon. Fluid levels are less numerous than in the distended small bowel, because only the cecum and ascending colon still contain semiliquid material.

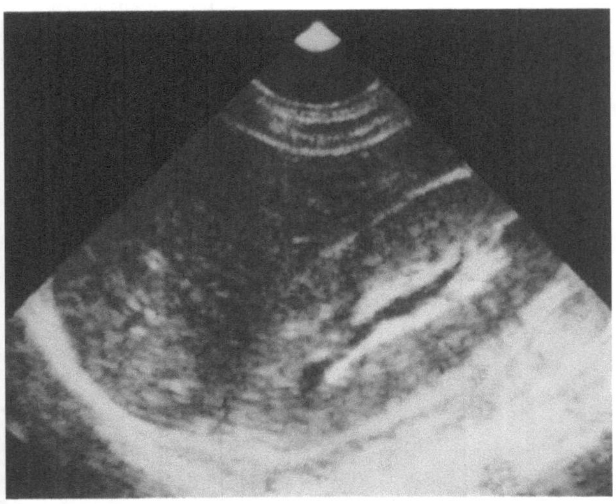
b

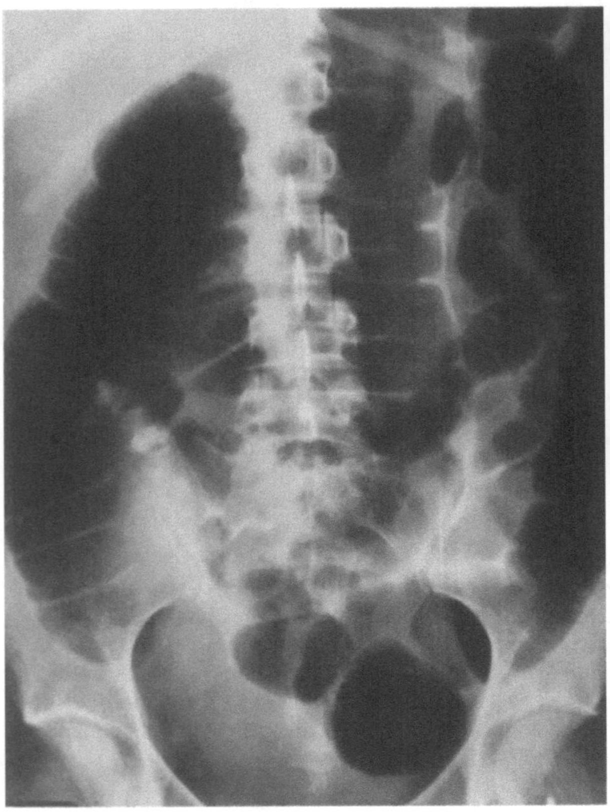
a

Fig. 25 a, b (Legend s. page 55)

Fig. 25a–d. Colonic distension secondary to retroperitoneal disease. Man, 49 years old, with recurring renal uric acid stones developed a right-sided colic radiating into the groin and testis. The right kidney area was tender to percussion, the abdomen was nonrigid, and peristalsis was absent.
a *Supine film* shows generalized colonic distension from the cecum to the rectum. A ureteral stone is not discernible. The left lateral film (not shown) displayed distension of the entire colon with minimal fluid levels and without small-bowel dilatation. **b** *Sonogram of the right kidney* shows slight splaying of the central echo by an outflow obstruction, probably caused by an ureteral stone. **c Paralytic ileus of the colon secondary to chemonucleolysis.** Woman, 55 years old, 3 days after undergoing chemonucleolysis at L2/3. Distended abdomen with diminished bowel sounds and inability to pass stool. Supine film shows isolated distension limited to the colon with slight, nonspecific distension of the small bowel. **d** *Left lateral film* shows colonic distension with individual fluid levels and no evidence of free air. The colon is gas-filled from the cecum to the rectum

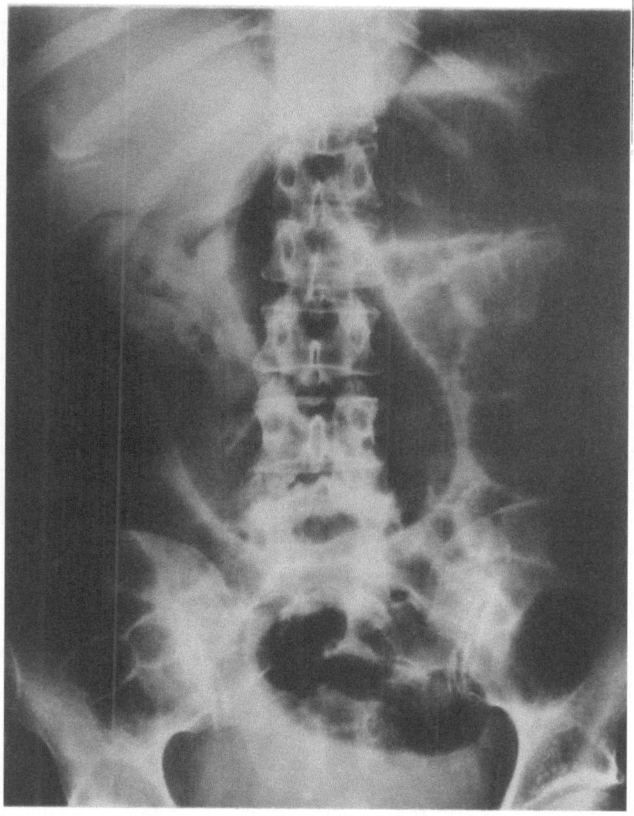

c

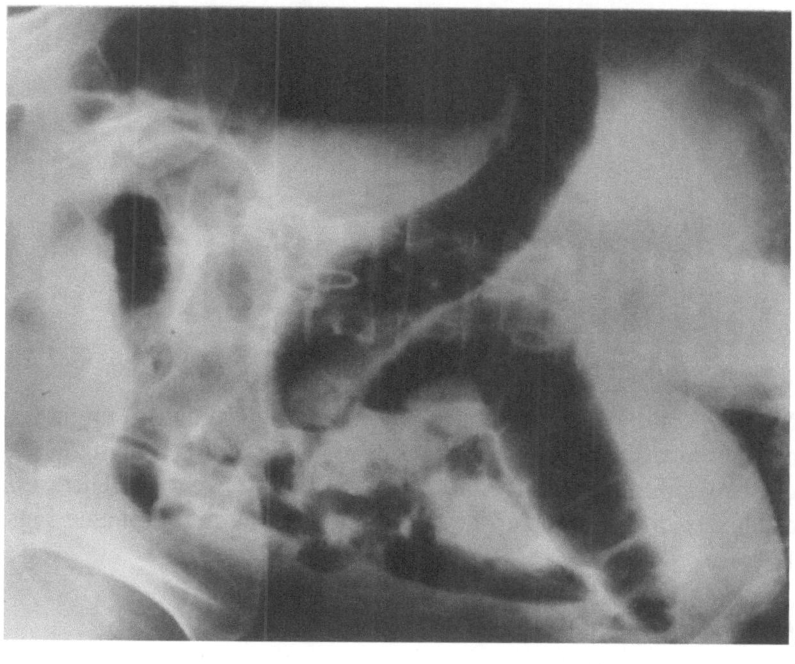

d

The *chronically* distended colon (tumor obstruction; fecal impaction Fig. 21b, 22) usually presents more fluid levels than the colon that is acutely distended by retro- or extraperitoneal disease (Fig. 24). The amount of cecal distension also depends on the function of the ileocecal valve.
Reflux may occur into the small bowel (see Combined Bowel Distension).

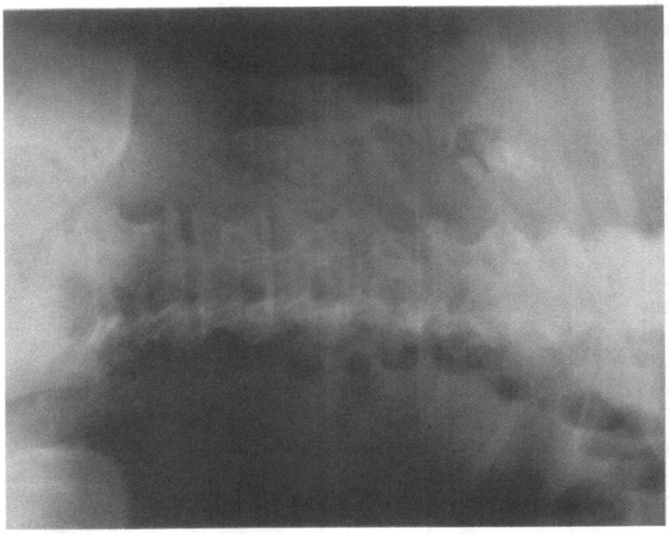

a

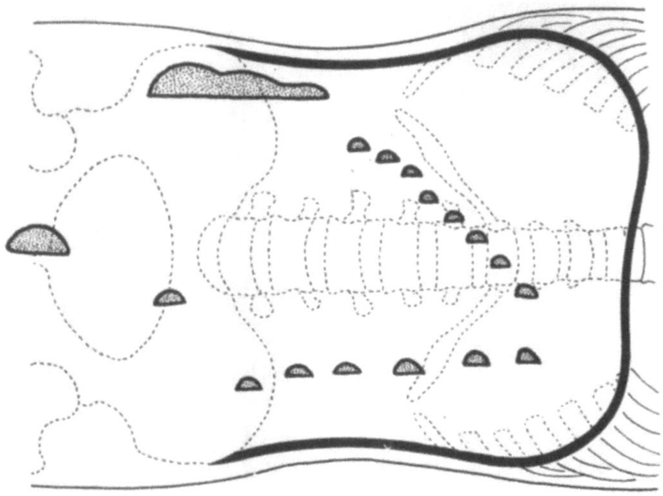

b

Fig. 26 a, b. Distension limited to the colon from low-grade entero-colitis. Man, 35 years old, presented with severe diarrhea and cramping abdominal pain, a soft abdomen with diffuse tenderness, and hyperperistalsis. **a** *Left lateral film* shows small gas collections in multiple haustra of the colon, especially the cecum, ascending and transverse colon, and proximal to the splenic flexure. Short fluid levels are visible in these haustra. There is no free air. **b** Limited colonic distension in inflammatory enterocolitis. *Left lateral film* shows a long fluid level in the cecum accompanied by multiple short levels in the haustra of the transverse and ascending colon

Sonography
Massive colonic distension makes sonography difficult. A target lesion may be seen near the cutoff of the gas column, signifying a malignant tumor growing circumferentially and infiltrating the bowel wall. Ultrasound may disclose a diverticulitic abscess in the lower left quadrant (see Figs. 146 d, 164 c).

Computed Tomography
Massive colonic distension also leads to artifacts on CT scans. The normal colon wall is less than 3 mm thick. The cause of the colonic distension may be apparent (tumor, diverticulitic abscess, pelvic abscess, retroperitoneal lesion). The main purpose of CT is to direct preoperative planning (see Fig. 146 c).

Note: Plain abdominal radiographs in two planes are far superior to sonography and CT in the evaluation of distension limited to the colon.

3.1.5 Combined Distension of the Small and Large Bowel

D. Beyer

Note: Combined distensions of the small and large bowel are the most difficult to evaluate! If the underlying cause acts on *both* bowel regions *and* the stomach it is usually extra-abdominal ("functional ileus") or relates to peritonitis (see Sect. 4.2.3). Differentiation in such cases must rely on *clinical symptoms*. A chest radiograph should always be obtained. If it is obvious that the distension predominantly affects either the small or large bowel, it should be interpreted as an "isolated bowel distension" (see Sect. 3.1.3–3.1.4).

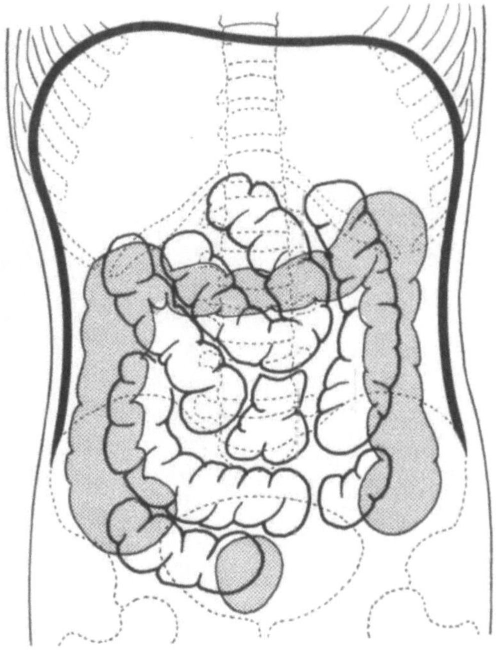
a

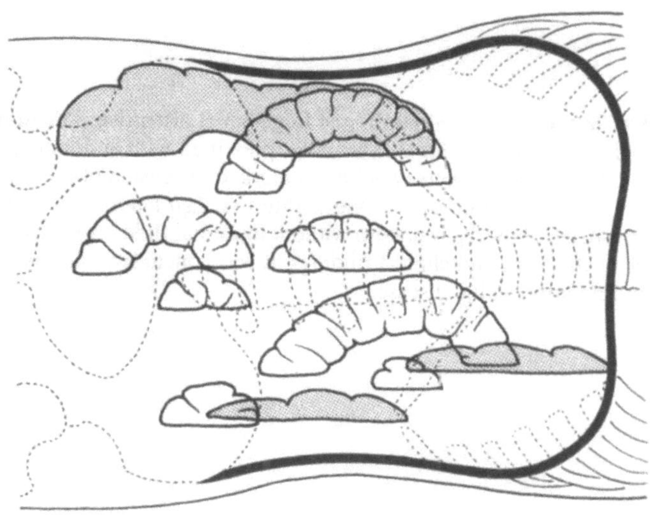
b

Fig. 27 a, b. Schematic illustration of **combined small- and large-bowel distension. a** *Supine film* shows combined gaseous distension of the more centrally positioned small bowel and the more peripheral, framelike colon.
b *Left lateral film* shows uncoiled, distended small-bowel loops with fluid levels. There is typical colonic distension with long fluid levels in the cecum and remaining portions of the colon

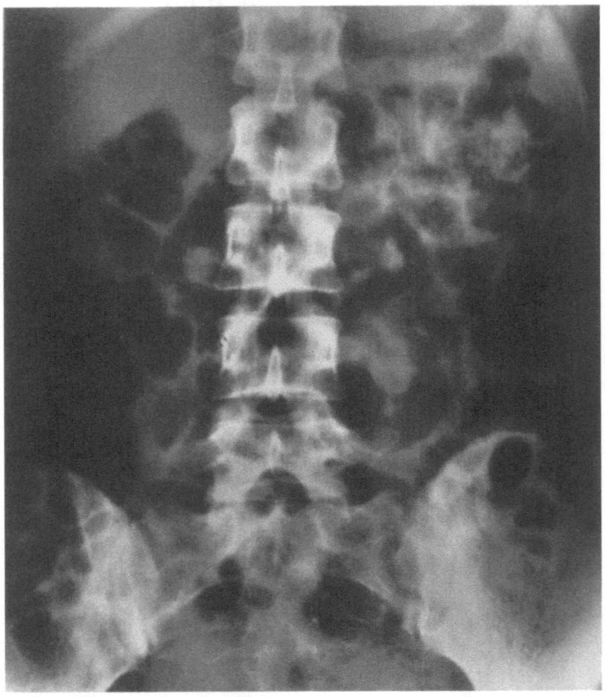

a

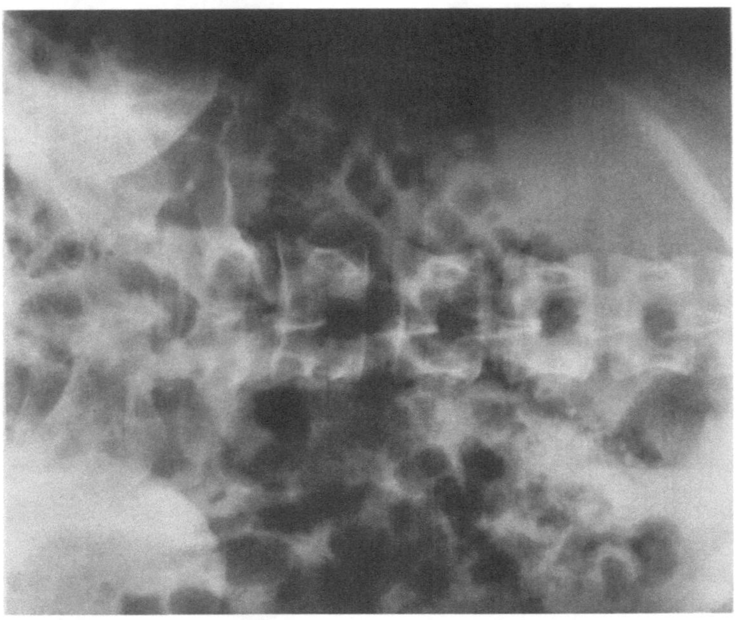

b

Fig. 28a–e. Combined small- and large-bowel distension without pathologic significance. Man, 35 years old, presented with abdominal pain and flatulence. **a** *Supine film* shows marked distension of the small and large bowel with no other abnormalities. **b** *Left lateral film* shows a nonspecific bowel gas pattern without intestinal fluid levels. On the basis of the films and clinical findings, it was concluded that the patient had no appreciable disease.

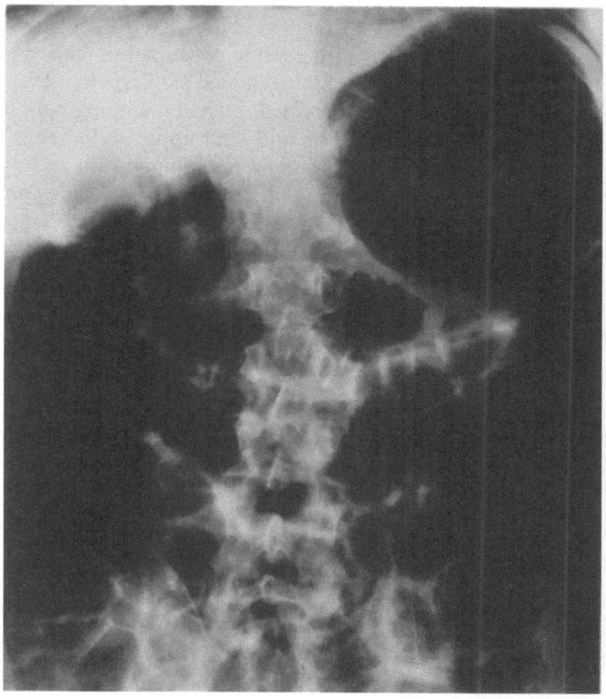

c

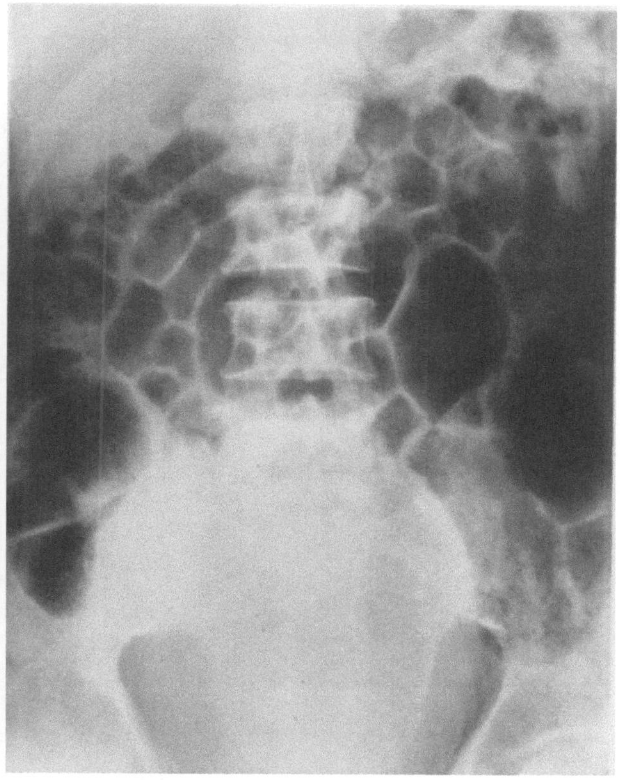

e

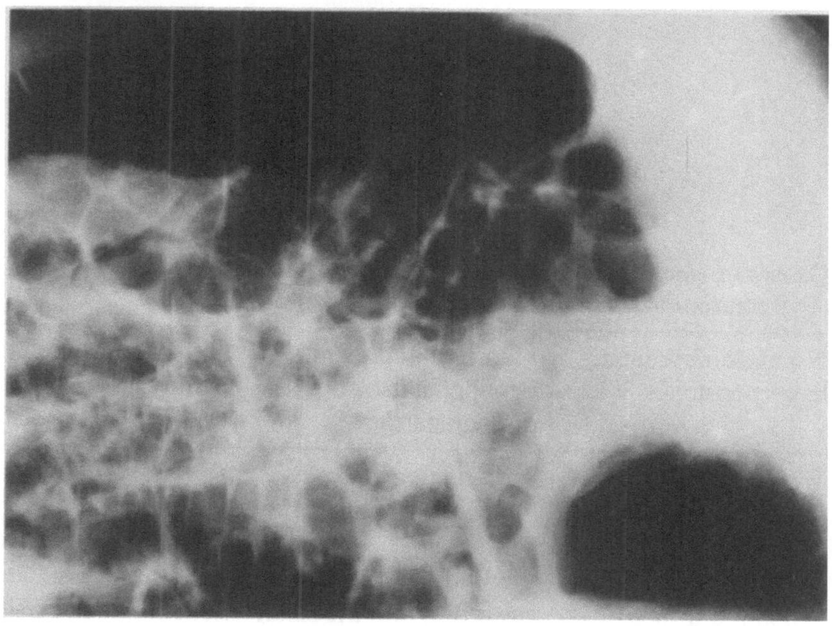

d

Fig. 28 (continued)
c Woman, 58 years old, presented with massive abdominal distension and cramping pains after gastroscopy. *Supine film* shows massive distension of the stomach, small, and large bowel caused by extensive insufflation of air. **d** *Left lateral film* shows no free air, with fluid levels in the stomach, small, and large bowel. After a short while the clinical symptoms resolved. **e** Man, 68 years old, with overflow incontinence from prostatic carcinoma presented with marked abdominal distension and a sensation of fullness. *Supine film* shows a large soft-tissue mass in the lower abdomen, identified by percussion and sonography as a large overflow bladder. The bladder displaced and compressed the distended loops of the small and large bowel. Symptoms regressed after catheterization

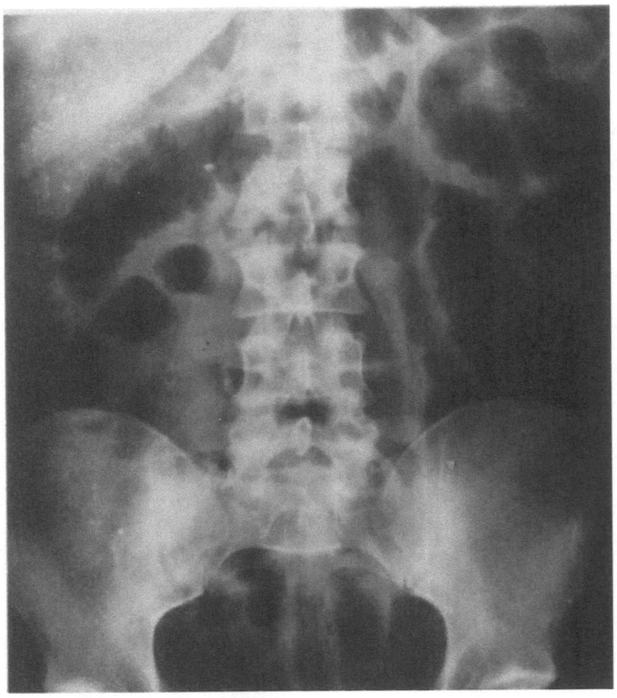
a

Fig. 29 a–d. Combined small- and large-bowel distension due to mechanical colonic obstruction by carcinoma. Man, 55 years old, had marked abdominal distension and increasing constipation with blood stained stools. When examined, he had cramping pain in the mid- and upper abdomen, a nonrigid abdominal wall, and normal peristalsis. **a** *Supine film* shows combined small- and large-bowel distension.

Causes of combined small and large bowel distension
(Differentiation by clinical symptoms)

Nonrigid abdomen, hyperperistalsis	Nonrigid abdomen, hypoperistalsis or aperistalsis	Diffuse abdominal rigidity, aperistalsis
With diarrhea Acute viral/bacterial or toxic gastroenteritis *Without diarrhea* Mechanical colon obstruction with consequent small-bowel distension and gas reflux through the ileocecal valve	*Exta-abdominal causes* ("intestinal pseudo-obstruction") *Toxic megacolon* with gas reflux into the small bowel without perforation *Postoperative state*	*Diffuse peritonitis* secondary to: a perforation of the intestinal tract, suture line leak, ischemia with bowel gangrene (late stage), an "old" mechanical bowel obstruction with wall infiltration, necrotizing enterocolitis, hematogenous spread of microorganisms (rare), (juvenile streptococcal and pneumococcal peritonitis)

Fig. 29 (continued)
b *Left lateral film* shows combined small- and large-bowel distension up to the splenic flexure with fluid levels in the ascending colon and small bowel. **c** *UGI series* with water-soluble contrast material shows dilated loops of small bowel and colon with cutoff of the contrast column a hand's width below the splenic flexure (➧). **d** *Spot film* shows marked dilatation of the proximal descending colon with cutoff at a thread-like stenosis (➧). Sonograms (not shown) demonstrated a target lesion in that area in addition to hepatic metastases. Findings were confirmed at operation

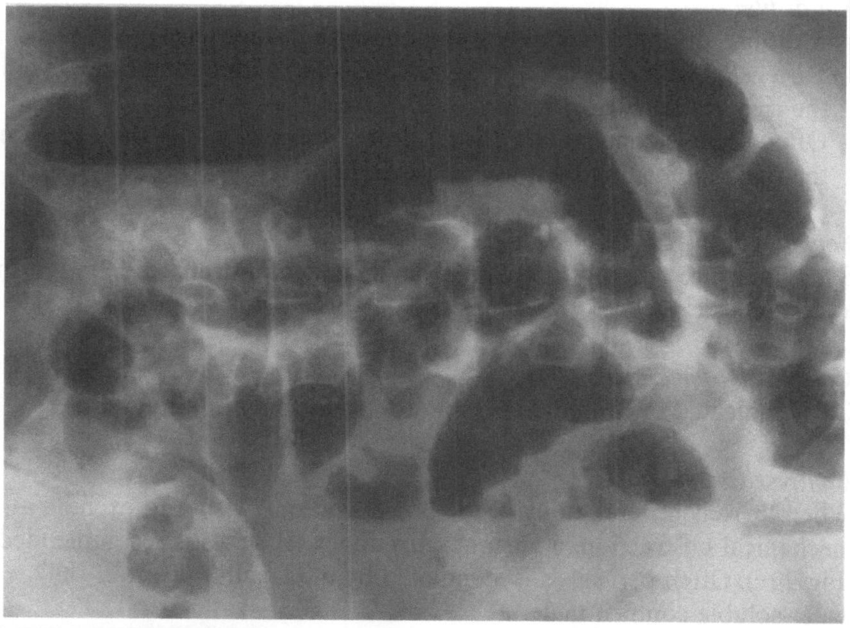
b

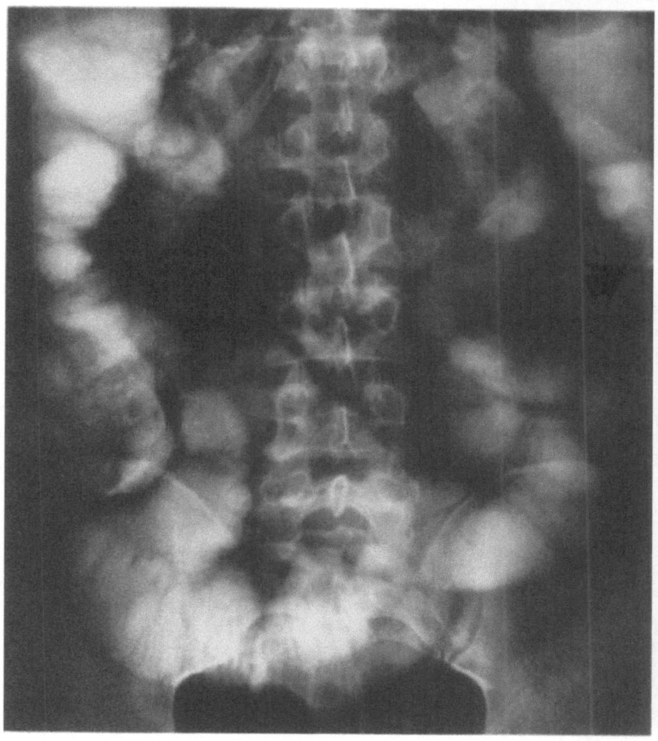
c

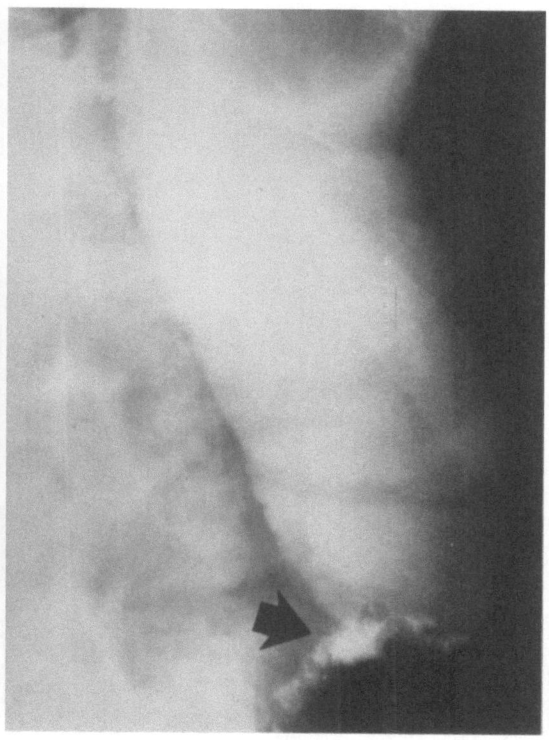
d

Radiologic Signs (Fig. 27)

Plain Radiographs
Supine film: Combined distension of the small and large bowel and often of the stomach, *without* a localized obstruction (Figs. 27 a, 30). Combined small- and large-bowel distension can also develop in the setting of a *mechanical colon obstruction* caused by an incompetent cecal valve. In this case the outflow obstruction in the colon often can be localized (Fig. 29).

L Lat film:
- Multiple, distended small-bowel loops with fluid levels (Fig. 29 b)
- Distension of the cecum and ascending colon with a long fluid level in the right flank (Figs. 29 b, 31 b, 32 c)
- Often there is concomitant gastric distension with a long fluid level in the midabdomen and left upper quadrant

Sonography
Sonograms are difficult to obtain. They may demonstrate free fluid in the abdomen as evidence of peritonitis.

Computed Tomography
CT is indicated in combined bowel distensions only in rare cases.

Contrast Examination
When there is general atony of the bowel and one wishes to exclude a mechanical obstruction, a Gastrografin upper GI series is recommended (Fig. 29 c). Often peristalsis is stimulated by the laxative effect of the water-soluble contrast material.

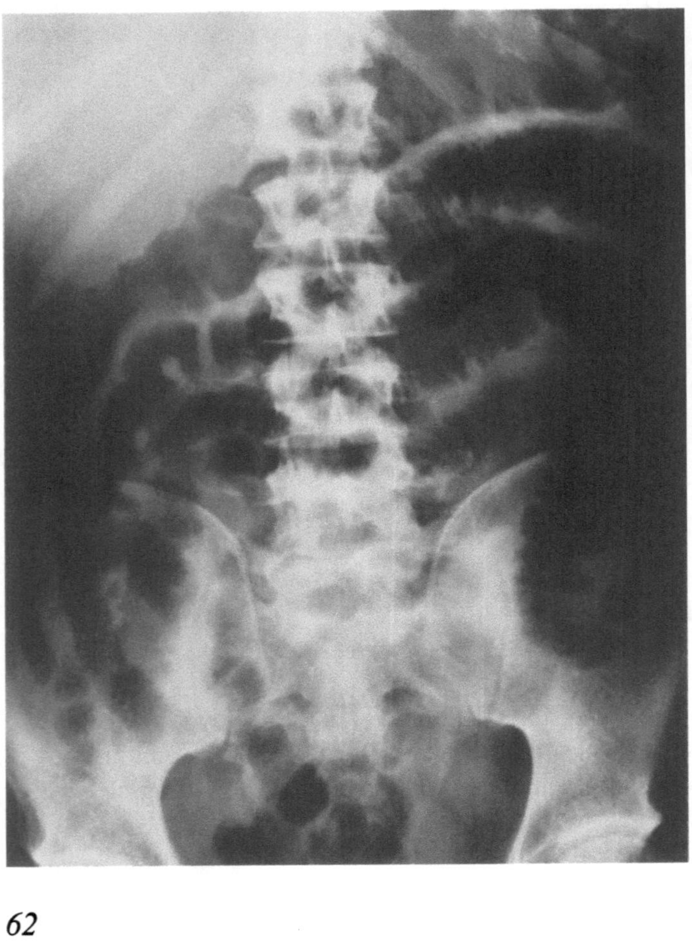

Fig. 30. Combined small- and large-bowel distension in necrotizing enteritis. Man, 39 years old, in poor general condition with marked tenderness and slight distension of the midepigastrium without rigidity. He had profuse, blood-stained diarrhea. *Supine film* shows generalized small- and large-bowel distension with marked widening of Kerckring's folds. The patient died in shock

Fig. 31 a, b. Combined small- and large-bowel distension due to post-operative paralytic ileus. Abdominal distension and aperistalsis developed in a man, 45 years old, following an appendectomy.
a *Supine film* shows massive combined distension of the small and large bowel without cutoff. **b** *Left lateral film* shows residual free air after surgery (▶). The cecum is greatly distended, and the cecum and transverse colon contain long fluid levels. There are multiple hairpinlike loops of small bowel with fluid levels. The symptoms regressed after therapy

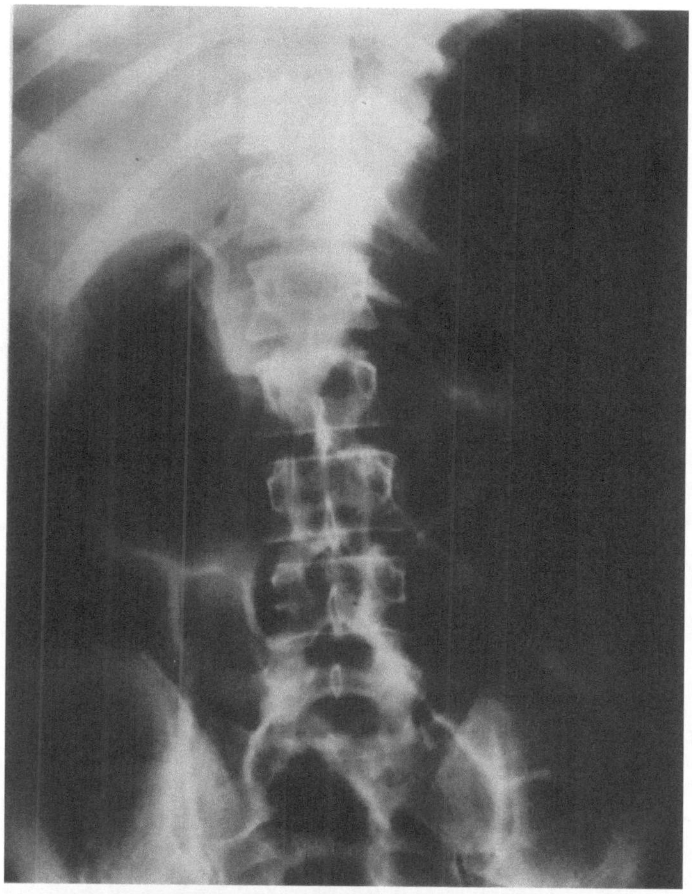
a

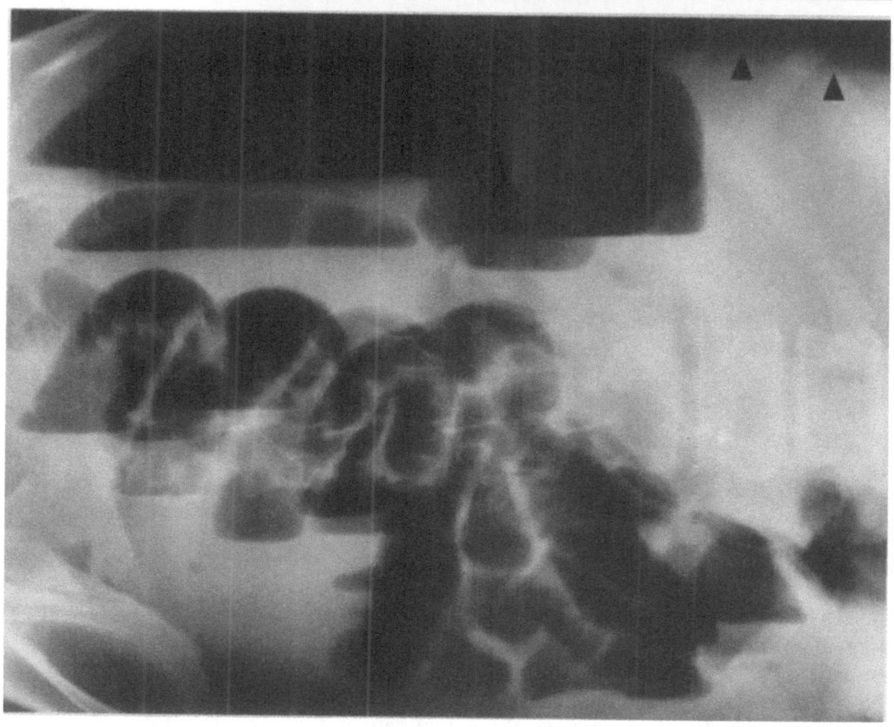
b

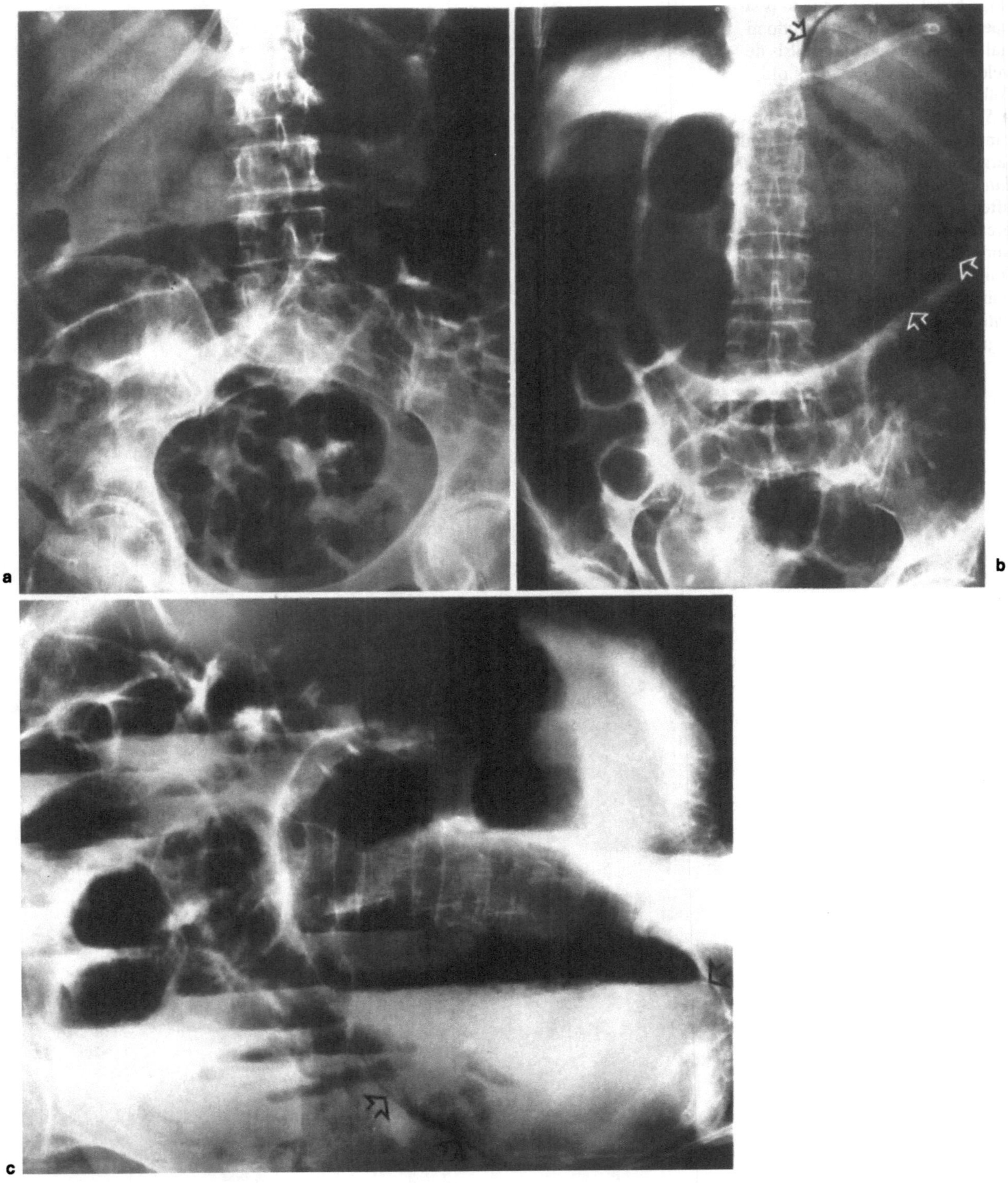

Fig. 32 a–c. Combined small- and large-bowel distension in advanced bowel ischemia with mesenteric infarction and diffuse peritonitis.
a Nonocclusive bowel ischemia, due to cardiac failure. Woman, 60 years old, had increasing abdominal pain and diarrhea for 3 days. She was being treated for a combined aortic-mitral valve disease, caused by endocarditis, with global cardiac failure. *Clinically* she exhibited abdominal distension and rigidity, a silent bowel, symptoms of shock, and leukocytosis. *Supine film* shows marked small-bowel distension with accompanying distension of the colon. The bowel loops are not separated. The *left lateral film* showed combined small- and large-bowel distension with fluid levels and no evidence of perforation. Patient was considered unable to tolerate surgery, and she died 7 h after admission. Autopsy disclosed subtotal, advanced infarction of the entire small bowel, ascending colon, and proximal half of the transverse colon. At autopsy there was no demonstrable thromboembolitic occlusion of the superior or inferior mesenteric artery and vein. Fibrinous peritonitis, shock kidney,

References

Beyer D (1983) Sonographie des Peritonealraumes. In: Bücheler E, Friedmann G, Thelen M (eds) Real-time-Sonographie des Körpers. Thieme, Stuttgart
Beyer D, Friedmann G (1983) Sonographie des Magen-Darm-Traktes. In: Bücheler E, Friedmann G, Thelen M (eds) Real-time-Sonographie des Körpers. Thieme, Stuttgart
Beyer D, Köster R (1980) Diagnostischer Wert von Abdomenübersichtsaufnahmen bei akuter Pankreatitis. Fortschr Röntgenstr 131/1: 9–15
Beyer D, Horsch S, Bohr M, Schmitz T (1980) Röntgensymptomatik der experimentellen Darmischämie beim Hund nach Ligatur der A. mesenterica superior. Fortschr Röntgenstr 4: 377–385
Beyer D, Köster R, Horsch S (1980) Radiologische Frühdiagnostik der akuten Darmischämie durch Nativaufnahmen des Abdomens und Angiographie. Experimentelle und klinisch-radiologische Ergebnisse. In: Müller-Wiefel H, Barras JP, Ehringer H, Krüger M (eds) Mikrozirkulation und Blutrheologie – Therapie der peripheren arteriellen Verschlußkrankheiten. Witzstrock, Baden-Baden Köln New York
Beyer D, Heuser L, Krestin GP (1984) Adjuvante sonographische Diagnostik bei Ileusverdacht. In: Lutz H (ed) Ultraschalldiagnostik 1983. Thieme, Stuttgart
Friedmann G, Wenz W, Ebel K-D, Bücheler E (1980) Emergency roentgen diagnosis. Thieme, Stuttgart
Frimann-Dahl J (1968) The acute abdomen. In: Strnad F (Hrsg) Röntgendiagnostik des Digestionstraktes und des Abdomens. Springer, Berlin Heidelberg New York (Handbuch der Med Radiol, Bd XI/2)
Govoni AF, Whalen JP (1981) The acute abdomen. In: Teplick JG, Haskin ME (eds) Surgical radiology. Saunders, Philadelphia
Hyson EA, Burell M, Toffler R (1983) Drug-induced gastrointestinal disorders. In: Meyers MA, Ghahreman GG (eds) Iatrogenic gastrointestinal complications. Springer, Berlin Heidelberg New York
McCort JJ (1981) Abdominal radiology. Williams & Wilkins, Baltimore
Meyers MA (1976) Dynamic radiology of the abdomen. Normal and pathologic anatomy. Springer, Berlin Heidelberg New York
Mindelzun RE, McCort JJ (1983) Acute abdomen. In: Margulis AR, Burhenne HJ (eds) Alimentary tract radiology. Mosby, St. Louis
Swart B (1968) Duodenum und Nachbarschaft. In: Strnad F (Hrsg) Röntgendiagnostik des Digestionstraktes und des Abdomens. Springer, Berlin Heidelberg New York (Handbuch der Med Radiol, Bd XI/2)
Swart B (1977) Leerbauchdiagnostik des rechten Oberbauches. In: Frommhold W, Gerhardt P (Hrsg) Erkrankungen der Organe des rechten Oberbauches – Klinisch-radiologisches Seminar. Thieme, Stuttgart
Swart B, Meyer G (1974) Die Diagnostik des akuten Abdomens bei Erwachsenen – ein neues klinisch-röntgenologisches Konzept. Radiologe 14: 1–57

◁ **Fig. 32** (continued)
toxic fatty infiltration of the liver with circulatory impairment, and lipoid release from the adrenal cortex were noted. Final diagnosis: nonocclusive gangrene of the bowel.
b, c Nonocclusive ischemia with gangrene of the stomach, small bowel, and ascending colon, and intramural gas in the gastric wall. The 74-year-old woman had been confined to a psychiatric ward for years with schizophrenia. She was bedridden and suffered cardiac insufficiency. She was referred with abdominal pain, distension, and vomiting. Clinically she had a massively distended, nonrigid, diffusely tender abdomen, and a pulse rate of 132. *Supine film* shows gaseous distension of the stomach, duodenum, small bowel, and colon and a linear gas collection in the wall of the fundus and greater curvature of the stomach (⇨). Nasogastric tube (**b**). *Left lateral film* shows massive gaseous distension of all gastrointestinal segments with multiple fluid levels. The position of the gas in the stomach wall remains unchanged (⇨); there is no free air. Exploratory laparotomy disclosed necrosis of the mucosal lining of the stomach, small bowel, and ascending colon, probably from nonocclusive ischemia. The patient died hours after the operation

3.2 Pathologic Thickening of the Bowel Wall - Separation of Gas-Filled Bowel Loops - Mucosal Alterations

D. BEYER, U. MÖDDER

Causes

Small bowel

- Bowel ischemia with edema secondary to direct mesenteric arterial or venous occlusion or extrinsic vasocompression by a volvulus, intussusception, strangulation, or incarceration (see Sect. 4.2.4)
- Spontaneous or trauma-induced hemorrhage into the bowel wall (anticoagulants, hemorrhagic diathesis due to coagulation defect, trauma) (see Sect. 4.3.3)
- Peritoneal carcinomatosis and pseudomyxoma (see Fig. 38) (from tumor imposition)
- Involvement of the bowel by malignant lymphoma
- Crohn's disease of the small bowel with transmural involvement (inflammation) (Fig. 36)
- Amyloidosis of the small bowel (Fig. 35)
- Radiation enteritis (Fig. 36)
- Idiopathic intestinal lymphangiectasis

Colon

- Toxic megacolon (see Sect. 4.2.5)
- Extrinsic vasocompression (sigmoid or cecal volvulus) (see Sect. 4.2.2)
- Local ischemia (see Sect. 4.2.4)
- Crohn's disease of the colon (see Sect. 4.2.2)

Radiologic Signs

Plain Radiographs

Supine film (Figs. 34–38):
Thickening of the bowel wall
Possible luminal narrowing
Separation of gas-filled bowel loops
Asymmetric change of inner wall contour due to mucosal swelling ("thumbprinting"), especially in the ileum and colon
Swelling of Kerckring's folds (especially in the jejunum)
L Lat film (Figs. 35, 174b): Immobility of thickened bowel loops with position change (rigid loop signs)

Note: Bowel wall thickening, separation, and inner wall contour changes are apparent only in connection with gaseous distension of the affected segment. Otherwise films show a "gasless abdomen" with a ground-glass haziness ("white abdomen" (see Fig. 173a). Bowel wall thickening is then confirmed by sonography (Fig. 173b).

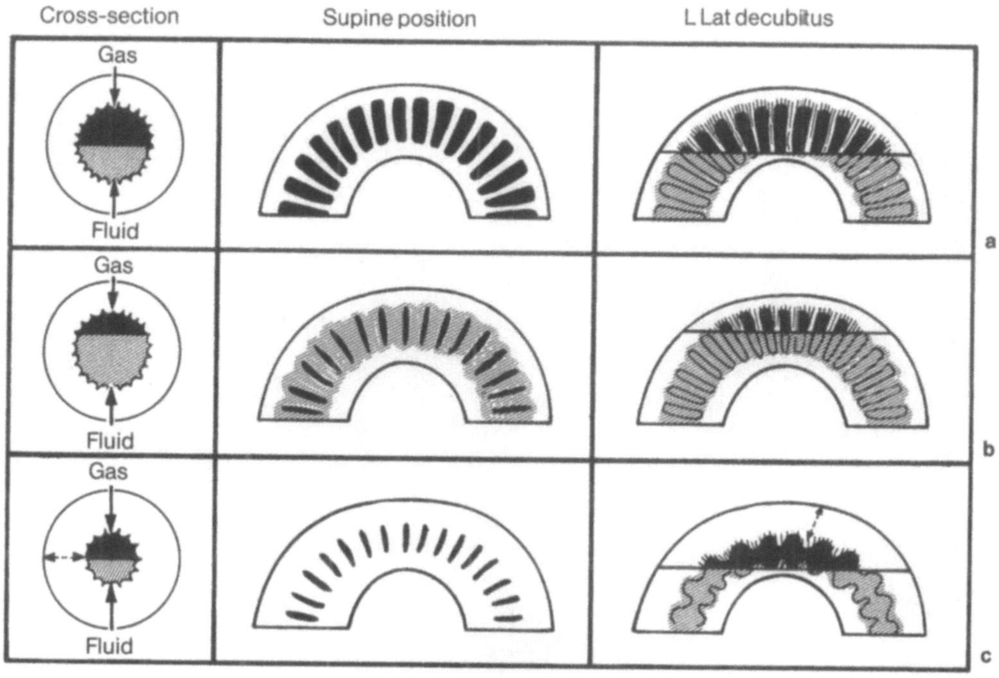

Fig. 33 a–c. Effect of fluid and gas in the bowel on the apparent thickness of the bowel wall on supine and left lateral radiographs.
a With a standard wall thickness and a gas-to-fluid ratio of at least 1:1, the bowel wall and Kerckring's folds present a normal width in both planes. A long fluid level appears in the left lateral position. **b** When the fluid content predominates (gas-to-fluid ratio less than 1:1), the bowel wall and Kerckring's folds appear thickened, especially on the supine film. The left lateral film shows a short fluid level but a normal wall thickness. Free intraperitoneal fluid can also simulate a thickening of the bowel wall. The actual wall thickness can be established by sonography. **c** A bowel wall thickened by edema, hemorrhage, or cellular infiltration shows a constant width on the supine and left lateral films, regardless of intraluminal fluid volume. Again, wall thickness is verified by sonography. (Modified from Mindelzun and McCort 1983)

Caution:
1. Wall thickening with separation can be mimicked by ascites or peritoneal pseudomyxoma (rare) between the bowel loops. Doubts are resolved by sonography (Figs. 37, 38).
2. Thickening of Kerckring's folds in the jejunum on the supine film can be mimicked by a predominant fluid content of the bowel loops (Fig. 33).

Further doubts can be resolved by the L Lat film and possibly by sonography.

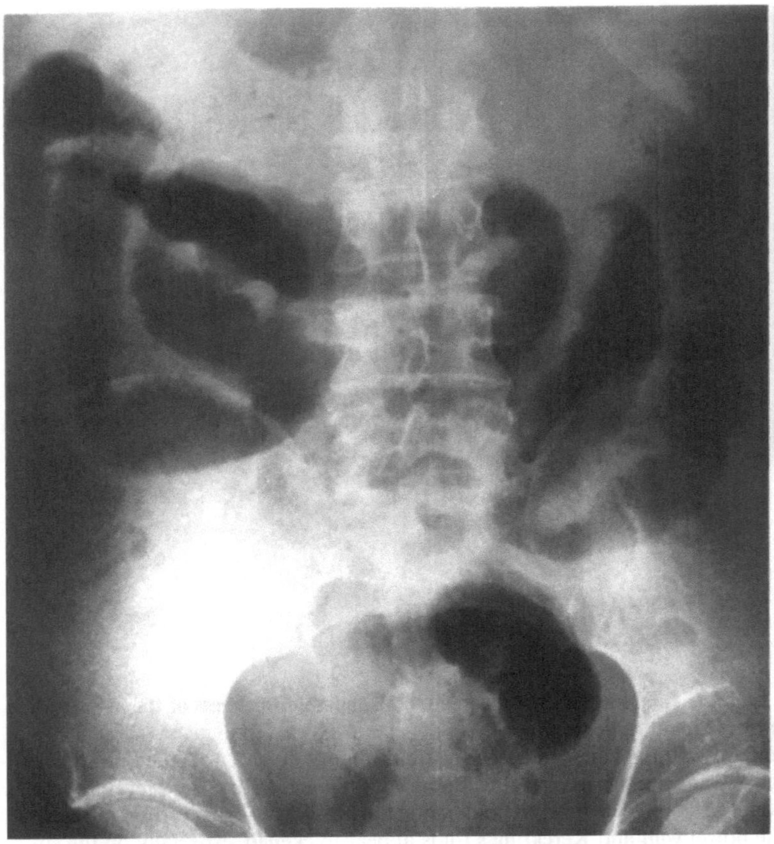

a

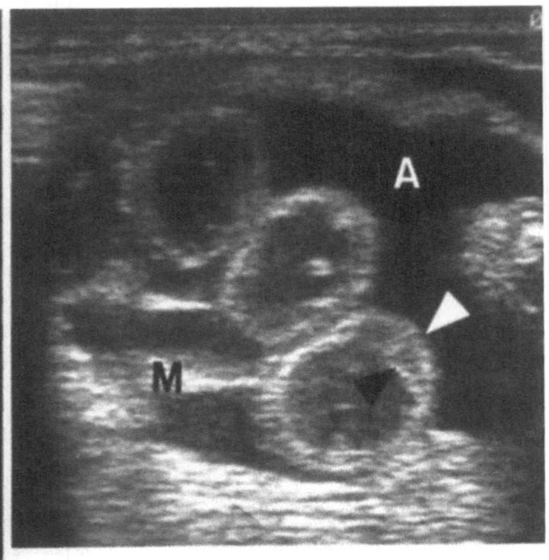

b

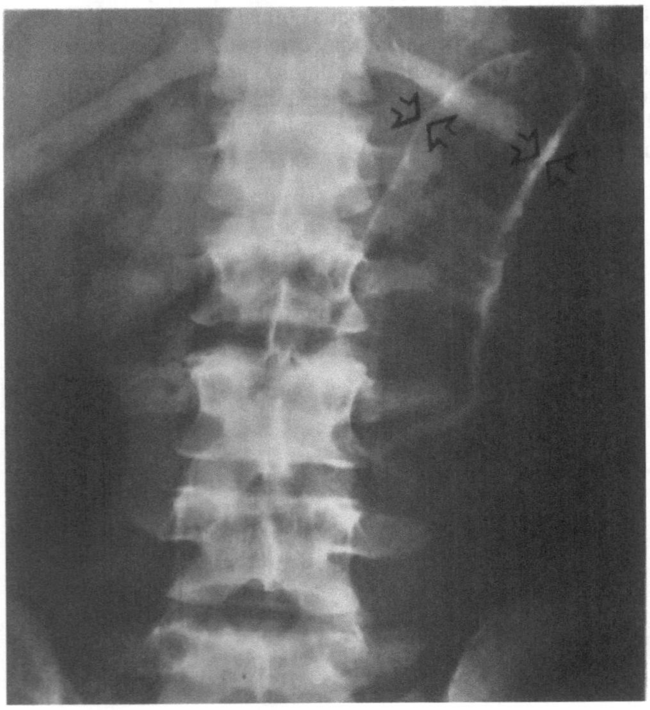

c

Fig. 34a–c. Pathologic thickening of the small-bowel wall secondary to ischemia (mesenteric venous thrombosis). Portal venous thrombosis complicated hepatic cirrhosis in this 53-year-old man, leading to thrombosis of the mesenteric vein. The patient, who also had a history of esophageal varices, had undergone splenectomy 2 years earlier because of thrombosis of the splenic vein. For 4 days before admission he experienced abdominal pain of increasing severity accompanied by bloody diarrhea. Clinical examination disclosed a distended and nonrigid abdomen, diffuse tenderness, aperistalsis, shock, and leukocytosis. **a** *Supine film* 4 days after onset of symptoms shows small-bowel distension with massive wall thickening, luminal narrowing at the flexures, and separation of adjacent loops. **b** *Sonogram* shows a markedly thickened wall (▷ ◁) of the fluid-filled small bowel, attached to an edematous mesentery *(M)*. There is concomitant ascites *(A)*. The patient's poor general condition precluded surgery. Autopsy 2 days later disclosed central mesenteric venous thrombosis secondary to thrombosis of the portal vein. The small bowel showed hemorrhagic infarction and gangrene. **c** For comparison, the *normal wall thickness* of the small bowel is shown in a *supine film* taken in a patient with gastric perforation. Intra- and extraluminal free air outlines the wall of the small intestine (⇨⇦)

Fig. 35a–c. Pathologic thickening of the small-bowel wall secondary to amyloidosis. Man, 66 years of age, with amyloidosis of the entire small bowel and colon. Amyloidosis had been confirmed before by rectal biopsy. For several days the patient had had profuse diarrhea and subsequently no bowel movement for 2 days. Clinical examination disclosed a massively distended, nonrigid, and nontender abdomen with aperistalsis; pulse rate was 88. **a** *Supine film* shows gaseous distension of the stomach and jejunum, swelling of Kerckring's folds (⇨), and marked separation of the gas-containing lumina (↔). **b** *Left lateral film* shows distension of the stomach, duodenum, and small bowel with multiple fluid levels, separation of loops, and swelling of Kerckring's folds. No free air is demonstrated. **c** *Sonogram,* longitudinal scan from the left flank, shows fluid-filled, wall-thickened, small-bowel loops without peristaltic activity. There is no ascites

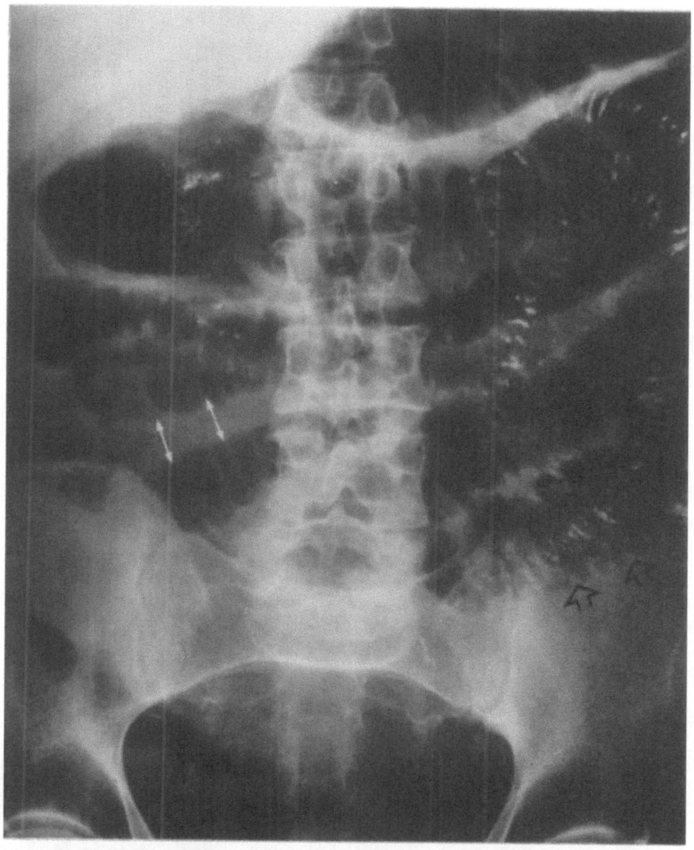

a

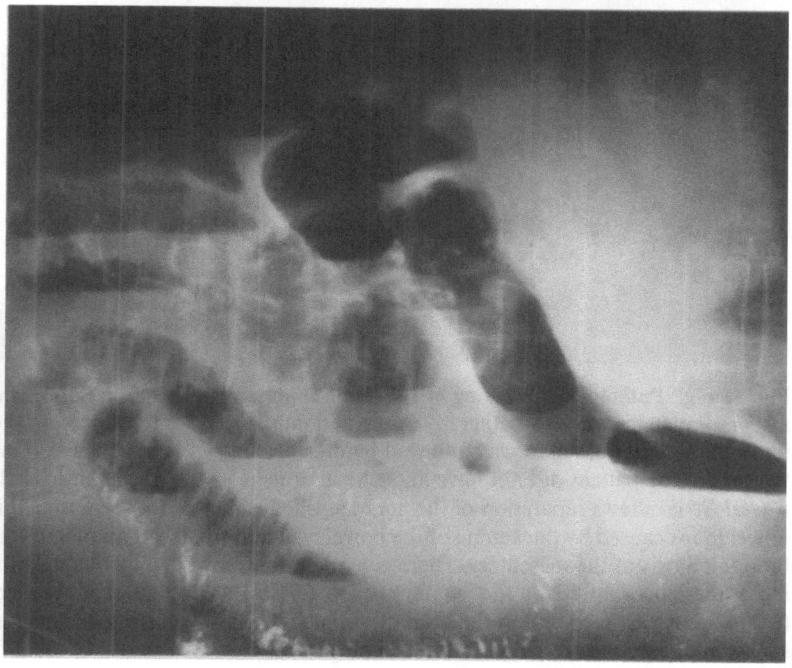

b

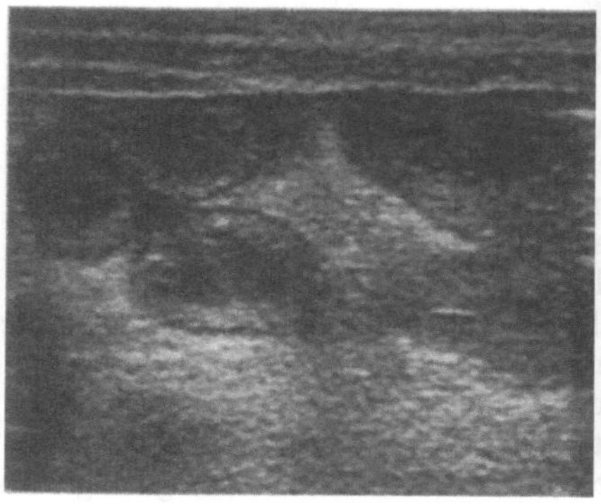

c

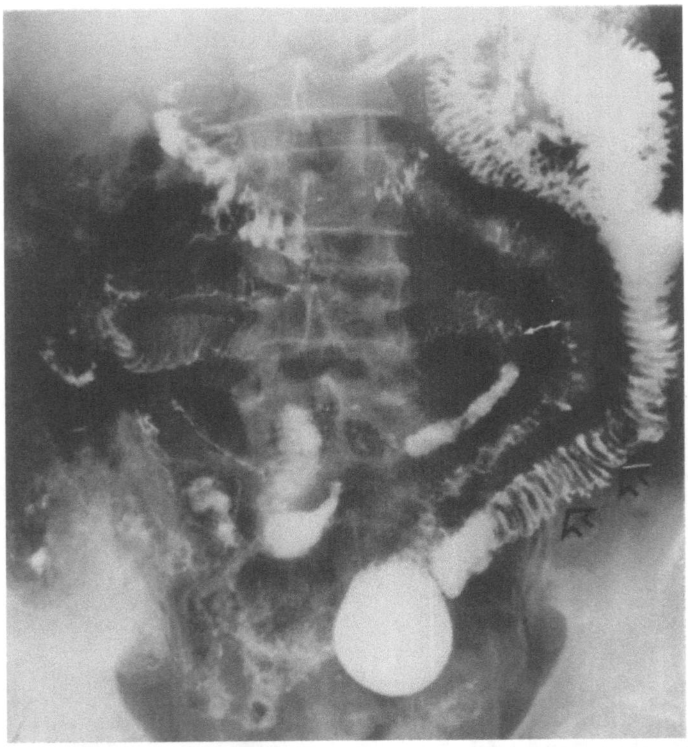

a

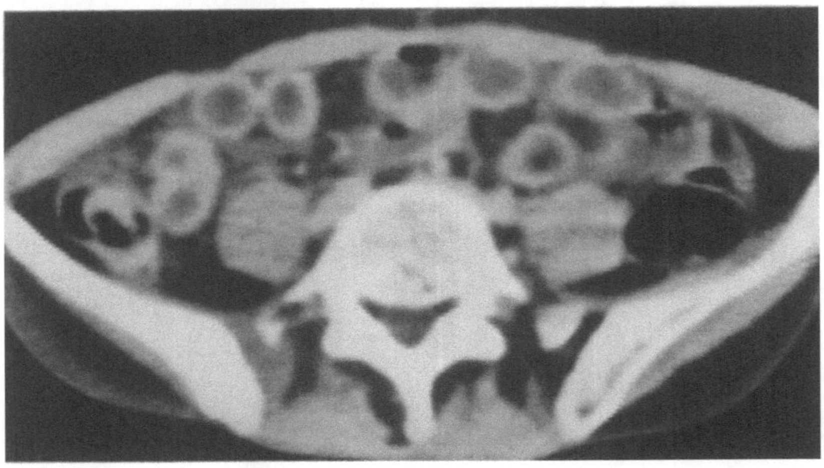

b

Fig. 36a–g. Pathologic thickening of the small-bowel wall after radiation therapy. Radiotherapy of the abdominal cavity in this 41-year-old man was followed by diarrhea and tenesmus. The patient did not have an acute abdomen. **a** *UGI-Series* shows separation of the contrast-filled, small-bowel loops caused by thickening of the bowel wall and fibrolipomatosis of the mesentery. There is marked thickening of the mucosal folds in the jejunum (⇨). **b** *CT scan* (without contrast medium) at the level of the iliac wings shows marked circumferential wall thickening of all the small-bowel loops depicted. The mesenteric markings appear accentuated. **c Pathologic thickening of the wall of the terminal ileum in Crohn's disease.** Woman, 20 years old, with acute appendicitis-like pain in the right lower quadrant. Sonogram shows an extended, hypoechoic wall thickening of the terminal ileum with narrowing of the central gas-filled lumen. **d** Small-bowel follow-through (after rectal air insufflation) shows narrowing of a long segment of the terminal ileum with a cobblestone appearance.
e Pathologic wall thickening of the sigmoid colon by acute diverticulitis in a 54-year-old man with fever, left lower quadrant tenderness, and leukocytosis. *Longitudinal sonogram* demonstrates the thick hypoechoic wall and narrow lumen of the affected bowel. **f** Transverse sonogram gives a clearer picture of the hypoechoic, wall-thickened sigmoid colon. **g** Contrast enema confirms the sonographic impression of sigmoid diverticulitis

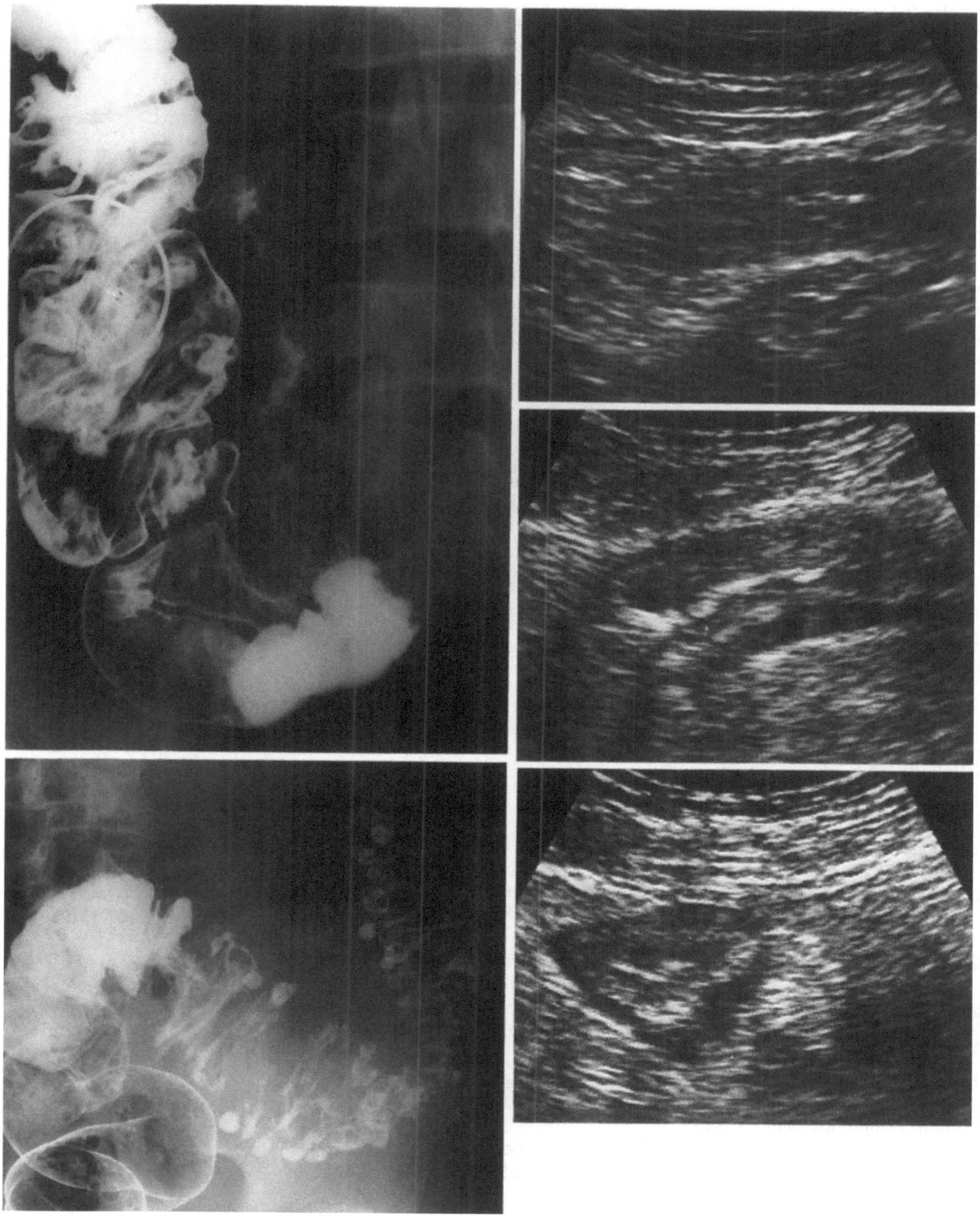

Fig. 36c–g (Legend see page 70)

Sonography
This study is best performed from the right or left flank to avoid the superimposition of bowel gas.
Findings: multiple "target lesions" in the affected bowel segment due to bowel wall thickening (Figs. 34–38)

Computed Tomography
CT scans show a concentric, soft-tissue-dense thickening of the bowel wall. If the affected segment is large, multiple "ring structures" may be visible on a single scan. Usually this is accompanied by luminal narrowing.
Attention should be given to possible involvement of the mesentery (weblike infiltration) (ischemia, Crohn's disease, radiation enteritis, peritoneal carcinomatosis).
CT can differentiate true bowel wall thickening from apparent thickening (due to ascites, peritoneal pseudomyxoma, paraluminal masses, etc.) (Figs. 36, 38).
CT always permits the concomitant evaluation of *all* neighboring structures including the abdominal wall and mesenteric fat. Pathologic changes can also be evaluated (tumor, lymphoma, hemorrhage, abscess, gas, etc.)

Note: The thickness of the bowel wall depends on its degree of distension. Local or diffuse thickening must be fairly massive before it can be demonstrated and evaluated with CT.

References

Beyer D, Horsch S (1980) Röntgendiagnostik bei akuter Darmischämie. Zentralbl Chir 105: 1005
Beyer D, Köster R (1984) Bildgebende Diagnostik akuter intestinaler Durchblutungsstörungen. Ein klinisch-radiologisches Konzept. Springer, Berlin Heidelberg New York Tokyo
Beyer D, Schultze P (1983) Sonographie des Magen-Darm-Traktes. In: Bücheler E, Friedmann G, Thelen M (eds) Real-time-Sonographie des Körpers. Thieme, Stuttgart
Beyer D, Horsch S, Bohr M, Schmitz T (1980) Röntgensymptomatik der experimentellen Darmischämie beim Hund nach Ligatur der A. mesenterica superior. Fortschr Röntgenstr 132/4: 377
Nelson SW, Eggleston W (1960) Findings on plain roentgengrams of the abdomen associated with mesenteric vascular occlusion with possible new sign of mesenteric venous thrombosis. AJR 83: 866
Swart B, Meyer G (1974) Die Diagnostik des akuten Abdomens beim Erwachsenen – Ein neues klinisch-radiologisches Konzept. Radiologe 14: 1

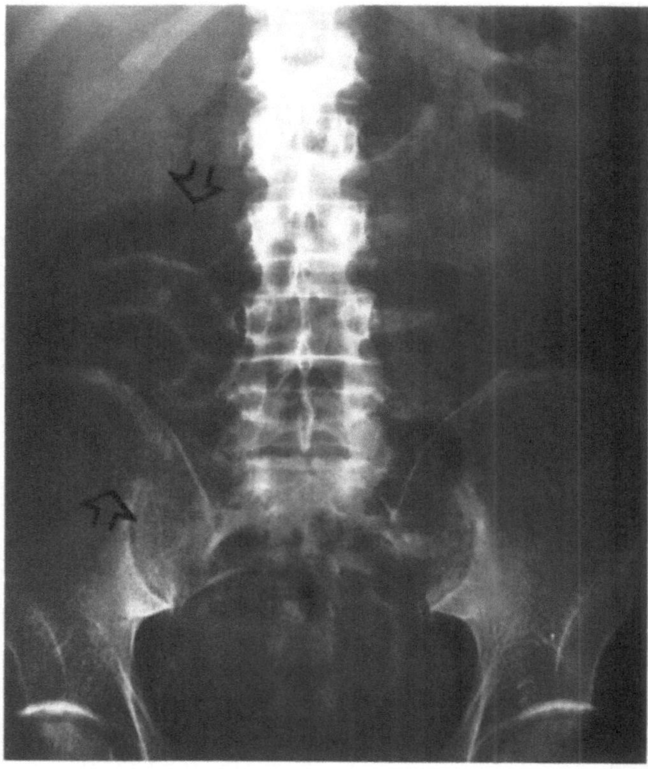

a

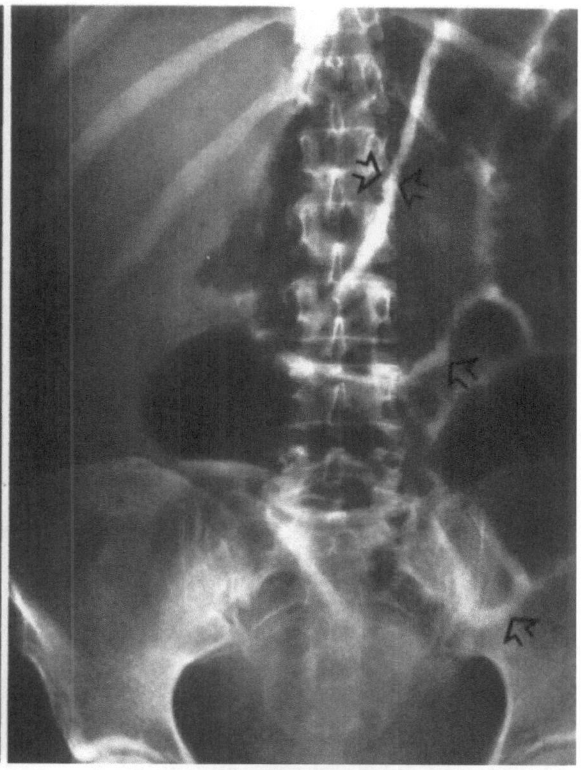

b

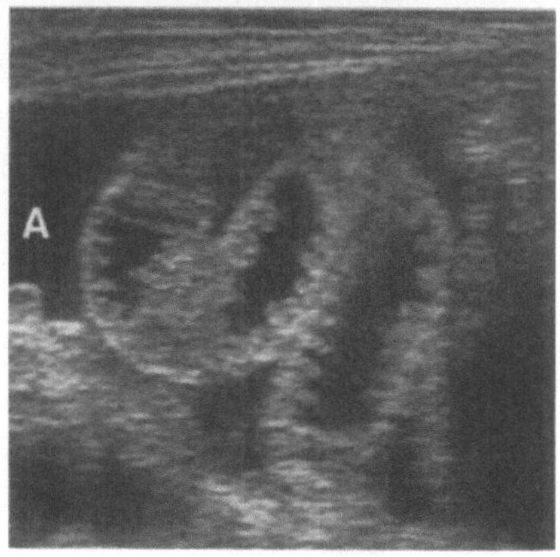

c

Fig. 37. a Bowel wall edema with loop separation in the right lower midabdomen (⇨⇦) mimicked by ascites associated with a known hepatic cirrhosis. Clinical symptoms were not consistent with infarcted bowel. **b** Simulation of bowel wall edema. Separation results from diffuse, operatively confirmed, peritoneal carcinomatosis from ovarian cancer with mechanical obstruction of the small bowel (⇨⇦). **c** *Sonogram* (left flank scan) shows a fluid-filled loop of jejunum with normal-sized Kerckring's folds and normal wall thickness; ascites *(A)* is present

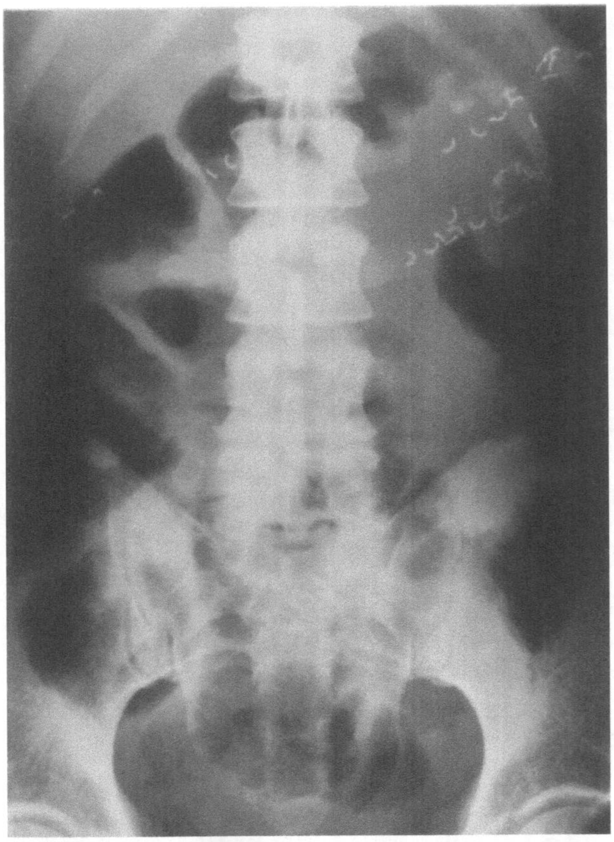

a

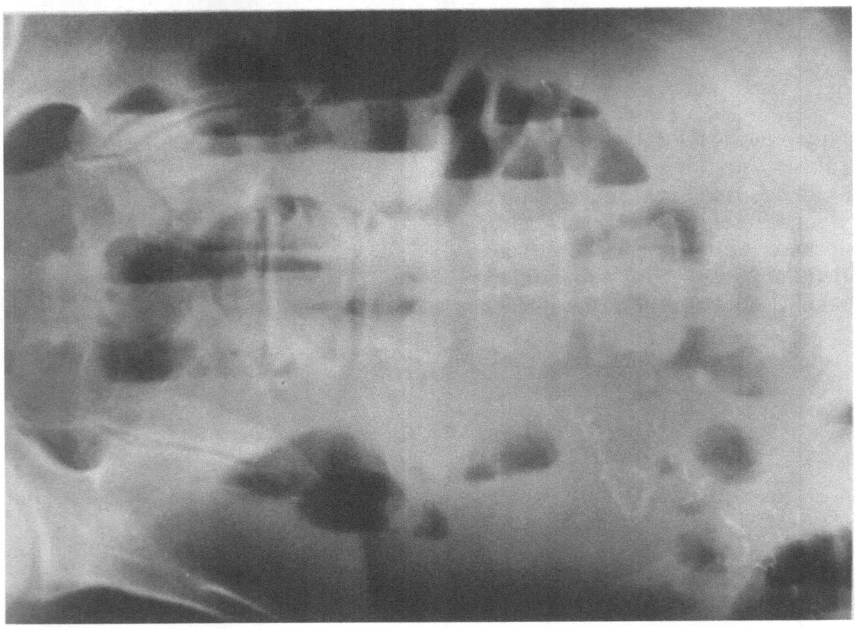

b

Fig. 38a–f. Simulation of bowel wall edema with separation by pseudomyxoma peritonei. The 42-year-old patient had a mucocele of the appendix removed 3 months earlier; he was surgically treated again 10 weeks later, at which time pseudomyxoma peritonei was diagnosed. The bulk of the pseudomyxoma was removed. Postoperatively the patient manifested pain, a distended, nontender abdomen, and alternation between diminished and increased bowel sounds. **a** *Supine film* shows combined small- and large-bowel distension with marked separation and uncoiling, especially of the distended small-bowel loops, as found in bowel wall edema. **b** *Left lateral film* shows combined small- and large-bowel distension with multiple short fluid levels. The separation of loops is not demonstrated in the cross-table view.

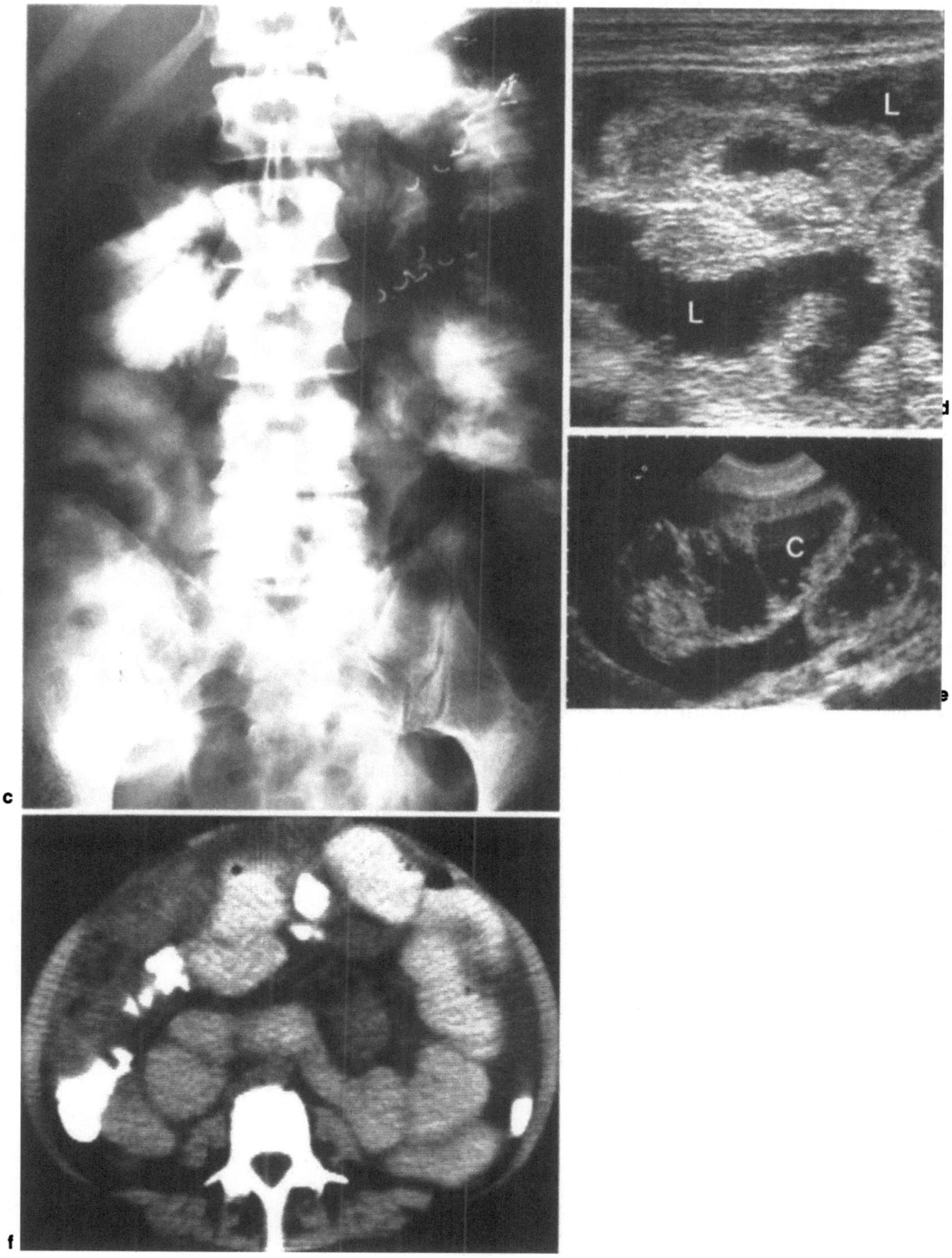

Fig. 38 (continued)
c *Gastrografin UGI series* shows alternating dilatations and stenoses of the small-bowel lumen, especially in the *left upper quadrant*. There is still obvious separation of bowel loops. **d** With *sonography* the small-bowel loops *(L)*, which are fluid filled, are separated by bizarre-shaped, hyperechoic, solid areas. **e** *Longitudinal sonogram* through the left upper quadrant shows the colon *(C)* also with marked fluid filling and wall thickening and the deposition of solid material. **f** On *CT scan* the small bowel, filled with diluted Gastrografin, appears as a dense structure containing little air. Luminal size is highly variable. The bowel loops are separated by low-density intraperitoneal masses (pseudomyxoma peritonei)

3.3 Intraperitoneal Fluid Collections

G. P. Krestin, D. Beyer

Free Intraperitoneal Fluid

Causes

Ascites

- Inflammatory diseases of the peritoneum:
  - Peritonitis
  - Bacterial infections, tuberculosis
- Venous stasis:
  - Portal venous thrombosis
  - Hepatic cirrhosis
  - Posthepatic congestion (due to tumors, thrombosis)
  - Budd-Chiari syndrome
  - "Right heart" failure
  - Constrictive pericarditis
- Chylous ascites
  - Congenital chylous ascites
  - Acquired obstruction of lymphatic drainage

  Lymph node enlargement

  Interruption of thoracic duct (tumor-related, traumatic)
- Peritoneal carcinomatosis
- Bile ascites (with biliary leakage), biloma
- Pancreatogenic ascites (pancreatitis, pancreatic tumors)
- Meigs' syndrome
- Hypoproteinemia

Note: The most common cause of ascites is malignancy (50%), followed by hepatic cirrhosis (30%), and heart disease (10%).

Hemorrhage into the peritoneal cavity

- Trauma-related:
  - Hepatic rupture
  - Splenic rupture
  - Mesenteric tear
- Tubal abortion
- Postoperative

Radiologic Signs

Plain Radiographs

Note: Small amount of free fluid are rarely appreciated on plain abdominal films. The major radiologic feature, regardless of location, is a homogeneous shadow of soft-tissue density.

Caution: The supine film is best for the detection of free fluid because displacement of the fluid in the lateral position ususally prevents recognition of pathologic changes.

Fluid collecting predominantly in the lesser pelvis (Figs. 39 a/b, 40, 41)
- Mostly seen in patients not on bed rest (because fluid seeks the lowest part of the peritoneal cavity)
- Sickle-shaped density with its convexity towards the pelvic floor (100-150 ml)
- Crescentic density on the pelvic floor (200-300 ml)
- Rounded density on the pelvic floor (over 400 ml)
- Separation of ileal loops
- Characteristic linear lucency between the fluid density and bony pelvic wall caused by pelvic fat (differentiate from tumor)
- Density may spread into the flank stripes

Caution: A full urinary bladder can hinder diagnosis!

Fluid collecting predominantly in the flanks (Fig. 39 b)
- Mostly seen after prolonged bed confinement
- Density has a sharp lateral border
- Density bordered medially by bowel gas (usually the ascending colon on the right side and the descending colon on the left side)
- Density may spread superiorly
- The inferior margin of the liver is obscured (Fig. 39 a, b)
- The outline of the spleen is indistinct

Fluid collecting in the midabdomen
- Usually associated with fluid in the flanks and/or pelvis
- Separation of bowel loops

  Broad line of density between the greater gastric curvature and the transverse colon (also characteristic of bleeding from a hepatic of splenic rupture)

Note: Gas-filled bowel loops facilitate the diagnosis. With fluid-filled bowel, differentiation is *not* possible on plain abdominal radiographs, and sonography has to be done.

a
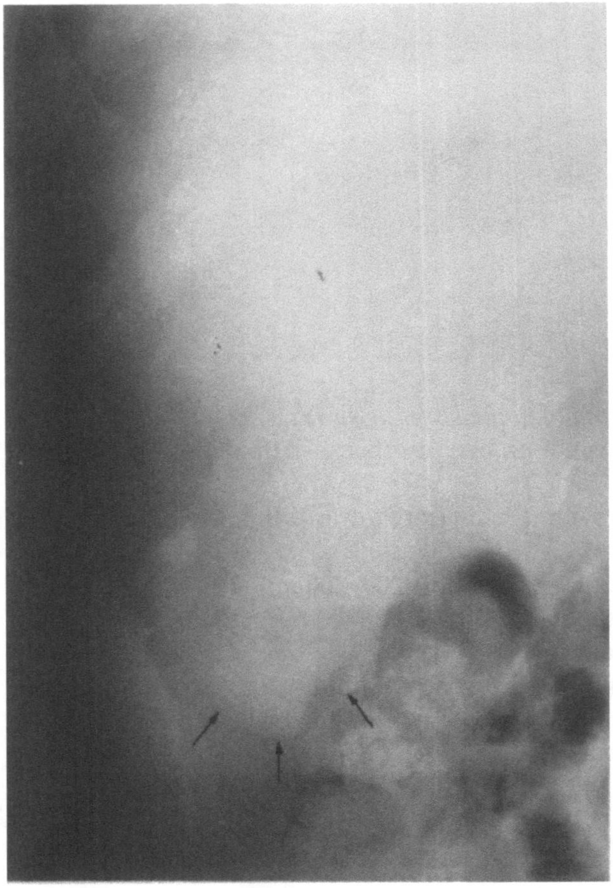

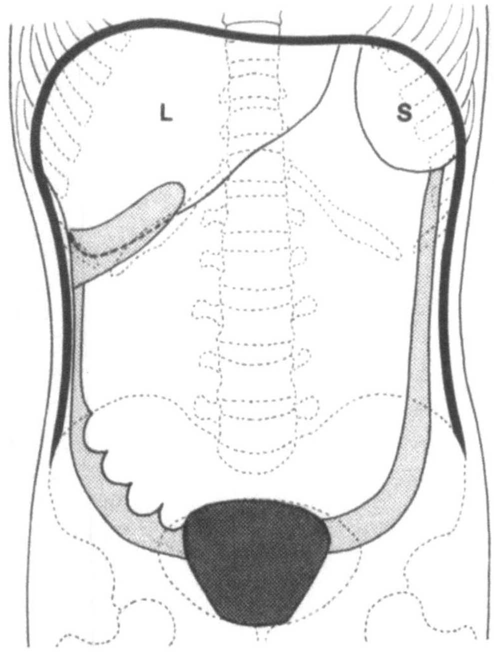

b

Fig. 39. a Normal anatomy: The right lower margin of the liver is clearly delineated (→). Even small amounts of fluid will obliterate its visible contour on the supine radiograph. **b Sites of collection of intraperitoneal fluid on the supine film:** the lesser pelvis, the flanks (paracolic gutters). The flank stripes and pelvic fat lines are preserved, while the inferior margin of the liver is obscured (fluid volume greater than 0.5 liter). *L*, liver; *S*, spleen

Sonography (Figs. 42, 43)

- Free fluid is mobile and echo-free
- Small amounts of fluid (30 ml or more) may be demonstrated behind the bladder and below the liver (Morison's pouch) and in the paracolic gutters
- With larger fluid volumes: freely floating small-bowel loops tethered at the mesenteric root ("sea anemone" pattern)
- Echo-free areas between the abdominal wall and liver or spleen or in Morison's pouch
- Ascites associated with peritoneal carcinomatosis is recognized by the simultaneous presence of tumor masses on peritoneal surfaces, perihepatic or the thickening of the greater omentum (Fig. 43 a)
- Floating echoes ("snowstorm" pattern) within the fluid: infectious ascites, hemorrhage, or fibrinous ascites in hepatic cirrhosis
- In many cases the cause of the ascites can be established (hepatic cirrhosis, tumor, cardiac congestion)

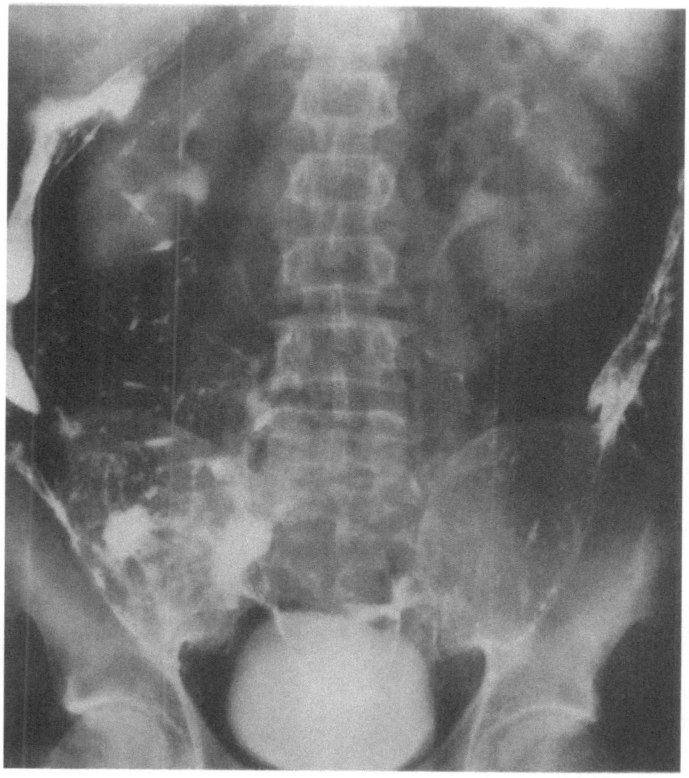

Fig. 40. Topography of the peritoneal space demonstrated by barium coating of the peritoneum and bowel. An iatrogenic rectal perforation during a barium enema led to extravasation of contrast material into the peritoneal cavity. The *urogram* shows barium sulfate in the lesser pelvis and paracolic gutters, extending up beneath the liver on the right side (Morison's pouch)

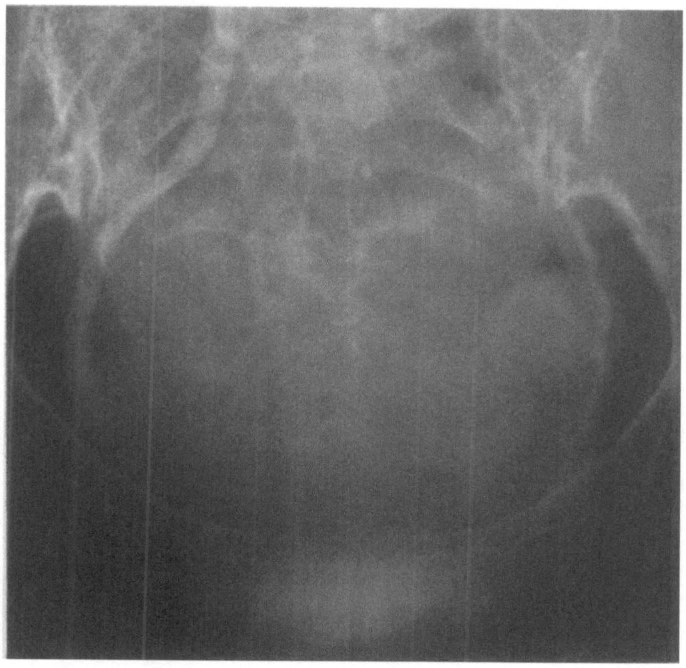

Fig. 41. Man, 68 years old, with known hepatic cirrhosis. **Ascites in the lesser pelvis** produces a homogeneous density with spreading of the ureters and caudad displacement of the bladder

Computed Tomography

- Ascites
  - Low-density margin around intraperitoneal organs with attenuation values of 5–20 Hn units
  - Eccentric bowel displacement by increased intraperitoneal pressure and ascites
  - Principal site of fluid collection is the cul-de-sac
  - Intraperitoneal fluid is easily distinguished from retroperitoneal collections
  - Solid tumor masses in peritoneal carcinomatosis are identifiable above a size of 1.5 cm
  - The cause of the ascites can often be demonstrated (tumor, pancreatitis)
  - Hemorrhage (see Fig. 193 a, b):
    Fresh blood presents as a high-density mass with attenuation values of 40–60 Hn units and can be clearly differentiated from ascites
    Hemorrhage after blunt trauma is localized to the area around the ruptured organ (liver, spleen) (see Fig. 196)

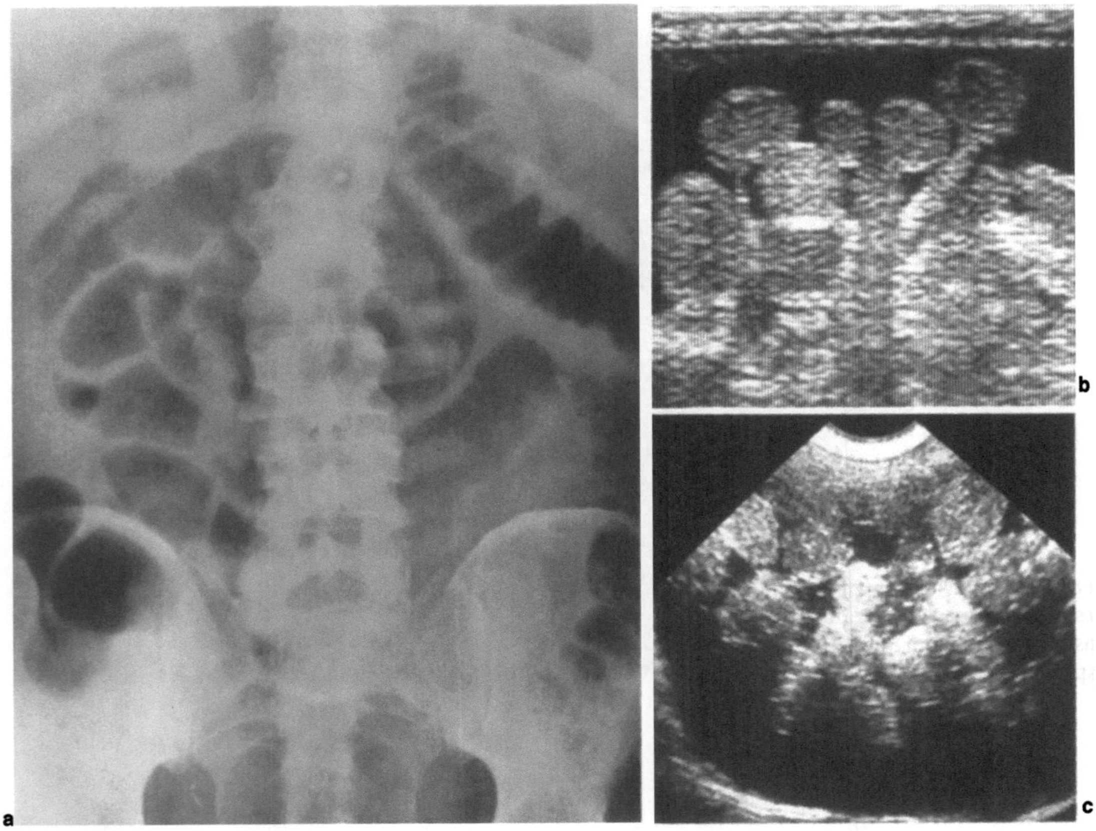

Fig. 42 a–c. Man, 76 years old, with **ascites** and known hepatic cirrhosis. **a** *Supine film* shows marked separation of air-filled bowel loops in the midabdomen, creating the impression of a thickened bowel wall. **b** *Sonogram* demonstrates free intraperitoneal fluid in which the small-bowel loops float freely, tethered by mesentery. **c** Woman, 54 years old, with an ovarian tumor. *Sonogram* shows a giant ovarian tumor, partly solid and partly cystic, filling the mid- and lower abdomen (do not mistake for ascites!)

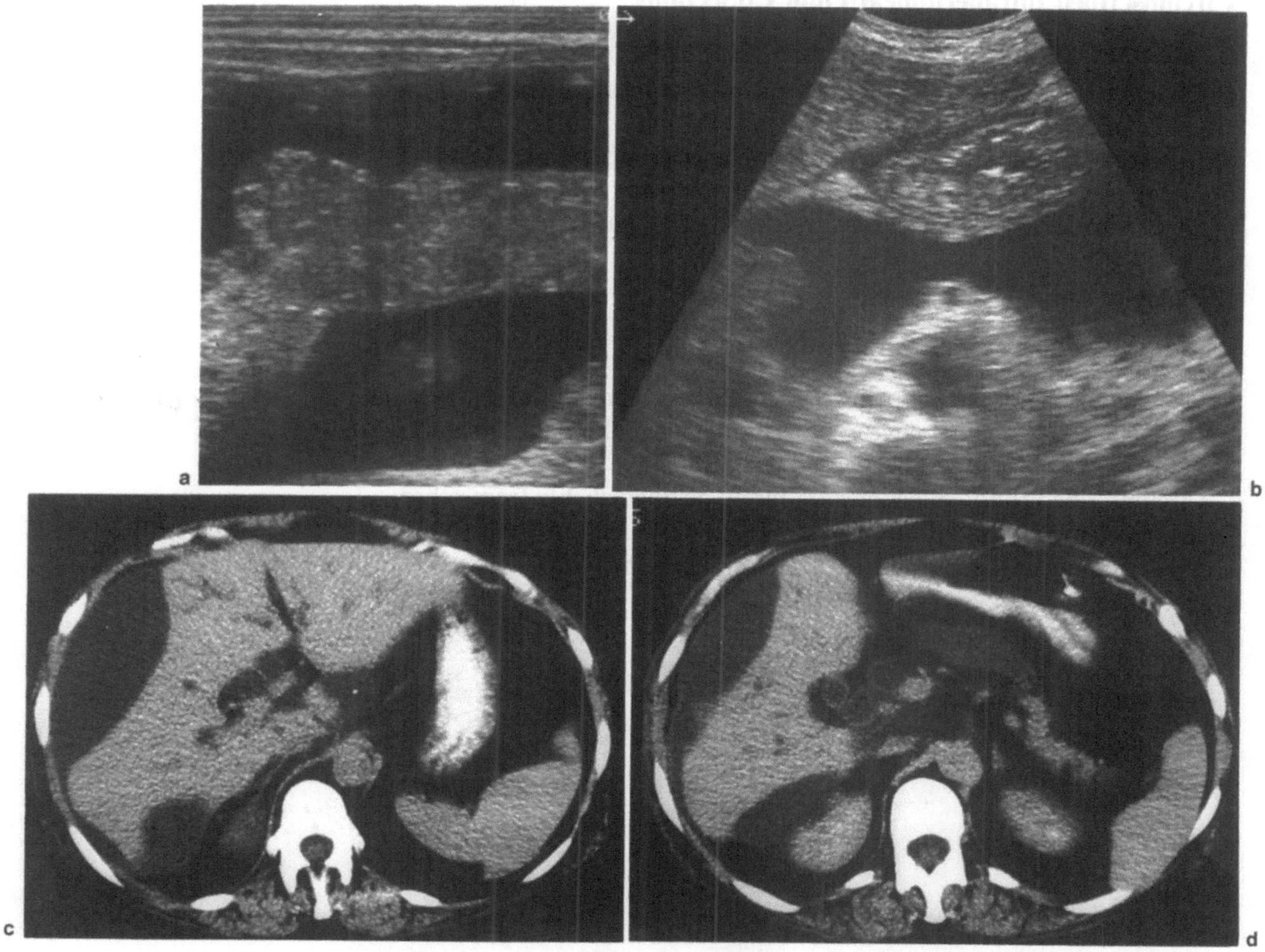

Fig. 43. **a** Woman with known **ovarian carcinoma, peritoneal carcinomatosis and ascites.** *Sonogram* shows large amounts of free fluid in the abdominal cavity. The greater omentum, widened by metastases, floats freely in the ascites. **b** Sonography demonstrates free fluid in the omental bursa behind the stomach. **c Biliomas** are seen in the peri- and subhepatic space, in the porta hepatis, and in the omental bursa **following gallbladder perforation** in a 52-year-old woman with a prepapillary calculus and jaundice. The patient had a 4-day history of biliary colic and slowly progressive icterus; she presented with increasing muscular rigidity in the right upper quadrant. *CT scan* (with continuous contrast infusion) shows fluid in the peri- and subhepatic spaces and porta hepatis, with dilatation of the intrahepatic bile ducts. **d Fluid in the omental bursa.** Small, collapsed bile ducts and dilatation of the common bile duct at the porta hepatis

Circumscribed Intraperitoneal Fluid Collections

Causes

Encapsulated ascites (after multiple punctures or local infection)
Abscess, circumscribed hematoma, biloma (Fig. 44)
Differential diagnosis: large organ cysts that protrude beyond organ boundaries into the peritoneal cavity, e.g., pancreatic pseudocysts, hepatic cysts, ovarian cysts, splenic cysts, mesenteric cysts, enterogenic cysts

Radiologic Signs

Plain Radiographs

- Presents like a space-occupying lesion (abscess, hematoma, cyst)
- Homogeneous density between bowel loops or in the flanks (Fig. 42)
- Fixed gas bubbles are indicative of abscess
- Circumscribed fluid collections are rarely distinguishable from other space-occupying lesions on plain radiographs
- Small amounts of encapsulated ascites are extremely difficult to recognize

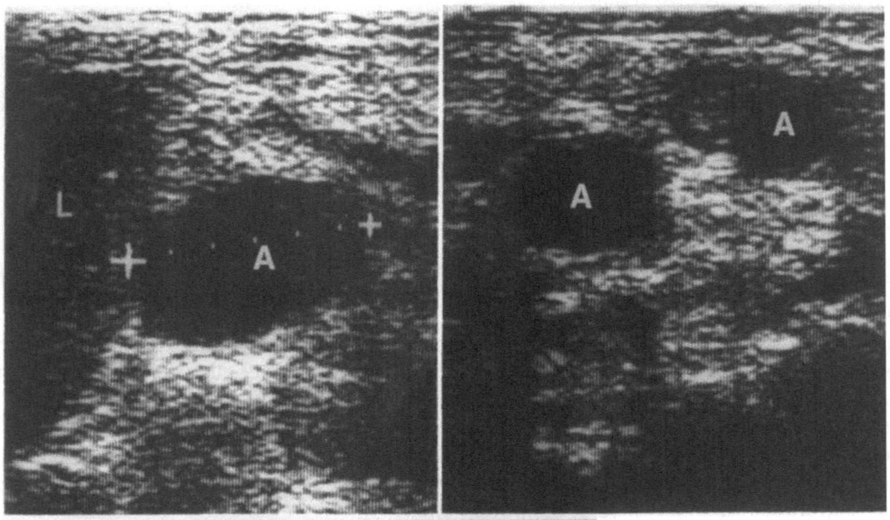

a

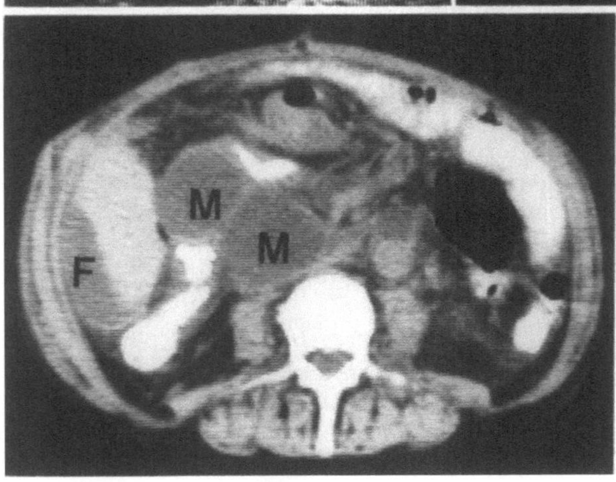

b

Fig. 44a–e. Biliomas. Man, 52 years old, exhibited signs of peritonitis after duodenopancreatectomy. **a** *Sonogram* (longitudinal scan) shows three anechoic, well-demarcated areas in the upper and midabdomen *(A); L,* left lobe of liver. **b** *CT scan* demonstrates free intraperitoneal fluid *(F)* and low-density, circumscribed masses *(M)* that represent encapsulated bilomas. *Diagnosis:* bilomas secondary to bile duct leak following duodenopancreatectomy.

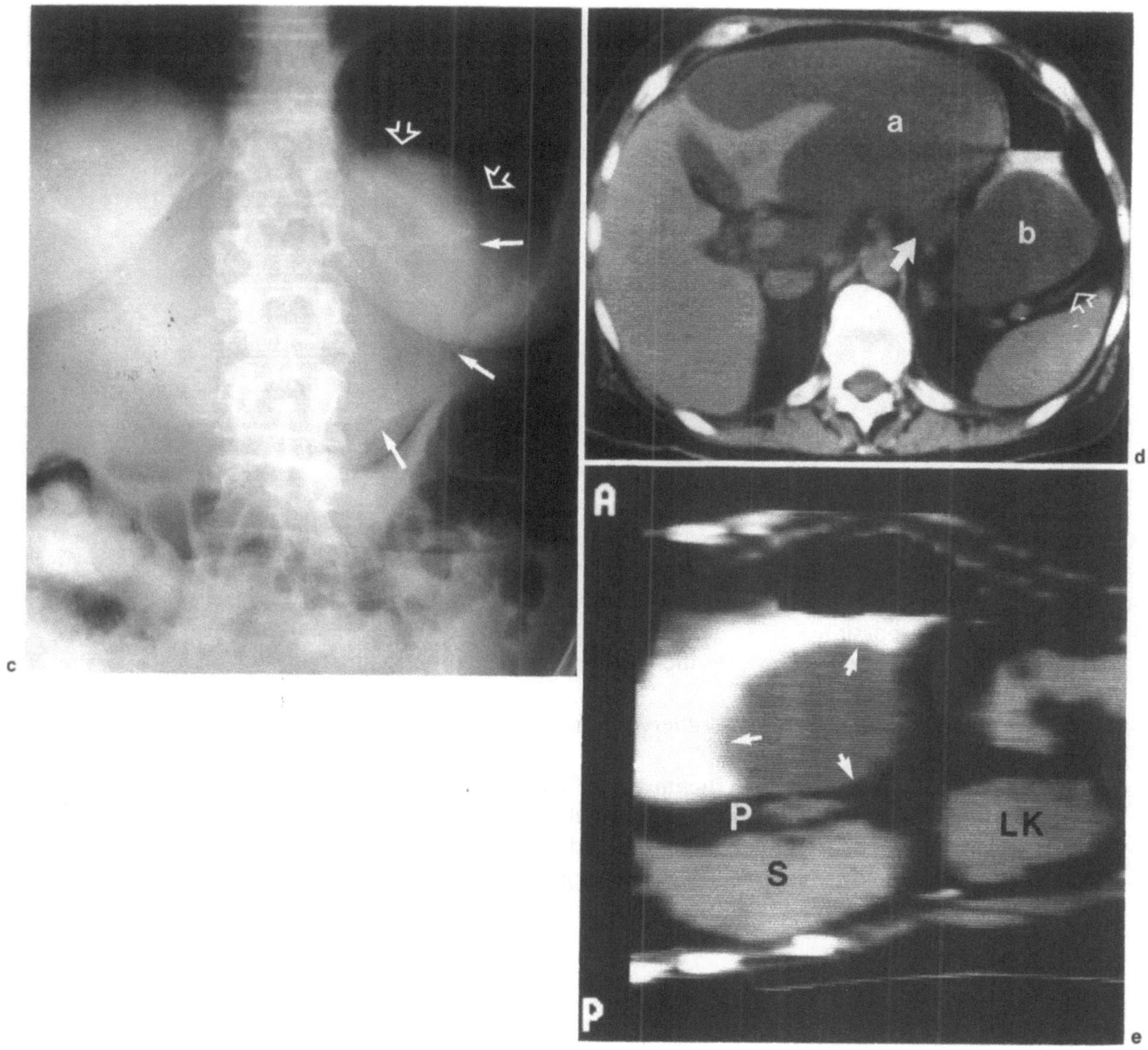

Fig. 44 (continued)
Bilioma in the subhepatic space and omental bursa of a 61-year-old woman who had undergone cholecystectomy and exploration of the common bile duct. On day 11 after operation the patient developed severe, spasmodic, upper abdominal pains that were treated conservatively. On day 18 the pains recurred, accompanied by a rise of alkaline phosphatase, bilirubin, and gamma-GT. **c** *Erect abdominal film* shows a mass in the epigastrium and left upper quadrant impressing on the lesser gastric curvature (⇨). The silhouette sign indicates the presence of a second, more posteriorly situated compartment in the mass (→). **d** *CT scan* at the level of the celiac trunk shows extensive fluid collections in the left perihepatic space *(a)* and in the splenic recess of the omental bursa *(b)*. Both fluid collections communicate through a narrow connection (➡). The gastrosplenic ligament (⇨) is tense. **e** Sagittal image reconstruction in the upper left quadrant shows the bilioma in the omental bursa impressing on the posterior aspect of the stomach (→) (*S*, spleen; *P*, tail of pancreas; *LK*, left kidney) (Prof. Dr. G. Schindler, Department of Diagnostic Radiology, University of Wurzburg)

Real-Time Sonography (Fig. 44a)
- A fluid collection larger than 2-3 cm in diameter is demonstrable as an echo-free zone
- Smooth-walled cysts can always te distinguished from abscesses with their irregular walls

- Floating echoes suggest infection (infected cysts, abscess) or old hematoma
- Floating echoes with reverberations and acoustic shadows suggest a gas-forming abscess
- Encapsulated ascites presents as an immobile, echo-free margin around organs
- Organ displacement can be demonstrated with abscesses, large cysts, and hematomas
- Accurate localization is possible

Caution: Older hematomas (especially when infected) are indistinguishable from abscesses. Ultrasound-guided, thin-needle aspiration, possibly with direct external drainage, can differentiate abscess from hemorrhage.

Computed Tomography (Fig. 44 b)
- Fluid collections are always distinguishable from solid masses
- Differentiation among biloma, encapsulated ascites, and old hematoma may not always be possible
- Mature abscesses frequently show an increased peripheral enhancement of i.v. contrast material ("rim sign")
- Cysts rarely show a rim sign but are otherwise difficult to distinguish from abscesses
- Gas can always be demonstrated in the interior of gas-forming abscesses
- Infected hematomas are indistinguishable from abscesses
- A fluid collection can be accurately localized and its extent ascertained
- Large cysts are more easily assigned to certain organs by CT (whole body cross-section) than by ultrasound

References

Bücheler E, Friedmann G, Thelen M (1983) Real-time-Sonographie des Körpers. Thieme, Stuttgart

Bundrick TJ, Cho S-R, Brewer WH, Beachley MC (1984) Ascites: Comparison of plain film radiographs with ultrasonograms. Radiology 152: 503

Federle MP, Jeffrey RB Jr (1983) Hemoperitoneum studied by computed tomography. Radiology 148: 187

Friedmann G, Bücheler E, Thurn P (1981) Ganzkörper Computertomographie. Thieme, Stuttgart

Hellmer H (1942) Die Konturen des rechten Leberlappens beim Ascites. Acta Radiol 23: 533

Jolles H, Coulam CM (1980) CT of ascites: differential diagnosis. AJR 135: 315

Jorulf H (1975) Roentgen diagnosis of intraperitoneal fluid. A physical anatomic and clinical investigation. Acta Radiol [Suppl] 343: 1

Love L, Demos TC, Reynes CJ (1977) Visualization of the lateral edge of the liver in ascites. Radiology 122: 619

Meyers MA (1976) Dynamic radiology of the abdomen. Springer, Berlin Heidelberg New York

Mueller P, Ferrucci JT Jr, Simeone JF, Butch RJ, et al. (1985) Lesser sac abscesses and fluid collections: drainage by transhepatic approach. Radiology 155: 615–618

Yeh H-C, Wolf BS (1977) Ultrasonography in ascites. Radiology 124: 783

3.4 Extraperitoneal Fluid Collections

F. E. Zanella, D. Beyer, R. Lorenz

Note: Unlike the peritoneal cavity, the retroperitoneum contains fixed layers of fibrous tissue which subdivide it into well-defined compartments and produce characteristic patterns of fluid accumulation.

Perirenal Space (Fig. 45): Predominantly fat-containing space between the renal capsule and renal fascia. The renal fascia envelops the kidney and adrenal.

Anterior Pararenal Space: Bounded by the posterior parietal peritoneum, the anterior renal fascia, and the lateroconal fascia.

Posterior Pararenal Space: Bounded by the posterior renal fascia and transverse fascia, communicates directly with the flank.

The major sites of pathologic fluid collection are as follows: *Perirenal space:* kidney, adrenal, ureter
Anterior pararenal space: duodenum, pancreas, ascending and descending colon, hepatic artery, splenic artery
Posterior pararenal space: abdominal aorta, lymphatic vessels, vertebral bodies, duodenum, pancreas, bile ducts, colon, retroperitoneal appendix, hepatic artery, splenic artery

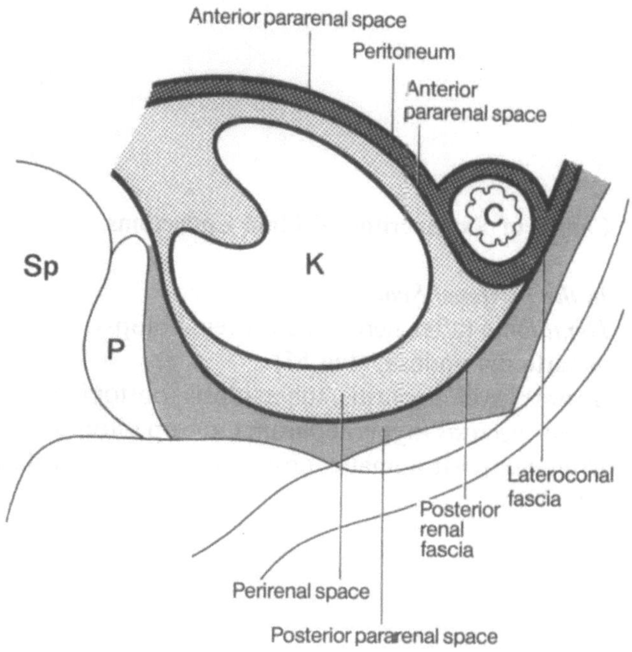

Fig. 45. Compartments of the right retroperitoneal space in cross section. *C,* colon; *K,* kidney; *P,* psoas muscle; *Sp,* spine

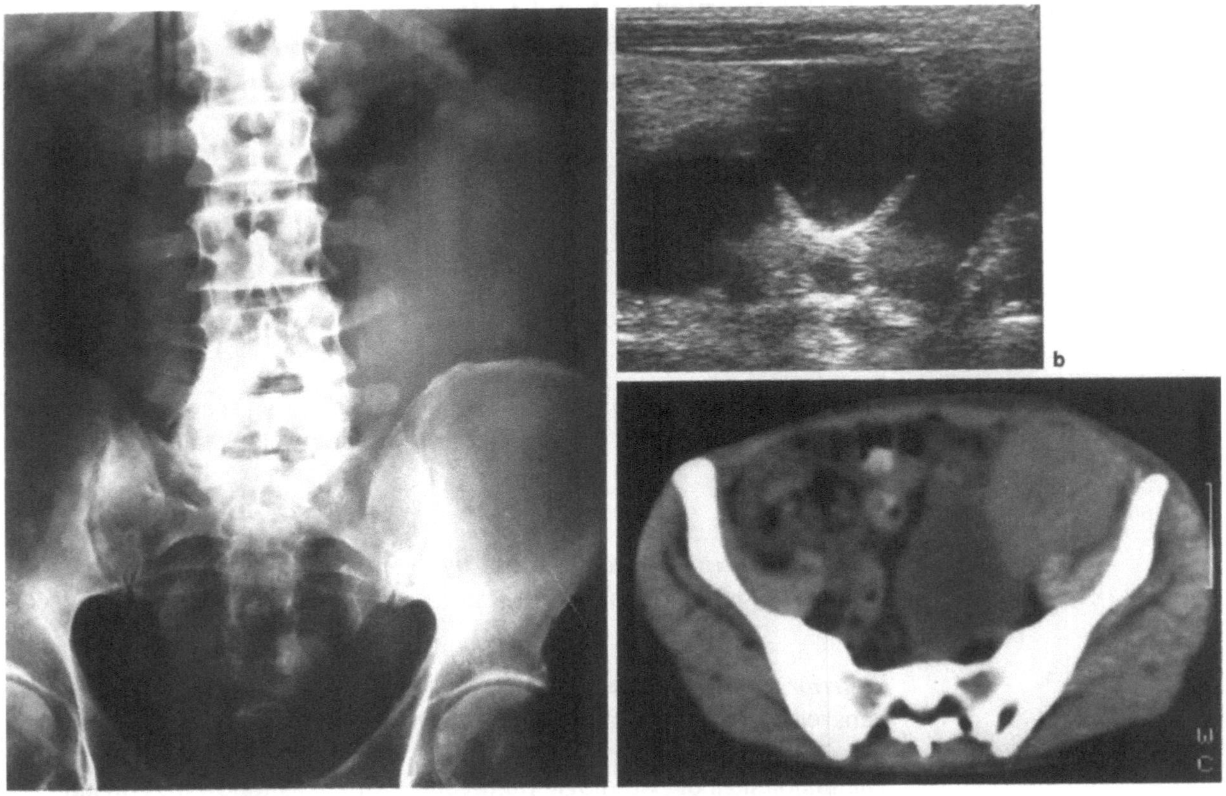

Fig. 46a–c. Lymphocele following renal transplantation. On the 2nd postoperative day the patient had increasing pain and a palpable mass in the left flank. **a** *Supine film* shows a soft-tissue mass in the left lower quadrant displacing adjacent bowel structures. The left psoas margin is obscured. **b** *Sonogram* (transverse scan) shows a lobulated, sharply marginated, almost echo-free structure with posterior acoustic enhancement. It is indistinguishable from an old hematoma. **c** *CT scan* shows a mass which exceeds 6 cm in its greatest diameter and directly adjoins the transplanted kidney. The low density of the mass expressed its liquid content

Note: The reaction of the retroperitoneum to pathologic processes is not as striking or as swift as that of the peritoneal cavity. Symptoms are often protracted and nonspecific and may include chills, vague abdominal or flank pains, nausea, vomiting, night sweats, and weight loss. Leukocytosis is variable, and the urine is usually normal.

Caution: Pressure on adjacent nerves may cause referral of pain to the groin, hips, thighs, or knees.

Causes of Extraperitoneal Fluid Collections

In the Perirenal Space

Hematoma (after percutaneous renal biopsy, trauma, tuberculosis, panarteritis nodosa) (Fig. 51)
Abscess (pyelonephritis, tuberculosis, postoperative infection) (Fig. 148)
Tumor necrosis (hypernephroma, retroperitoneal metastases)
Urinoma (posttraumatic, postoperative, acute with ureteral obstruction) (Fig. 48)

Caution: Urinomas may become manifest after a latent period of 1–4 months.

In the Anterior Pararenal Space
Hematoma (after abdominal or back trauma, e.g., with perforation of the duodenum or pancreas; perforated aneurysm of the hepatic or splenic artery)
Abscess (after duodenal rupture, pancreatitis, nephrectomy, cholecysto-choledocho-duodenostomy, fistula after spontaneous discharge of a stone) (see Fig. 144)
Tumor necrosis (lymph node mass under cytostatic therapy, deficient blood supply to center of tumor)

In the Posterior Pararenal Space
Hematoma (after translumbar angiography, post-traumatic perforation of aneurysm of abdominal aorta, hepatic artery, or splenic artery)
Abscess (posttraumatic, e.g., rupture of rectum in pelvic fracture, spondylodiscitis or spondylitis, retrocecal appendicitis, Crohn's disease, colitis, perforating colon cancer, postoperative infection, e.g., prosthetic infection)
Aneurysm (aneurysm or suture aneurysm of abdominal aorta) (Fig. 49)
Lymphocele (incidence of about 25%-30% following extensive lymphadenectomies)
Tumor necrosis (lymph node metastases under cytostatic therapy or tumor progression with central ischemia)

Radiologic Signs

Plain Radiographs

Table 3.1. Localizing radiologic signs of extraperitoneal fluid collections

Radiologic feature	Anterior pararenal space	Perirenal space	Posterior pararenal space
Perirenal fat and renal outline	Preserved	Obliterated	Preserved
Axis of density	Vertical	Vertical	Parallel to psoas muscle
Kidney displacement	Lateral and superior	Anterior, medial, and superior	Anterior, lateral, and superior
Psoas muscle outline	Preserved	Upper half obliterated	Obliterated throughout
Displacement of ascending or descending colon	Anterior and lateral	± Lateral	Anterior and medial
Displacement of descending duodenum or duodenojejunal junction	Anterior	Anterior	± Anterior
Flank stripe	Preserved	Preserved	Obliterated

* Based on data from Meyers MA: Semin Roentgenol 8: 445, 1973. From Thornbury JR: Perirenal anatomy: normal and abnormal. Radiol Clin North Am 17: 321, 1979

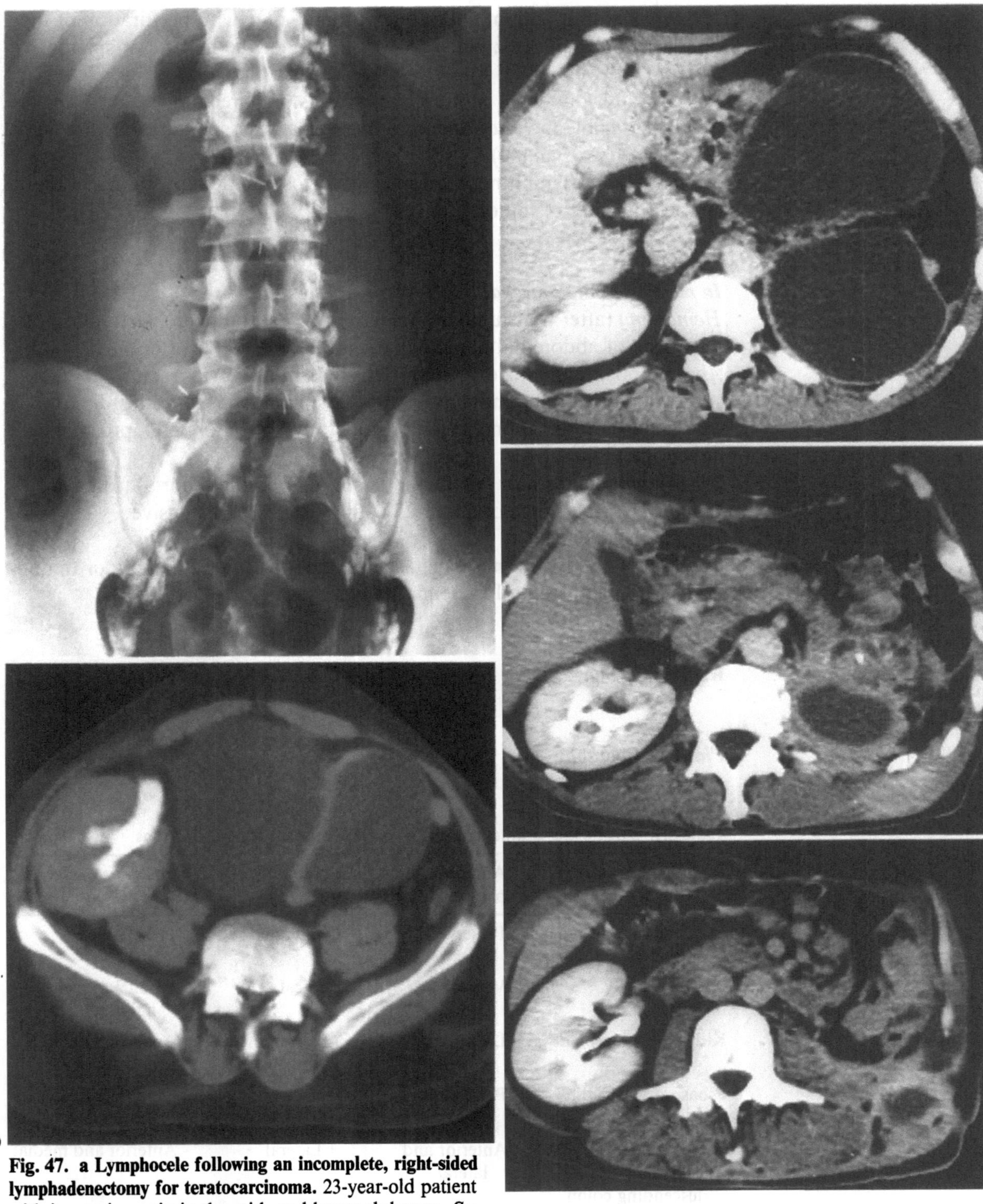

Fig. 47. a Lymphocele following an incomplete, right-sided lymphadenectomy for teratocarcinoma. 23-year-old patient with increasing pain in the mid- and lower abdomen. *Supine film* (following lymphography) shows absence of the right psoas margin and a right paravertebral soft-tissue mass extending into the lesser pelvis. Several metallic clips are visible following lymphadenectomy. **b Lymphocele after renal transplantation.** *CT scan* shows compression of and stasis in the ureter of the transplanted kidney in relation to a low-density, 8-cm mass in the lesser pelvis. The lymphocele displaces the bladder (not opacified) laterally. **c–e Retroperitoneal fluid collection due to a pancreatic fistula. c** *CT scan* shows posttraumatic pancreatic pseudocyst, which had been known for several years. Repeated puncture attempts failed. **d, e** *CT scan* taken after surgery. There was development of septic fever, pain, and inflammation of the left flank. CT demonstrates fluid collections in the left retroperitoneal space and dorsal abdominal wall. Intravenous bolus injection reveals enhancement of the wall marginating the fluid collections. Surgical diagnosis was pancreatic fistula with peripancreatic effusions

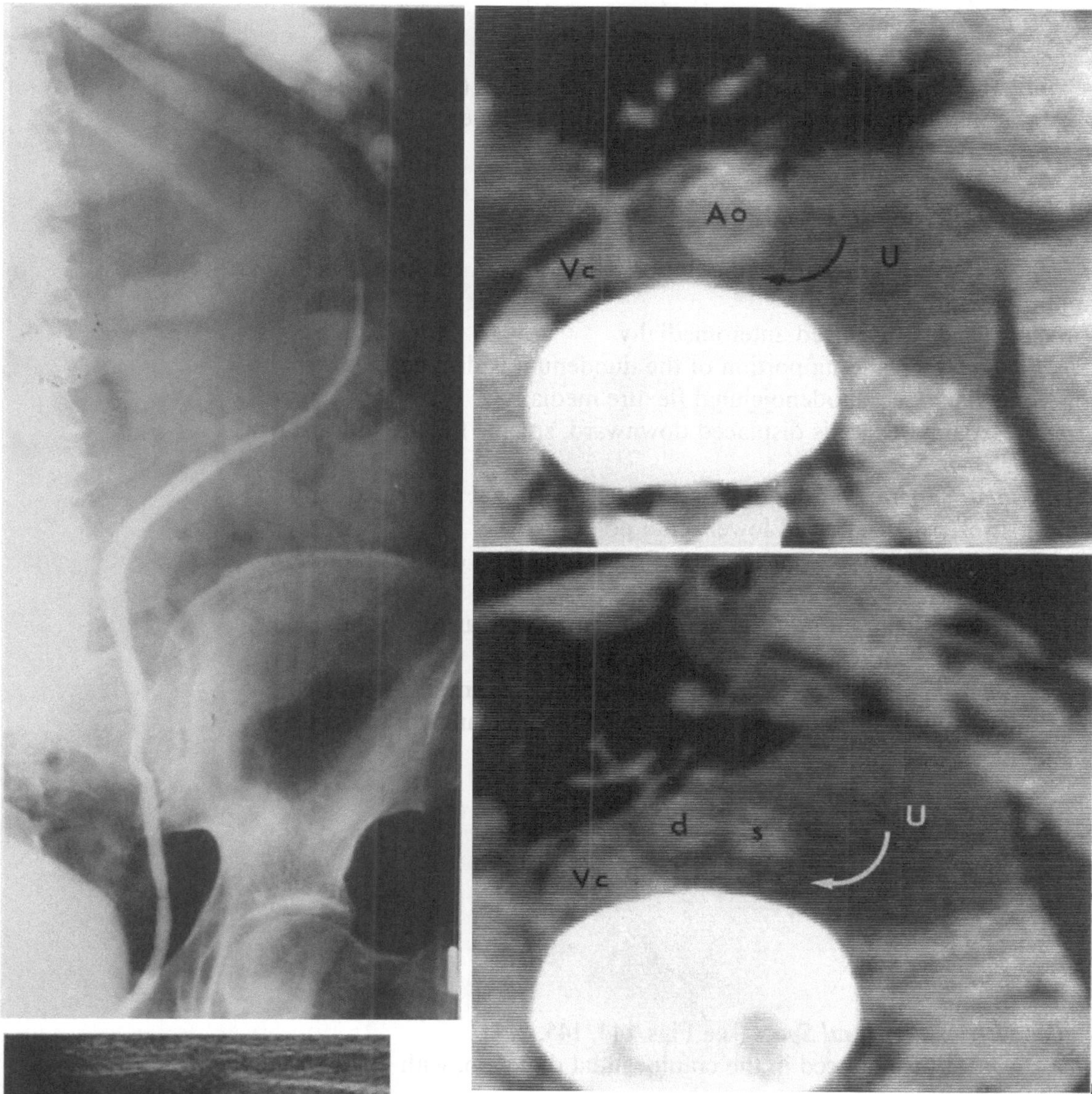

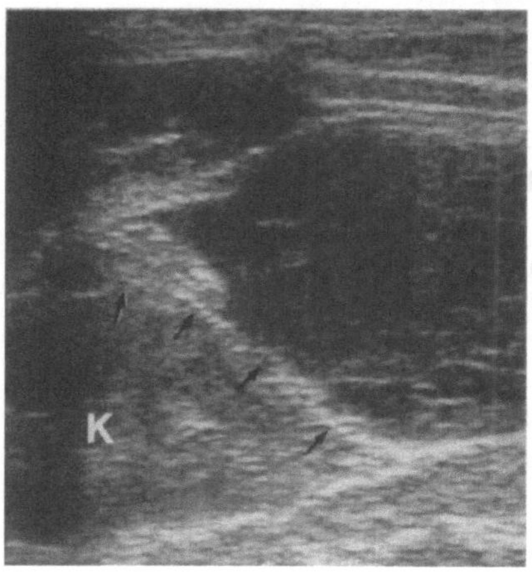

Fig. 48a–d. Urinoma in a woman whose left ureter was operatively splinted 3 weeks earlier. She presented with increasing flank pains. **a** *Left retrograde pyelography* shows craniolateral displacement and axial rotation of the left kidney. The proximal ureter is bowed laterally by an extensive soft-tissue mass. The left psoas margin is obscured. **b** *Sonogram* (longitudinal scan) shows a hypoechoic mass caudal to the upward and anteriorly displaced kidney *(K)*. **c Urinoma secondary to lymphadenectomy.** *CT scan* at the level of the lower abdominal aorta shows the urinoma *(U)* lying in front of the left psoas muscle, extending to the vertebral column, and enveloping the aorta *(Ao)* (*Vc*, inferior vena cava). **d** CT scan below the aortic bifurcation shows the urinoma *(U)* also surrounding the right *(d)* and left *(s)* common iliac arteries (**c, d,** courtesy of Prof. Dr. G. Schindler, Department of Diagnostic Radiology, University of Wurzburg)

In All Compartments
- Soft tissue density (Figs. 46-48)
- Displacement of adjacent organs (Fig. 48)
- Obliteration of characteristic outlines and fat stripes (Figs. 46, 47)
- Absent of diminished respiratory motion of the kidney

In the Perirenal Space (Figs. 48, 51 b, 207 c, d)
Displacements:
Kidney is displaced upward and anteriorly (lateral film confirms rotation about longitudinal axis).
Ureter is usually displaced anteromedially.
Small bowel: Descending portion of the duodenum is displaced anteromedially, the duodenojejunal flexure medially.
Colon: Hepatic flexure is displaced downward, splenic flexure upward or downward.
Obliterated: Superior border of psoas muscle, perirenal fat stripe (early sign: loss of visualization of lower renal pole).
Enlargement of intrinsic renal shadow: Projection effect due to anterior displacement.
Rounding and separation of the normally acute angle at which the renal fascia fuses inferiorly signifies a large fluid collection.
Subcapsular fluid collection: Renal border is displaced inward because of the rigid capsule. Usually there is associated flattening and compression of the kidney.

> *Note:* In an acute process, the shadow usually has a convex inferior border and often extends down beyond the iliac crest; in a chronic process, the shadow conforms to the shape and position of the perirenal space.

In the Anterior Pararenal Space (see Figs. 144, 145, 201)
Density: most pronounced in the craniocaudal direction, with extension to the iliac fossa.
Displacement: Usually the *kidney* is displaced laterally and superiorly.
Small bowel: The descending duodenum may be displaced anteriorly (especially with duodenal perforation).
Colon: Ascending or descending colon is displaced anteriorly and laterally.
Obliterated: Medial border of liver or spleen.

> *Note:* Masses in the anterior pararenal space tend to protrude into the peritoneal cavity, displacing loops of small bowel. The flank shadows and upper renal shadow are preserved.
>
> *Caution:* Accompanying changes are often present at the splenic flexure due to spread via the phrenicocolic ligament.

In the Posterior Pararenal Space (see Fig. 201)
Density: Most pronounced in the laterocaudal direction, parallel to the psoas muscle.
Displacement: The *kidney* is displaced anteriorly, laterally, and superiorly.
Colon: Ascending or descending colon is displaced anteriorly and medially (with a large fluid volume).
Obliterated: Outline of the psoas muscle, possibly the flank shadow (with a large fluid volume).

Note: The perirenal fat and kidney borders are usually preserved. An extension to the lesser pelvis along the ureter is possible.

Sonography

In All Compartments (Figs. 46–50)
Hematoma: Fresh hematoma is echo-free or hypoechoic; older hematomas are more echogenic and frequently show septation.
Abscess: Predominantly hypoechoic, although hyperechoic areas may occur. Air inclusions, which may appear as mobile echoes with acoustic shadowing and reverberation, are nearly pathognomonic.
Tumor necrosis: Usually appears as a hyperechoic mass with an echo-free or hypoechoic center.
Position changes do not cause significant fluid displacement.

In the Perirenal Space
Urinoma: Usually appears as an extensive echo-free mass in close proximity to the kidney. Larger collections are located at the inferior pole.

Caution: Accurate anatomic localization can be difficult with a large urinoma.

In the Anterior Pararenal Space

Note: Fluid in the anterior pararenal space usually cannot be distinguished from fluid collections in the posterior pararenal space.

In the Posterior Pararenal Space
Lymphocele: Echo-free mass occupying a typical location (para-aortic, paracaval, iliac).

Note: Older lymphoceles are more echogenic and may contain mobile septa and posterior sedimentation.

Caution: Sudden enlargement with the appearance of sedimentation is indicative of infection.

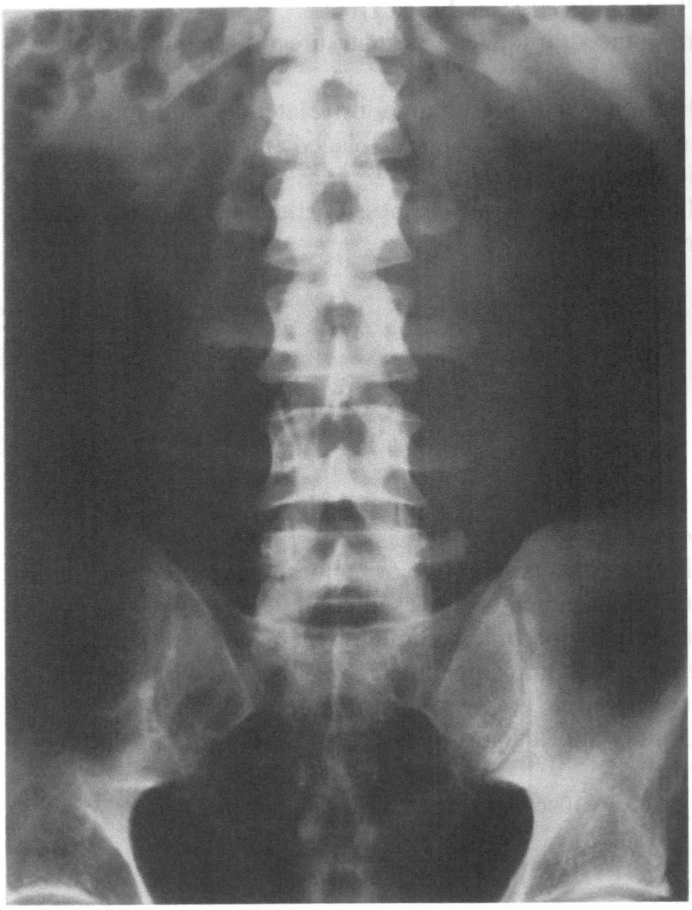
a

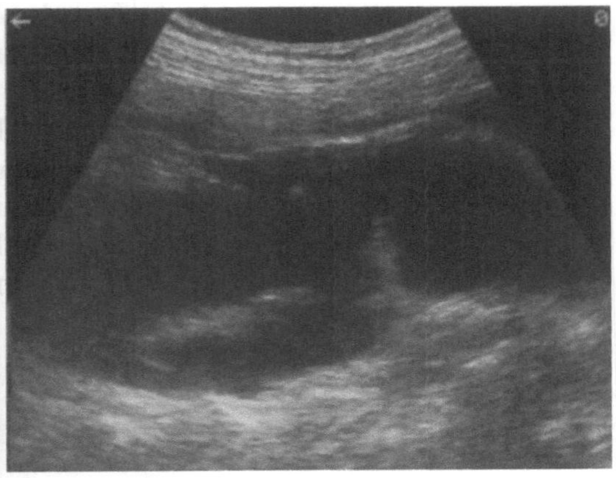
b

Fig. 49 a, b. Retroperitoneal hemorrhage after surgery for an abdominal aortic aneurysm. The patient presented with increasing pain, febrile episodes, and a falling hemoglobin level. **a** *Supine film* shows a soft-tissue density in the left lower quadrant (?). The left psoas margin is not visible. There is accompanying colonic distension. **b** *Sonogram* (longitudinal scan) shows a large, hypoechoic retroperitoneal mass starting just caudal to the inferior renal pole and extending into the lesser pelvis. The multiple, fine, septalike, echogenic, internal structures are commonly seen in older hematomas

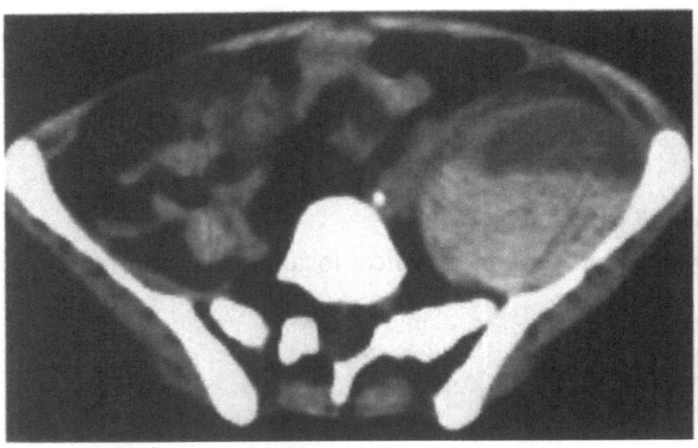
a

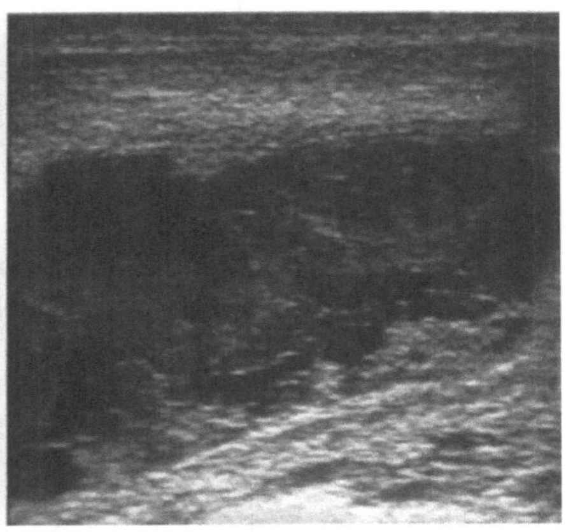
b

Fig. 50 a, b. Retroperitoneal, intramuscular hematoma after a fall at home. **a** *CT scan* shows extensive bleeding into the left iliac muscle. The age of the hemorrhage is evidenced by "fluid levels" caused by the sedimentation of hemoglobin-containing material. There is no coexisting fracture. **b** *Sonogram* (longitudinal scan) shows extensive hypoechoic structures in the area of the left iliac muscle. The septation and echogenic features are characteristic of organized hematoma

Abdominal aortic aneurysm without perforation: Lumen is echo-free or hypoechoic; surrounding thrombus is more echogenic.
Suture aneurysm: Dilatation at the level of prosthetic attachment.
Bleeding aneursysm: Hypoechoic paravascular mass.
Abscess: With processes arising from the spine, it may be difficult or impossible to distinguish the great abdominal vessels.

Caution: Prosthetic infections are diagnosable only if fluid surrounds the implant.

Advantages of sonography:
- Evaluation of dynamic processes (e.g. intestinal peristalsis)
- Demonstration of coexisting urinary stasis
- Monitoring of process easily accomplished

Computed Tomography

In All Compartments (Figs. 46-51, 144, 145, 148)
Hematoma: irregular, homogenous soft tissue mass; fresh hematoma is hyperdense, older hematoma is hypodense.

Caution: Differentiation from a solid retroperitoneal mass or abscess may be difficult, depending on the age of the hemorrhage.

Abscess: An older abscess presents as a low-density mass with peripheral enhancement. The presence of gas is nearly pathognomonic.
Tumor necrosis: Usually a high-density mass with a low-density center.

In the Perirenal Space
Urinoma: Generally hypodense and well-delineated. The site of the extravasation can be demonstrated with contrast medium.
Hematoma: The border lines of the kidney and psoas muscle are lost. With intramural bleeding, the walls of the renal pelvis and ureter are thickened.

Note: CT is the method of choice for differentiating between a subcapsular and perirenal fluid collection.

In the Anterior Pararenal Space
Pancreatitis: Permanent thickening of the renal fascia is possible (see Sect. 4.1.2).

Note: Necrotizing pancreatitis, unlike the uncomplicated form, is generally accompanied by a spread of abscess formation to *both* sides.

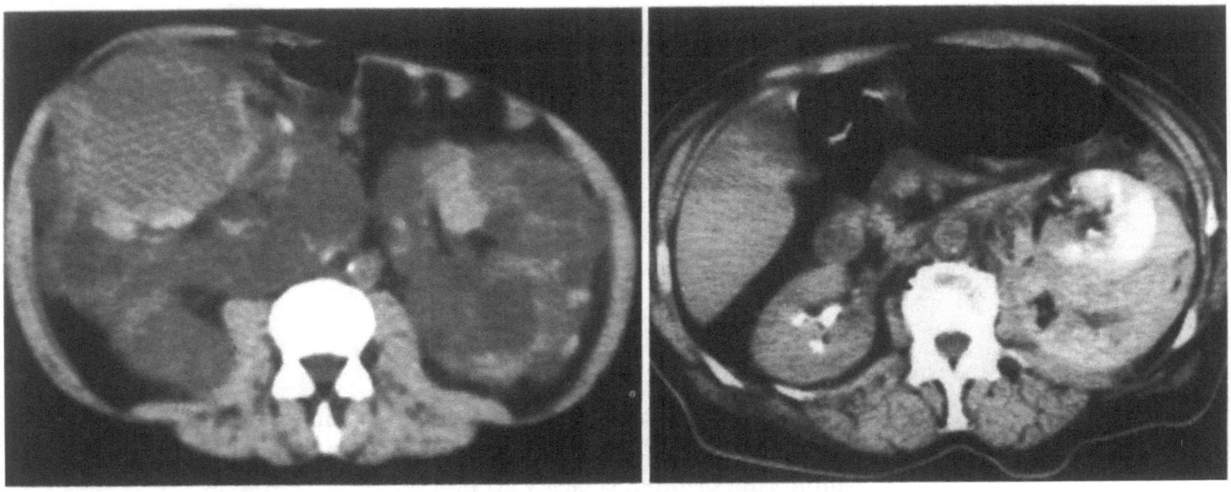

a b

Fig. 51 a, b. Retroperitoneal hematomas. a Bleeding into renal cysts in a 44-year-old woman. *CT scan* shows multiple, low-density masses associated with polycystic renal degeneration. The masses contain high-density areas that represent bleeding into the cysts. Even with CT, it is not possible to localize the lesions to a specific compartment. **b Renal hemorrhage** in a 56-year-old woman taking anticoagulants. *CT with bolus injection* shows a large, high-density mass in the perirenal space and posterior pararenal space. The relatively heavy opacification of the left kidney signifies delayed outflow. There is accompanying bowel distension

In the Posterior Pararenal Space

Lymphocele: Low-density, sharply marginated mass accupying a typical location. Often there is no displacement of retroperitoneal organs.

Abscess: With prosthetic infection, very fine gas collections are seen in the aortic bed around the prosthesis.

Bleeding aneurysm: Fresh bleeding produces a high-density, paravascular mass that does not require contrast application. In doubtful cases an i.v. bolus is given, and sequential scans are obtained (extravasation of contrast medium?). In a dissecting aneurysm, differentiation between the true and false lumen is possible.

Note: A fresh hemorrhage may require i.v. contrast medium for differentiation from aorta and vena cava.

Advantages of CT:

- Staging of retroperitoneal tumors (e.g., hypernephroma)
- Excretory function of kidney or urinary stasis
- Skeletal changes (e.g., in hypernephroma, spondylodiscitis)
- Foreign bodies (e.g., as cause of abscess)

Clinical Evaluation of Questionable Retroperitoneal Fluid Collections

- *History:* congenital disorders (systemic diseases, panarteriitis nodosa, lupus erythematosus, hemophilia)
  Acquired disorders (inflammation, malignancy)
  Medications (anticoagulants, cytostatics)
  Iatrogenic changes (surgery, needle aspiration)
  Trauma
- *Clinical examination:* inspection (scars, stomas, external sequelae of trauma)
  Palpation
  - no abnormalities on palpation
  - abnormality on palpation (tenderness to pressure, soft, elastic, fluctuating, pulsating; enlargement)

  Auscultation (murmurs, bowel sounds)

Note: The clinical manifestation of abnormal retroperitoneal fluid collections are frequently nonspecific or even misleading. Often the first symptom is unilateral urinary stasis caused by ureteral compression. The history is crucial.

References

Beyer D, Friedmann G (1983) Retroperitoneale Raumforderungen. In: Bücheler E, Friedmann G, Thelen M (eds) Real-time-Sonographie des Körpers. Thieme, Stuttgart

Donovan PJ, Zerhouni EA, Siegelmann SS (1981) CT of the psoas compartment of the retroperitoneum. Semin Roentgenol 16: 241-250

Lorenz R, Beyer D, Peter PE (1984) Detection of intraperitoneal bile accumulations: significance of ultrasonography, CT and cholescintigraphy. Gastrointest Radiol 9: 213-217

Marks SC Jr, Raptopoulos V, Kleinmann P, Snyder M (1986) The anatomical basis for retrorenal extensions of pancreatic effusions: the role of the renal fasciae. SRA 8: 89-97

McCullogh DL, Leopold GR (1976) Diagnostic of retroperitoneal fluid collections by ultrasonography: a series of surgically proved cases. J Urol 115: 656

Meyers MA, Whalen JP, Peelle K, Berne AS (1972) Radiologic features of extraperitoneal effusions. Radiology 104: 249-257

Morettin LB, Kumar R (1981) Small renal carcinoma with large retroperitoneal hemorrhage: diagnostic considerations. Urol Radiol 3: 143-148

Schmidt R, Schindler G, Gutzeit B (1986) Bilom in Spatium subhepaticum und in der Bursa omentalis nach Choledochusrevision. Fortschr Roentgenstr 145 (5): 601-603

Spring DB, Schroeder D, Babu S, Agee R, Gooding G (1981) Ultrasonic evaluation of lymphocele formation after staging lymphadenectomy for prostatic carcinoma. Radiology 141: 479

3.5 Pathologic Gas Collections

3.5.1 Free Intraperitoneal Gas (Pneumoperitoneum)

D. BEYER, G.P. KRESTIN

Causes of Free Air in the Peritoneal Cavity
(arranged by peritoneal portal of entry)

1) Perforation of a Hollow Viscus

- Perforation of a gastric or duodenal ulcer (most common cause)
- Perforation in inflammatory bowel disease (appendicitis, Crohn's disease, diverticulitis, typhus, Meckel's diverticulum, toxic megacolon)
- Suture line leak
- Iatrogenic perforation (endoscopy, biopsy, cleansing enema, contrast enema, endoscopic polyp removal)
- Rupture of a hollow viscus after blunt abdominal trauma
- Ischemic disease culminating in gangrene and perforation
- Overdistension of the intestinal tract (in colon obstruction, toxic megacolon)
- Neoplastic disease
- Foreign bodies ingested or inserted rectally
- Pneumatosis intestinalis (without peritonitis!)

2) Transperitoneal Origin

- Usually without peritonitis
  - Postoperative (residual air is absorbed in 1-24 days after surgery, depending on its volume; 4-5 days is normal; less time is needed in asthenic patients; an increasing air volume is abnormal!)
  - Iatrogenic after laparoscopy, needle puncture
  - From the chest cavity (often iatrogenic from positive pressure ventilation, intubation, after pneumomediastinum or pneumothorax). In this case pneumoperitoneum and pneumomediastinum always coexist
- With peritonitis
  - From the retroperitoneum (perioperative, abscess perforation); always combined with retroperitoneal gas
  - Penetrating abdominal trauma
  - Gas gangrene and kindred gas-forming infections

3) Intraperitoneal Origin

Gas-forming abscess, gas-forming peritonitis

4) Entry of Air Through the Female Genital Tract

- Usually without peritonitis
  - Iatrogenic after uterus perforation, after examination in the knee-elbow position, after tubal insufflation, after hysterosalpingography
  - Postpartum
  - After douching, sexual intercourse
  - Rarely after athletic activities (horseback riding, water skiing, high diving)

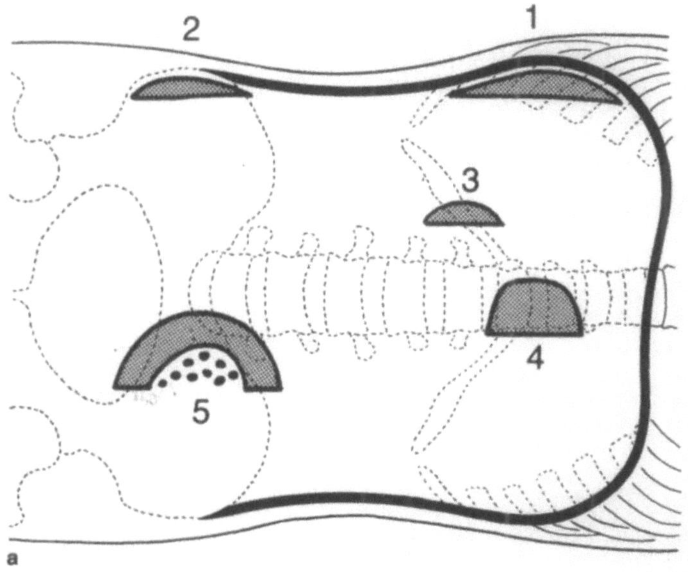

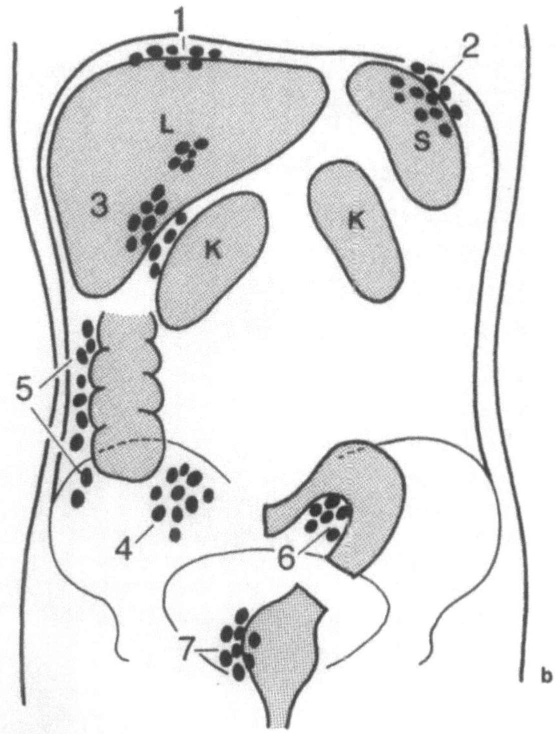

Fig. 52. a Sites of collection of *free* intraperitoneal gas in the abdomen on the left lateral film: *1*, between liver and chest wall; *2*, under right lateral abdominal wall at the level of the iliac crest; *3*, in Morison's pouch; *4*, in the omental bursa; *5*, between bowel loops. *Note:* Free gas moves when the patient is repositioned! **b Sites of collection of *fixed* intraperitoneal gas on a supine film:** *1*, right subphrenic space; *2*, left subphrenic space; *3*, Morison's pouch; *4*, paracecal space in right lower quadrant; *5*, paracolic gutter; *6*, between bowel loops; *7*, apparently pararectal (extraperitoneal) gas collection in the prevesical space (intraperitoneal). *L*, liver; *K*, kidneys; *S*, spleen.
Note: Fixed gas does *not* move when the patient is repositioned

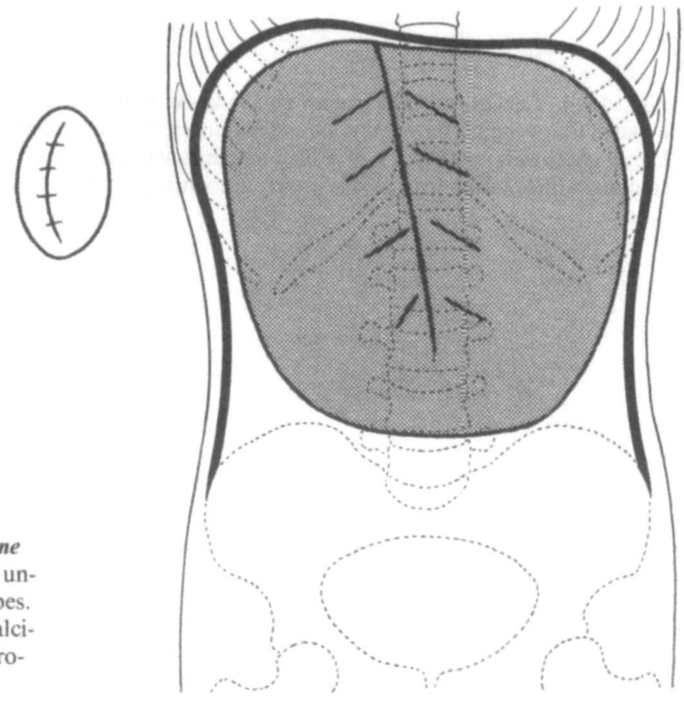

Fig. 53. Schematic representation of *free air* on the *supine film*. "Football" sign: large, oval-shaped gas collection under the abdominal wall extending out to the flank stripes. The "laces" of the football are formed by the visible falciform ligament and appear as thin, cordlike shadows projected over the liver to the right of the spine

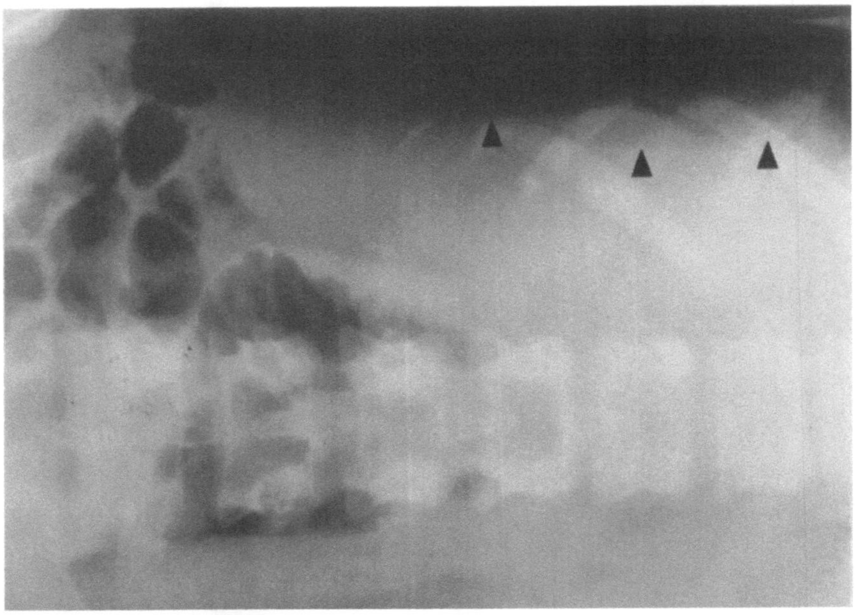

a

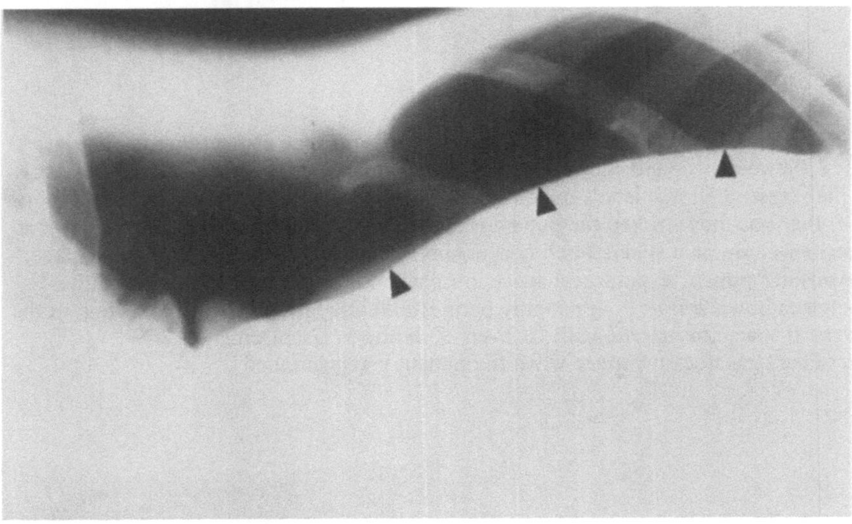

b

Fig. 54 a–d. Configuration of free air on *left lateral radiographs.*
a Status following perforation of a duodenal ulcer. Free air is demonstrated between the lateral chest wall and liver (▶). **b** Pneumoperitoneum in the *left lateral position*. The smooth surface of the liver (▶) is clearly recognized on the underexposed film.

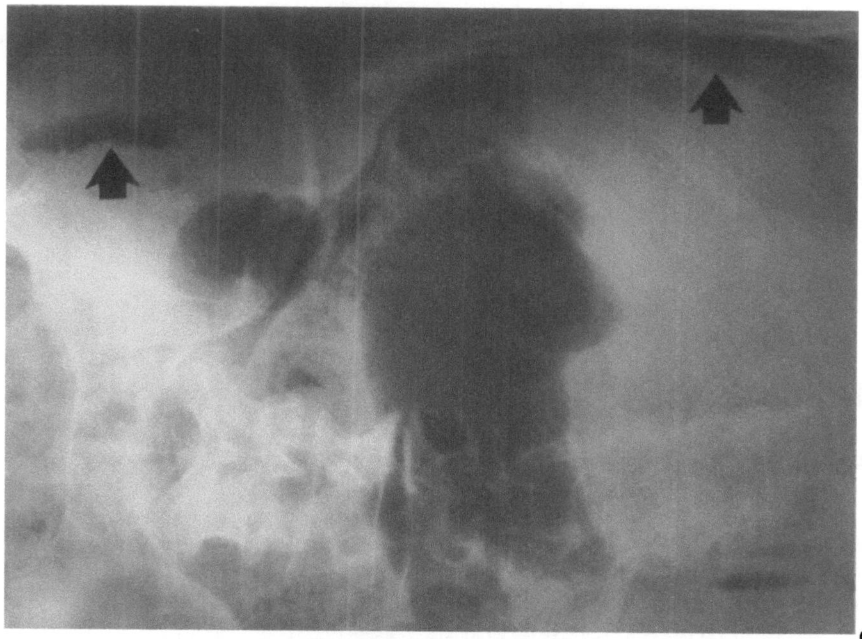

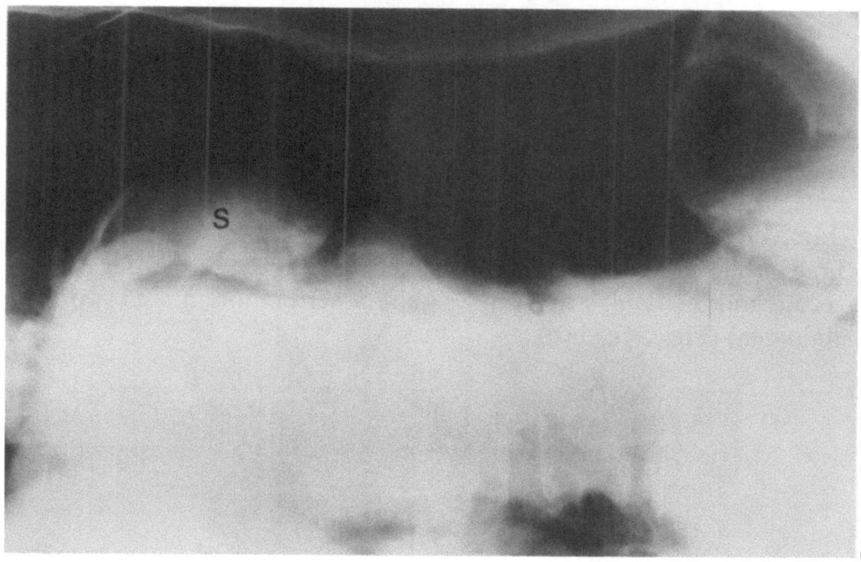

d

Fig. 54 (continued)
c Following perforated appendicitis, a large amount of free air is observed below the lateral abdominal wall projected over the right iliac crest (➧). A smaller collection of air is seen between the right lateral chest wall and liver (➧). **d** *Right lateral film* shows a huge pneumoperitoneum following positive-pressure ventilation of a patient who attempted suicide. The spleen *(S)* is markedly displaced from the left lateral chest wall, as are the bowel loops

Note: Between 10% and 35% of all perforation of hollow viscera show *no* free air. Patients should be kept in the L Lat position for a longer period of time before the X-ray is taken. Sometimes only free intraperitoneal fluid can be demonstrated (sonography). If doubt exists and clinical symptoms are unclear, oral Gastrografin is given, and leakage of contrast material is sought under flouroscopy (usually necessary in the postoperative period). Bowel gas can rarely pass through the normal intestinal mucosa in patients with jejunal diverticula or gastric distension.

Radiologic Signs

Plain Radiographs

Note: Free gas always collects at the highest point in the abdomen!

Caution: Overexposed L Lat films can mask small amounts of free air! For a left lateral decubitus view the central beam should be centered at the level of the free air, otherwise, small amounts of free air will *not* be visualized. Adhesion between the liver and diaphragm *prevent* free air from collecting in typical sites

Free air on the L LAT film (cross-table projection) (Fig. 52a)
- Free air between the right lateral chest wall and liver (1-2 ml or more) (Fig. 54a, b)
- Free air in the right paracolic space between the lateral border of the cecum and the flank stripe (may signify a perforation in the lower abdomen) (Figs. 54c, 55b).

Note: Free air from the perforation of a hollow viscus is often combined with free fluid in the peritoneal cavity! Sonographic evaluation is necessary if findings are equivocal.

Free air on the supine film (vertical projection) (Figs. 52b, 53)
- The "football sign" (more common in small children): large, oval-shaped collection of gas under the anterior abdominal wall, extending to the flank stripe (Figs. 53, 56). Differentiation from massive gastric dilatation in required
- Visible falciform ligament (the "laces" of the football): thin, cordlike shadow projected over the liver to the right of the spine (Figs. 56a, 57b, c)
- Visible gastrointestinal wall (Rigler's sign): intra- and extraluminal gas outlines both the outer and inner walls of the bowel (Figs. 55, 56a)
- Gas in the hepatorenal recess (Morison's pouch): usually this is triangular in outline and projected over the superior pole of the right kidney (see Fig. 140a)
- Para- and prehepatic gas (Fig. 56a)
- Inverted V sign: gas under the abdominal wall outlines the remnants of the umbilical arteries on one or both sides; the apex of the V points to the umbilicus

Fig. 55 a, b. Rigler's sign (outlining of the gastrointestinal wall). **a** *Supine film* in a 36-year-old man with a perforated duodenal ulcer shows the bowel wall clearly outlined by intra- and extraluminal gas. The small bowel wall (→←) and colonic wall (⇨⇦) are visible in their normal thickness, much as they might appear in a contrast examination. **b** *Left lateral film* in a 24-year-old woman with a duodenal ulcer who had a barium swallow examination; the ulcer had perforated 2 h previously. The film shows an obvious pneumoperitoneum between the chest wall and liver surface with a visible diaphragm (*D* ➧). Air is also noted in the right lower quadrant, where the walls of the cecum are visible (Rigler's sign) (➧). There is residual contrast medium in the ascending colon

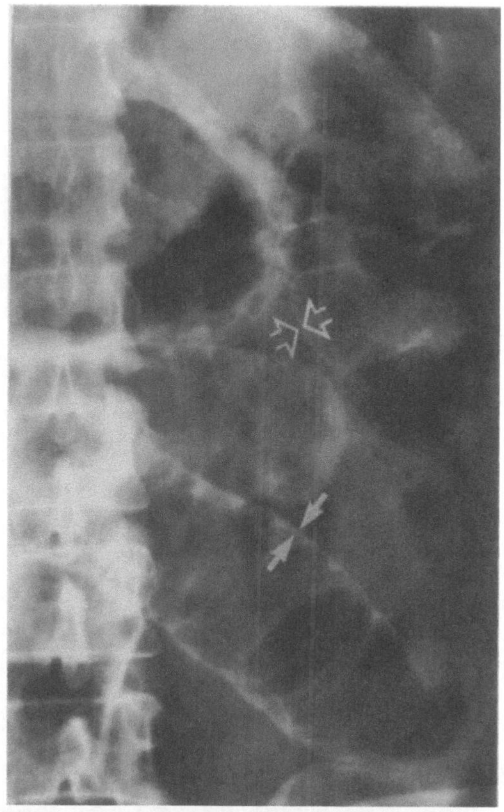

a

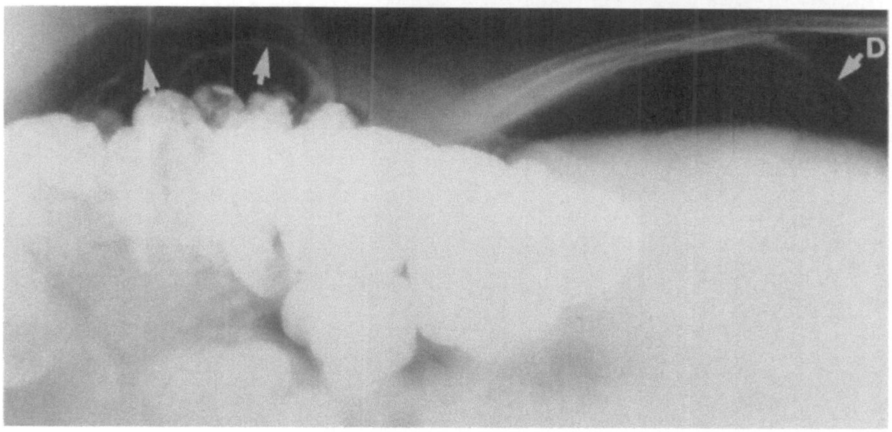

b

- Gas in the retrogastric omental bursa from a posteriorly perforating ulcer; communicates with other parts of the peritoneal cavity through the epiploic foramen (Fig. 58)

Note: The *L LAT film* is the *most important* radiographic view for the demonstration of fee air! Overexposure should be avoided. An additional erect or cross-table supine radiograph is rarely necessary to confirm free air.

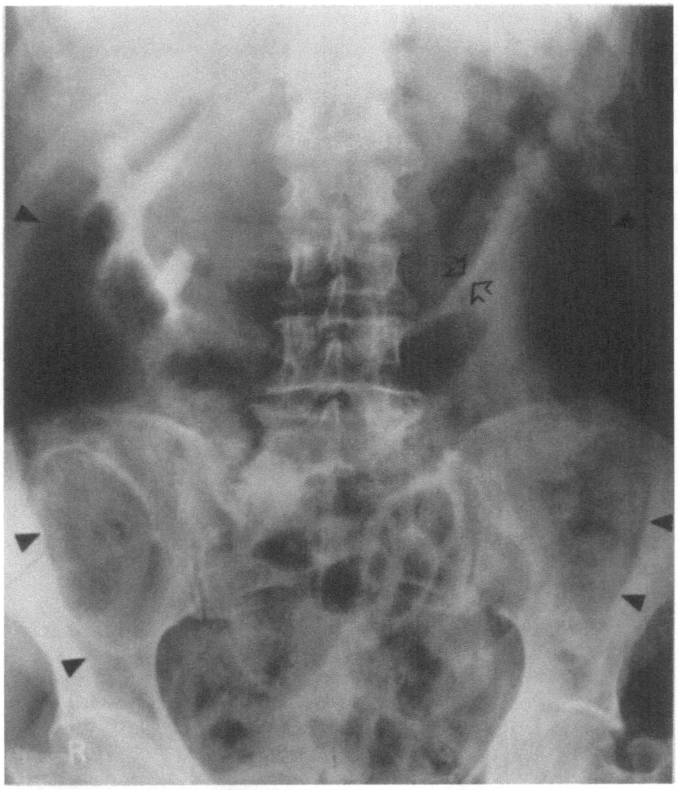

a

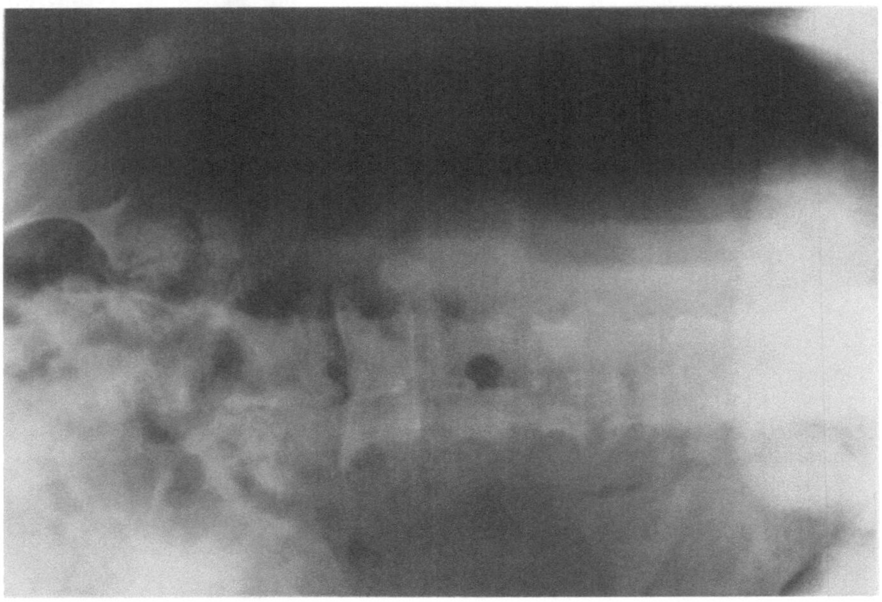

b

Fig. 56a, b. "Football" sign. a *Supine film* shows a huge, rounded gas collection under the abdominal wall that extends to the flank stripes (▶). Outlining of the stomach wall (Rigler's sign) is also apparent (⇨⇦). **b** *Left lateral film* shows a giant pneumoperitoneum extending from the lower abdomen to the diaphragm and displacing all intraperitoneal organs medially and to the left

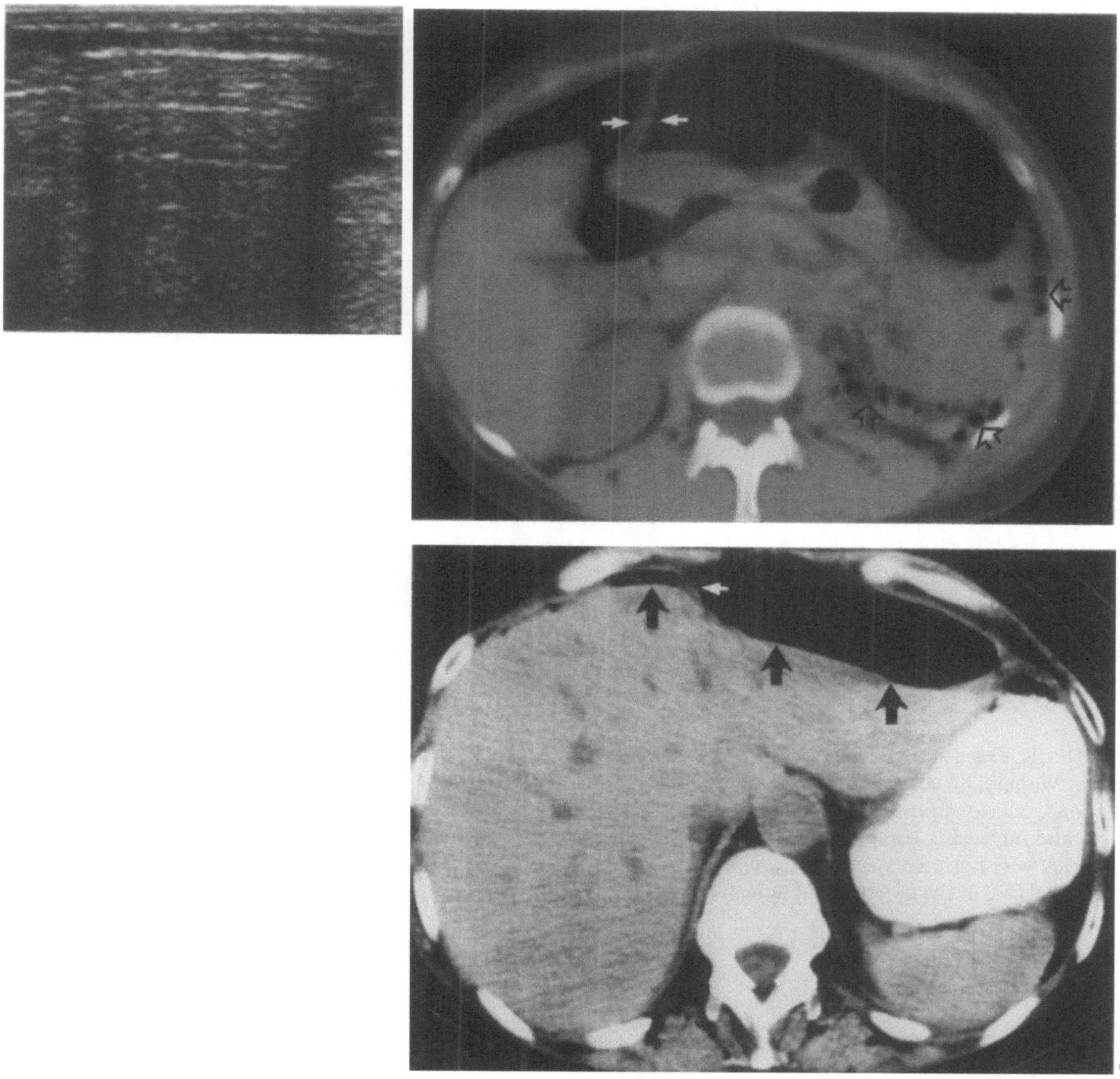

Fig. 57 a–c. Sonographic and CT demonstration of free air (pneumoperitoneum).
a Postoperative pneumoperitoneum: *sonogram* (left paramedian longitudinal scan) shows an elongated echo front behind the abdominal wall with marked reverberations and acoustic shadowing. **b** Residual peritoneal gas (⇨) in a 36-year-old woman operated for stenosis at the ureteropelvic junction. The peritoneal space was inadvertently opened at operation, and pneumoperitoneum ensued. *CT scan* shows marked posterior displacement of organs in the peritoneal cavity. The tense falciform ligament stretches between the liver and upper abdomen (→←). **c** *CT scan* appearance of pneumoperitoneum from perforated sigmoid diverticulosis. A transverse scan was performed through the upper abdomen to search for abscess. The pneumoperitoneum displaces the left lobe of the liver from the abdominal wall (➡), stretching the falciform ligament (➡)

Sonography
Sonography is *not* the initial diagnostic procedure of choice in the search for free peritoneal air, although free air is often noted as an incidental finding. In the supine patient free air produces a linear echo front under the abdominal wall with reverberations, or between the abdominal wall and the anterior aspect of the left lobe of the liver (Fig. 57 a).

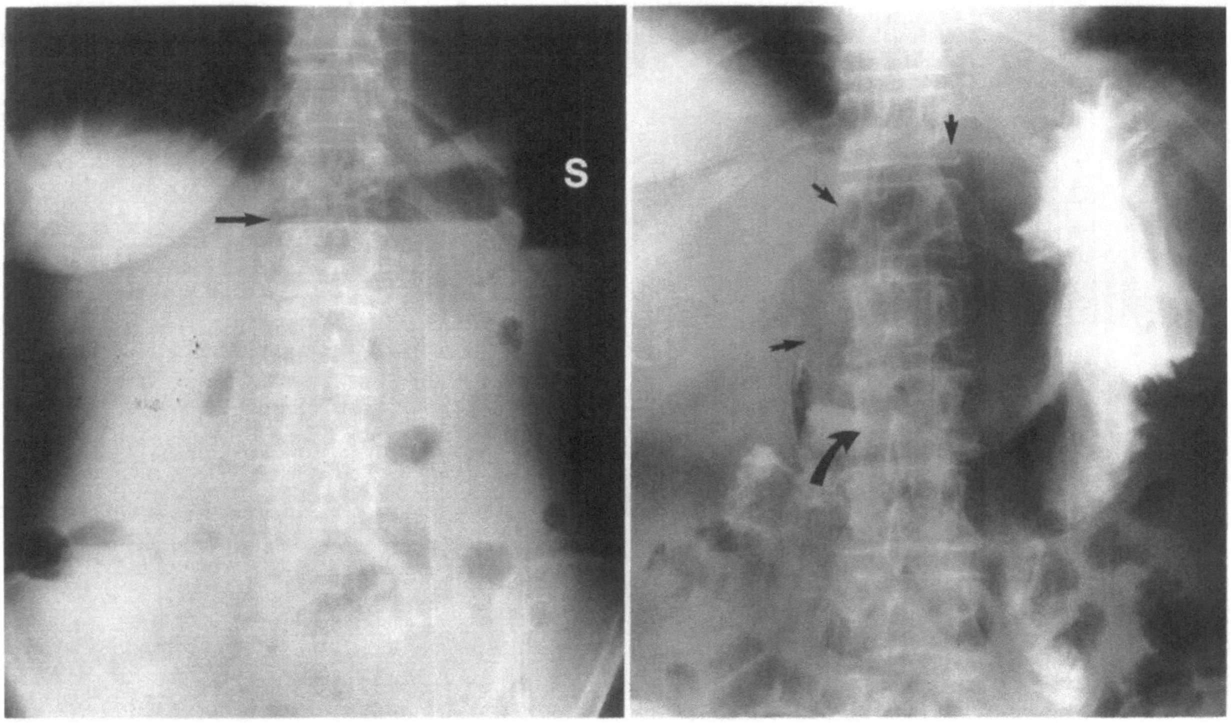

a b

Fig. 58 a, b. Duodenal ulcer perforating into the omental bursa. Woman, 86 years old, with general malaise, postprandial, colicky, upper abdominal pain, a nonrigid abdomen, and increasing leukocytosis. Hepatic and pancreatic enzymes were normal. **a** *Erect abdominal film* shows an air-fluid level (→) in the upper midabdomen next to the stomach *(S)*. There is no evidence of subphrenic air. **b** *UGI series* with water-soluble contrast medium shows perforation of the duodenal ulcer into the omental bursa (↗). Note the extensive air collection (→) in the omental bursa medial and posterior to the stomach (Priv. Doz. Dr. B. Kurtz, Department of Radiology, University of Tübingen)

Computed Tomography
Small amounts of free air may be overlooked on CT scans unless they are specifically sought! Free air collects between the anterior abdominal wall and the usually distended bowel loops (center and window setting for soft-tissue diagnosis), displacing the liver from the anterior abdominal wall; the falciform ligament is tense (Fig. 57 b, c).

Causes of "Pseudopneumoperitoneum" (plain radiographs)
1. Gas-forming, encapsulated subphrenic abscess
2. Extraperitoneal gas collections in the flank stripe
3. Gas-containing diaphragmatic hernia
4. Chilaiditi' syndrome: gas-filled bowel between the liver, diaphragm, and abdominal wall
5. Interposed greater omentum (fat!) between the liver, diaphragm, and lateral abdominal wall
6. Subdiaphragmatic fat collections
7. Pneumothorax
8. Low basal atelectasis with aerated lung between the atelectasis and diaphragm
9. Gas-containing superior gastric diverticulum

Note: Differentiate between pneumoperitoneum and pseudopneumoperitoneum by repositioning the patient. *Free* air will move with a position change!

References

Chandler, JG, Berk RN, Golden GT (1977) Misleading pneumoperitoneum. Surg Gynecol Obstet 144: 163
Felson B, Wiot JF (1973) Another look at pneumoperitoneum. Semin Roentgenol 8: 437
Frimann-Dahl J (1968) The acute abdomen. In: Strnad F (ed) Röntgendiagnostik des Digestionstraktes und des Abdomens. Springer, Berlin Heidelberg New York (Handbuch der medizinischen Radiologie, vol 11/2)
Greenstein AJ, Mann D, Sachar DB, Aufses AH (1985) Free perforation in Crohn's disease: a survey of 99 cases. Am J Gastroenterol 80: 682-689
McCort JJ (1981) Abdominal radiology. Williams & Wilkins, Baltimore
Menuck L, Siemers PZ (1976) Pneumoperitoneum: importance of right upper quadrant features. AJR 127: 753
Miller RE, Becker GJ, Slabaugh RD (1980) Detection of pneumoperitoneum: optimum body position and respiratory phase. AJR 135: 487
Mindelzun RE, McCort JJ (1983) Acute abdomen. In: Margulis AR, Burhenne HJ (eds) Alimentary tract radiology, vol 1. Mosby, St. Louis
Rice RP, Thompson WM, Gedgaudas RK (1982) The diagnosis and significance of extraluminal gas in the abdomen. Radiol Clin North Am 20/4: 819
Swart B, Meyer G (1974) Die Diagnostik des akuten Abdomens beim Erwachsenen - ein neues klinisch-radiologisches Konzept. Radiologe 14: 1-57

3.5.2 Extraperitoneal Gas Collections

G. P. Krestin, D. Beyer, U. Mödder

Causes

Perforation of retroperitoneal hollow viscera

- Rectal perforation (iatrogenic, foreign body)
- Low perforation on the sigmoid colon (diverticulum, diverticulitis, tumor, iatrogenic)
- Perforation of the appendix (acute appendicitis) - in retroperitoneally seated retrocecal appendix
- Perforation of the duodenum (ulcer of posterior wall of bulb, rupture)
- Trauma (rupture, perforating injury, iatrogenic)

Mediastinal emphysema - spreading into the posterior pararenal space

Gas-forming abscesses

- Pancreatic abscess (usually after acute pancreatitis)
- Renal abscess (pyelonephritis with abscess formation)
- Paracolic abscesses (e.g., diverticulitis complicated by abscess)
- Psoas abscess (e.g., in spinal tuberculosis)
- Retrorectal abscess (postoperative, postendoscopy, perforation)
- Abdominal wall abscess (after surgery in area of the wound)
- Gluteal abscess (e.g., intramuscular injection)
- Postoperative retroperitoneal abscesses (Fig. 61)

Necrotic tumor degeneration with gas formation

- Pancreatic carcinoma (Fig. 63)
- Renal tumors (also after therapeutic embolization)
- Uterine tumors
- Rectal tumors

Gas gangrene (Fig. 65)

Note: Every retroperitoneal gas collection is pathologic, except for collections in the early postoperative period.

Caution: Clinical symptoms from retroperitoneal gas collections are usually nonspecific and less acute than those associated with abnormal gas collections in the peritoneal cavity.

Radiologic Signs

Note: Radiologic signs are determined by the tendency of gas to collect in the various compartments of the retroperitoneum. The location of the collection provides important etiologic clues (Fig. 59).

Plain Radiographs

Gas in the posterior pararenal space (Figs. 59, 60 a, b)

- Gas does *not* pass medially beyond the lateral psoas border.
- Gas may spread into the flank stripes.
- Gas may spread into the mediastinum.

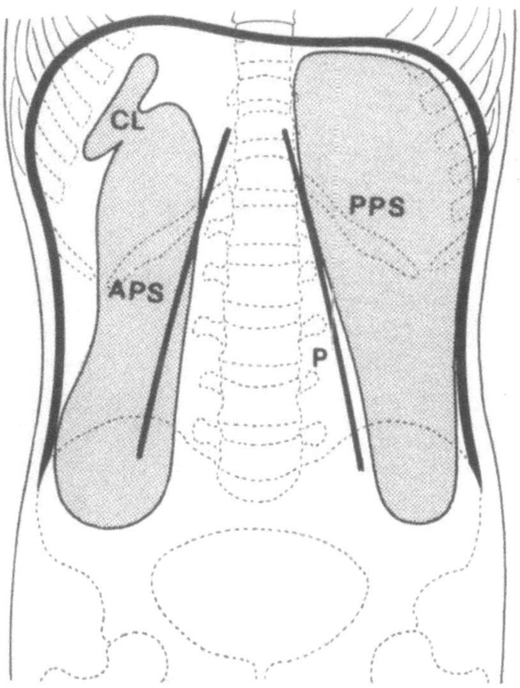

Fig. 59. Characteristic spread and configuration of extraperitoneal gas in the anterior *(APS)* and posterior *(PPS)* pararenal spaces. *P*, psoas margin; *CL*, coronary ligament of the liver

Gas in the perirenal space (Figs. 57 b, 60 c)
- Gas collection is unilateral in most cases.
- Renal contours are accentuated or superimposed.
- Gas may spread into the soft tissues of the lesser pelvis.

Gas in the anterior pararenal space (Figs. 59, 64)

- Gas may be demonstrated on *both* sides of the spine.
- Gas projects beyond the lateral border of the psoas.
- The flank stripe is preserved.

Note: Retroperitoneal gas usually appears in the form of bubbles or linear collections along fascial planes. It shows little or no movement when the patient is repositioned. An accompanying mass usually signifies an abscess.

Caution: Retroperitoneal gas is detected on plain radiographs in only about 50% of cases. It is demonstrated more clearly on CT scans. Localization on plain film is possible only with a characteristic pattern of spread.

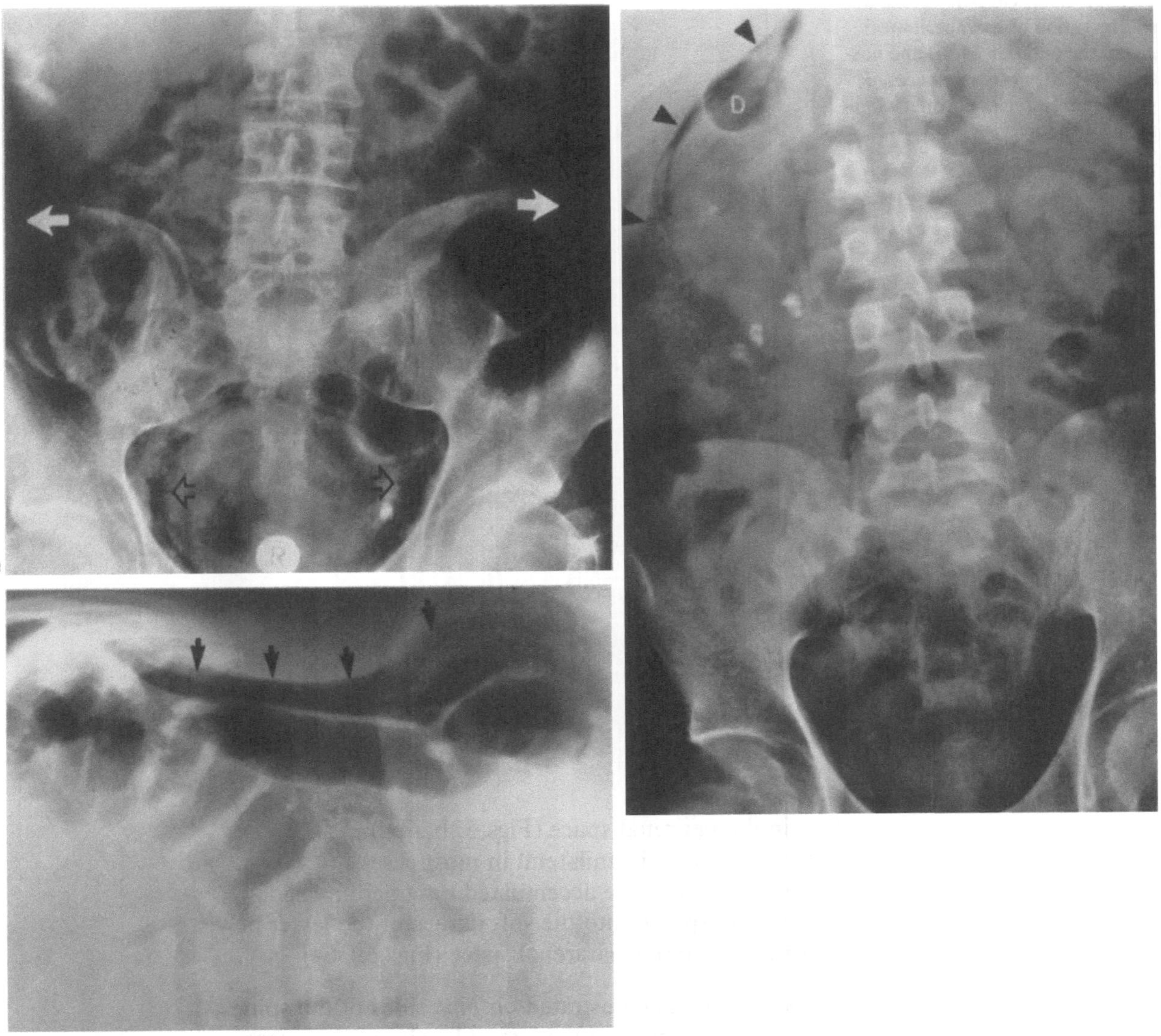

a b c

Fig. 60 a–c. Extraperitoneal gas collections. Man, 50 years old, who had undergone retroscopic removal of a small pedunculated polyp 12 cm into the rectum. The procedure was followed by pain in the lower abdomen and slowly progressive, muscular defence.
a, b *Supine and right lateral films* depict retroperitoneal gas collections in the perivesical space (⇨) and paracolic gutters (➡) signifying perforation into the posterior pararenal space. Retroperitoneal iatrogenic perforation was diagnosed at operation. **c** Man, 62 years old, who had undergone endoscopic removal of a rectal polyp but did not experience pain until about 10 h after surgery. *Supine film* shows small amounts of retroperitoneal gas in the right perirenal area (▶) and traces in the perivesical area. The rounded gas collection projected over the upper renal pole represents the gas-filled duodenal bulb *(D)*. The patient was treated conservatively

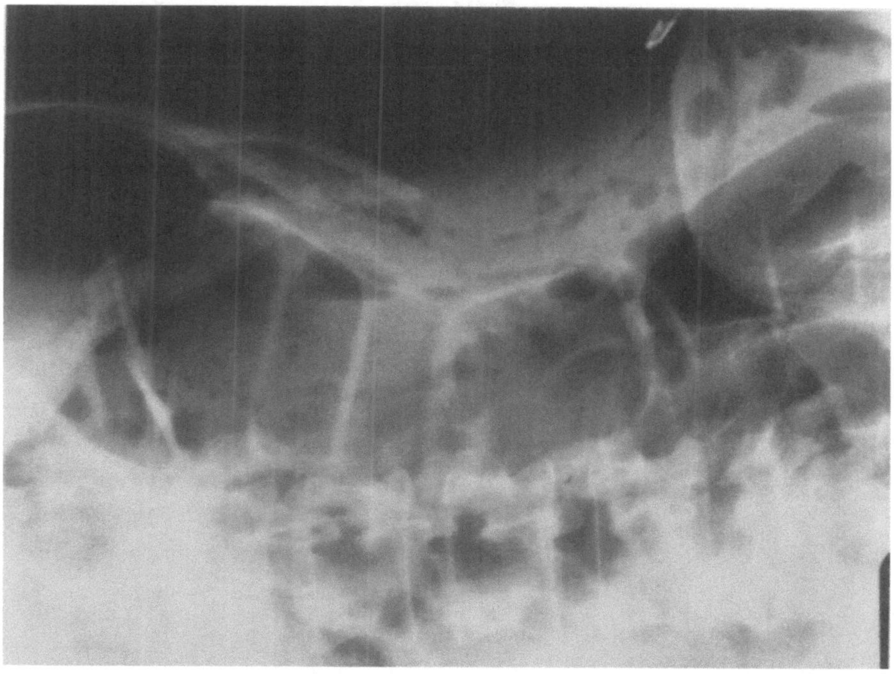

Fig. 61. Extraperitoneal gas. Man, 52 years old, who had undergone left nephrectomy for hypernephroma. He developed a fever 2 days postoperatively. ***Right lateral film*** shows fixed gas bubbles projected over the soft tissues of the left flank, extending into the anterior abdominal wall and left flank. Three days later the abdominal survey film showed no abnormalities, proving that the patient had a surgery-related, self-limiting retroperitoneal gas collection without pathologic significance

Sonography
Echogenic structures with acoustic shadows and/or reverberations within or in proximity to retroperitoneal organs are suggestive of retroperitoneal gas collections (Figs. 62, 145 c). Sonograms often show associated displacement of retroperitoneal organs by an abscess (kidney). The *positive demonstration* of a gas collection is necessary to confirm the diagnosis.

Computed Tomography (Figs. 64 d, 63 c, 144 c, 147 b)
- CT is markedly superior to plain radiographs.
- Even small amounts of retroperitoneal gas can *always* be visualized.
- Accompanying soft-tissue masses are demonstrated (abscess).
- The fascia and compartments can be evaluated, and accurate localization is usually possible.
- Pathways of spread can be identified.
- Organ assignment is possible.
- Intravenous administration of contrast material aids differentiation.
- The etiology of the gas collection can be established in approximately 90% of cases.

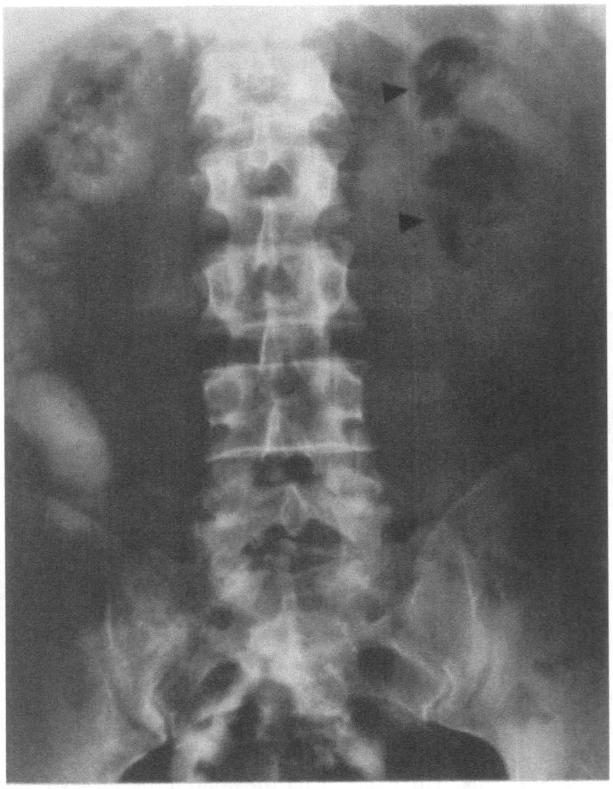

a

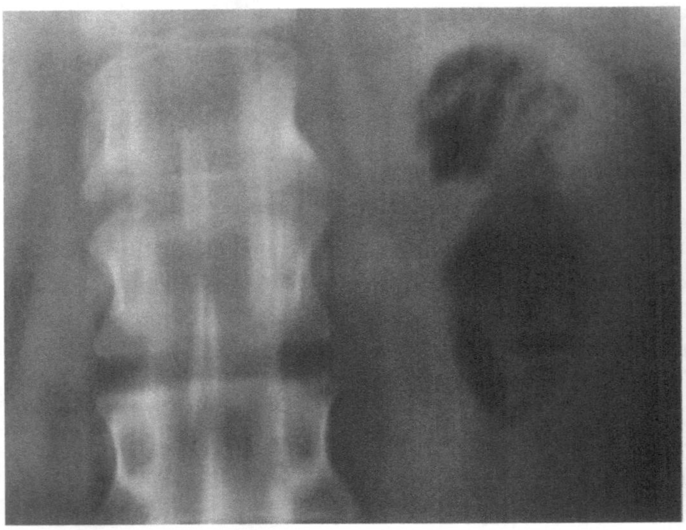

b

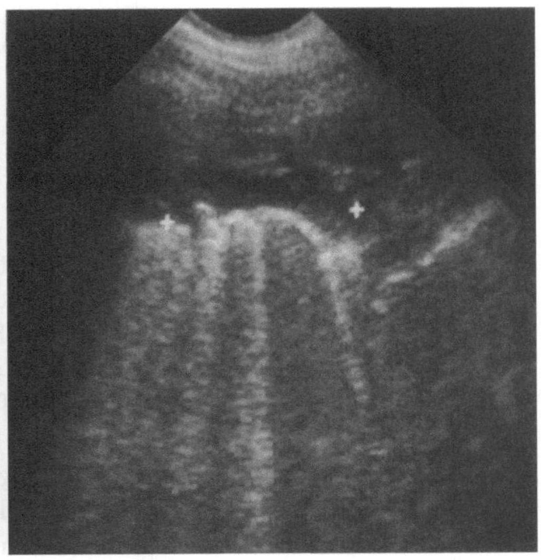

c

Fig. 62 a–c. Gas-forming abscess after nephrectomy. Man, 50 years old, who had undergone left nephrectomy for hypernephroma. Eight days postoperatively he developed pain in the left flank and fever; the operative scar showed no signs of irritation. *Supine film* (**a**) and *plain tomogram* (**b**) show a large, fixed gas collection in the left renal bed (▶). **c** *Sonogram* shows a thick-walled area with scalloped contours (+ +) and posterior acoustic shadowing in the region of the left renal bed. Operation disclosed a gas-forming abscess in the left renal compartment following nephrectomy

Fig. 63a-c. Gas in a retroperitenal tumor. Woman, 66 years old, who experienced an increasing sensation of fullness and epigastric discomfort for several months. Amylase and lipase values were within normal limits. **a** *Supine film* shows a large soft-tissue mass in the left upper quadrant with central, fixed gas bubbles (➡). **b** *CT scan* demonstrates a mass 10 cm in diameter in the tail of the pancreas, consistent with a gas-containing abscess or a centrally necrotic tumor. Operation disclosed a carcinoma of the tail of the pancreas with central, gas-containing necrosis. **c** *Upper GI series* (lateral projection) shows a large retrogastric mass that displaces the stomach anteriorly and contains central gas bubbles

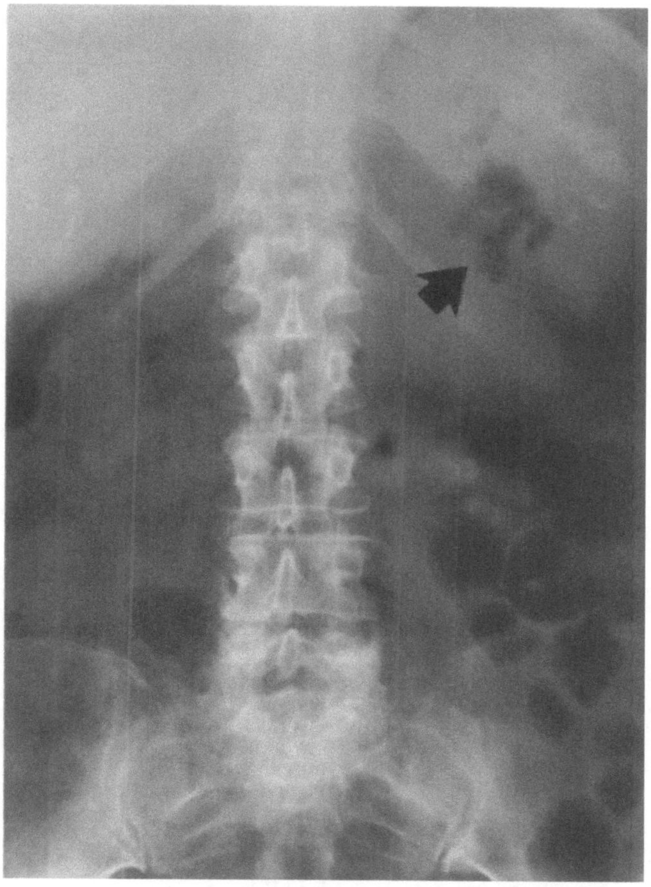

a

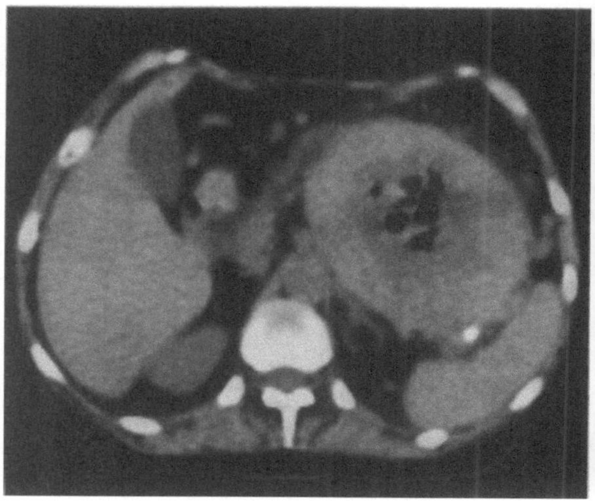

b

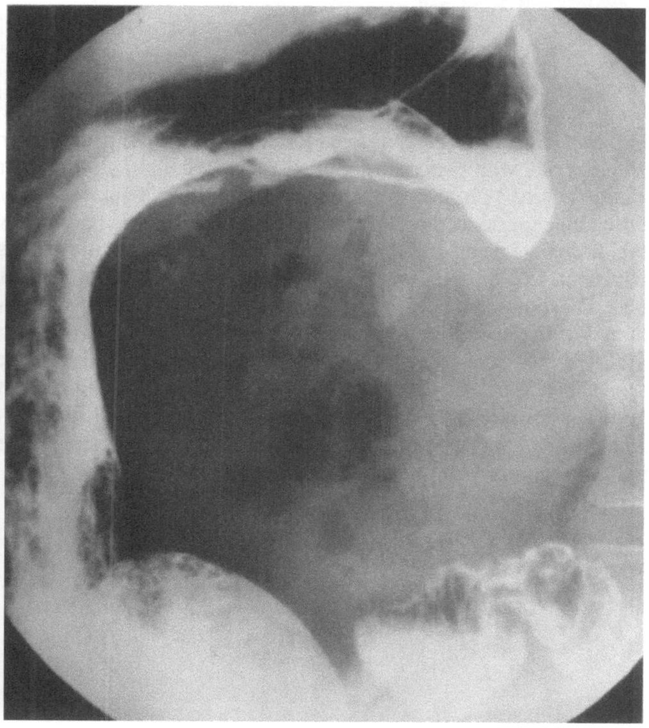

c

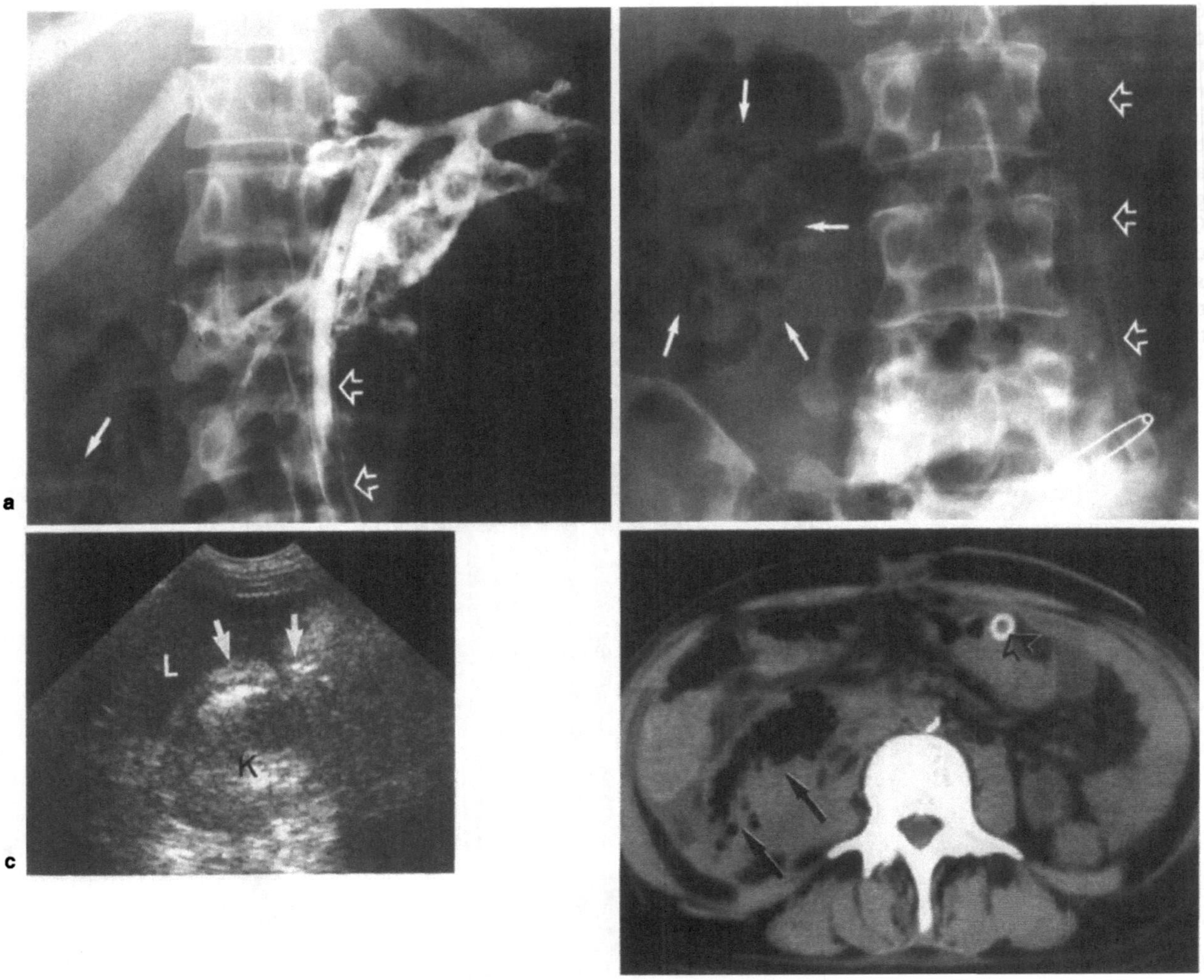

Fig. 64a-d. Gas-forming abscess following traumatic pancreatic rupture. Woman, 24 years old, with pancreatic rupture following blunt abdominal trauma. Extensive pancreatic necrosis prompted the insertion of a drain. One week later the patient became febrile and experienced midepigastric pain. **a** *Instillation of water-soluble contrast* through the drain (⇒) demonstrates extensive cavity formation in the presumed pancreatic compartment. Gas bubbles are also projected over the region of the right kidney (→). **b** *Supine film* shows a cluster of gas bubbles to the right of the spine (→) which are not contained in the bowel and are not related to the drain itself (⇒). **c** *Sonogram of the right kidney* shows gas (→) in front of the right kidney *(K)* with reverberations (*L*, liver). **d** *CT scan* shows a pancreatic abscess adjacent to the indwelling drain (⇒). There is also a large gas-forming abscess in the right anterior pararenal space (→). Operation disclosed an abscess in the right anterior pararenal space and pancreatic necrosis with abscess formation secondary to traumatic pancreatic rupture

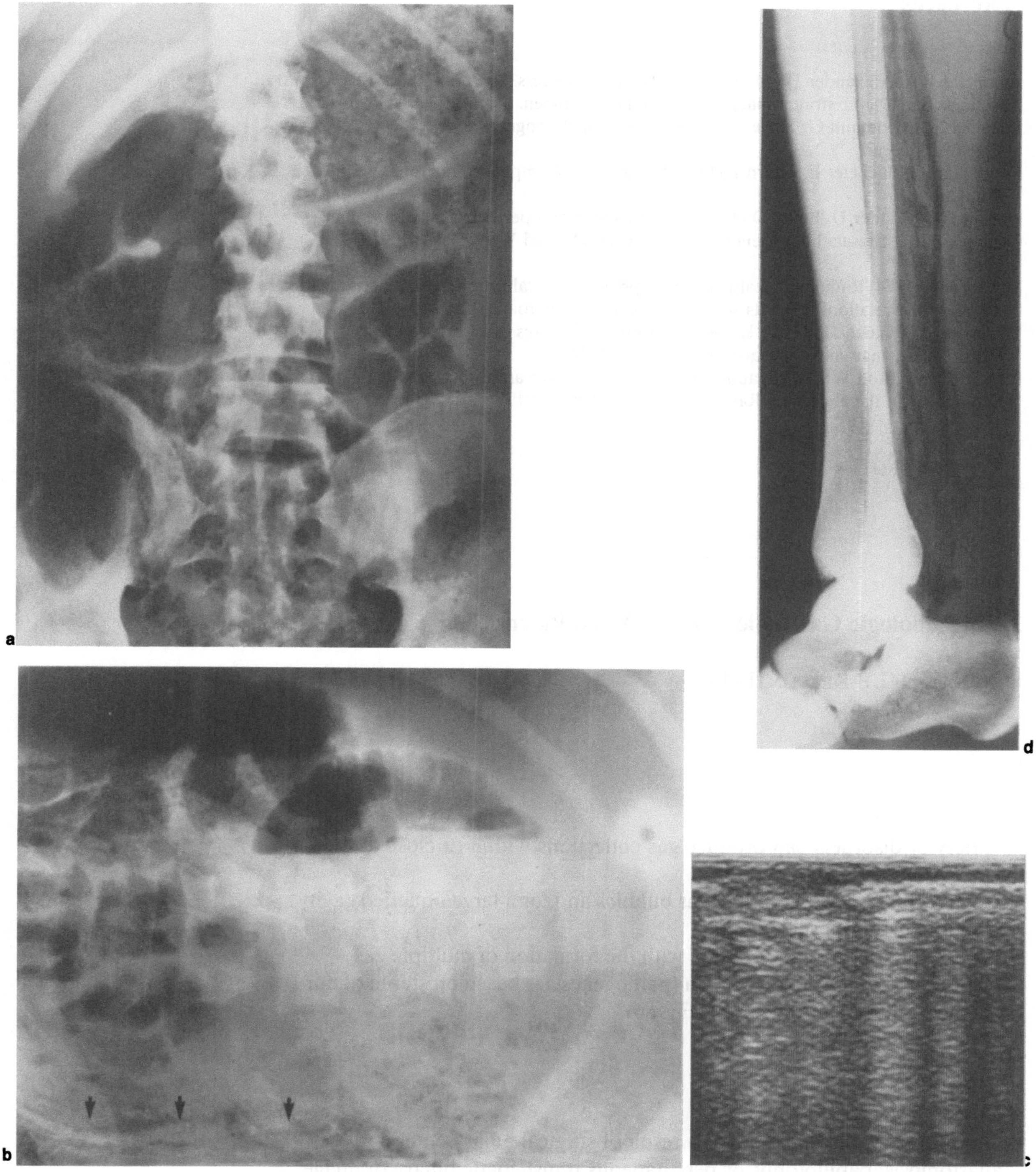

a
d
b
c

Fig. 65a–d. Gas gangrene. Man, 33 years old, with known chronic lymphocytic leukemia, leukopenia, and thrombocytopenia. For days he experienced acute abdominal complaints and had significant pain in the left calf with crepitations on palpation. *Supine film* (**a**) and *left lateral film* (**b**) show small, fixed gas bubbles projected over the left epigastrium and midabdomen that extend beyond the gastric contours. The left lateral film also shows gas bubbles in the abdominal wall and flank stripe (→). **c** *Sonogram* of the upper abdomen shows multiple acoustic shadows under the abdominal wall due to gas bubbles in the soft tissues. **d** *Lateral view* of the left lower leg shows streaky lucencies in the area of the calf muscles, consistent with a gas-forming inflammation. Diagnosis at autopsy: gas gangrene

References

Altemeier WA, Alexander JW (1961) Retroperitoneal abscess. Arch Surg 83: 512
Anschuetz SL (1984) Extraluminal gas in the upper abdomen. Semin Roentgenol 19: 255
Bücheler E, Friedmann G, Thelen M (1983) Real-time-Sonographie des Körpers. Thieme, Stuttgart
Friedmann G, Bücheler E, Thurn P (1981) Ganzkörper-Computertomographie. Thieme, Stuttgart
Krestin GP, Mödder U, Beyer D (1984) Die Diagnose retroperitonealer Gasansammlungen durch Einsatz bildgebender Verfahren. Dtsch Med Wochenschr 109/35: 1313-1318
Meyers MA (1974) Radiologic features of the spread and localization of extraperitoneal gas and their relationship to its source: an anatomic approach. Radiology 111: 17
Meyers, MA, Whalen JP, Peelle K (1972) Radiologic features of extraperitoneal effusions: an anatomic approach. Radiology 104: 249
Rice RP, Thompson WM, Gedgaudas RK (1982) Diagnosis and significance of extraluminal gas in the abdomen. Radiol Clin North Am 20: 819

3.5.3 Pathologic Gas Collections in Organ Parenchyma

U. Mödder, G. P. Krestin, D. Beyer

Causes

Hepatic Parenchyma
A variety of disorders can produce gas collections within or close to the liver.
- Hepatic abscess with multiple gas bubbles and/or a large liquefied cavity with an air-fluid level (Fig. 68)
- Sequela of arterial embolization, with the formation of multiple gas bubbles in a tumor-involved area (pathogenesis is based on sterile tumor necrosis rather than infection) (Fig. 66)
- Tumor necrosis (Fig. 67)

Bile Ducts (see Sect. 3.5.4)
- Gas may enter the bile ducts as a result of surgical biliary-enteric anastomosis, papillotomy, or percutaneous transhepatic biliary drainage (see Fig. 78 a)
- Emphysematous cholangitis
- Emphysematous cholecystitis (see Fig. 114)

Portal Vein (see Sects. 3.5.4, 4.2.4)
The most common causes of portal venous gas are mesenteric venous thrombosis and mesenteric arterial occlusion, pneumatosis intestinalis, gastroenterocolitis, and mucosal necrosis due to chemical agents (see Figs. 79, 80).

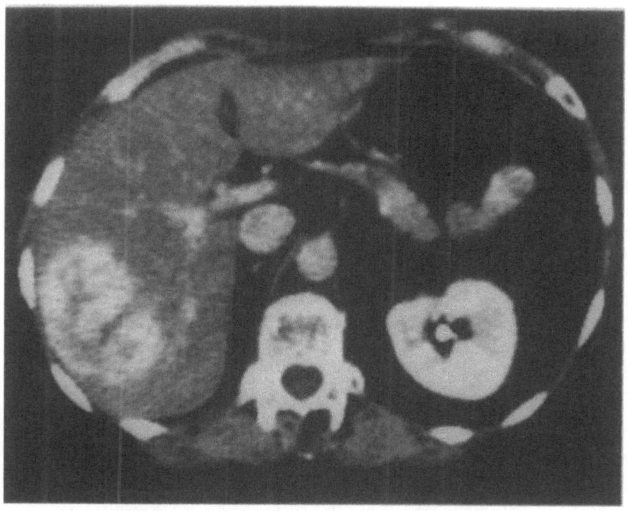

a

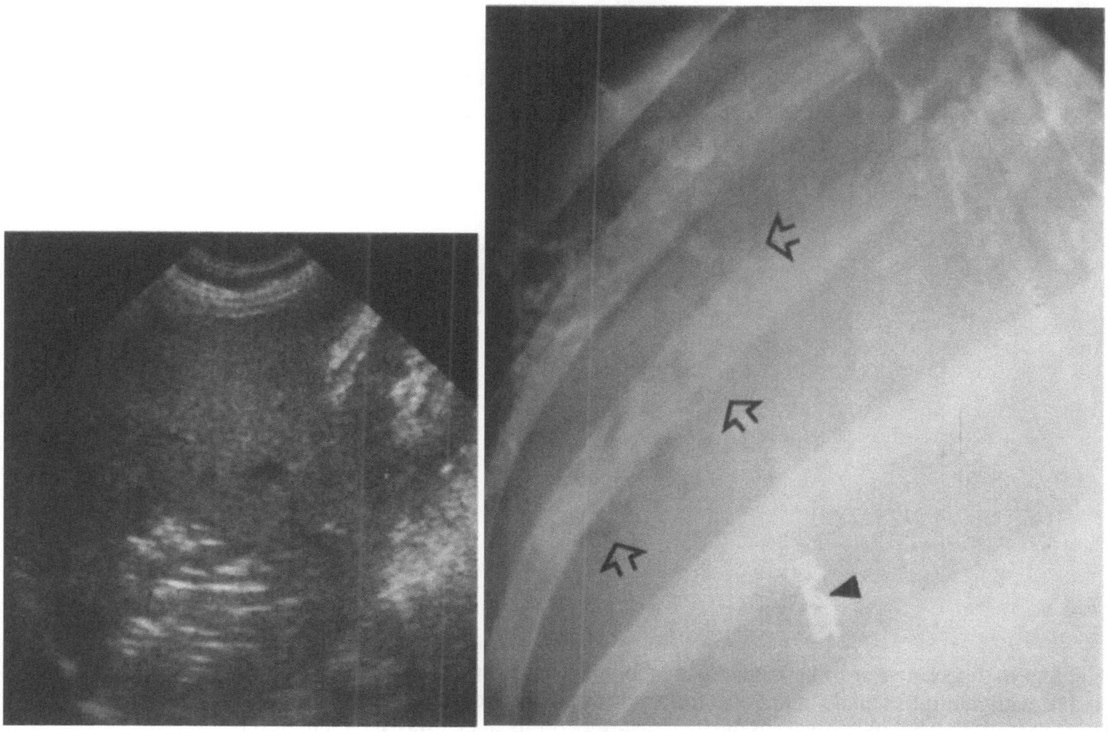

c b

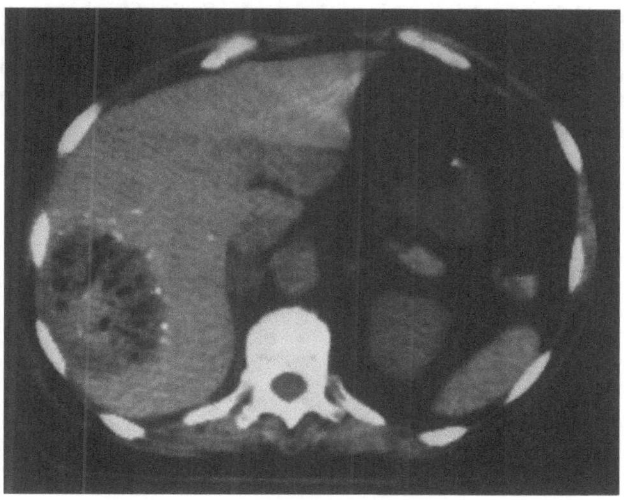

d

Fig. 66a–d. Gas formation in a liver metastasis after embolization. Thyroid carcinoma with known metastasis in the right lobe of the liver. **a** *Initial CT scan* showed a richly vascularized metastasis in the right hepatic lobe. **b** *Supine film,* following embolization with Histoacryl and a Gianturco coil (⇒), shows fixed gas bubbles projected over the right hepatic lobe (▶) **c** *Sonogram* shows an echogenic lesion with canalicular internal echoes and a hypoechoic margin as evidence of necrosis with gas formation. **d** *CT scan* also shows sign of necrosis and gas formation within the metastasis. High-density embolization material is visible at the periphery of the lesion

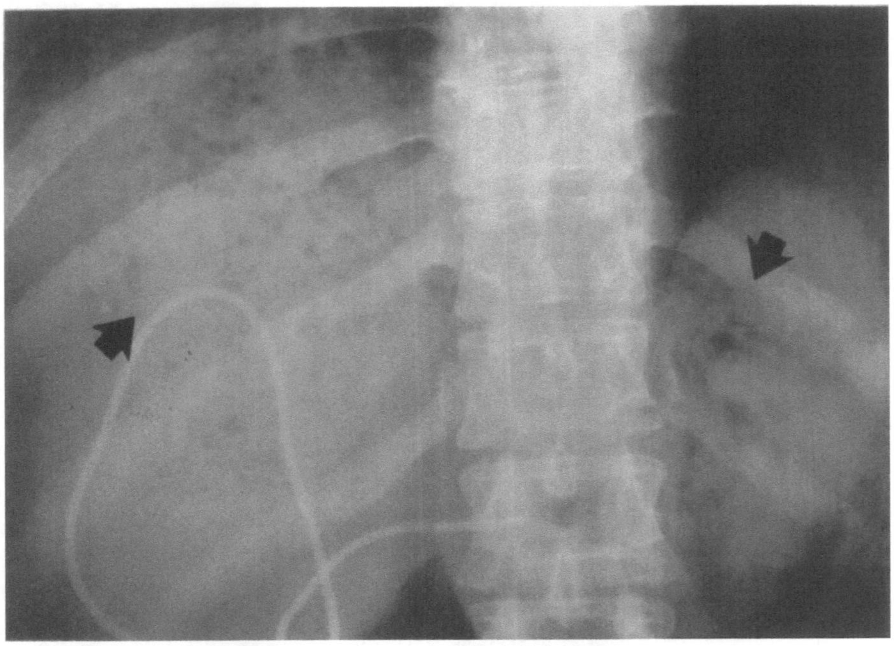

a

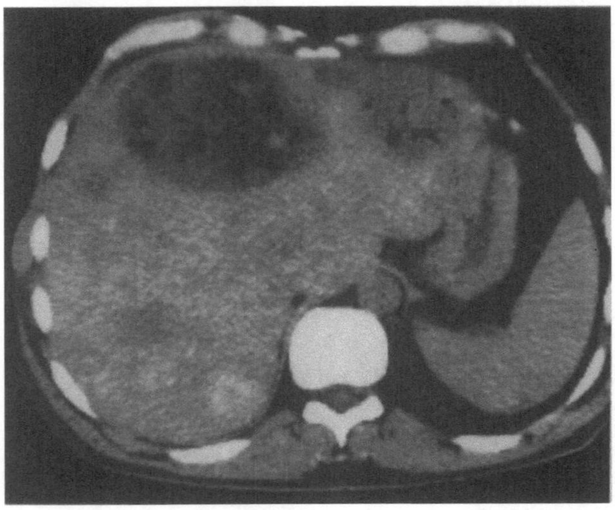

b

Fig. 67 a, b. Infected necrosis in two metastases following cytostatic therapy. Man, 42 years of age, with multiple hepatic metastases from colorectal carcinoma. A perfusion catheter had been inserted by operation into the hepatic artery for local cytostasis. Patient developed fever and epigastric tenderness. **a** *Supine film* shows multiple gas bubbles projected over the left hepatic lobe (➡). The right hemidiaphragm is elevated. The indwelling catheter is projected over the hilus of the liver. **b** *CT scan* shows diffuse hepatic metastases consisting of large, low-density areas with massive gas accumulation in the left and quadrate lobe

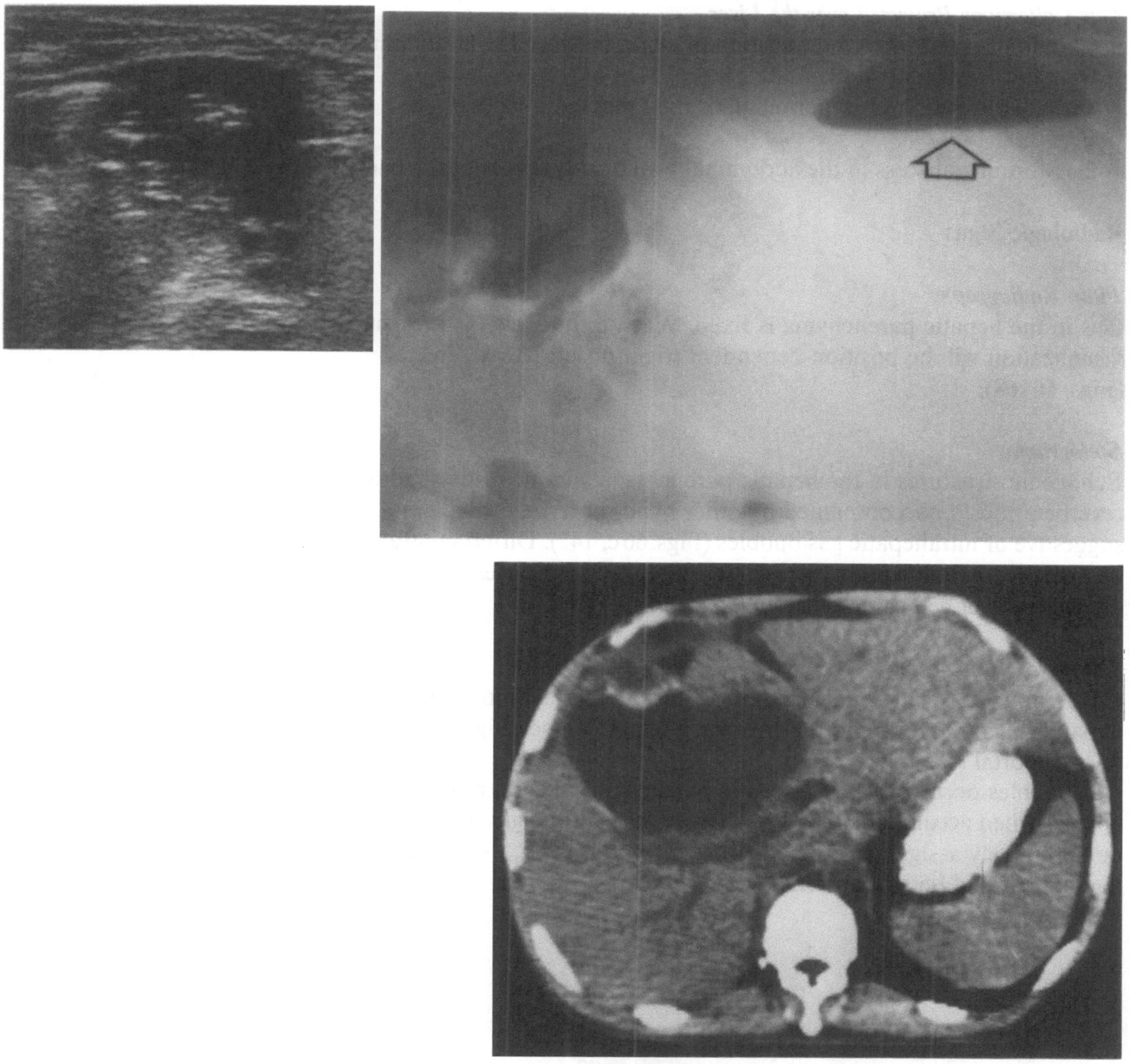

Fig. 68 a–c. Pathologic postoperative gas collections.
a, b Turkish man, 42 years of age, who received surgery for an echinococcal cyst, which was filled with hyperosmolar NaCl solution. **a** *Left lateral film* shows an air-fluid level 4 days postoperatively (⇒). **b** *CT scan* shows a partially collapsed, fluid-filled mass with movable air bubbles near the anterior abdominal wall. This represents a postoperative state rather than an abscess. **c** Woman, 44 years old, developed fever and tenderness in the right upper quadrant after cholecystectomy. *Sonogram* (longitudinal scan through the right hepatic lobe and gallbladder bed shows a fluid collection at the lower edge of the right hepatic lobe with multiple floating echo complexes with associated shadows and reverberations. Operation disclosed a gas-forming parahepatic abscess after cholecystectomy

Gas Collections Projected over the Liver

- Chilaiditi's syndrome (interposition of colon between the abdominal wall and liver; innocuous finding)
- Perihepatic, subphrenic, perirenal, or right paracolic abscess (see Figs. 138, 140)
- Gas-forming abscess in the abdominal wall or soft tissues of the back

Radiologic Signs

Plain Radiographs

Gas in the hepatic parenchyma is fixed. When a fluid level is present, visualization will be position-dependent (right or left lateral, erect) (Figs. 66-68).

Sonography

Echogenic structures in the hepatic parenchyma with acoustic shadows or reverberations, unaccompanied by other hypo- or hyperechoic areas, are suggestive of intrahepatic gas bubbles (Figs. 66c, 142). Differentiation must be made from intrahepatic calcifications (hepatic metastases, Echinococcus alveolaris, liver cell carcinoma).

Computed Tomography

CT permits the accurate localization of gas bubbles as: intra- or extrahepatic (Figs. 66d, 67b), intra- or extracholangiolar (see Fig. 82d), or intra- or extraportal (see Fig. 80c).

Gas bubbles occurring in the hepatic parenchyma suggest a diagnosis of abscess when accompanied by low-density areas. If the gas bubbles cannot be definitively assigned to the bile ducts or portal veins, i.v. contrast medium should be administered.

Note: Sonography and CT facilitate interventional procedures, such as puncture or drainage of an intra- or perihepatic abscess.

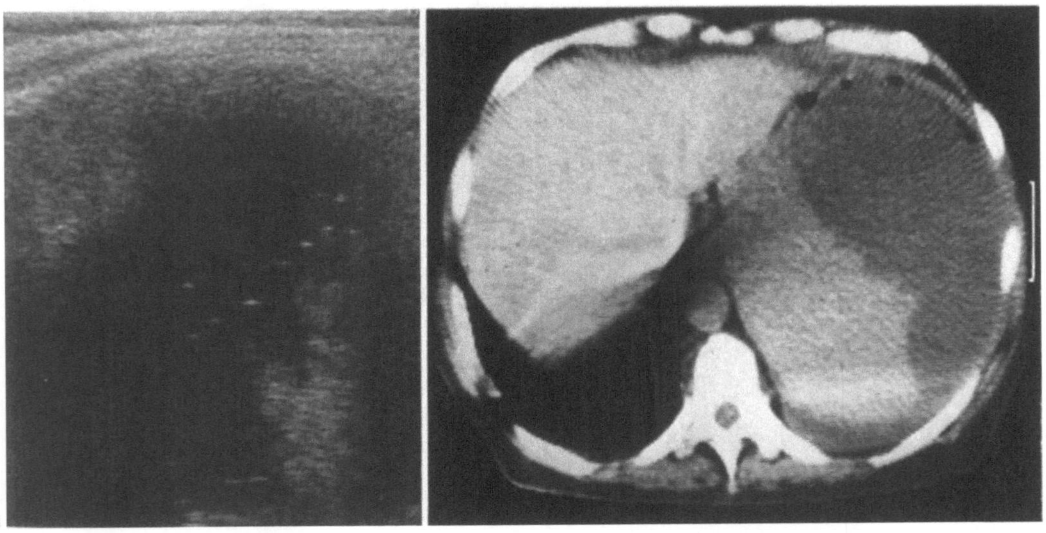

a b

Fig. 69a, b. Splenic abscess after radiotherapy. Man, 42 years old, with chronic lymphocytic leukemia. He had received radiation of the spleen because of hypersplenism. Febrile episodes developed during therapy. **a** *Sonogram* shows central anechoic and peripheral hypoechoic areas with floating gaseous inclusions within the enlarged spleen. **b** *CT scan* depicts a large, low-density area with gas bubbles anteriorly; splenomegaly

Pancreas

Causes

- Complication of acute pancreatitis (suppurative pancreatitis) (see Fig. 122a)
- Septic thrombosis
- Bacterial inflammation of a pancreatitis or pseudocyst
- Tumor necrosis (see Fig. 63)

Radiologic Signs

Plain Radiographs

- Gas bubbles projected over the pancreas (air-fluid level may be noted on L LAT and erect films) (see Fig. 64a)
- Left renal contour and left psoas border are obscured (see Fig. 63a)
- Stomach is displaced anteriorly, and the duodenojejunal flexure and transverse colon are displaced downward (see Fig. 63b).

Caution: In rare cases fluid levels in the stomach, in a hernia, or in a diverticulum can mimic an abscess in the retroperitoneal space.

Note: A subphrenic or perinephritic abscess is often indistinguishable from a pancreatic abscess on abdominal plain films. Further evaluation with sonography and CT is required.

a 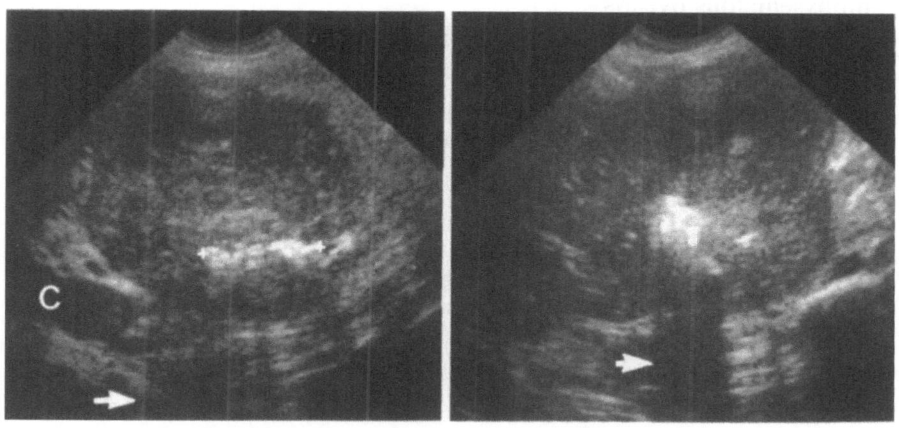 b

Fig. 70a, b. Retroperitoneal sarcoma with central necrosis, gas formation, and abscess. Woman, 62 years of age, with an increasing sensation of epigastric fullness for several weeks and a palpable mass. **a** *Sonogram,* longitudinal scan through the inferior vena cava *(C),* shows a large, precaval mass extending to the anterior abdominal wall. Posteriorly there is a wide echo front (+ +) with acoustic shadowing and reverberations (→). **b** A *transverse sonogram* through the lesion shows marked gas collection in the interior of the mass with acoustic shadowing (→) and abscess

Sonography

- Evidence of pancreatitis with widening and swelling of the head and tail of the pancreas and increased sonolucency due to edema (see Figs. 119, 120)
- Widening of the retroperitoneal space (usually on the left side with pancreatic abscess formation)
- Reverberations associated with the presence of gas bubbles (Fig. 70); they require differentiation from calcifications associated with chronic pancreatitis (see Fig. 95 b)
- With a fluid-filled pancreatic abscess, echo-free or hypoechoic areas with sedimentation of cellular material may be demonstrated.

Computed Tomography

- Permits definitive assignment to the pancreas, kidney, retroperitoneal space, splenic compartment, or left lobe of the liver (see Figs. 122 a, 64 d, 63 b)
- Besides gas bubbles, CT can demonstrate widening of the organ and exudation into the peripancreatic compartments (right and left pararenal space, omental bursa) (see Figs. 119–122)

Note: In acute pancreatitis and pancreatitis with abscess formation, the entire abdomen should be surveyed by CT due to the possible spread of the inflammatory process along typical necrotic tracks (see Sect. 4.1.2).

Kidneys (Renal Transplants) Ureters, Urinary Bladder

Causes

Inflammation:

- Renal abscess, which is especially common in diabetics. Multiple septic-pyemic abscesses may permeate both kidneys
- Emphysematous pyelitis
- Emphysematous pyelonephritis (main causative organisms: E. Coli, Proteus, Clostridium) (see Fig. 147)
- Cystic pyeloureteritis with subepithelial cysts in the renal pelvis and proximal ureter. The pathogenesis is unclear; there is no bacterial inflammation

Note: The spinal column and intervertebral discs should always be evaluated in patients with renal abscess. A pararenal abscess may be secondary to a spondylitis or spondylodiscitis.

Tumor:

- Hypernephroma or metastasis with tumor necrosis (Fig. 70)
- Perforation of a colon carcinoma with urointestinal fistula

Trauma:

- Penetrating injury and possible secondary inflammation of a hematoma or urinoma

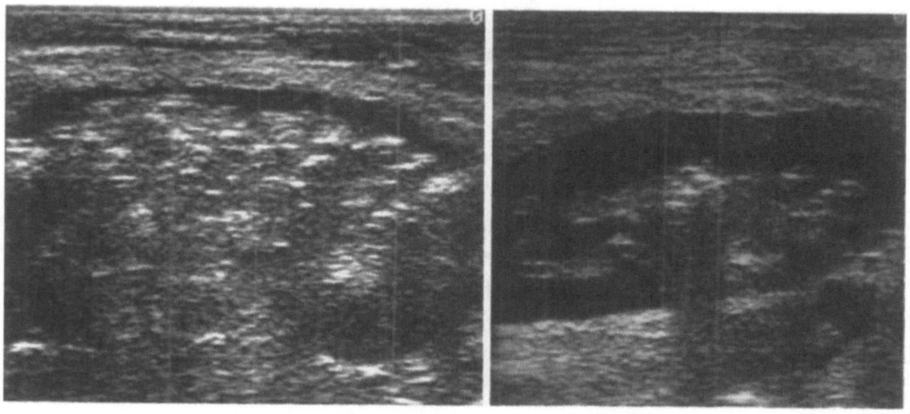

a b

Fig. 71 a. Gas collections in renal transplants. Man, 31 years of age, who had undergone a renal transplantation experienced a rejection crisis with fever. The transplant was tender to pressure. *Sonogram* shows narrowing of the parenchymal margin and multiple gaseous inclusions in the renal parenchyma with faint acoustic shadows and reverberations. *Diagnosis:* emphysematous pyelonephritis associated with rejection (confirmed after surgical removal of the transplant). **b** Routine follow-up *sonogram* of a 28-year-old woman who had undergone renal transplantation. The scan shows gas bubbles in the pyelocaliceal system which move with position changes. The transplant appears normal. *Diagnosis:* postoperative gas residue in the renal pelvis without pathologic significance. The gas bubbles persisted for 4 days

Postoperative:
- Urointestinal fistula
- Implantation of a ureter in the rectosigmoid
- Gas formation in a tumor area following transcatheter embolization

Spontaneous urointestinal fistulas:
- Perforation of a sigmoid diverticulum
- Fistula formation in Crohn's disease

Ureterovaginal fistulas:
- Congenital, postoperative, after perforation of a carcinoma

Ureterocutaneous fistulas:
- Perforating trauma, postoperative, ectopic opening of ureter into the vulva, perineum, or scrotum

Radiologic Signs

Plain Radiographs

- Radially streaked, reticulated, or bullous collection of air in the renal parenchyma and/or perirenal space (Fig. 147)
- Concomitant isolated colonic distension as evidence of a retroperitoneal process
- With renal abscess, elevation of the diaphragm and compensatory scoliosis, obliteration of psoas margin, enlargement of the renal shadow, or possibly the presence of a "renal bulge."
  The kidney may be displaced laterally, anteriorly, or inferiorly (see Fig. 147).
  Differential diagnosis: retroperitoneal inflammatory process, acute pancreatitis.

Urography

- Intrarenal gas collection with expanding process → tumorlike displacement, deformation, or compression of calices, of caliceal necks, or of renal pelvis
- Peri- or pararenal gas collection → peri- or paranephritic abscess with displacement of the renal shadow and obliteration of the psoas border and/or the flank shadow (see Fig. 145)
- Abscess communicates with the renal pyelocaliceal system → retrograde filling of the abscess cavity from the pyelocaliceal system (irregular inner contour with fresh abscess, smooth inner contour with chronic abscess)
- Multiple septic-pyemic abscesses may permeate both kidneys

Sonography

Renal abscess presents as a liquid or semiliquid area with indistinct margins and acoustic enhancement. Gas bubbles appear as echogenic areas with reverberation echoes (Figs. 71, 145 c).

Differential diagnosis: necrotic hypernephroma, possibly with central hemorrhage

- Hematoma
- Hemorrhagic infarction associated with renal vein thrombosis

Computed Tomography

CT permits an accurate topographic assignment of gas collections (peri- or pararenal; intrarenal; renal pelvis, ureter, or bladder wall) (see Figs. 57 b, 147).

The following signs are characteristic of abscess:

- Isodense or hypodense area in the renal parenchyma with decreased central contrast enhancement
- After bolus injection, enhancement of the abscess wall in the early arterial phase (see Fig. 148 e)
- Mottled, nonhomogeneous enhancement is characteristic of multiple septic-pyemic abscesses

Differential diagnosis:

- Necrotic tumor; evidence of a mass lesion in the kidney, possible penetration of the capsule, invasion of the renal vein or inferior vena cava, enlarged lymph nodes, distant metastases

History should be checked for prior embolization of a renal tumor, an old hematoma, or perforating trauma.

Note: CT of the kidneys should be done initially without employing a renally excreted i.v. contrast medium. When contrast medium is administered, the bolus technique is preferred.

Spleen

Causes

- Splenic abscesses (echinococciasis, tuberculosis, histoplasmosis, brucellosis, sepsis); most common in patients with generally low resistance
- Splenic infarction; accompanies splenomegaly; major causes are leukoses lymphoma and endocarditis
- Prior embolization (indication: hypersplenism); excessive embolization also carries a danger of abscess formation

Radiologic Signs

Plain Radiographs

Circumscribed subphrenic gas bubbles located outside the bowel lumen which do not move with position changes. Possible pleural effusion on the left side.
With splenomegaly, the kidney is displaced downward and medially.
Concomitant, isolated colonic distension suggest a retroperitoneal process.

Sonography

Circumscribed, generally hypoechoic mass with irregular margins located in the splenic parenchyma (see Fig. 69 a).
Large gas inclusions lead to acoustic shadows.
An intra-abdominal, parasplenic fluid collection may form as a localized response.

Computed Tomography

- Gas inclusion are pathognomonic of hepatic abscesses, except after embolization (see Fig. 69 b).
- Densitometry permits differentation from fresh hemorrhage (see Figs. 205 e, 194, 196).
- Intravenous bolus injection helps to differentiate perfused from unperfused, pathologic areas of the spleen.

Note: A mottling of the parenchyma may appear shortly after the i.v. bolus injection of renally excreted contrast medium as an expression of compartmentalization of the contrast-containing blood in the splenic trabeculae; pseudoparenchymal defects are caused by time differences in the perfusion of the splenic trabeculae and pulp.

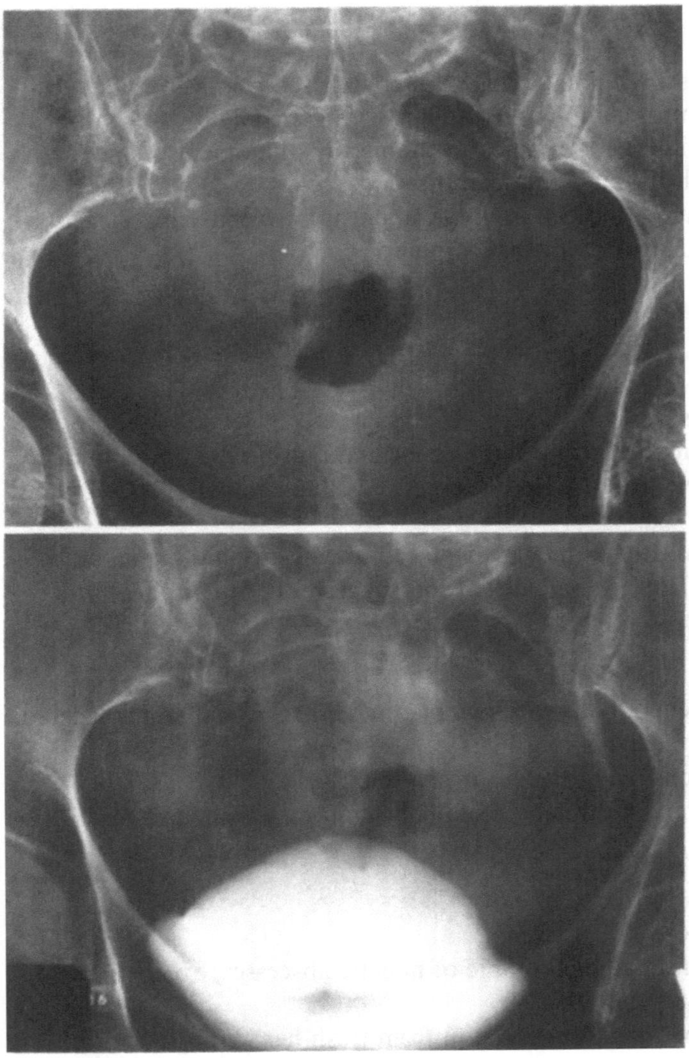

a

b

Fig. 72a, b. Uterine carcinoma with central necrosis and gas formation. Woman, 64 years of age, with known uterine carcinoma. **a** *Preoperative urogram and supine radiograph* show an irregular gas collection projected over the urinary bladder that has no apparent relation to the rectum or sigmoid colon. **b** *Urogram* shows the gas collection positioned behind the bladder and surrounded by a soft-tissue mass. Operation disclosed central tumor necrosis with gas formation in a large, degenerating uterine carcinoma

Uterus

A gas-forming inflammation (see Fig. 224) or tumor necrosis (Fig. 72) causes gas collections to be projected over the uterus. Sonography and CT can establish the intracavitary or intramural location of uterine gas (Fig. 224).

Gas in the Vaginal Wall

Causes

Most common in pregnant women and in drug addicts with severe vaginal infections caused by Candida, Trichomonas, or E. coli.

Radiologic Signs

Plain Radiographs

Plain films show a tubular arrangement of gas bubbles in the vaginal position (spreading downward and projected over the symphysis. Differential diagnosis: gas containing tampon (see Fig. 111 a).

Computed Tomography

If necessary, CT can establish the location of the gas and confirm its intramural position.

References

Callen PW (1979) Computed tomographic evaluation of abdominal and pelvic abscesses. Radiology 131: 171

Krestin GP, Mödder U, Beyer D (1984) Retroperitoneale Gasansammlungen: Diagnose durch Einsatz bildgebender Verfahren. Dtsch Med Wochenschr 109: 1313-1318

Lange S (1983) Niere und ableitende Harnwege. Thieme, Stuttgart

Lorenz R, Beyer D, Friedmann G, Mödder U (1983) Grenzen der Differenzierung fokaler Milzläsionen durch Sonographie und Computertomographie. Fortschr Roentgenstr 138: 447-452

Rehwald U, Heckemann R (1983) Die sonographische Untersuchung der Milz. Radiologe 23: 114-120

Rösch J (1973) Röntgendiagnostik des Pankreas. In: Strnad F (ed) Röntgendiagnostik des Pankreas und der Milz. Springer, Berlin Heidelberg New York (Handbuch der medizinischen Radiologie, vol 12/2)

Rupp N (1976) Die Nativdiagnostik der Lebererkrankungen im Röntgenbild. In: Heuck F (ed) Röntgendiagnostik der Leber und der Gallenwege. Springer, Berlin Heidelberg New York (Handbuch der medizinischen Radiologie, vol XII/1)

Swart B, Meyer G, Herrmann FJ (1976) Röntgendiagnostik der Gallenblase und Gallenwege. In: Heuck F (ed) Springer, Berlin Heidelberg New York (Handbuch der medizinischen Radiologie, vol 12/1)

3.5.4 Intraluminal and Intramural Gas Collections in Canalicular Structures and Hollow Viscera

D. BEYER, U. MÖDDER

Note: A gas collection in a canalicular structure (blood vessel, bile duct, urinary tract, vagina) or hollow viscus (gallbladder, bowel wall, urinary bladder) (Fig. 73), if not the result of a previous operation or diagnostic procedure, nearly always signifies a highly acute process and urgently requires further evaluation.

Intramural Gas in the Bowel Wall (Pneumatosis Intestinalis)

Causes

Gastrointestinal causes

Necrotizing enterocolitis (Fig. 78 d, e)
Acute or protracted intestinal gangrene (Figs. 76, 78 a, b)

Intestinal obstruction, possibly with ischemia:
- Mechanical bowel obstruction (Fig. 78 a, b)
- Gastric outlet obstruction
- Hypertrophic pyloric stenosis
- Gastric volvulus
- Imperforate anus
- Hirschsprung's disease

Caustic injury to the gastrointestinal wall
Iatrogenic or pharmacologic causes:
- Previous operation (bowel anastomosis, jejunoileal bypass)
- Previous endoscopy (stomach/colon)
- High-dosage steroid therapy

Collagen diseases
- Systemic lupus erythematosus
- Scleroderma
- Rheumatoid arthritis

Inflammations
- Phlegmonous gastritis
- Acute or chronic enteritis, gastritis, appendicitis
- Diverticulitis, perforated diverticulum
- Ulcerative colitis
- Acute pancreatitis

Peptic ulcers, carcinomas of the gastrointestinal tract, abdominal trauma, Whipple's disease, intestinal parasite infestations

Other causes

Acute or chronic obstructive airway disease, pneumomediastinum

Idiopathic pneumatosis intestinalis

(especially cystic pneumatosis of the colon) (Figs. 74, 75)

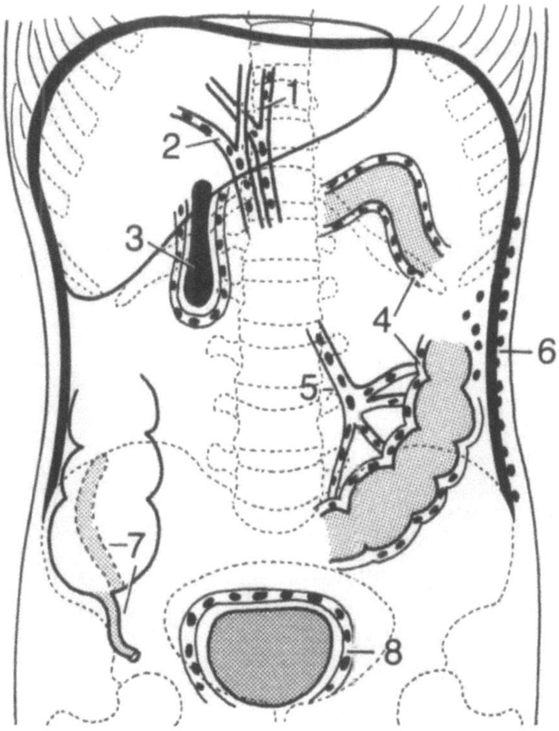

Fig. 73. Sites of intraluminal gas collection in tubular structures and hollow viscera: *1*, gas in the bile ducts; *2*, gas in the portal vein; *3*, gas in the lumen and wall of the gallbladder in emphysematous cholecystitis; *4*, intramural gas in the bowel wall; *5*, gas in the mesenteric veins; *6*, gas in the flank stripe (in contradistinction to *4* and *5*); *7*, gas in retrocecal appendicitis; *8*, gas in the wall and lumen of the urinary bladder

Radiologic Signs

Plain Radiographs (Fig. 73)
Linear or cystlike gas collections in the wall of the stomach, small bowel, or colon (Fig. 75).
The position of the gas bubbles is constant on both planes. If the X-ray beam strikes a bowel loop with intramural gas in orthograde fashion, a circumferential lucency is produced that can be very difficult to interpret (Fig. 76 a, b).
Particular attention should be given to simultaneous gas collections in the mesenteric and portal veins (L LAT film) (Figs. 78, 79).

Caution: Gas bubbles in the stool can mimic intramural gas, especially with fecal impaction. Differentiate by Gastrografin enema (Fig. 77)!

Sonography
Intramural gas can usually be diagnosed only in conjunction with the abdominal plain films.
Ultrasound scans show string-of-bead gas collections in the bowel wall with acoustic shadowing and reverberations (Fig. 75 a). Free intra-abdominal fluid may be observed.

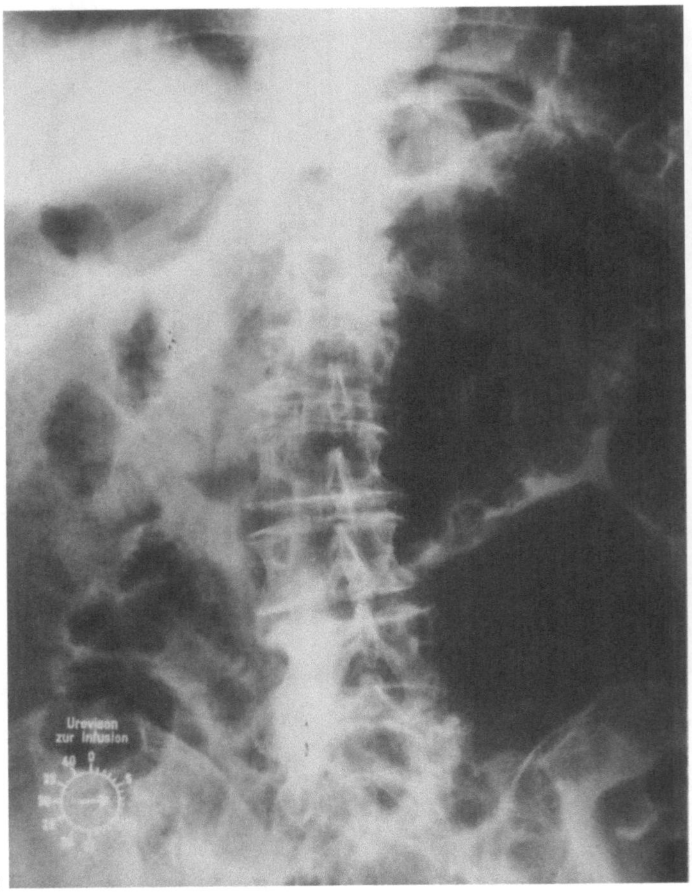

a

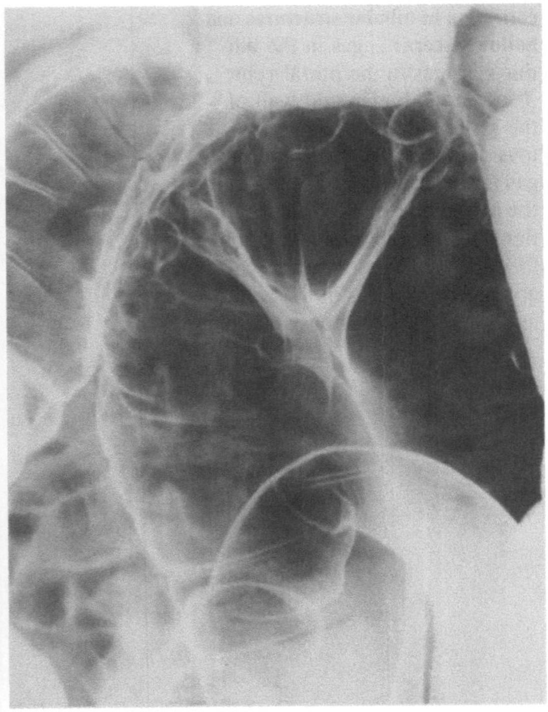

b

Fig. 74a, b. Asymptomatic pneumatosis cystica coli. Man, 86 years old, with prostatic adenoma, no abdominal complaints, and no stool irregularities. **a** Supine film (urogram) shows massive colonic distension with multiple, tangentially imaged gas bubbles in the bowel wall. **b** Contrast enema shows that the pneumatosis cystica is confined to the elongated and dilated loop of sigmoid colon (Dr. K. Korth, Dr. D. Ross, Department of Radiology, St. Ansgar Hospital, Hoxter)

Fig. 75a–e. Intramural gas collections in the colon (pneumatosis cystoides coli). The small bowel of this 64-year-old man had been completely removed 4 weeks earlier because of mesenteric venous thrombosis; an ascendo-duodenostomy was constructed. The patient was hospitalized and placed on total parenteral nutrition for short bowel syndrome. Clinical examination showed a soft, nontender abdomen, normal peristalsis (?), a pulse rate of 88, and no fever or leukocytosis. **a** *Sonogram,* longitudinal scan through the right lower quadrant, shows gas *(G)* in the anterior and posterior wall of the ascending colon (→); etiology is unclear. Therefore: **b** *supine film* shows distension limited to the colon and linear gas collections (→) in the wall of the cecum, extending from the ascending colon to the midportion of the transverse colon. There are also gas bubbles adjacent to the colon wall, probably in the mesentery or the mesenteric veins (⇒). **c** The *CT scan scout-view* demonstrates the intramural gas collection more clearly (→). Otherwise findings are the same as on the plain film. ▷ **d** *CT scan* through the role of the cecum shows a conspicuous, crescentic gas collection in the posterolateral portion of its wall (→). Gas bubbles *(G)* are seen anterior to the psoas muscle and in the region of the mesentery (→). Because of the increasing volume of intramural gas on the plain films and the patient's history of mesenteric venous thrombosis, a laparotomy was performed despite an absence of clinical symptoms. Resection was not performed. Multiple submucosal gas bubbles were found in the area examined radiologically. In the 8 months since the laparotomy the patient's condition has been stable. **e Intramural gas in the ileum secondary to mesenteric embolism.** *CT scan* shows string-of-beads gas bubbles in the intestinal wall with distension of the small bowel (**e** courtesy of Prof. Dr. W. Wenz, Department of Diagnostic Radiology, Albert-Ludwig University, Freiburg)

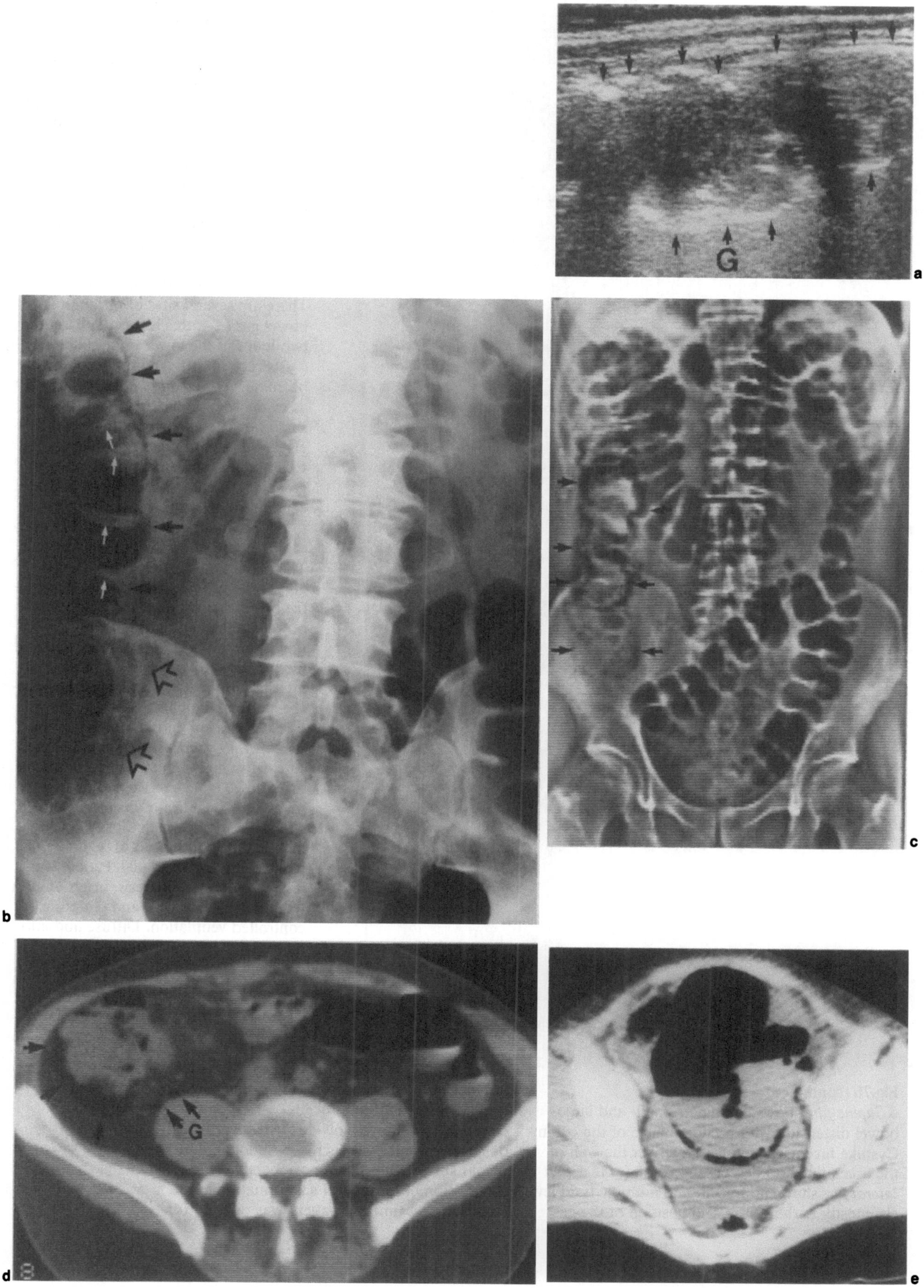
G
a
b
c
G
d
e

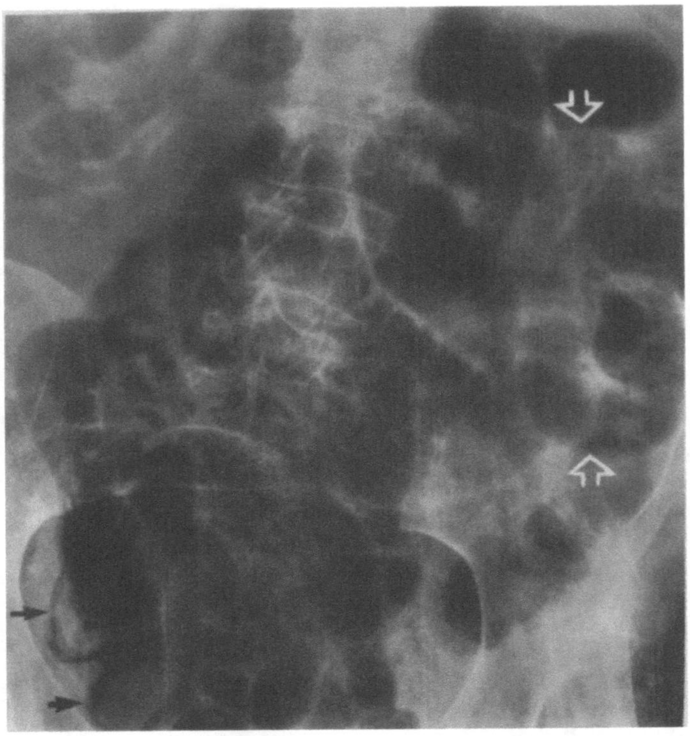

a

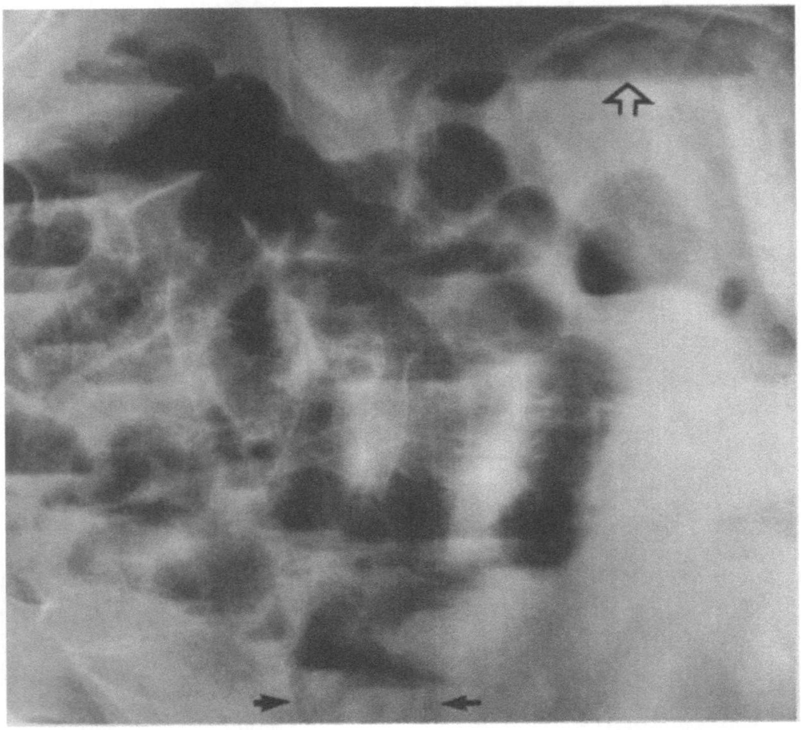

b

Fig. 76a–e. Gas in the bowel wall after mesenteric ischemia.
a, b Mesenteric arterial thrombosis with intramural gas and perforation in a woman 73 years old. For 1 day prior to admission the patient had pain throughout the abdomen most pronounced in the right lower quadrant; she also presented with vomiting and bloody diarrhea. Clinical examination disclosed boardlike abdominal rigidity, aperistalsis, a pulse rate of 110, and cyanosis; the patient's general condition was extremely poor. **a** *Supine film* shows predominant distension of the small bowel. There are several sites of intramural bowel gas (⇒); this is most apparent in two loops in the lower right quadrant (→) struck in orthograde fashion by the beam. **b** *Left lateral film* depicts free air as evidence of a perforation (⇒). The small bowel contains multiple fluid levels, and intramural gas is visible (→←). Exploratory laparotomy disclosed gangrene of the entire small bowel and ascending colon with a free perforation into the peritoneal cavity and diffuse peritonitis; there was gas in the bowel wall. The patient died a few hours after surgery. Autopsy disclosed diffuse peritonitis, hemorrhagic infarction of the small bowel and ascending colon with perforation; there was gas in the bowel wall and mesenteric veins. *Diagnosis:* mesenteric arterial thrombosis. **c, d Nonocclusive ischemia from digitalis poisoning with colonic necrosis and intramural gas formation.** The 19-year-old woman attempted suicide by ingesting 80 0.2-mg tablets of digoxin, 20 tablets of isosorbide dinitrate, and 20 tablets of bromazepam. *Clinical examination* disclosed septic temperatures of around 41 °C and a white cell count of 21000. Patient was treated by plasmapheresis, insertion of a temporary pacemaker, and temporary controlled ventilation. Diffuse abdominal rigidity and aperistalsis were noted on day 7 after the suicide attempt.

Fig. 76 (continued)
c *Supine film* shows combined small- and large-bowel distension with predominance of the colon. Cystlike lucencies are projected over the wall of the ascending and descending colon (⇒). **d** *Left lateral film* shows no free air and multiple fluid levels, mostly in the colon. The position of the gas bubbles in the descending colon is unchanged, signifying fixed intramural gas (⇒). Operation disclosed a small-bowel volvulus *without* gross evidence of colonic wall necrosis. Abdominal biplanar survey films taken postoperatively showed progression of intramural gas formation in the colon. At that time the patient was referred for

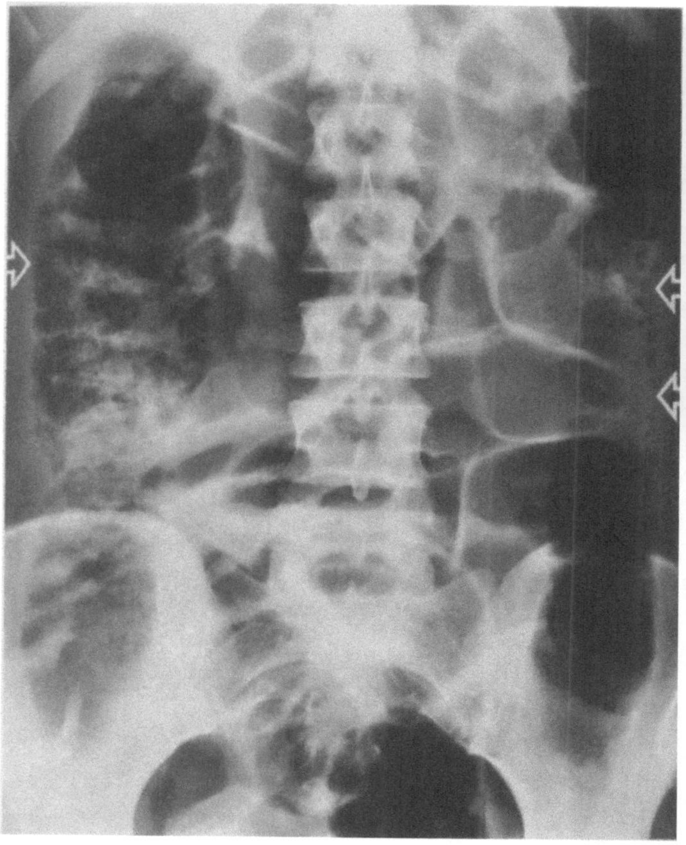

c

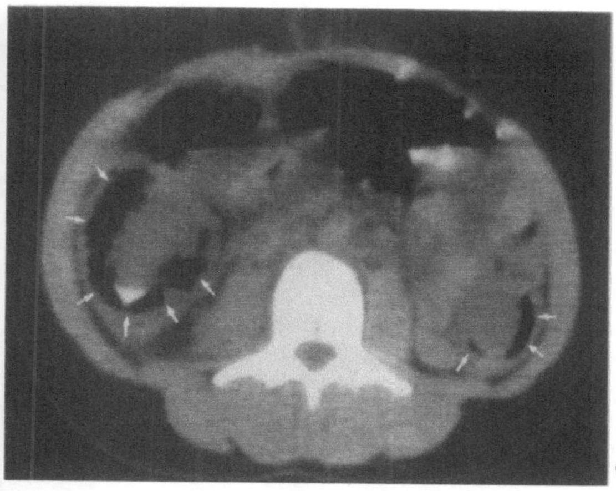

e

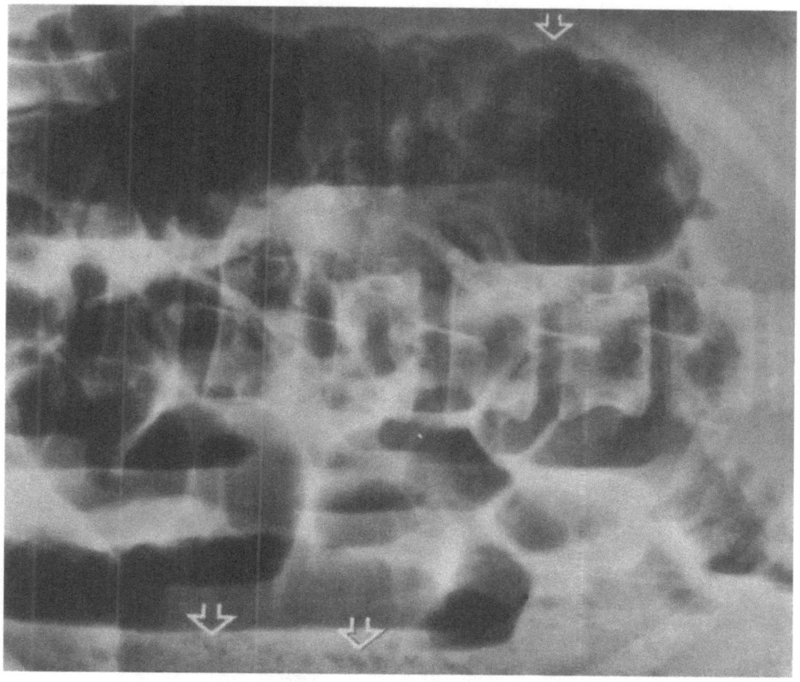

d

Fig. 76 (continued)
e *CT scan* (at the level of the 2nd lumbar vertebra), which shows a hugely dilated ascending colon (10 cm in diameter) with partly crescentic and partly cystlike intramural lucencies in the ascending and descending colon having the density of air (→). This confirmed the plain film diagnosis. A second operation was performed 2 days after CT examination; the patient was still febrile. The anterior portions of the colon wall appeared grossly normal. It was only *after* the colon was opened that obvious mucosal necrosis and intramural gas were found. A colectomy and ileosigmoidostomy were carried out. *Histologic examination* showed necrosis of the mucosa and submucosa and incipient necrosis of portions of the muscularis. Vascular occlusions were not observed. *Diagnosis:* nonocclusive ischemia secondary to digitalis toxicity. The patient survived

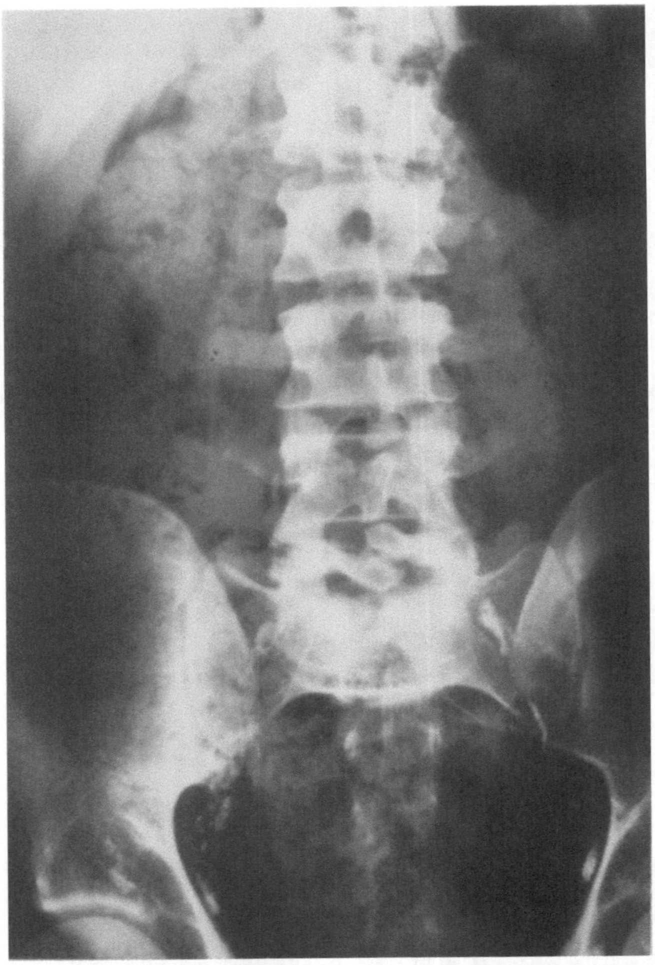
a

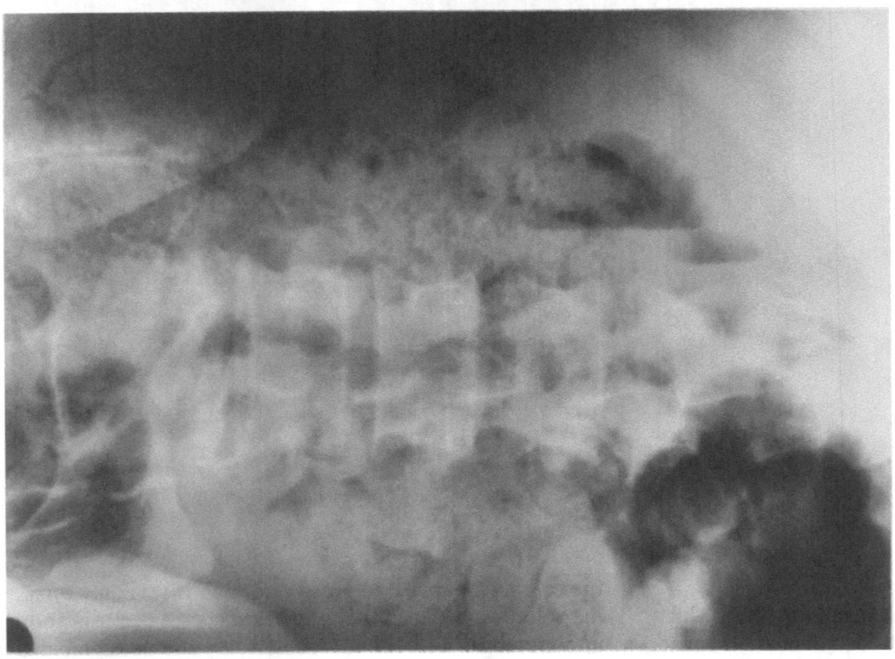
b

Fig. 77 a, b. Intramural or intravascular gas simulated by inspissated feces intermixed with gas. The *supine film* (**a**) and *left lateral film* (**b**) show soft-tissue densities intermixed with small gas collections projected over the colon. This pattern represents inspissated feces with gas bubbles and has no pathologic significance

Computed Tomography

CT is superior to plain radiography in differentiating intramural from intraluminal gas (Figs. 75 d, f, 76 e). Even the scout-scan (longitudinal scan) is diagnostic in many patients (Fig. 75 c). Gas in the mesenteric and portal veins is very clearly demonstrated with CT (Fig. 79 d).

Gas in the Mesenteric and Portal Veins

Causes

Same as for intramural gas. Intramural gas can enter the portal vein through the mesenteric veins.

Radiologic Signs

Plain Radiographs

Plain films show multiple tubular gas collections in the portal vein and its side branches (Figs. 78, 79). Unlike gas in the bile ducts, portal gas forms a ramifying pattern that radiates towards the periphery of the liver owing to the centrifugal flow of portal venous blood. It is appreciated most clearly on the L LAT film. Gas in the mesenteric veins is difficult to recognize. It is characterized by a fingerlike pattern of tubular gas collections in the mesentery which unite at the portal vein.

Sonography

Mesenteric and portal venous gas appears as canalicular, gas filled structures in the periportal field with acoustic shadowing and reverberations. It is difficult to distinguish from gas in the bile ducts (flow phenomena).

Computed Tomography

Canalicular structures having the density of air can be clearly identified and anatomically localized (Fig. 79 d).

a
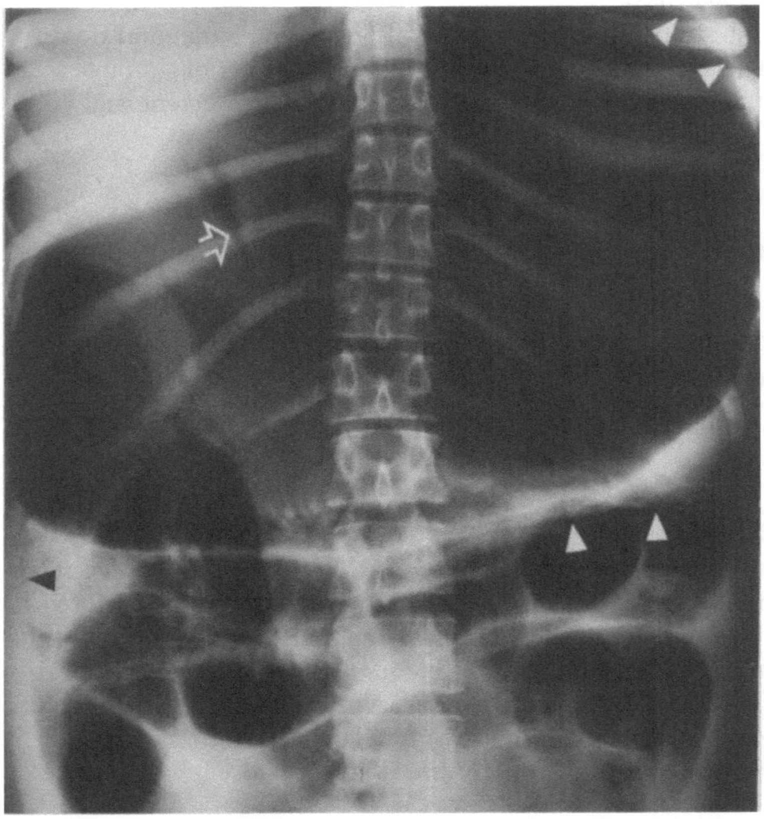

b
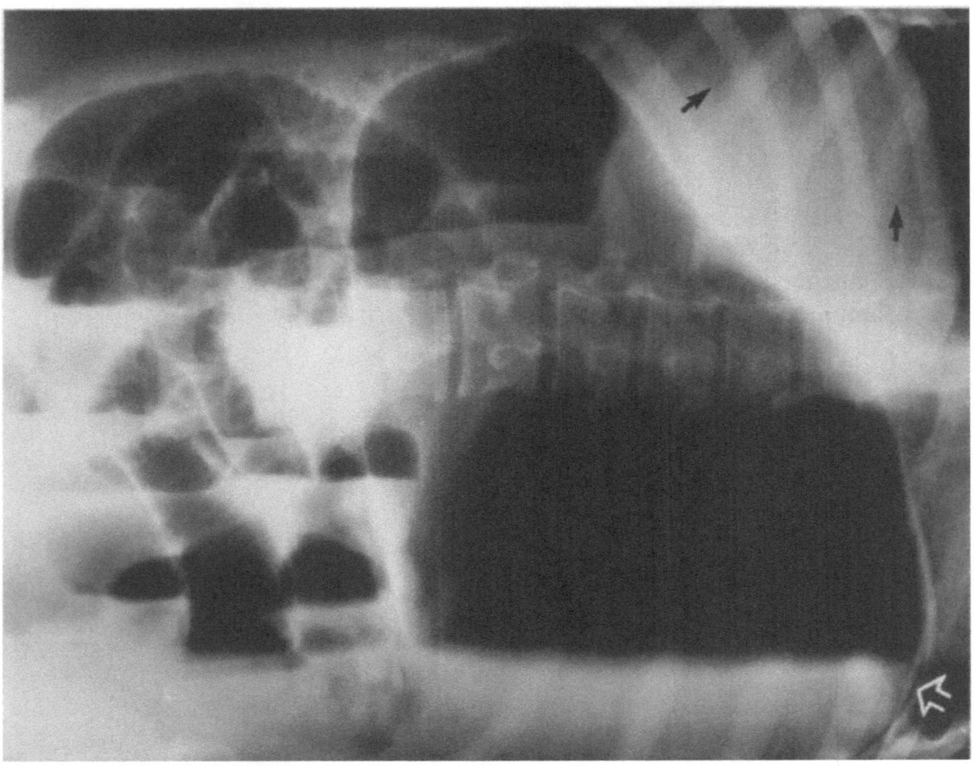

Fig. 78 a, b (Legend see page 135)

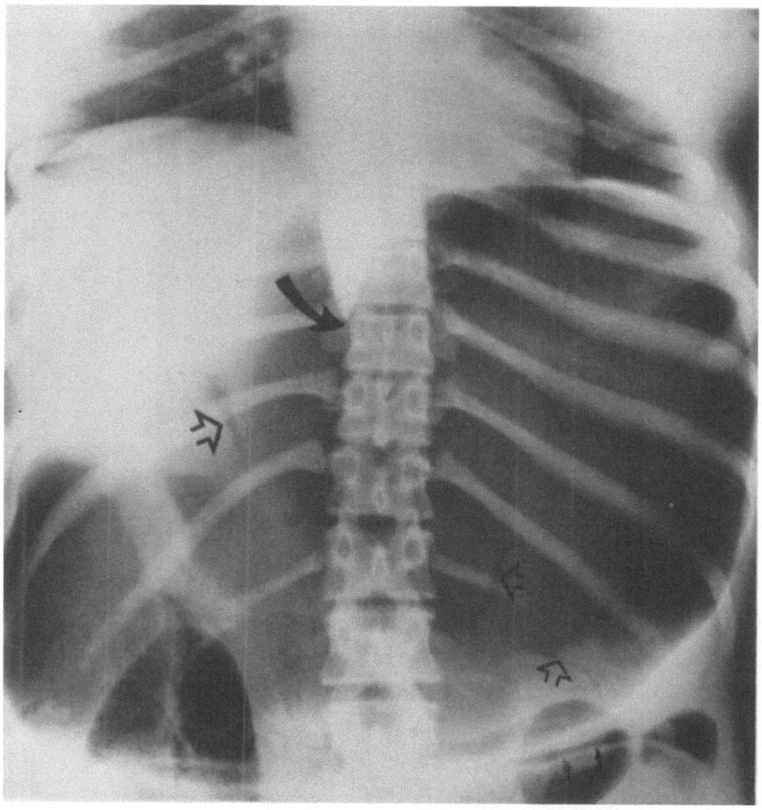

c

Fig. 78a–e. Intramural gas and portal venous gas in intestinal gangrene. **a–c** Intestinal gangrene caused by mesenteric arterial and venous thrombosis associated with an old strangulated obstruction. Girl, 13 years old, with a virtually complete cauda equina lesion below L2 resulting from a congenital, operatively treated lumbosacral myelomeningocele. A colon conduit was constructed 1 year earlier for neurogenic bladder dysfunction and left hydronephrosis. Over a 3-day period the patient developed increasing abdominal distension and marked abdominal rigidity. *Clinical examination* showed meteoritic abdominal distension and aperistalsis; tenderness was elicited only by deep palpation. Leukocyte count was 30000. **a** *Supine film* shows grotesque gastric dilatation, distension of the entire small bowel, intramural gas in the stomach and small bowel (▶) and intravascular gas in the mesenteric veins and portal vein (⇒). **b** *Left lateral film* shows absence of free air, massive dilatation of the stomach, duodenum, and small bowel, and intramural (⇒), intravascular, and intraportal gas (⟶). **c** *Abdominal survey after Gastrografin swallow.* A nasogastric tube could not be inserted. Obstruction proximal to the cardia is evident in the Gastrografin-filled esophagus (⤻); there is no entry of contrast material into the stomach. The stomach exhibits intramural gas (➧), and gas fills the mesenteric and gastric veins (⇒); portal venous gas is also noted (⇒). Operation (exploratory laparotomy) revealed diffuse peritonitis associated with an old, strangulated, small bowel obstruction caused by an adhesive band in the terminal ileum; there was total necrosis of the stomach, duodenum, and small bowel down to the ileocecal valve; the colon appeared normal. The mesenteric arteries and veins were thrombosed. Autopsy disclosed hemorrhagic gangrene of the stomach, duodenum, and small bowel; gas in the stomach and bowel walls; blood-stained gastrointestinal contents; blood-stained ascites; thrombosis of the mesenteric arteries and veins; bilateral pleural effusion; and hepatic edema with foci of necrosis.

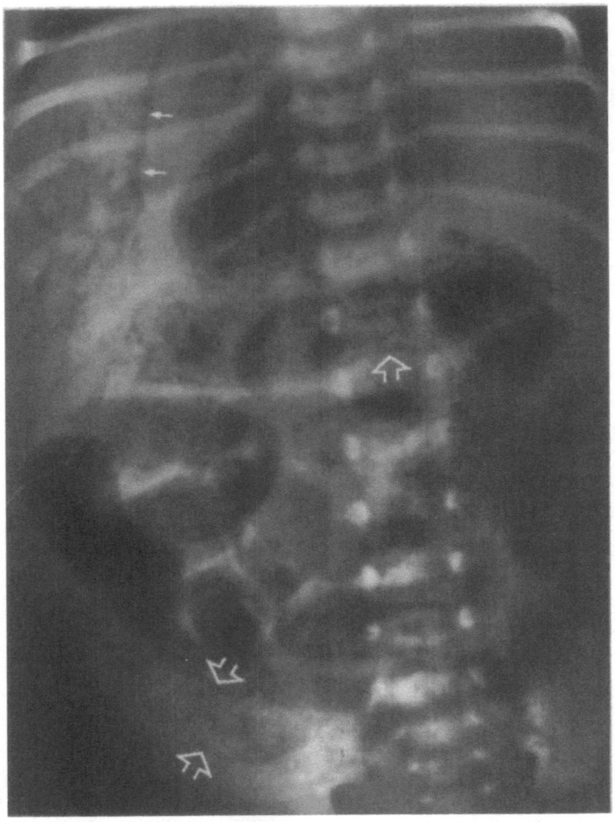

d

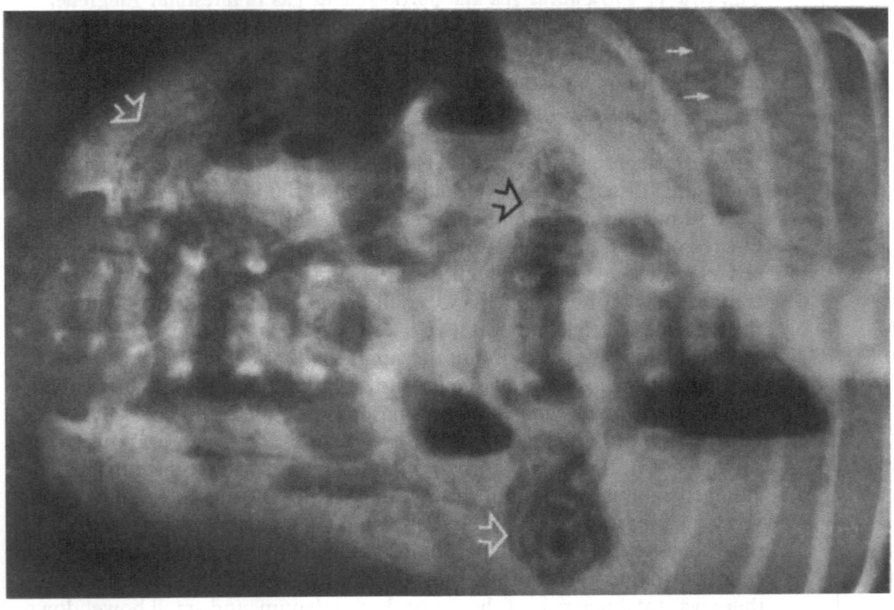

e

Fig. 78 (continued)
d, e Necrotizing enterocolitis in a male infant with Down's syndrome, birthweight 2300 g, body length 46 cm, Apgar score 9. On day 10 the infant was referred to the pediatric unit for failure to thrive and recurrent, copious vomiting after feeding. Two days after admission there was a sudden, severe deterioration of the infant's condition with abdominal distension, absent bowel sounds, watery, blood-tinged feces, and coffee-ground vomitus. **d** *Supine film* shows combined small- and large-bowel distension and double contouring of the transverse colon wall with string-of-beads gas collections (⇒). Massive amounts of gas in the portal vein branches can be traced to the periphery (→). **e** *Left lateral film* findings are the same as in the supine film. Additionally there is double contouring of the ascending colon with intramural, string-of-beads gas collections (⇒). There is massive gas accumulation in the intrahepatic portal vein branches (→). *Diagnosis:* necrotizing enterocolitis

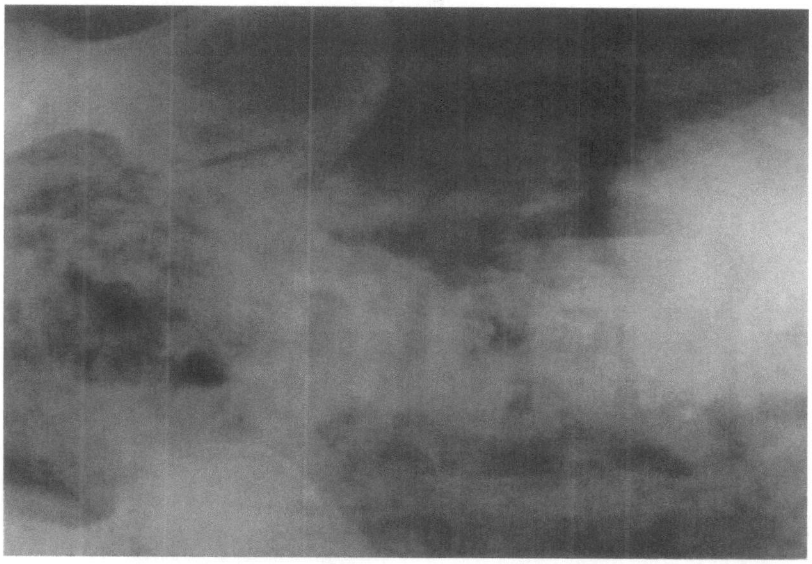

a

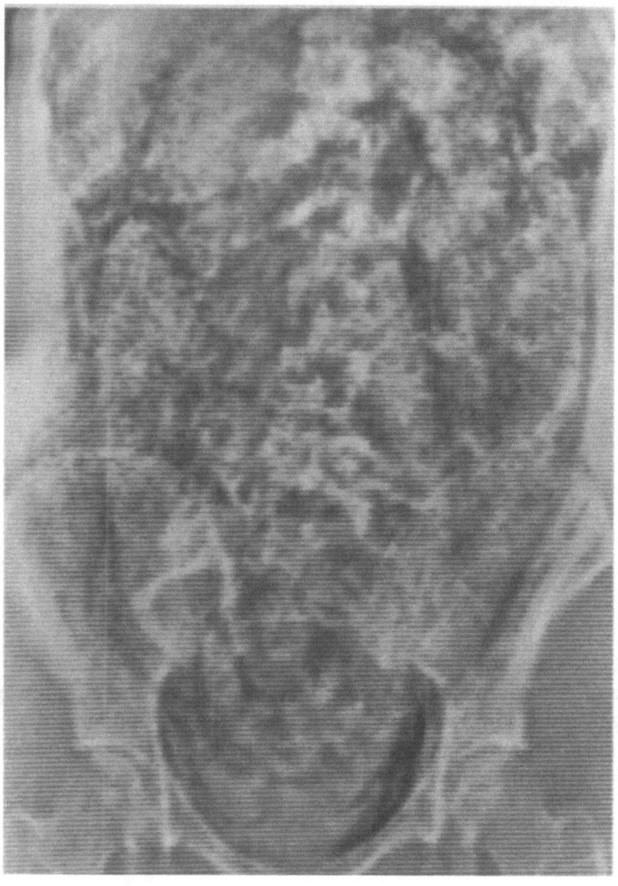

b

Fig. 79 a–d. Intra- and retroperitoneal, intramural, and intravascular gas collections in gas gangrene. The 38-year-old woman had an IUD-related endometritis and adnexitis with a mixed infection by gas-forming bacteria. She had undergone a Billroth II gastric resection 3 weeks earlier and experienced sudden lower abdominal pain 5 days after discharge. She was admitted with a presumptive diagnosis of adnexitis. The IUD, in place for about a year, was removed by a gynecologist. The gynecologic diagnosis was endometritis. When shock symptoms became more severe, the patient was taken to intensive care. She was comatose with a boardlike abdomen, aperistalsis, leukocyte count 1000, temperature 35.5 °C, Quick value 13%, PTT >2 min. **a** *Left lateral film* shows a massive gas collection projected over the entire abdomen. It is uncertain whether the collection is intraluminal or free, or whether it is intra- or extraperitoneal. **b** *CT scan scout-view* shows a massive gas collection in the peritoneal space and lesser pelvis.

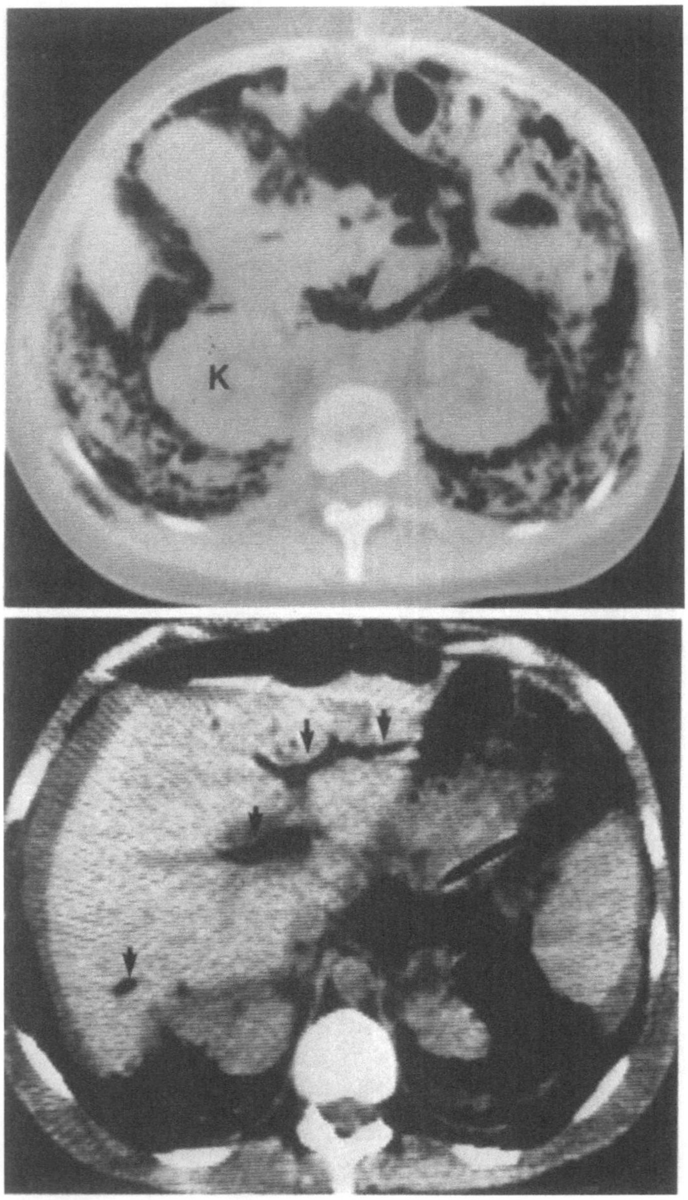

c

d

Fig. 79 (continued)
c *CT scan* at the level of the kidneys *(K)* shows intra- and retroperitoneal gas, intramural gas in the bowel wall, and gas in the mesentery and mesenteric vessels. **d** *CT scan* at the level of the liver shows ascites, free intra- and retroperitoneal air, and portal venous gas (→). The patient died in shock

Gas in the Gallbladder

Causes

- Perforation of the gallbladder into the bowel (gallstone, inflammation, tumor, trauma), usually accompanied by air in the bile ducts
- Emphysematous cholecystitis (gas in the lumen or wall), possibly accompanied by air in the bile ducts
- After surgery or papillotomy

Radiologic Signs

Plain Radiographs

Films in both planes show gas in the lumen and/or wall of the enlarged gallbladder. With a patent cystic duct, there will also be air in the bile ducts (Figs. 80a, 114a, b).

Sonography

Sonograms show a wide echo front in the gallbladder position with acoustic shadowing and reverberations. A string-of-beads pattern is characteristic of intramural gas.

Computed Tomography

CT clearly demonstrates the intramural or intracavitary gas collection and enables its assignment to the gallbladder.

Gas in the Bile Ducts

Causes

Communication between the biliary system and gastrointestinal tract

- Postoperatively after choledochoduodenostomy, choledochojejunostomy, cholecystoenterostomy
- After endoscopic or operative papillotomy
- Air injected during endoscoping retrograde cholangiography
- Gallstone perforation into the bowel (gallstone ileus?)
- Perforation of a hepatic flexure carcinoma into the gallbladder
- Trauma
- Emphysematous cholecystitis
- Bronchobiliary fistula after thoracic infection (rare)
- Ascending gas-forming cholangitis (rare)

Radiologic Signs

Plain Radiographs

Plain films usually show central, linear gas collections located in the porta hepatis, with gas also filling some bile duct branches, especially on the L LAT film. Owing to the centripetal flow of bile, gas does not collect in the periphery of the liver (permits differentiation from portal venous gas) (Fig. 80a).

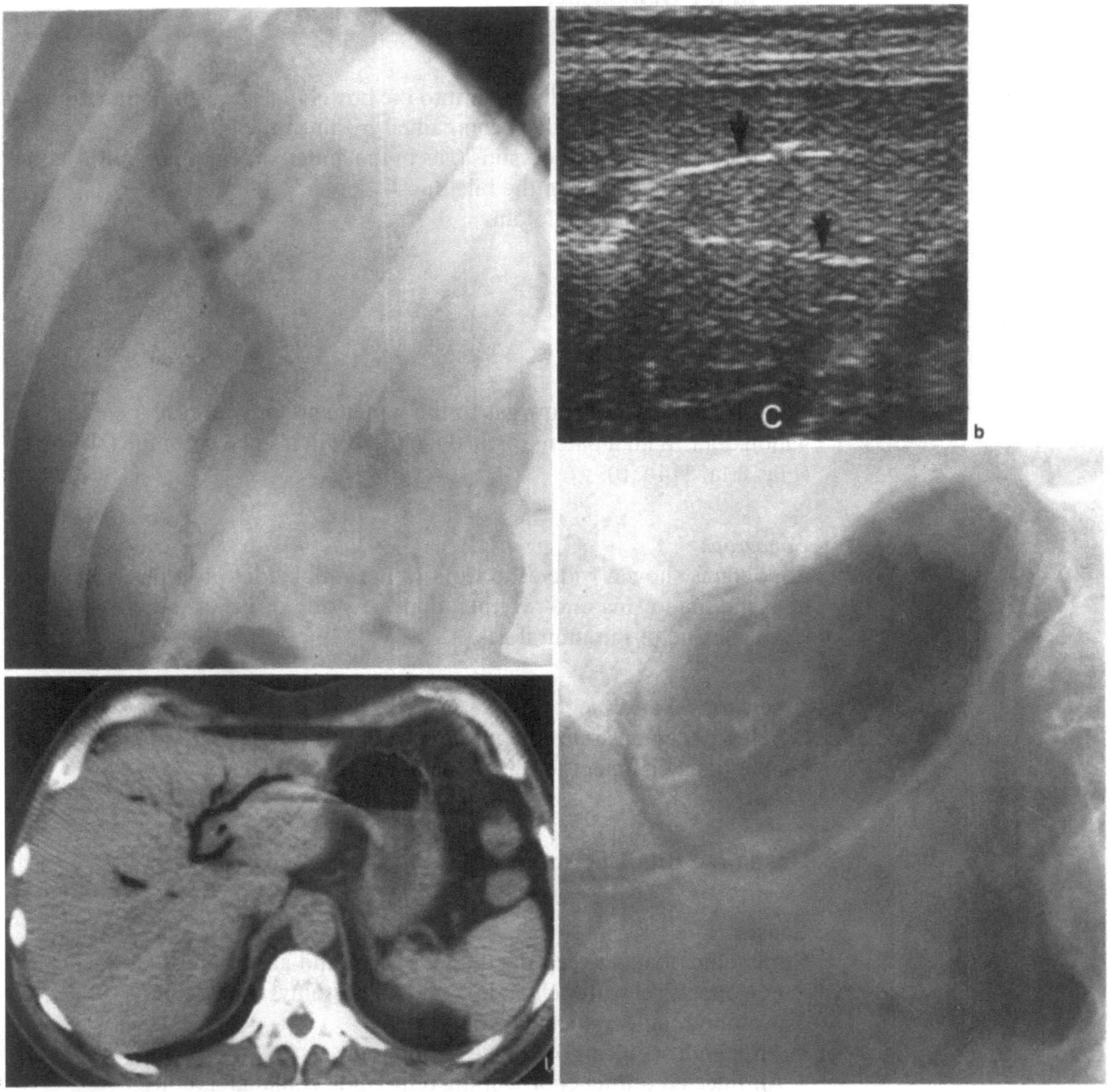

a b c d

Fig. 80 a–d. Gas in the bile ducts and gallbladder.
a *Supine film* following a biliary-enteric anastomosis demonstrates gas filling the central portions of the biliary system. **b** *Sonogram* transverse scan through the left hepatic lobe anterior to the inferior vena cava *(C);* the air-filled bile ducts appear as echogenic cords (→) with faint posterior acoustic shadowing. **c** *CT scan* clearly demonstrates the gas-filled bile ducts; note that the gas does not extend into the periphery. **d** Gas in the gallbladder wall and lumen in a 72-year-old woman with poorly controlled diabetes, fever, and tenderness in the right upper quadrant of the abdomen. *Supine film* shows a linear gas collection in the gallbladder wall and lumen associated with emphysematous cholecystitis

Sonography
Sonograms show canalicular, gas-filled structures in the periportal field with acoustic shadowing and reverberations and a normal appearance of the peripheral portal branches (Fig. 80b)

Computed Tomography
Scans show canalicular, air-dense structures in the periportal field and gas in the common bile duct (Figs. 80c, 114c).

Gas in the Renal Pelvis and Ureter

Causes
Usually the collection is iatrogenic following retrograde pyelography or surgery. Gas-forming pyelonephritis is an infrequent cause.

Radiologic Signs

Plain Radiographs
Plain films show a gaseous "cast" of the renal pelvis or ureter, or gas bubbles projected over these structures. When gas bubbles are seen, differentiation must be made between peri- and pararenal gas collections.

Sonography
Sonograms show gas in the renal pelvis with acoustic shadowing and reverberations. Gas in the ureter is not visualized with sonography (see Fig. 71).

Computed Tomography
CT clearly demonstrates gas collections in the renal pelvis and ureter, which are distinguishable at once from peri- or pararenal collections. CT is the best method for the detection and anatomic localization of the gas.

Gas in the Urinary Bladder

Causes
- Usually iatrogenic following cystoscopy or bladder catheterization
- Fistula formation between bladder and bowel in Crohn's disease, diverticulitis, postradiation, and from a bowel tumor invading the bladder
- Emphysematous cystitis (rarely in diabetic females) (Fig. 81)

Radiologic Signs

Plain Radiographs
Plain films in emphysematous cystitis show intramural gas bubbles with a polypoid configuration. The gas bubbles are immobile. Intravesical gas creates air-fluid levels on the L LAT film → urography.

Sonography
Usually sonograms show a gas collection of unknown cause in the position of the bladder with acoustic shadowing and reverberations.

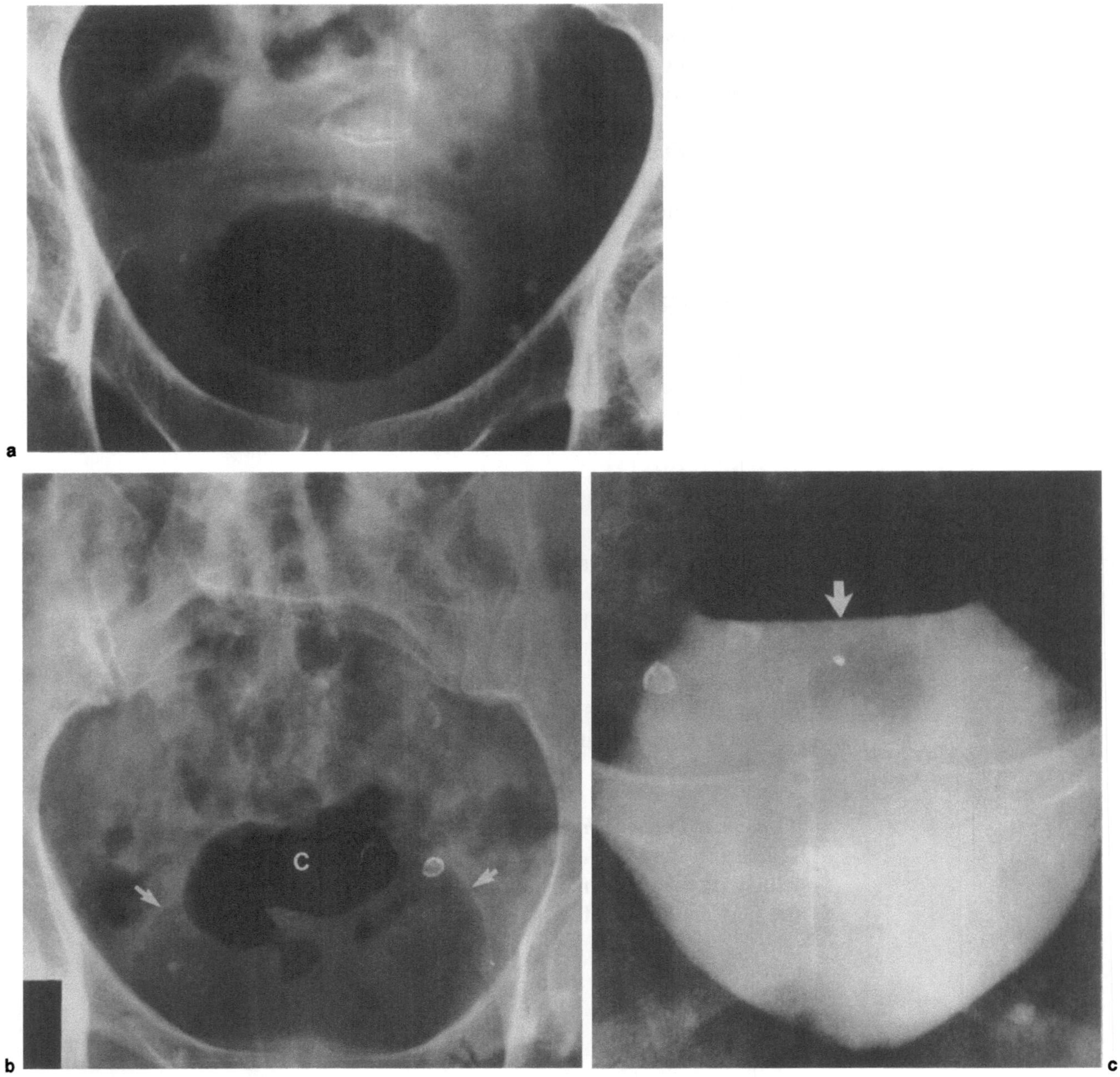

Fig. 81 a–c. Emphysematous cystitis. Woman, 89 years old, with insulin-dependent diabetes and clinical signs of cystitis. **a** *Urogram* (detail) shows a gas-filled urinary bladder without prior manipulation. There is also evidence of intramural gas. **b, c Acute perforation of sigmoid diverticulitis into the bladder.** Woman, 68 years old, with history of left lower quadrant tenderness for several months, suddenly noticed passage of air during micturition. **b** *Supine film* (detail) shows a gas-filled urinary bladder (↙) and partial gas filling of the rectosigmoid *(c)*. **c** *Urogram* (detail, erect) shows a depressed bladder floor, an air-fluid level between the contrast-opacified urine and gas (←), and no retrograde filling of the perforation

Computed Tomography

CT clearly demonstrates gas in the wall or lumen of the urinary bladder. It reliably establishes the location of the gas as intramural, intracavitary, or paravesical.

References

Beyer D, Köster R (1984) Bildgebende Diagnostik akuter intestinaler Durchblutungsstörungen. Ein klinisch-radiologisches Konzept. Springer, Berlin Heidelberg New York

Gruenberg JC, Grodsinsky C, Ponka JL (1979) Pneumatosis intestinalis: a clinical classification. Dis Colon Rectum 22: 5

Kelvin FM, Korobkin M, Rauch FR, Price RP, Silverman PM (1984) Computed tomography of pneumatosis intestinalis. J Comput Assist Tomogr 8: 276-280

Meyer MA, Ghahremani GG, Clements JL jr, et al. (1977) Pneumatosis intestinalis. Gastrointest Radiol 2: 91

Nelson SW (1972) Extraluminal gas collections due to diseases of the gastrointestinal tract. AJR 115: 225

Radin DR, Rosen RS, Halls JM (1987) Acute gastric dilatation: a rare cause of portal venous gas. AJR 148: 279-280

Rice RP (1980) Extraluminal gas in the abdomen. Diagnosis and implications. Pract Gastroenterol 4: 53

Rice RP, Thompson WM, Gedgaudas RK (1982) The diagnosis and significance of extraluminal gas in the abdomen. Radiol Clin North Am 20/4: 819

3.6 Intra-abdominal Masses

G. P. KRESTIN, D. BEYER

Causes

Note: An abdominal mass may be important or irrelevant for the etiology and pathogenesis of an acute abdomen, i.e., it may represent an incidental finding!

Masses that have major relevance in the acute abdomen

Benign masses:

- Abscesses
- Hematomas
- Lymphocele
- Urinoma
- Biloma
- Encrusted ascites
- Isolated fluid-filled bowel loops in volvulus
- Intussusception
- Benign intramural tumors and enterogenic cysts of the gastrointestinal tract
- Inflammatory tumors in Crohn's disease
- Gallbladder hydrops
- Pancreatic pseudocyst
- Overdistended urinary bladder (Fig. 82)

Malignant masses:

- Carcinoma of the stomach
- Carcinoma of the colon
- Carcinoma of the small intestine (rare)
- Retroperitoneal lymphomas

Masses that have limited relevance for the acute abdomen

Benign masses:

- Hepatomegaly
- Splenomegaly
- Cysts (ovarian, mesenteric)
- Uterine myomas
- Cystic kidneys
- Adrenal adenoma
- Retroperitoneal fibrosis (Ormond's disease)

Malignant masses:

- Primary hepatic tumors and metastases
- Splenomegaly in malignant lymphoma
- Hypernephroma
- Adrenal carcinoma
- Pancreatic tumors
- Ovarian carcinoma
- Bladder carcinoma
- Peritoneal carcinomatosis (with ascites)
- Intra-abdominal metastases

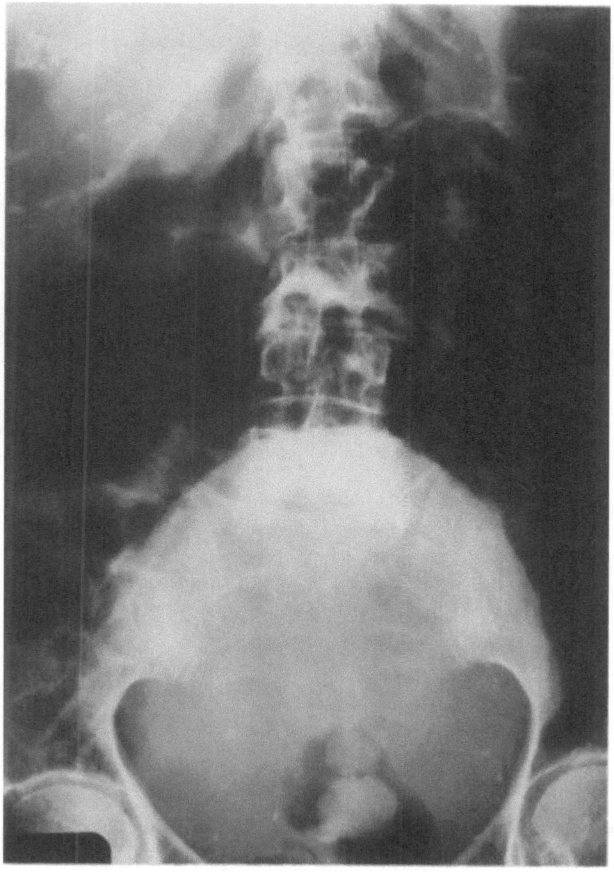

Fig. 82. Overflow incontinence secondary to prostatic hypertrophy. Man, 78 years old, with increasing pain in the lower abdomen and hypoperistalsis. *Supine film* shows a large, rounded soft-tissue mass in the lesser pelvis displacing small-bowel loops. The mass represents the overdistended urinary bladder (sonography)

Masses that have no relevance for the acute abdomen
- Riedel's lobe of the liver (Fig. 83)
- Large accessory spleen
- Renal dystopia, horseshoe kidney

Radiologic Signs

Plain Radiographs

Note: Masses are characterized on plain films by the displacement of organs, the obliteration of normally visible organ contours, and changes of the borders of gas-containing organs. Only displacement of normally visible organs and their most frequent causes have to be considered. Nonvisualization does not exclude a space-occupying lesion.

a
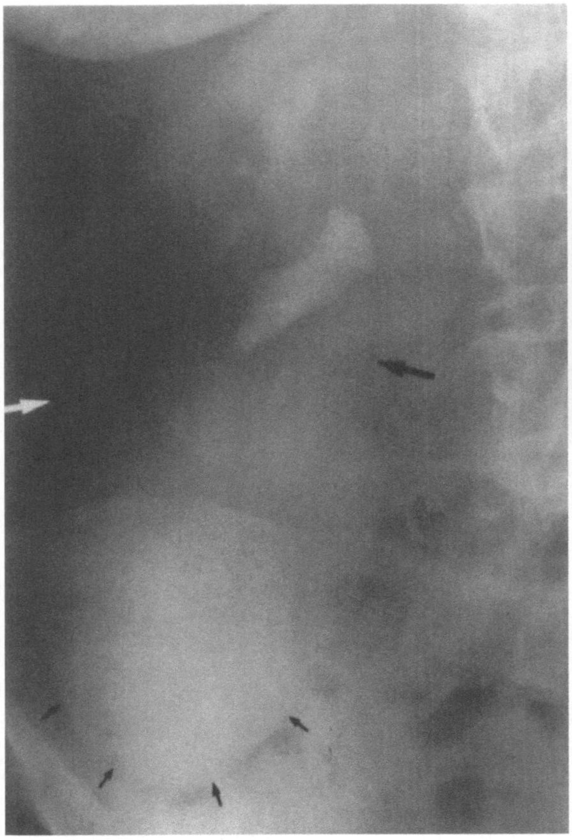

b
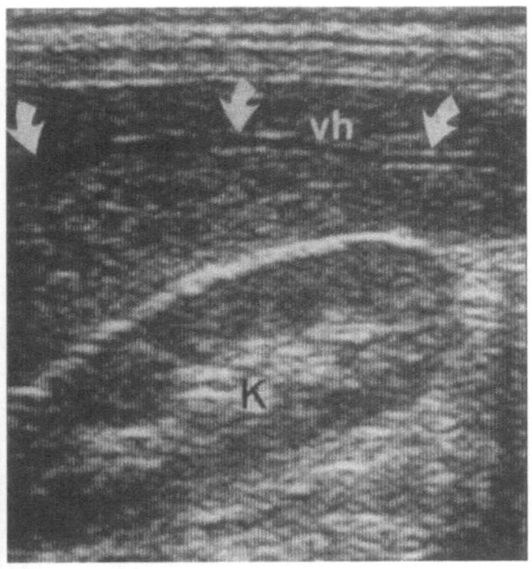

Fig. 83a, b. Riedel lobe of the liver. Woman, 75 years old, with acute epigastric pain. **a** *Supine radiograph* (urogram) shows an elongated mass with sharp margins in the right midabdomen which is oriented craniocaudally and is not easily distinguished from the liver (→). **b** *Sonogram* shows a Riedel lobe anterior to the right kidney *(K)* (*vh,* hepatic vein ➧)

a
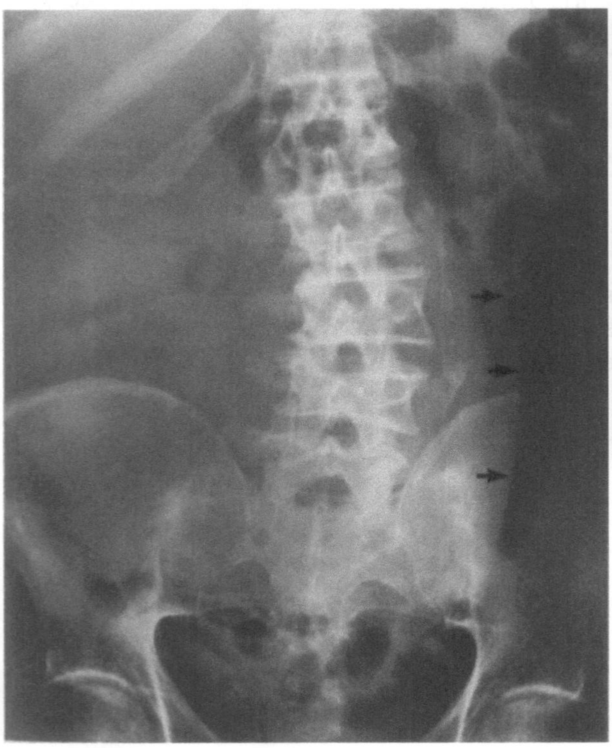

b
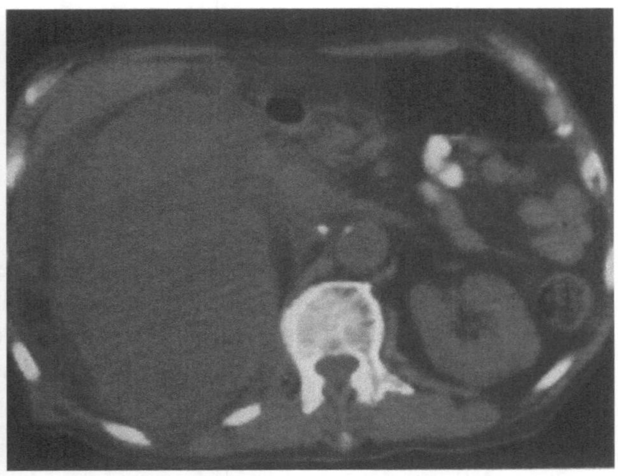

Fig. 84a, b. Pyonephrosis. Man, 76 years old, with known bladder carcinoma presented with severe right flank pain radiating to the lesser pelvis and fever. **a** *Supine film* shows a large soft-tissue mass in the right midabdomen markedly displacing the entire colon (→) to the left. The right psoas shadow is obscured. **b** *CT scan* shows a massive liquid mass on the right side caused by hydronephrosis secondary to bladder carcinoma (not presented here). *Diagnosis:* bladder carcinoma, silent right kidney with pyonephrosis

Displacements of Radiopaque or Gas-Containing Organs

Pathologic changes of position and axial alignment

- Displacement of the stomach by:
  - Splenomegaly
  - Tumor (Fig. 86)
  - Abscess (subhepatic, lesser sac, subphrenic) (see Fig. 7)

- Displacement of the colon by:
  - Perityphlitic abscess (see Figs. 130-133)
  - Diverticulitic abscess (Figs. 88, 146)
  - Tumor
  - Hepatomegaly and gallbladder hydrops (see Fig. 112)
  - Splenomegaly
  - Inflammatory mass (Fig. 87)
  - Large ovarian cysts

- Displacement of the small bowel by:
  - Midabdominal abscesses
  - Ovarian cysts or distended urinary bladder (Fig. 82)
  - Malignant tumors
  - Expansion of the duodenal C loop by pancreatitis or pancreatic tumor (see Sect. 4.1.2)
  - Lymphomas, inflammatory mass in Crohn's disease

- Displacement of the kidney by:
  - Retroperitoneal abscesses (see Fig. 145)
  - Retroperitoneal tumors
  - Retroperitoneal hematomas (see Fig. 201)
  - Retroperitoneal fibrosis
  - Lymphomas

Organ displacements that do not have pathologic significance: Chilaiditi's syndrome, malrotation, situs inversus, Riedel's lobe of the liver (Fig. 83), accessory spleen, duplex kidney, pelvic kidney, horseshoe kidney

Caution: Organ displacements without pathologic significance are the ones most likely to be misdiagnosed. Plain radiographs should be supplemented by sonograms.

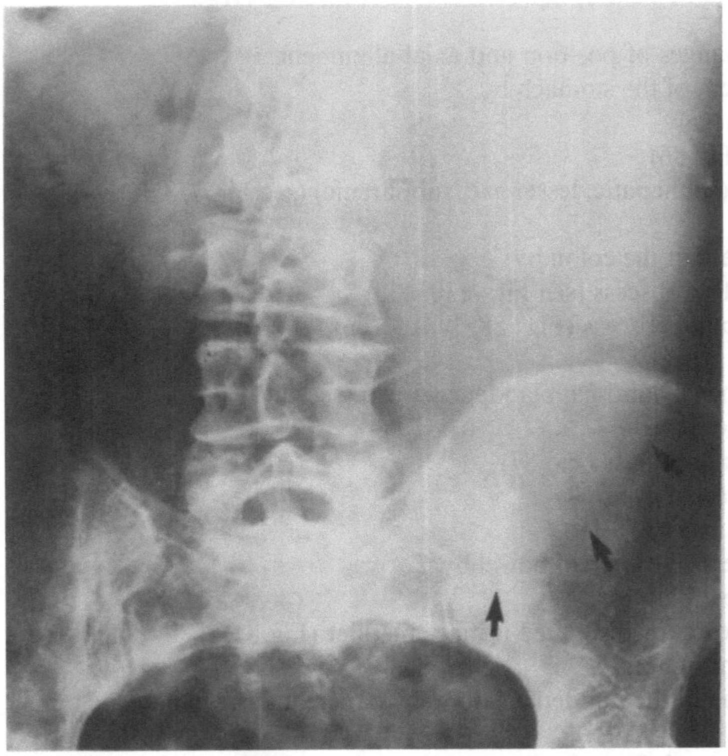

a

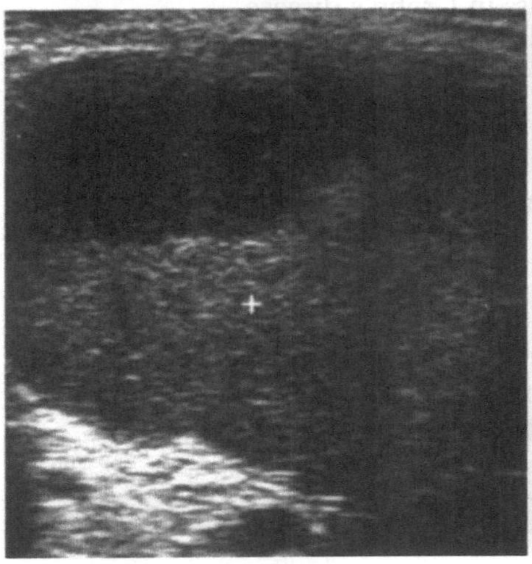

b

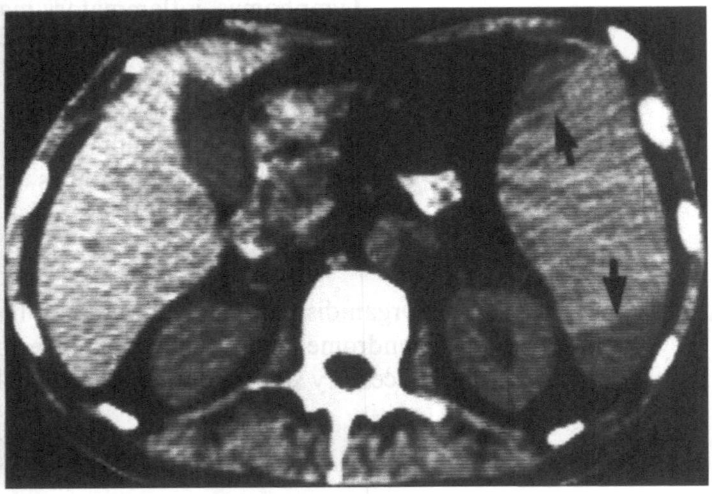

c

Fig. 85a-c. Multiple splenic infarctions associated with splenomegaly. Man, 48 years old, with known Waldenstrom's macroglobulinemia, presented with acute pain in the left upper quadrant. **a** *Supine film* shows a large mass with a sharp caudal margin (→), probably caused by splenomegaly. **b** *Sonogram* shows a large, rounded, hypoechoic, subcapsular mass in the spleen. Differentiation among infarction, nodular lymphomatous infiltration, metastasis, or abscess cannot be made. **c** *CT scan* demonstrates two, low-density, wedge-shaped foci (→) in the anterior and posterior portions of the spleen. Their shape identifies them as areas of splenic infarction

Loss of Normally Visible Contours

Inferior margin of the liver may be obscured by:
- Ascites, hemorrhage (see Figs. 39b, 209)
- Paracolic abscesses
- Subhepatic abscesses
- Tumors of the right colic flexure
- Gallbladder hydrops (see Fig. 112)
- Tumors of the lower right hepatic lobe (Fig. 83)

Inferior contour of the spleen may be obscured by:
- Ascites, hemorrhage
- Left paracolic abscesses
- Left subhepatic abscesses
- Tumors of the left colic flexure

Caution: Even with good image quality, the inferior margin of the liver and of the spleen are visible in only about 60% and 30%, respectively, of *normal* individuals.

Psoas contours may be obscured by:
- Paravertebral abscess
- Psoas abscess
- Lymphomas
- Renal tumor or hydronephrosis (Fig. 84)
- Retroperitoneal fibrosis
- Pancreatic abscess (see Fig. 64)
- Pancreatic tumor (see Fig. 63)
- Retroperitoneal hematoma, lymphocele, urinoma (see Figs. 46-48)

Note: The psoas contours may be obscured by any lesion of the *anterior* pararenal space, lesions intrinsic to the psoas muscle, or by infiltrative processes of the posterior pararenal space. The psoas contours are *not affected* by fluid collections in the *posterior* pararenal space.

The flank stripes may be obscured by:
- Abscesses (see Fig. 146)
- Hematomas (see Fig. 200)
- Perforations of retroperitoneal hollow viscera (rectal perforation (see Figs. 60, 61)

Note: The flank stripes are obscured *only* by lesions of the posterior pararenal space or by lesions infiltrating into the flanks.

Nonvisualization *of renal contours* may be caused by:
- Renal tumor
- Perirenal abscess or hematoma (see Figs. 145, 207 e)
- Polycystic kidneys (see Fig. 200 b)
- Duplex kidney
- Splenic impression (no pathologic significance) (Fig. 85 a)
- Fetal lobulation (no pathologic significance)

Note: Renal contour changes are usually demonstrable only in the "gasless" or "nearly gasless" abdomen. Urography or sonography is indicated.

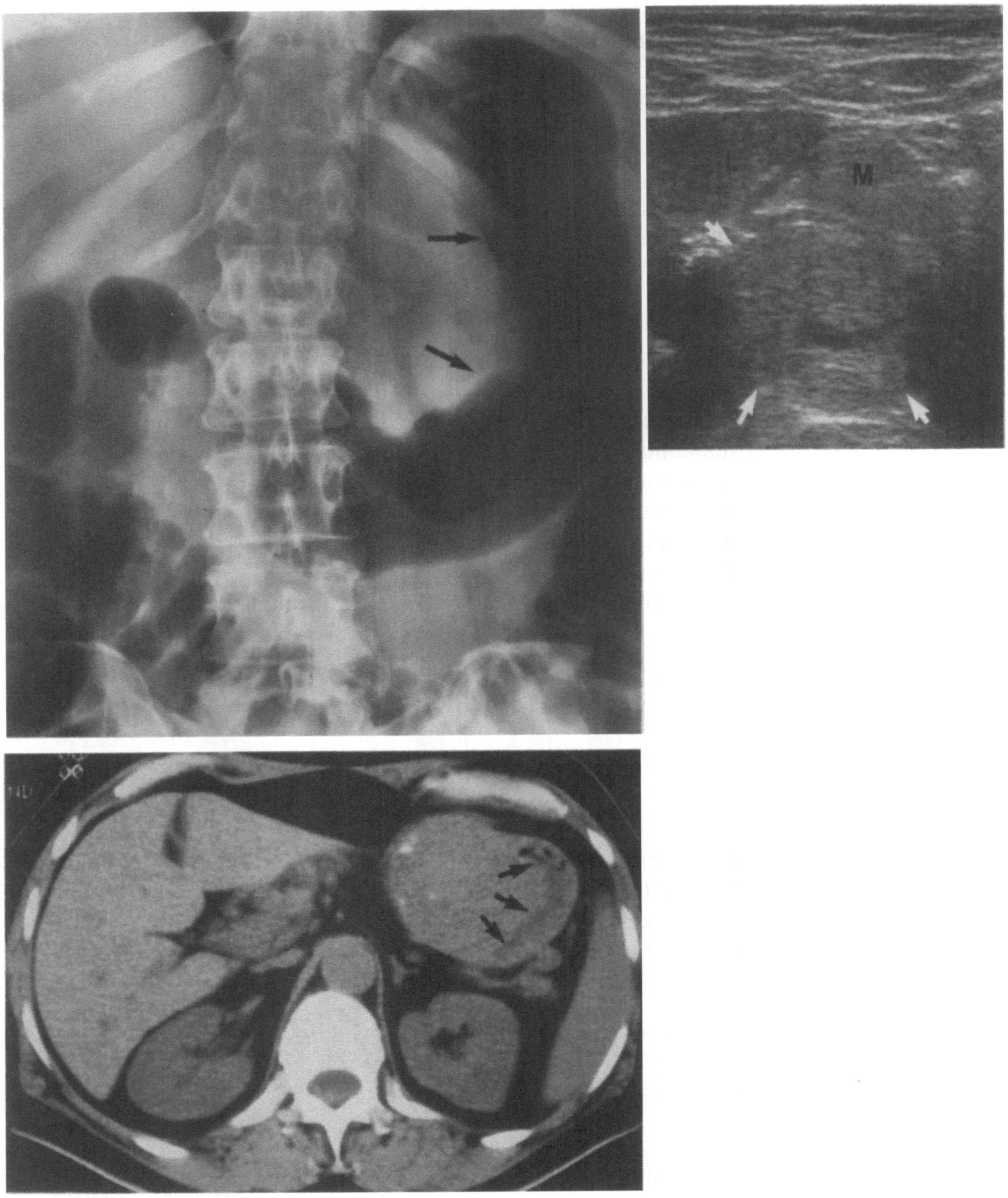

a b c

Fig. 86a–c. Gastric neurinoma. Man, 46 years old, with epigastric pain and vomiting, a nontender abdomen, and normal peristalsis. **a** *Supine film* shows a markedly gas-filled stomach with double contouring of the lesser curvature produced by an extragastric mass (→) displacing the stomach to the left. **b** *Sonogram* shows a retrogastric mass (→) with displacement of the normal gastric target pattern *(M)* (*L*, left lobe of liver). **c** *CT scan* discloses a soft-tissue density (→) in the gastric wall with small calcifications

Changes in the Contours of Hollow Viscera

Note: Circumscribed contour changes in gas-filled hollow viscera are indicative of disease.

Stomach:
- Intramural tumors (leiomyoma, lipoma, lymphoma) (Fig. 86)
- Gastric carcinoma (see Fig. 100a)
- Absceses (omental bursa) (see Fig. 7)
- Pancreatic tumor
- Costal impression (no pathologic significance)

Small bowel:
- Overdistended bladder (see Fig. 82)
- Intussusception (see Figs. 157, 247)
- Tumors (intramural, adjacent organs)
- Lymphomas
- Crohn's disease

Large bowel (Fig. 89):
- Colon tumor (Fig. 87a)
- Abscess (Fig. 87b, c)
- Intussusception
- Crohn's disease
- Gallbladder impression (hydrops) (see Fig. 112c)
- Diverticulitis (Fig. 88, 146)

Caution: Contour changes are always suspicious for disease and should be investigated by sonography or appropriate contrast examination.

Note: The signs listed above are often of minor diagnostic importance in patients with acute abdomen. At the same time, a large mass should *not* be overlooked in the evaluation of these patients. It may become necessary to exclude a secondary disease. Further investigations should consist of sonography, CT, urography, and contrast studies of the GI tract if time permits.

Radiologic Signs

Sonography

- Sonography is markedly superior to plain radiography in the evaluation of masses.
- The following types of masses can be accurately diagnosed:
- Riedel's lobe, hepatomegaly (see Fig. 83)
- Accessory spleen, splenomegaly (see Fig. 85)
- Gallbladder hydrops (see Figs. 111, 112)
- Renal tumors (see Fig. 84)
- Polycystic kidneys (see Fig. 200a)
  Cysts (ovarian) (see Fig. 42c)
  - Fluid collections are readily distinguishable from solid masses.
  - Large masses are *always* demonstrable under suitable examining conditions.
  - Advanced malignant tumors of hollow viscera are identified by the presence of a "target" pattern.

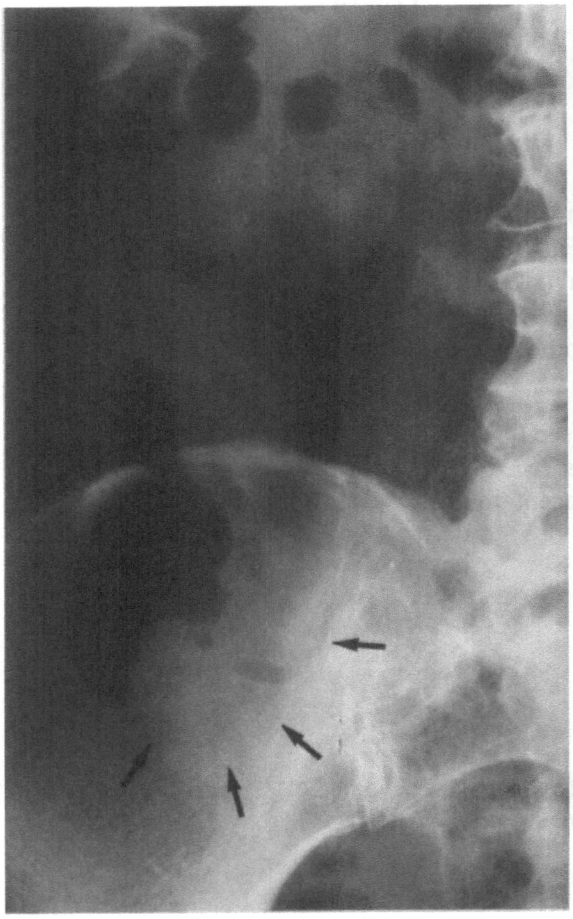
a

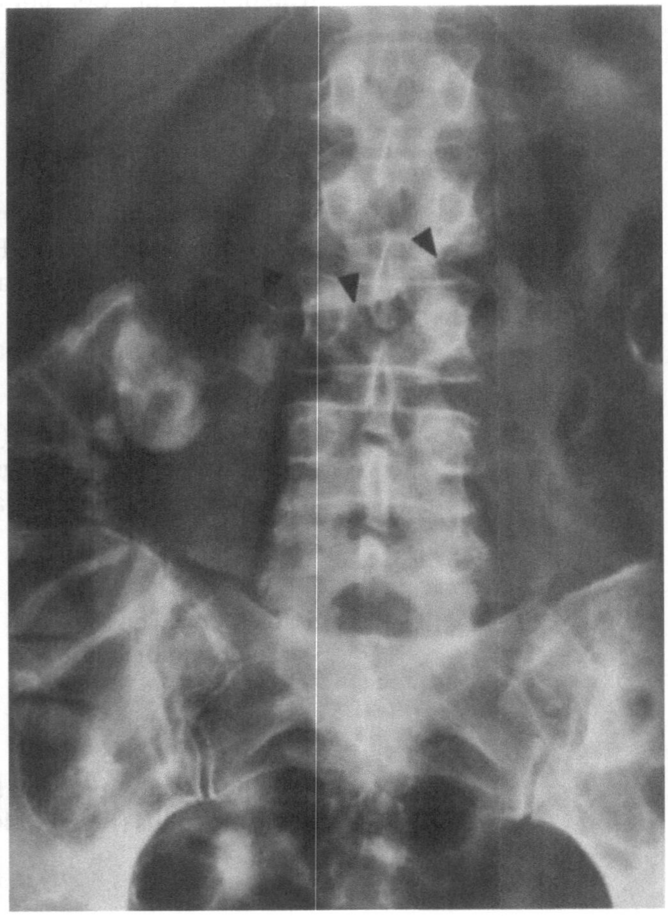
b

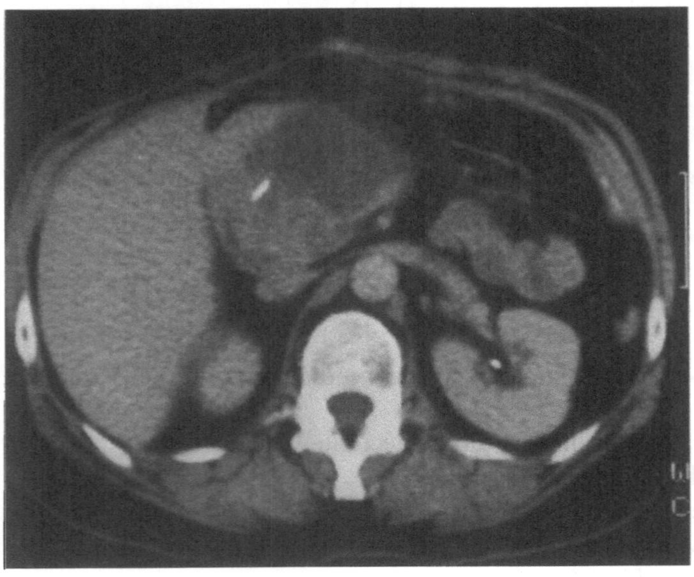
c

Fig. 87a–c. Cecal carcinoma. Man, 72 years old, with right lower quadrant pain and symptoms of partial intestinal obstruction. **a** *Supine film* shows a soft-tissue mass in the right lower quadrant indenting the air-filled cecal pole (→). **b Postoperative abscess in the head of the pancreas with secondary inflammatory involvement of the transverse colon.** Woman, 51 years old, who had undergone gastrectomy 10 years ago, presenting with fever. *Supine film* (24 h after oral water-soluble contrast) shows an (about 10 cm long) eccentric stenosis in the area of the transverse colon (▶). Sonograms (not shown) depicted a complex midabdominal mass that could not be accurately localized. **c** *CT scan* shows marked widening of the region of the pancreatic head, which presents unsharp boundaries and contains a central low-density area after contrast enhancement

Fig. 88a, b. Abscess in the left side of the lesser pelvis and fistula formation associated with Crohn's disease. Woman, 22 years old, with known Crohn's disease developed pain in the left lower quadrant and fever. **a** *Supine film* shows irregular contours of the air-filled large bowel at the junction of the sigmoid and descending colon (→), with a gasless rectum. A soft-tissue mass presents in the left portion of the lesser pelvis. **b** Enema by water-soluble contrast medium demonstrates sigmoid stenosis with a fistula. Small-bowel loops are displaced by a paracolic soft-tissue mass (→)

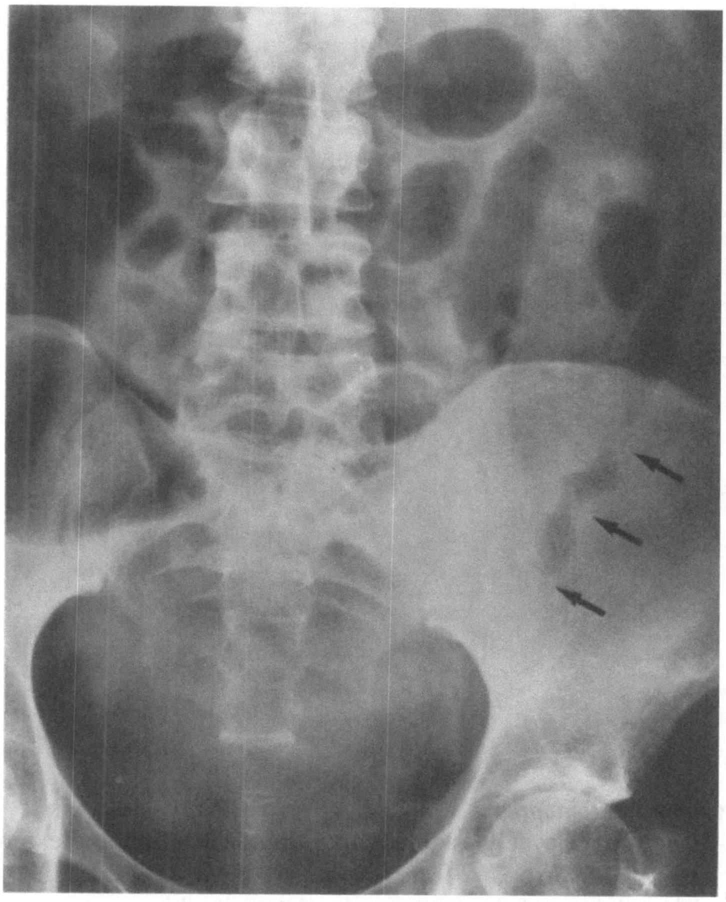

a

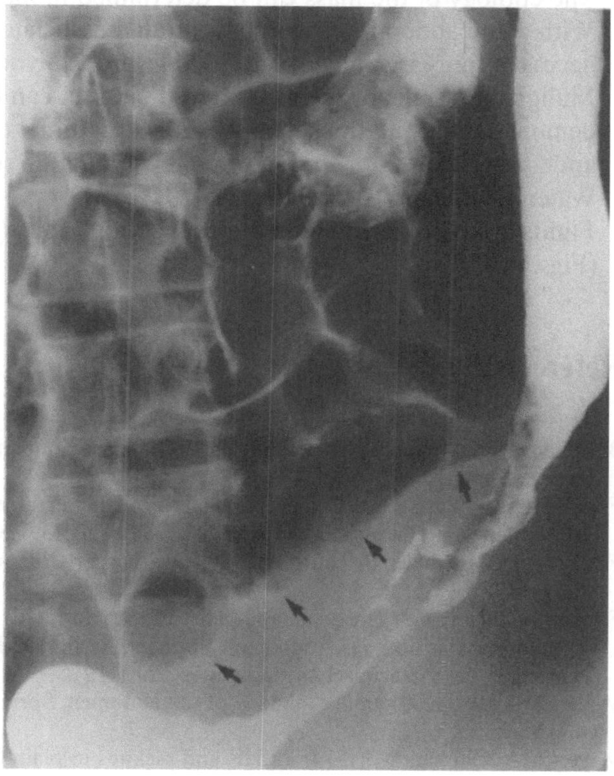

b

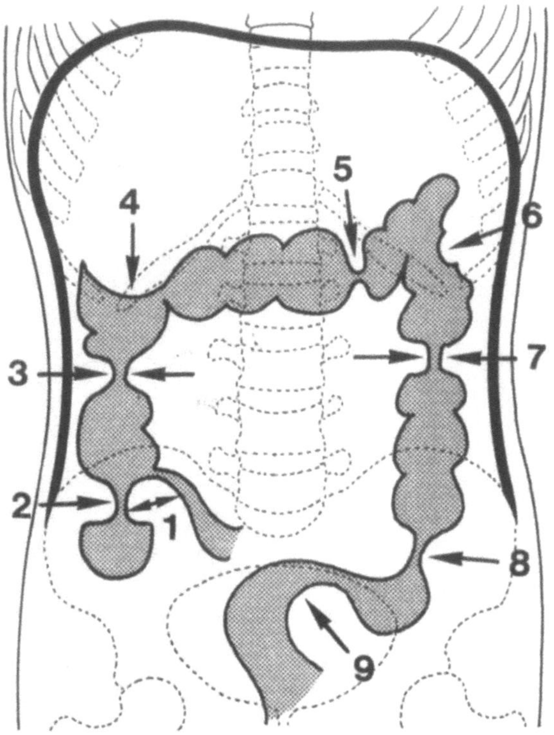

Fig. 89. Possible deformations and contour changes of the gas-filled large bowel caused by adjacent masses and lesions intrinsic to the colon. *1,* Crohn's disease, cecal tumor; *2,* perityphlitic abscess; *3,* carcinoma with abscess formation; *4,* gallbladder hydrops, gallbladder carcinoma, hepatomegaly; *5,* stenosis (inflammatory, neoplastic, vascular); *6,* splenomegaly, pancreatitis, pancreatic tumor; *7,* stenosis (inflammatory, neoplastic, vascular); *8,* diverticulitis, secondary tumor infiltration; *9,* cul-de-sac abscess, peritoneal carcinomatosis

Computed Tomography

- CT can accurately establish both the localization and extent of a mass lesion (Fig. 86c).
- The etiology of the mass can be determined in most cases (Fig. 84b).
- With acute abdominal symptoms and an associated mass, CT is necessary only if sonographic findings are equivocal.
- Malignant lesions of the gastrointestinal tract can be diagnosed only by demonstrating wall thickening or an extraluminal tumor extent after oral and/or rectal administration of contrast medium (e.g., Gastrografin = Water-soluble amidotrizoate).
- Fluids are easily differentiated from solid lesions (densitometry) (Figs. 84b, 85c).

References

Bücheler E, Friedmann G, Thelen M (1983) Real-time Sonographie des Körpers. Thieme, Stuttgart

Frick MP, Feinberg SB (1982) Deceptions in localizing extrahepatic right-upper-quadrant abdominal masses by CT. AJR 139: 501

Friedmann G, Bücheler E, Thurn P (1981) Ganzkörper Computertomographie. Thieme, Stuttgart

Frimann-Dahl J (1968) The acute abdomen. In: Strnad F (ed) Röntgendiagnostik des Digestionstraktes und des Abdomens. Springer, Berlin Heidelberg New York (Handbuch der medizinischen Radiologie, vol 11/2)

Meyers MA (1976) Dynamic radiology of the abdomen. Springer, Berlin Heidelberg New York

Meyers MA, Oliphant M (1974) Pitfalls and pickups in plain-film diagnosis of the abdomen. Current problems in radiology, vol 4/2. Year Book Medical, Chicago

Wolf BS, Khilnani MT, Lautkin A (1960) Diagnostic roentgenology of the digestive tract without contrast media. Grune & Stratton, New York

3.7 Calcifications

R. LORENZ, D. BEYER, U. MÖDDER

Prerequisites for the Evaluation of Abdominal Calcifications and Calcific Shadows

History: stone disease (kidney, gallbladder), gross hematuria, surgery, neoplasia (metastases), time spent in the tropics, calcifications known since previous examinations? Prior radiation therapy?
Inspection: scars, birthmarks, external foreign material
Palpation: resistance in surgical scars, tender gluteal area after i.m. injection, palpable mass (movable/fixed)
Laboratory values: hyperuricemia, hypercalcemia, hyperphosphatemia, cholestasis, microscopic hematuria

Classification of Calcifications

Localization:
- intra-abdominal
  - → intraperitoneal
    - → extraluminal
    - → intraluminal
  - → extraperitoneal
- extra-abdominal
  - → abdominal wall
  - → dorsal soft tissues
  - → skeleton

Topography
1. Wall calcification (vessel, duct system, hollow viscus, cyst) (Fig. 90 c)
2. Intraluminal calcification = calculus (hollow viscus, duct system, vessel) (Fig. 90 a)
3. Parenchymal or soft-tissue calcification (Fig. 90 b)

Morphology
1. Margins: distinct - indistinct
2. Definite geometric structure - amorphous
3. Rounded - polygonal
4. Linear - tubular - ringlike
5. Scattered or diffuse - follows course of preexisting structures
6. Structured (bone)
7. Not classifiable

Classification of Abdominal Calcifications in Adults

1. Right Upper Quadrant

Lesions That Are Common and Relevant to Diagnosis in Patients with Acute Abdomen

Gallstones (Fig. 90a, 91)
Only 10%-30% are calcified! Geometric structure or layering; facetting and motility are seen with multiple stones. Absence of motility may signify impaction in the cystic duct. Stones in hemochromatosis are extremely dense (iron-containing).

Stone(s) in the Common Bile Duct (Fig. 90a)
Only 2% are radiopaque! Most are solitary. Occur close to the vertebral column; transverse process may be superimposed.

Caution: Bile duct stones can simulate renal calculi or pancreatic calcifications.

Note: Bile duct stones are difficult to diagnose on abdominal plain films, and sonographic evidence is often indirect (dilated bile ducts without a mass in the hilus of the liver or head of the pancreas). The stone itself may be directly visible on the abdomen plain film or CT scan.
In doubtful cases: i.v. cholangiography

Renal Calculi (Figs. 90a, 197a)
Urolithiasis: stones in the renal collecting system including the ureter - solitary, multiple, pelvic stone, staghorn calculus (stony cast of the collecting system), caliceal stone. Most are radiopaque because they contain calcium. Uric acid stones, xanthine stones, and cystine stones are radiolucent!

Note: Calculi on the abdominal survey can be difficult to assign to the kidney, so oblique films or conventional tomograms are needed when sonograms do not confirm nephrolithiasis. Small calculi and especially ureteral stones are usually not demonstrated with ultrasound, and so urography is indicated.

Lesions That Are Uncommon but Relevant to Diagnosis in Patients with Acute Abdomen

Porcelain Gallbladder (Fig. 90e)
A sign of chronic cholecystitis, old empyema (differential diagnosis: calcified hepatic cyst)

Milk of Calcium Bile (Limy Bile) (Fig. 90e)
A sign of chronic cholecystitis (fluid level, change on repositioning)

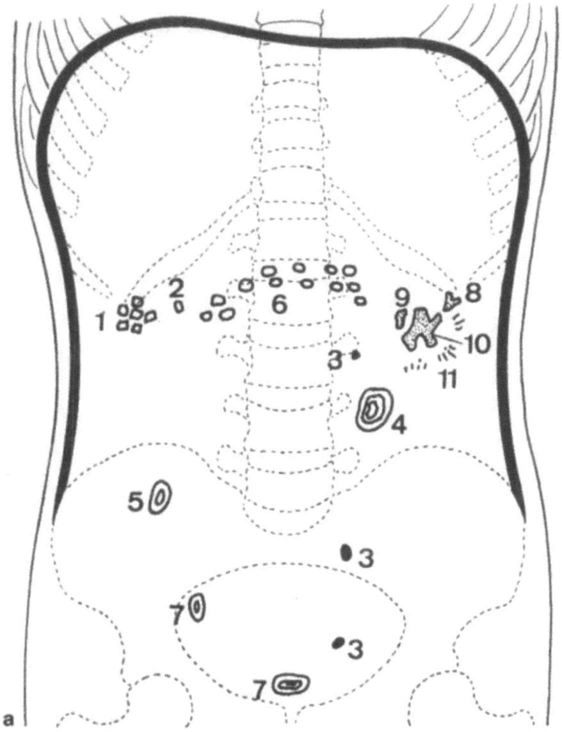

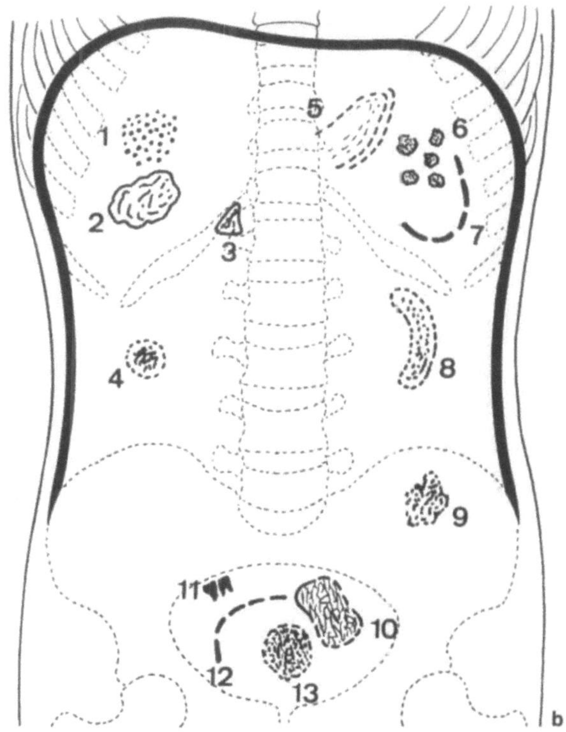

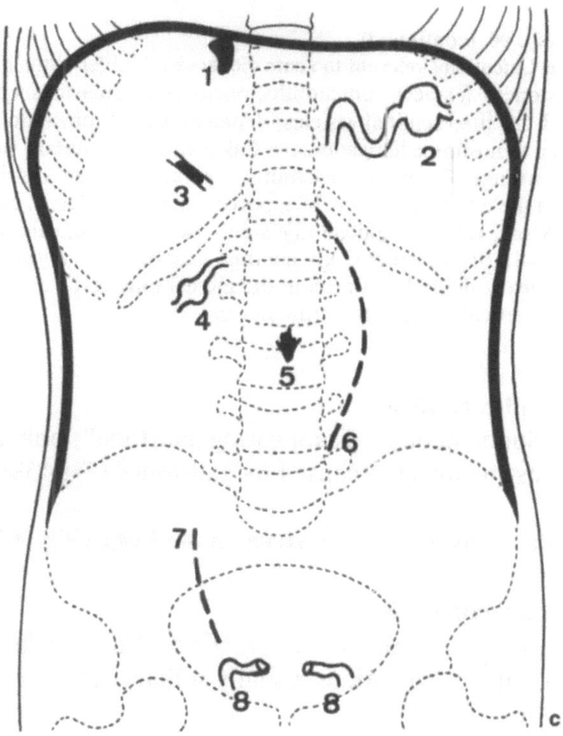

Fig. 90. a Calculi that are relevant to acute diagnosis: *1*, stones in the gallbladder; *2*, common duct stone; *3*, ureteral stone; *4*, enterolith; *5*, appendicolith; *6*, pancreatic calcification; *7*, bladder stone; *8*, calcifying papillary necrosis; *9*, caliceal stone; *10*, staghorn calculus; *11*, medullary sponge kidney with streaklike calcifications in the collecting ducts. **b Parenchymal calcifications relevant to acute diagnosis:** *1*, calcified hepatic metastasis; *2*, calcifying hepatic abscess; *3*, calcifying adrenal tumor (e.g., pheochromocytoma); *4*, hypernephroma; *5*, calcifying gastric carcinoma (mucinous adenocarcinoma); *6*, brucellosis of the spleen; *7*, perisplenitis calcarea after inflammation; *8*, nephrocalcinosis; *9*, calcifying colon carcinoma; *10*, calcifying ovarian carcinoma; *11*, teeth in a dermoid cyst; *12*, cystitis calcarea; *13*, rectal carcinoma. **c Vascular calcifications:** *1*, vena cava thrombus; *2*, splenic arterial aneurysm; *3*, portal venous thrombosis; *4*, renal arterial aneurysm; *5*, plaque in the aorta; *6*, abdominal aortic aneurysm; *7*, ureteritis calcarea; *8*, calcified vas deferens in chronic renal failure (not relevant to acute diagnosis).

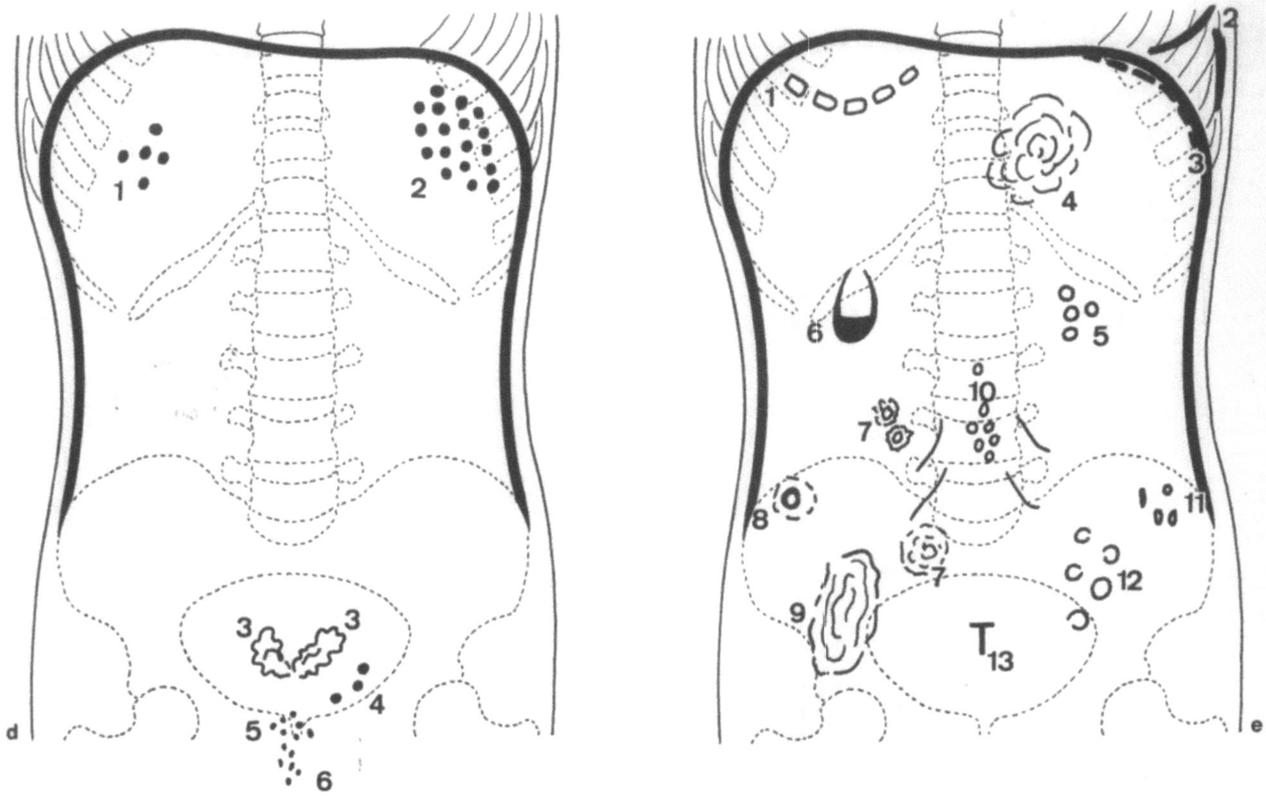

Fig. 90 (continued)
d Calculi not relevant to acute diagnosis: *1,* phleboliths in the liver, intrahepatic bile duct stones; *2,* spleen: phleboliths, previous toxoplasmosis or tuberculosis (both inactive); *3,* calcified seminal vesicles; *4,* phleboliths; *5,* prostatic calcifications (stones); *6,* corpus cavernosum calcifications. **e Calcifications important for differential diagnosis:** *1,* costal cartilage; *2,* pleural thickening; *3,* pleuritis calcarea; *4,* bezoar in the stomach; *5,* tablets in the intestine; *6,* limy bile, porcelain gallbladder; *7,* calcified mesenteric lymph nodes; *8,* old, calcified, gluteal injection abscess; *9,* old, calcified hematoma of the abdominal wall; *10,* intraspinal, oily contrast material after myelography; *11,* cysticercosis with linear calcified cysticerci in the gluteal muscles; *12,* barium contrast medium in colonic diverticula; *13,* intrauterine device

Gallstone Ileus
"Spontaneously disappearing gallstone"; only about 1% of all bowel obstructions are caused by gallstones (Fig. 158).

Parenchymal Calcifications in the Liver (Fig. 90b)

Echinococciasis
Frequent cause, 10% calcified; oval or circular calcifications are typical; arclike calcifications, usually solitary, are seen in the early stages (Figs. 92, 94c).

Brucellosis
Multiple punctate calcified granulomas; foci are somewhat larger than in histoplasmosis and tuberculosis (similar foci are common in the spleen; Fig. 94a). The latter do not have acute pathologic significance.

Amebiasis, Gummata of the Liver
Rare; calcified granulomas (Fig. 93a)

Calcified Metastases
All hepatic metastases may become calcified, especially those from colorectal carcinoma, ovarian carcinoma, breast carcinoma, and medullary thyroid carcinoma. These calcifications tend to have a granular appearance (Fig. 93 b).

Hepatocellular and Cholangiocellular Carcinoma (Fig. 90 b)
Calcifications associated with these lesions are also granular and may form small coalescent patches or clumps.

Note: Besides calcified hepatic metastases, ovarian carcinoma may be accompanied by calcified peritoneal metastases associated with peritoneal carcinomatosis.

Cavernous hemangioma
"Sunburst" pattern, usually without nodular foci as in other organs. Can simulate a malignant tumor.

Thorotrastosis
Multiple punctate or patchy densities caused by Thorotrast deposits in the Kupffer cells. This condition is not significant in itself but may lead to hemangiosarcoma after 20–30 years, so tumor exclusion is necessary. Densities may also occur in the spleen and parapancreatic lymph nodes.

Vascular Calcifications: Hepatic Arterial Aneurysm (Fig. 90 c)
Eggshellike calcifications that resemble cysts; 75% are extrahepatic (differential diagnosis: gallbladder, echinococciasis, abscess, intrinsic renal disease). This aneurysm is very prone to rupture, and so the prognosis is poor.
Renal arterial aneurysm (approx. 50% calcified); calcified renal aneurysms rarely rupture.

Parenchymal Calcifications in the Kidney (Fig. 90 a)
Papillary necrosis (ringlike calcification)
Tuberculosis: flecks of calcification in the papillary region, later replaced by clumpy, amorphous calcifications
Abscess (clumpy)
Tumor calcification (up to 40% of cases): reticular pattern, but also plaquelike (differential diagnosis: retroperitoneal tumor, bony lesion)

Parenchymal Calcifications in the Adrenal (Fig. 94 c, d, e)
Carcinoma (10%–20% bilateral): granular calcification, solitary clumpy or plaquelike calcification
Pheochromocytoma (rare): granular, ringlike (*caution:* mimicks gallstone!)
Differential diagnosis: costal cartilage, lymph nodes, tuberculosis or lithiasis of the upper pole of the kidney, paravertebral or pararenal abscesses, vascular calcification, pleural plaque, osteochondroma of the 12th rib
Echinococciasis (rare): bleeding into the hydatid cyst can lead to complaints!

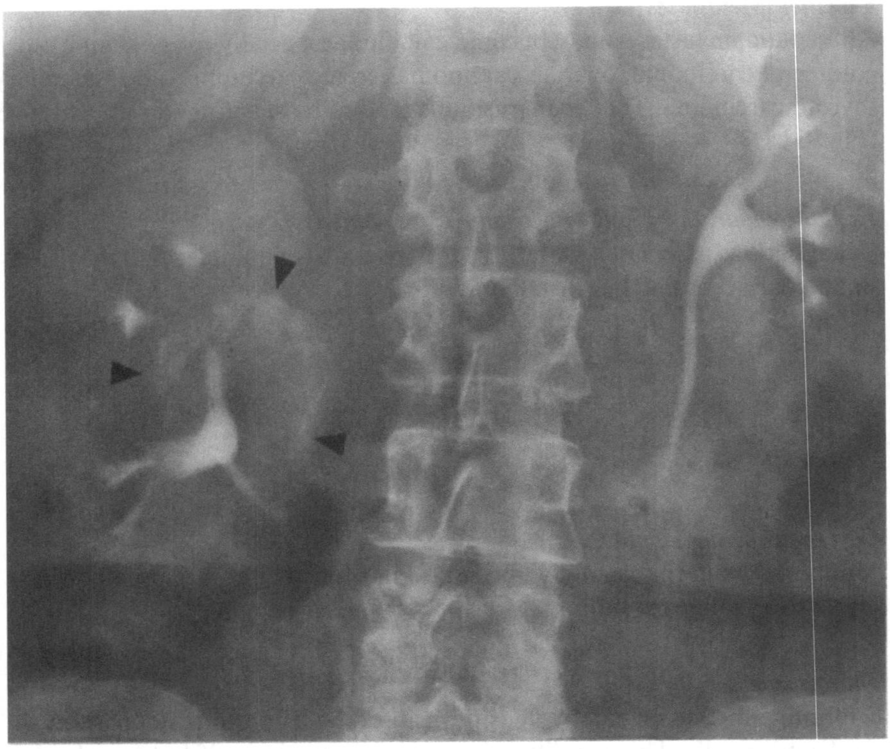

a

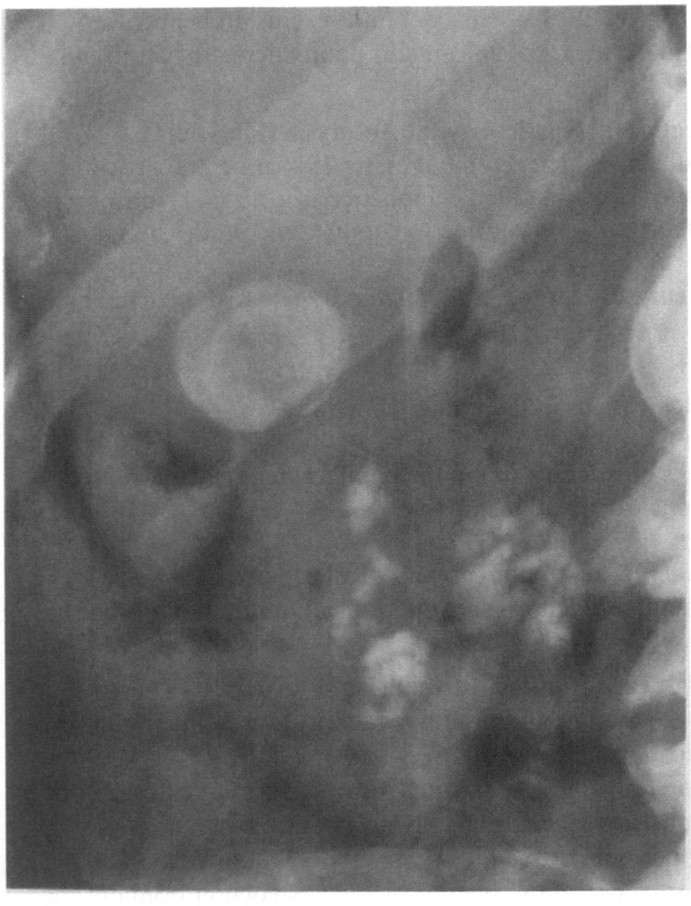

b

Fig. 91 a, b. Stones in the gallbladder. **a** Large stone in the gallbladder presenting a roughly circular outline (►) and projected over the right renal pelvis (general enteroptosis). Differentiation from an intrinsic renal tumor is required; this may be accomplished with lateral radiographs or by sonography. **b** Concentrically calcified gallstone, below which are calcified, clumpy lymph nodes projected over the renal shadow

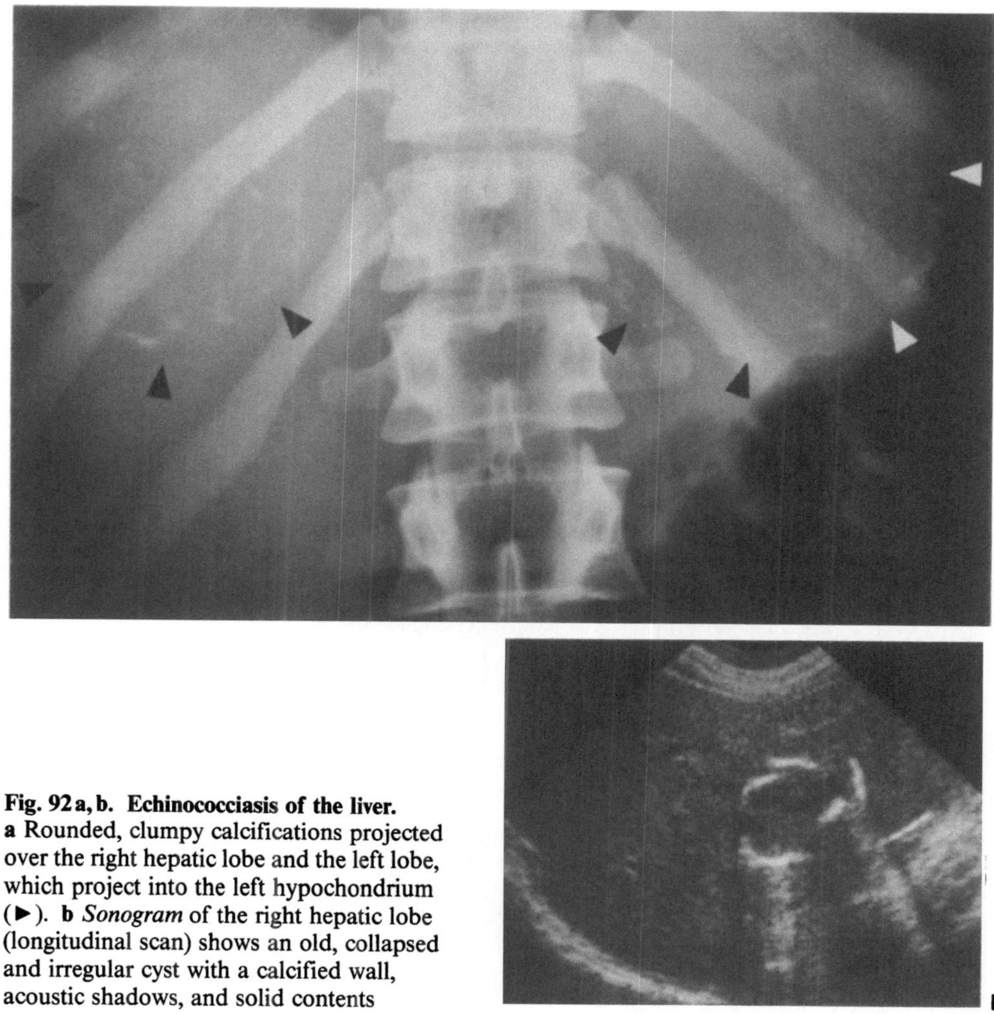

a

b

Fig. 92a, b. Echinococciasis of the liver.
a Rounded, clumpy calcifications projected over the right hepatic lobe and the left lobe, which project into the left hypochondrium (►). **b** *Sonogram* of the right hepatic lobe (longitudinal scan) shows an old, collapsed and irregular cyst with a calcified wall, acoustic shadows, and solid contents

Lesions not Relevant to Diagnosis in Patients with Acute Abdomen

Adrenal Cyst (one-third calcified, 15% bilateral)
Pseudocysts, cystic adenomas, polycystic changes, echinococciasis extremely rare
Traumatic pseudocysts are most common (Fig. 94c, d).

Calcified Lymph Nodes (Fig. 91b)

Intrahepatic Calculi
In the bile duct system

Stone Formation in the Ureteral Stump
After nephrectomy leaving a long residual ureter (see Fig. 96e) (differential diagnosis: ossifying tumor)

Caution: Calcified basal pulmonary metastases can mimic abdominal calcifications. Doubts are resolved by chest X-ray and/or fluoroscopy.

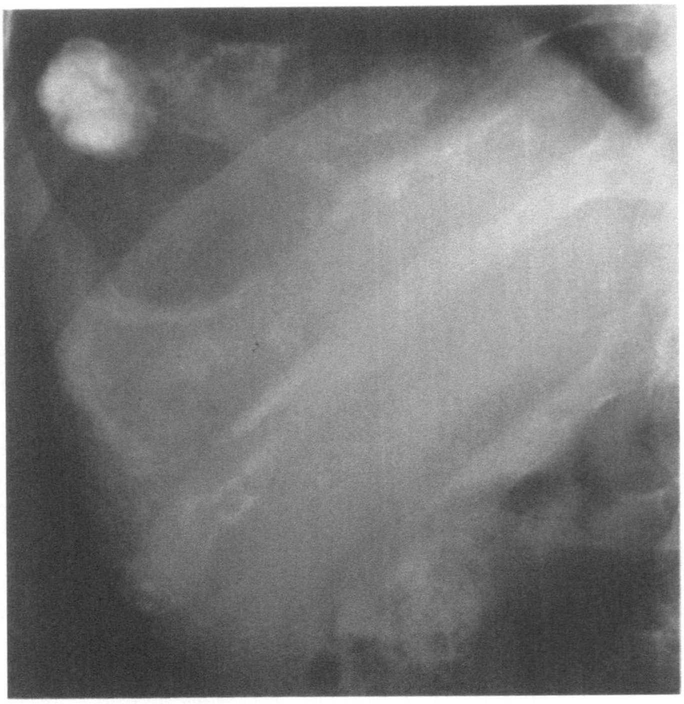

a

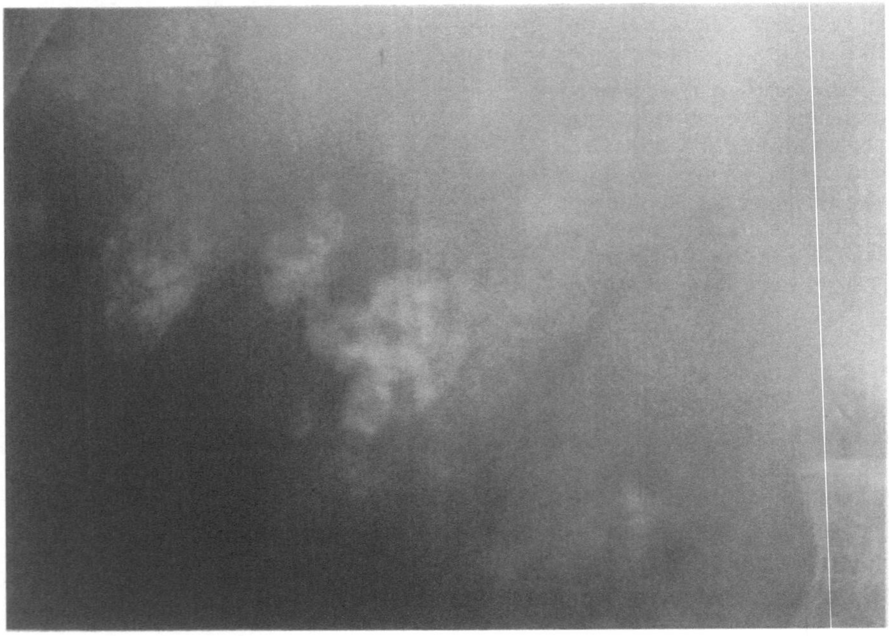

b

Fig. 93a, b. Calcifications of the hepatic parenchyma. a Old calcified hepatic abscess, requires differentiation from old hematoma. **b** Flocculent, partly coalescent calcifications in metastases from medullary thyroid carcinoma

2. Left Upper Quadrant

Lesions That Are Common and Relevant to Diagnosis in Patients with Acute Abdomen

Splenic Arterial Aneurysm (Fig. 90c)
Serpiginous course; saclike aneurysms can mimic cysts.

Note: Most ruptured aneurysms of the splenic artery are *not* calcified!

Kidney (see Right Upper Quadrant)
Adrenal (see Right Upper Quadrant)
Tail of pancreas (see Midline and Paramedian Region)

Lesions That Are Uncommon but Relevant to Diagnosis in Patients with Acute Abdomen

Splenic Cyst
Two-thirds are parasitic (only 2% of all echinococciases lead to splenic involvement) (Fig. 94b–e).
Pseudocysts are four times more common than true cysts, and most are posttraumatic.
True cysts (rare): lymphangioma, angiomatous cyst, dermoid.
Nonparasitic cysts calcify in about 9%–20% of cases.

Note: Rupture of a cyst (posttraumatic, spontaneous) should always be considered in the differential diagnosis of acute abdomen with calcification.

Brucellosis of the Spleen
Calcified nodules about 1 cm in diameter that consist of smaller foci and display a snowflakelike pattern. Some have a translucent rim (multiple granulomas or abscesses) indicating that the lesion is still active, in contrast to the smaller calcific foci of tuberculosis and histoplasmosis (differential diagnosis: phleboliths), which are inactive and have no pathologic significance (Fig. 94a).

Kidney (see Right Upper Quadrant)

Adrenal (see Right Upper Quadrant) (Fig. 94c–e)

Stomach
Calcified adenocarcinoma (mucinous): stippled or plaquelike calcifications arranged in a cluster (calcification pattern is identical to leiomyoma) (Fig. 100a).

Note: Very rarely a perforating gallstone may migrate proximally into the stomach or may perforate directly into the stomach. Thus, with corresponding clinical signs and gas in the bile ducts, one should not just search the distal portions of the bowel for a calculus.

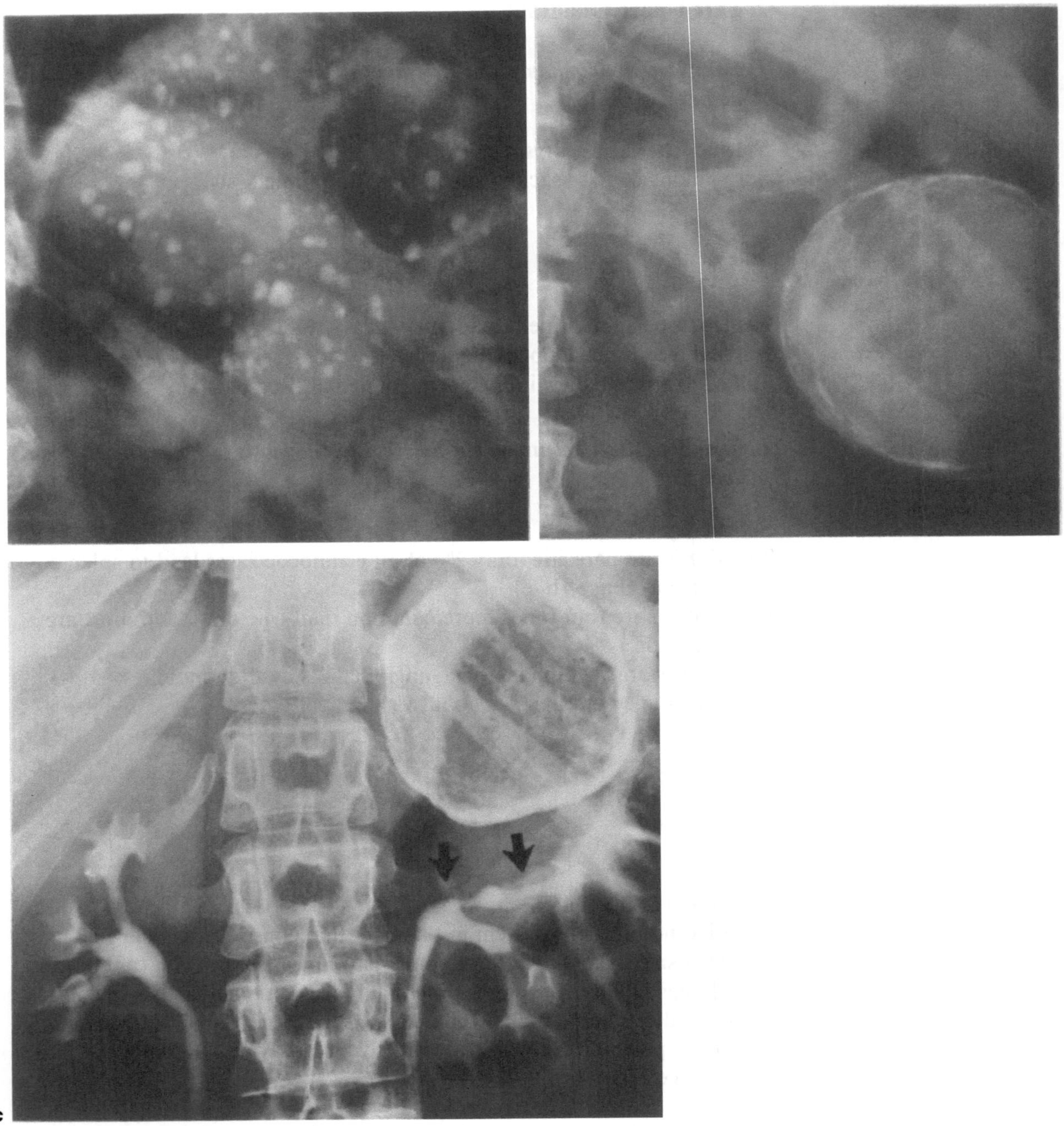

a b c

Fig. 94a–e. Calcifications projected over the splenic region.
a Multiple small nodular calcifications. Differential diagnosis: phleboliths, histoplasmosis, tuberculosis (both inactive). **b** Calcified posttraumatic splenic cyst (not echinococciasis!). **c** Calcified adrenal echinococciasis. Displacement of the left kidney and its opacified collecting system (➡) signifies a retroperitoneal process, i.e., one occurring in the region of the adrenals.

Fig. 94 (continued)
d Calcified, posttraumatic, loculated adrenal cyst (film tomography) *A1*, splenic artery imaged in cross section). **e** Corresponding CT slice at the level of the left adrenal shows a large, loculated, partially calcified cystic mass *(Z)* having no relation to the spleen *(S)* or left kidney. The right adrenal *(RA)* appears normal

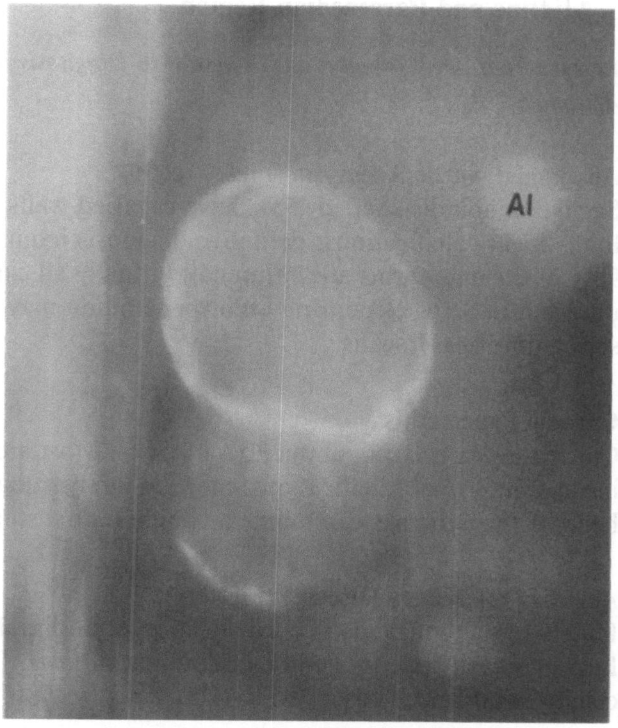

d

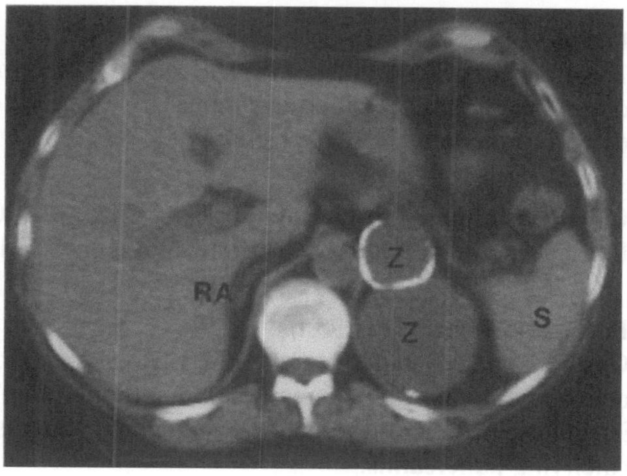

e

Lesions Not Relevant to Diagnosis of Acute Abdomen

Splenic phleboliths (differential diagnosis: tuberculosis, histoplasmosis - no acute pathologic significance) (Fig. 94 a)
Acute infarction of the spleen: wedge-shaped
Antecedent perisplenitis: linear or shellike calcifications (Fig. 90 b)
Old splenic hematoma: plaquelike or amorphous calcifications (differential diagnosis: calcified splenic abscess - rare)
Thorotrastosis: multiple punctate nodules scattered throughout the parenchyma (no clinical significance, but predisposes to eventual hepatic angiosarcoma)

3. Midline and Paramedian Region

Lesions That Are Common and Relevant to Diagnosis in Patients with Acute Abdomen

Abdominal Aortic Aneurysm (Figs. 90 c, 96)
Saclike or spindle-shaped; 55% have calcified walls, but only 10% have long, linear calcifications; definitive diagnosis requires sonography. Over 90% of the aneurysms are infrarenal; virtually all can be diagnosed with ultrasound. Signs of perforation or penetration may be visible on sonograms or CT scans.

Chronic Pancreatitis
Calcifications occur in about 30% of cases. Most are duct stones or intraparenchymal calcifications; they are rarely solitary. Calcification in the head of the pancreas can mimic a common duct stone (Fig. 95).

Aortitis (Takayasu's Disease) (Fig. 90 c)
Platelike; there may also be calcification of an intraluminal thrombus. Lesion is easily overlooked on abdominal surveys. The entire aorta may calcify in advanced cases.

Portal Venous Thrombosis (Fig. 90 c)
Tortuous, tubular paramedian calcification at the level of the porta hepatis, or an intraluminal calcified thrombus. In advanced cases findings may extend to the hilus of the spleen.

Calcified Thrombus of the Inferior Vena Cava (Fig. 90 c)
Extremely rare in adults; see Calcifications in Children

Pancreatic Tumors (Fig. 90 a)
Cystadenoma, cystadenocarcinoma, islet cell carcinoma, lymphangioma, adenocarcinoma. *All* pancreatic tumors, though rarely, may undergo irregular calcification; thus they *cannot* be distinguished from chronic calcifying pancreatitis.

Tuberculous Paraspinal Abscess
Calcification follows the course of the psoas muscle, may extend into the lesser pelvis and to the lesser trochanter. Bone changes are evident in the vertebral column.

Lesions Not Relevant to Diagnosis in Patients with Acute Abdomen

Arteriosclerosis
All intra-abdominal arterial vessels may calcify, especially the main trunks arising from the aorta (Fig. 96 a).

Calcified Nucleus Pulposus (ochronosis)

Lesions of the Abdominal Wall and Back (see Sect. 4.7) (Fig. 99)

4. Right Lower Quadrant

Lesions That Are Common and Relevant to Diagnosis in Patients with Acute Abdomen

Appendicolith
About 10% of patients with acute appendicitis exhibit coproliths in this region. The reported incidence of accompanying peritonitis is 50%–90%. Thus, when a stone is demonstrated and typical complaints are present, an indication exists for appendectomy (see Sect. 4.1.4) (Figs. 90a, 130). The stone may calcify in a homogeneous, diffuse, or layered fashion; facetting may be evident in multiple adjacent stones.

Caution: Appendicolith can mimic a stone in a low-lying gallbladder in enteroptosis (females) or a perforated gallstone (most common in the terminal ileum) (see Right Upper Quadrant).

Stone in Meckel's Diverticulum
The location is variable (small bowel): right paramedian or even in the left lower quadrant. Calcification of the stone may be homogeneous or layered. The diagnosis is suggested by a previous appendectomy and a "stoneless" gallbladder, though again confusion with a perforating gallstone is possible (see Right Upper Quadrant) (Fig. 90a).

Lesions That Are Uncommon but Relevant to Diagnosis in Patients with Acute Abdomen

Calcified Mucocele of the Appendix
Features are the same as in porcelain gallbladder.

Abscess After Confined Perforation of the Appendix
Amorphous, partly plaquelike structure

Older Hematoma
Soft tissues or bowel wall (hemophilia)

Lesions Not Relevant to Diagnosis in Patients with Acute Abdomen

The most common source of calcifications in this region are calcified *mesenteric lymph nodes*. They need to be distinguished from intraosseous lesions of the iliac wing (see Fig. 91b).

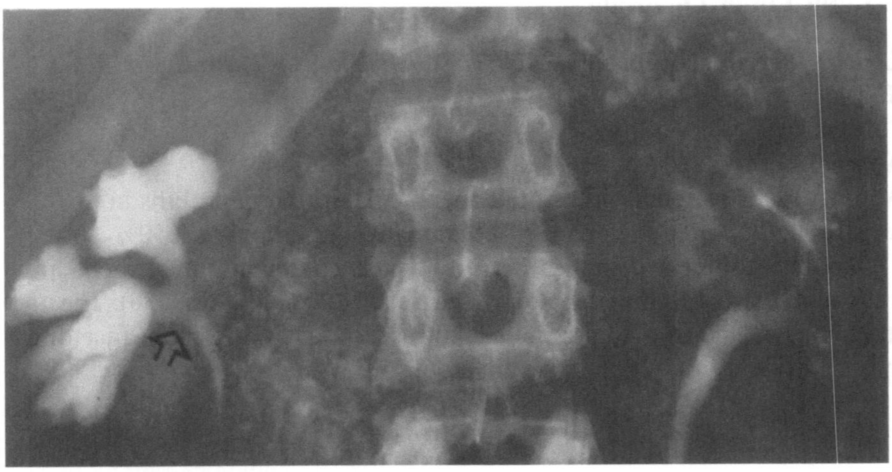

a

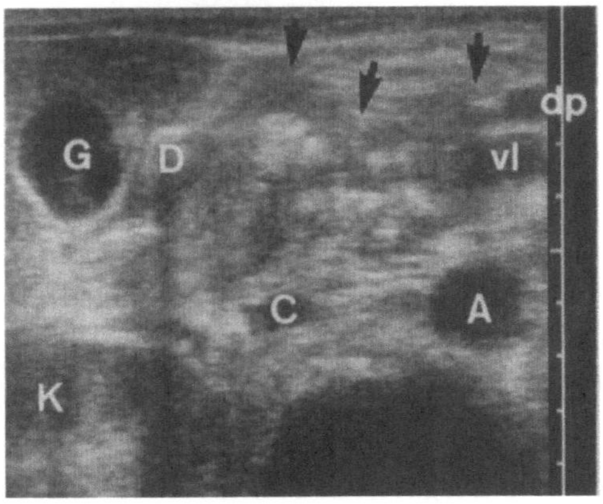

b

Fig. 95 a, b. Pancreatic calcifications in chronic, recurring pancreatitis.
a Stippled to clumped calcifications are scattered throughout the organ. There is compression of the right renal pelvis (⇨) with associated outflow obstruction caused by a pseudocyst in the head of the pancreas. **b** *Sonogram* shows multiple, echogenic, clumped calcifications in the enlarged head of the pancreas (➡) and an obstructed pancreatic duct *(dp)*; *G*, gallbladder; *D* duodenum; *CV*, inferior vena cava; *A*, aorta; *K*, right kidney

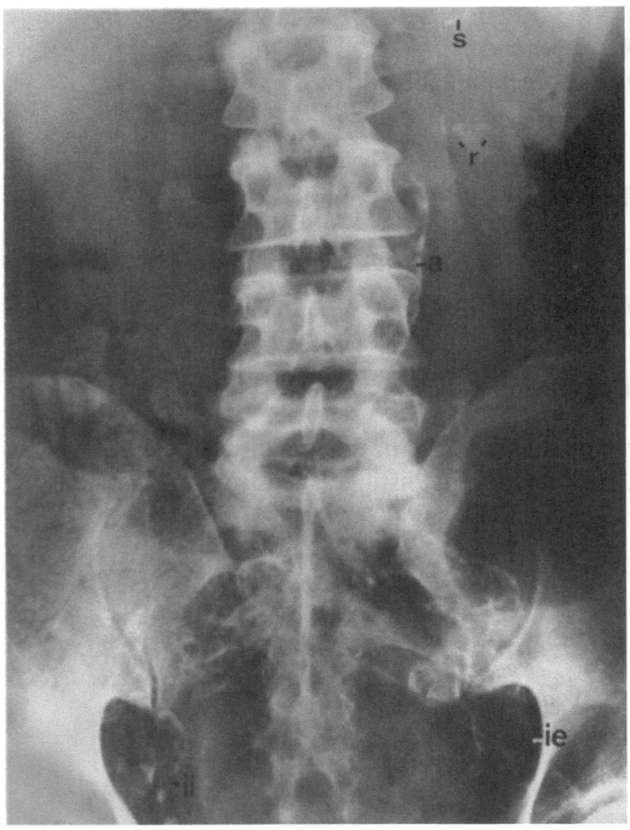

a

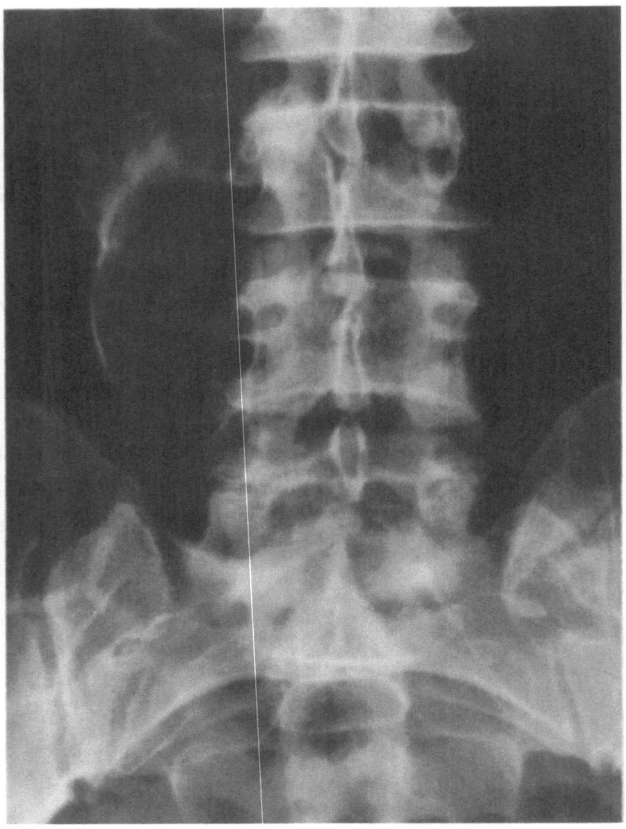

b

Fig. 96 a–e (Legend see page 169)

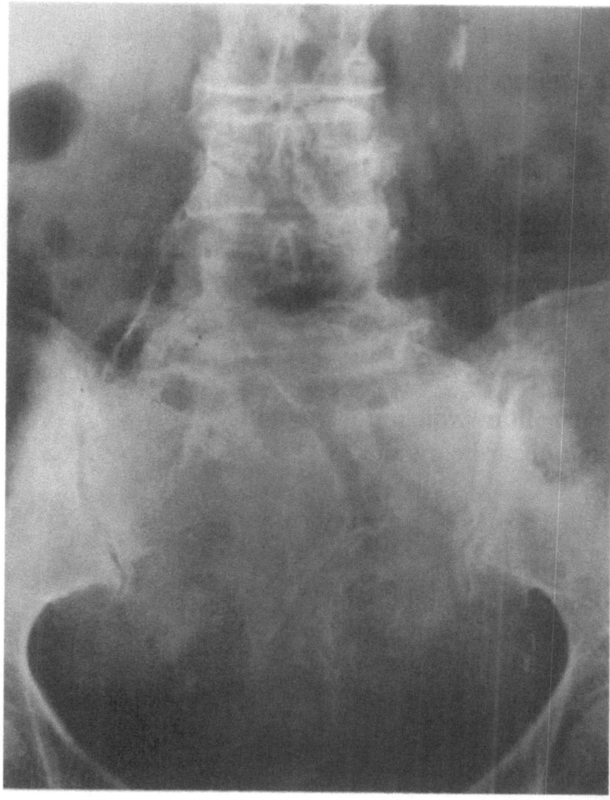

c

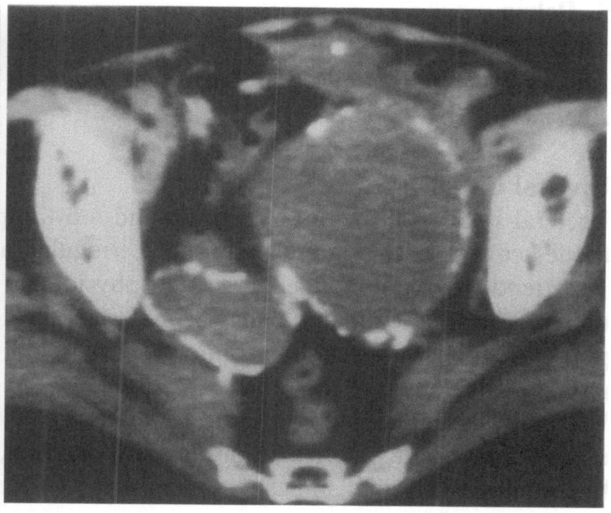

d

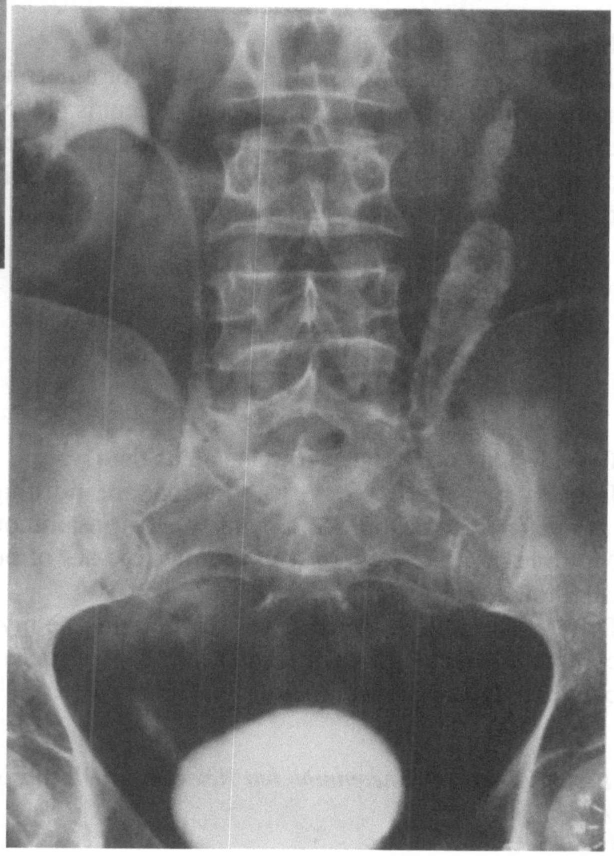

e

Fig. 96a–e. Calcifications of vessels and tubular structures. **a** Vascular calcifications associated with general arteriosclerosis: *s*, splenic artery; *r*, renal artery, *a*, abdominal aorta; *ii*, internal iliac artery; *ie*, external iliac artery. **b** Circumscribed right-sided (rare) saccular aneurysm of the abdominal aorta. **c** Conspicuous saccular aneurysm of the common iliac artery. **d** Corresponding *CT scan* shows two rounded aneurysmal sacs with calcified walls The markings anterior to the large aneurysmal sac on the left side reflect perianeurysmal fibrosis. **e** Calculus forming a long, post nephrectomy ureteral stump

5. Pelvis

Lesions That Are Common and Relevant to Diagnosis in Patients with Acute Abdomen

Ureteral Calculi
Ureteral stones are the most common and most important calcifications in the lesser pelvis. They are usually small, irregular, and lightly calcified. They tend to become lodged at sites of physiologic constriction - the ureterovesical junction and pelvic brim. Ureteral calculi occur in the medial part of the pelvis above a line connecting the ischial spines. Their long axis parallels the course of the ureter (see Fig. 90a).
Ureteral calculi mainly require differentiation from **phleboliths,** which are usually larger and spherical, more heavily calcified, and occur below the line joining the ischial spines.

Bladder Calculi
These may be single or multiple, layered or amorphous. Free intraluminal stones will change position when the patient is moved. A stone in a bladder diverticulum usually occurs laterally, close to the pelvic wall; some are dumbbell-shaped with one end lodged in the diverticulum and the other projecting into the bladder (see Fig. 97c).

Note: In the acutely traumatized patient, a *change in the position of phleboliths* within the lesser pelvis over time is suggestive of hematoma from soft-tissue injury!

Cystadenoma or Cystadenocarcinoma of the Ovary
Initially there are fine calcifications that are indistinguishable from other intrapelvic calcifications. Calcium spheres: psammomatous bodies. Multiple peritoneal deposits are found in cases of peritoneal carcinomatosis. Calcified cysts.
Differentiation is required from calcified uterine myomas (the most common gynecologic calcification in the lesser pelvis), which presents a clumped, typical appearance.

Lesions That Are Uncommon but Relevant to Diagnosis in Patients with Acute Abdomen

Rectal Carcinoma (see Fig. 100b)
Fine, granular foci similar to ovarian carcinoma. Requires differentiation from osseous lesions (e.g., chondrosarcoma of sacrum, chordoma, retrorectal soft-tissue sarcoma); also from calcified coprolith, residual barium in the sigmoid, and older calcified hematoma.

Cystitis
Nonspecific calcifying cystitis, radiation cystitis, bladder carcinoma

Caution: Do not confuse with cystic ovarian process (usually eccentric).

Schistosomiasis (Bilharziosis)
Calcium in the wall of the distal ureter and bladder. Can mimic calcification of the iliac arteries. The bladder wall may undergo a shell-like or cystlike calcification, but it retains its motility, so that the size of the cystic feature varies with the state of bladder fullness.
This contrast with:

Tuberculosis of the Urinary Bladder
Fixed, rigid, calcified bladder wall

Salpingitis (also tuberculous)
Bilateral intramural calcifications having a string-of-beads appearance; intraluminal "calculi" in pyosalpinx with obstruction

Prostatic Tuberculosis
Indistinguishable from prostatic stones of other etiology (see below)

Calcification of Seminal Vesicle (Fig. 97 d)
Tuberculosis, gonorrhea, nonspecific. Pattern of calcification is indistinguishable from other lesions and can mimic ureteral stones.

Ovarian Dermoid Cyst (Fig. 97 a, b)
Contains skin, teeth, hair, and possibly bone

Ovarian Calcification After Torsion
Autoamputation with infarction

Ovarian Tuberculosis
Calcification pattern resembles that of a lymph node.

Lithopedion
Calcified ectopic pregnancy (fetal death after 3rd month of gestation): If calcification is confined to the fetal membranes, it is indistinguishable from tumor calcification.

Lesions Not Relevant to Acute Diagnosis but Important in Differential Diagnosis

Uterine Myomas (see above)
Calcification of Seminal Vesicle (see above; Fig. 97 d)
Prostatic Calculi (see above)
Calcified Vas Deferens (in about 10% of all diabetics)
Tubular structures occupying a typical anatomic position; rare in tuberculosis (see Fig. 90 c)

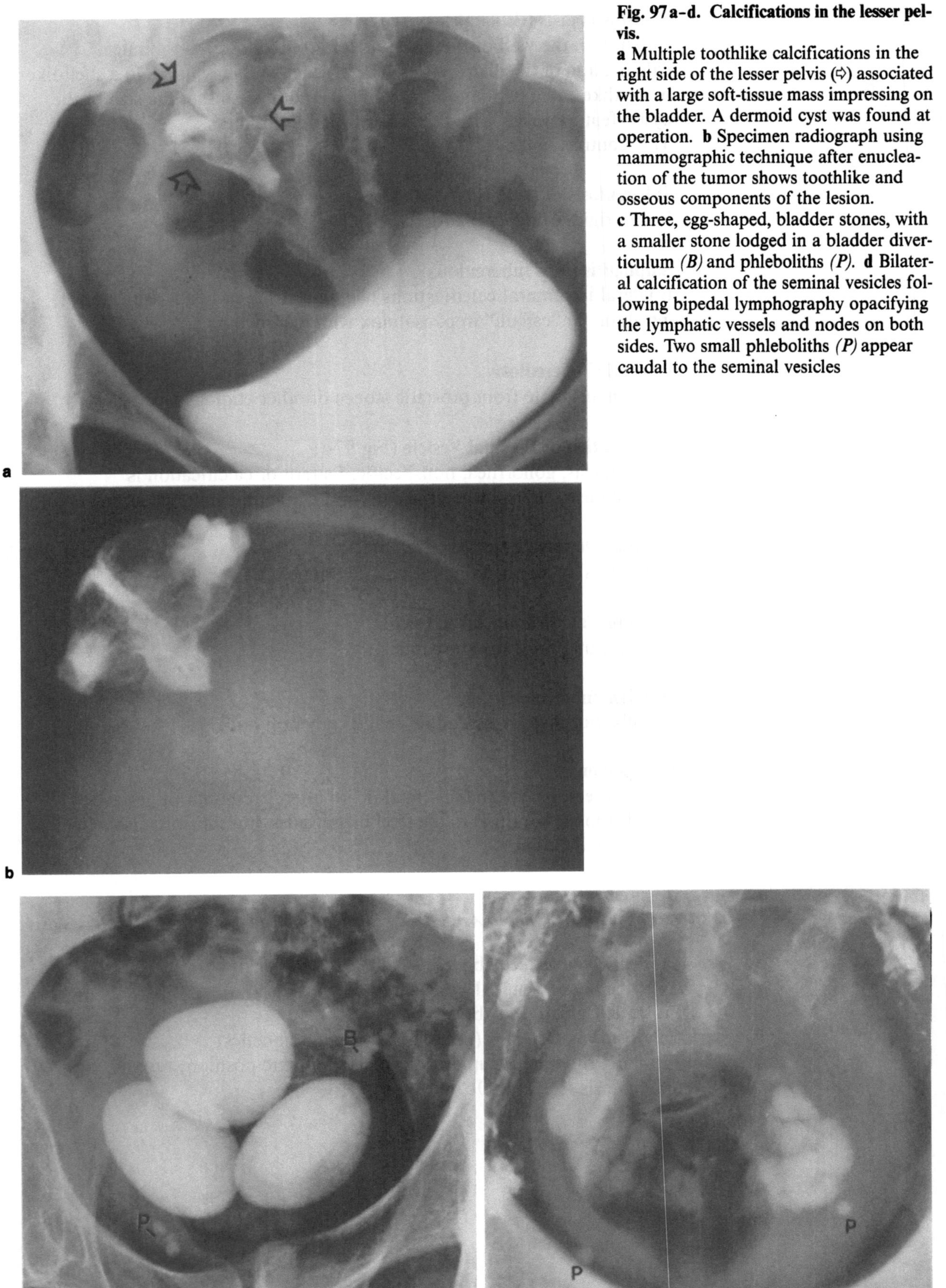

Fig. 97 a–d. Calcifications in the lesser pelvis.
a Multiple toothlike calcifications in the right side of the lesser pelvis (⇨) associated with a large soft-tissue mass impressing on the bladder. A dermoid cyst was found at operation. **b** Specimen radiograph using mammographic technique after enucleation of the tumor shows toothlike and osseous components of the lesion.
c Three, egg-shaped, bladder stones, with a smaller stone lodged in a bladder diverticulum *(B)* and phleboliths *(P)*. **d** Bilateral calcification of the seminal vesicles following bipedal lymphography opacifying the lymphatic vessels and nodes on both sides. Two small phleboliths *(P)* appear caudal to the seminal vesicles

6. Calcifications Occurring Without Sites of Predilection (Fig. 98)

Calcified Lymph Nodes

Calcified Appendices Epiploicae

Caution: Acute abdomen may be secondary to torsion with infarction.

Free calculus in the abdominal cavity (Fig. 98)
Enterogenic cysts
Require differentiation from other cystic structures, q. v.

Enteroliths
Can occur practically anywhere in the bowel. Always consider stenosis or aganglionic segment as causes.

Gallstones
(Passed physiologically, perforated). Can occur virtually anywhere in the bowel lumen. Motility! For differential diagnosis, see Right Lower Quadrant.

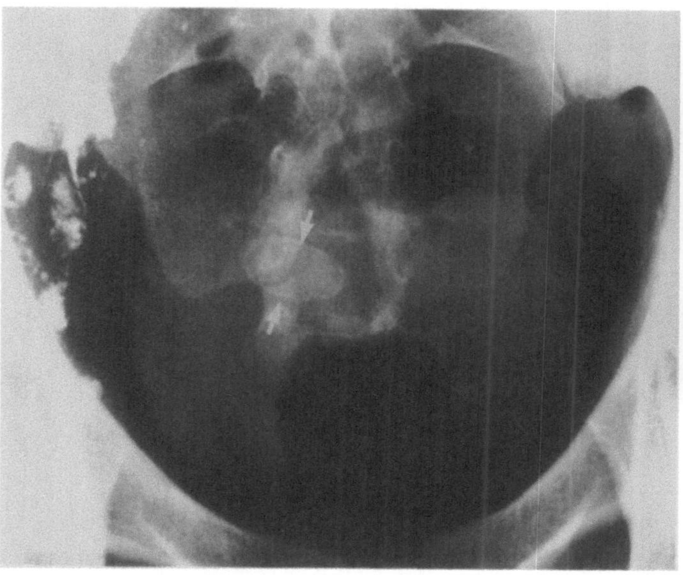
a

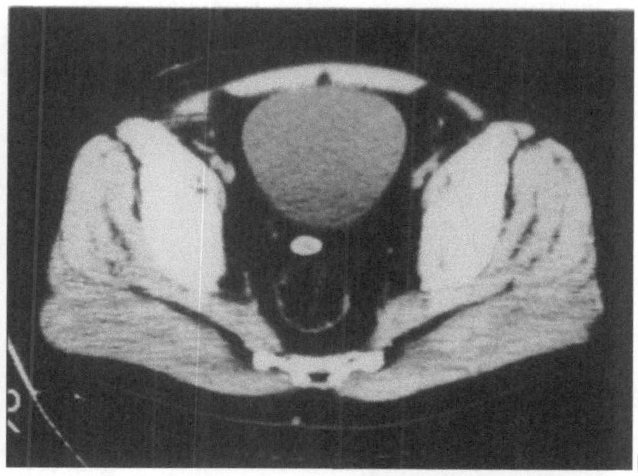
b

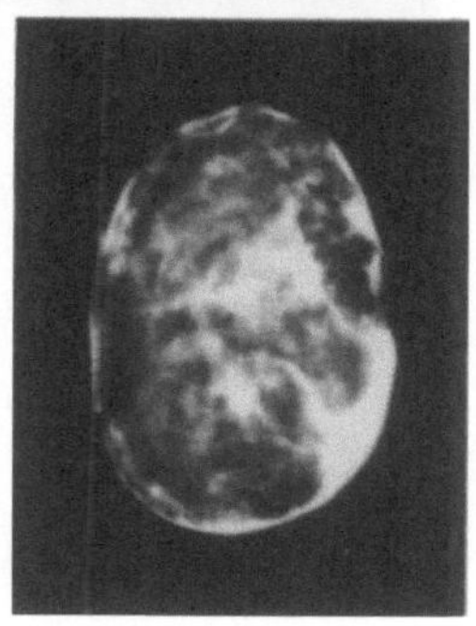
c

Fig. 98 a–c. Free calculus in the abdominal cavity as an incidental finding.
Man, 42 years old, who had undergone a right semicastration for embryonal testicular carcinoma. Before undergoing a scheduled transperitoneal lymphadenectomy, he was referred for lymphography. **a** Survey film during lymphography shows an oval, smoothly marginated, heterogeneously calcified, midline structure projected onto the sacrum. **b** *CT scan* localizes the calcified structure to the cul-de-sac. The free calculus was removed at operation. **c** Grossly, the mass measured 1.8 × 1.4 cm, had a smooth surface, showed a patchy yellow-brown coloration, and was friable internally. Chemical analysis revealed amorphous calcium phosphate and protein ("protein calculus") (Dr. F. Christ, Department of Radiology, University of Bonn)

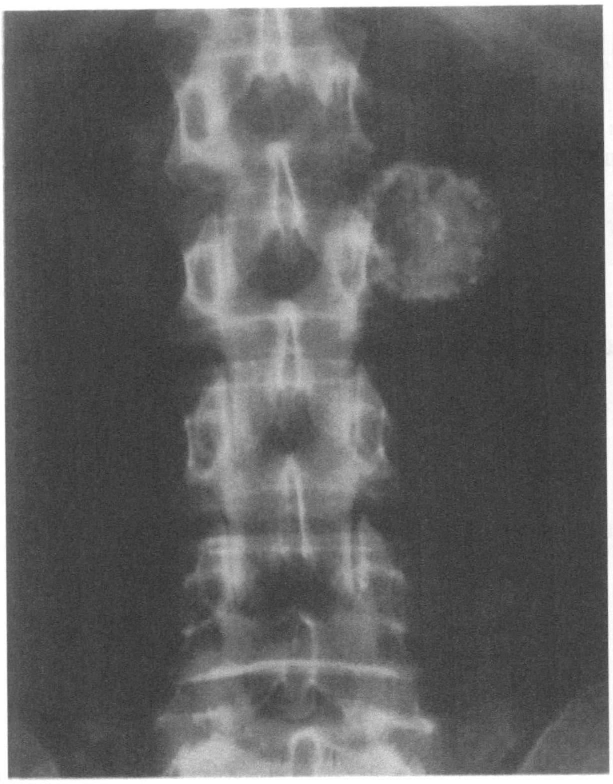

a

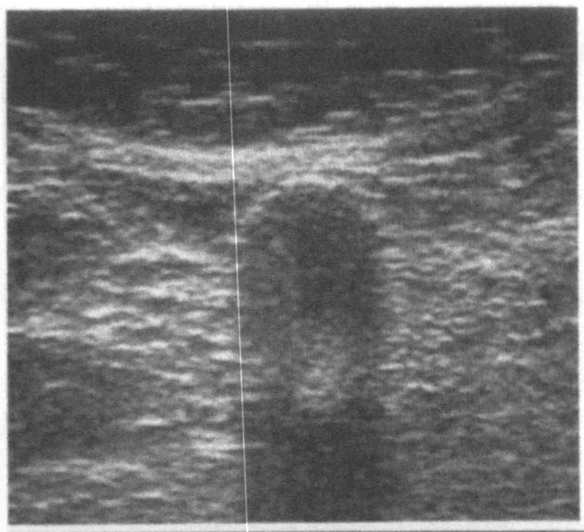

b

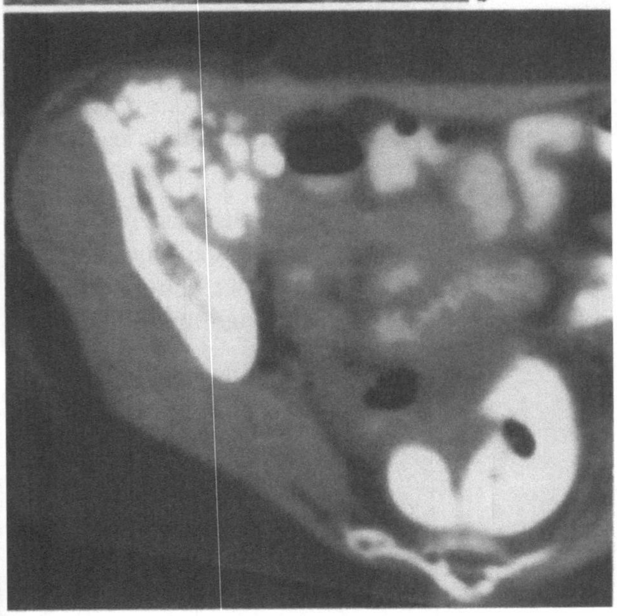

d

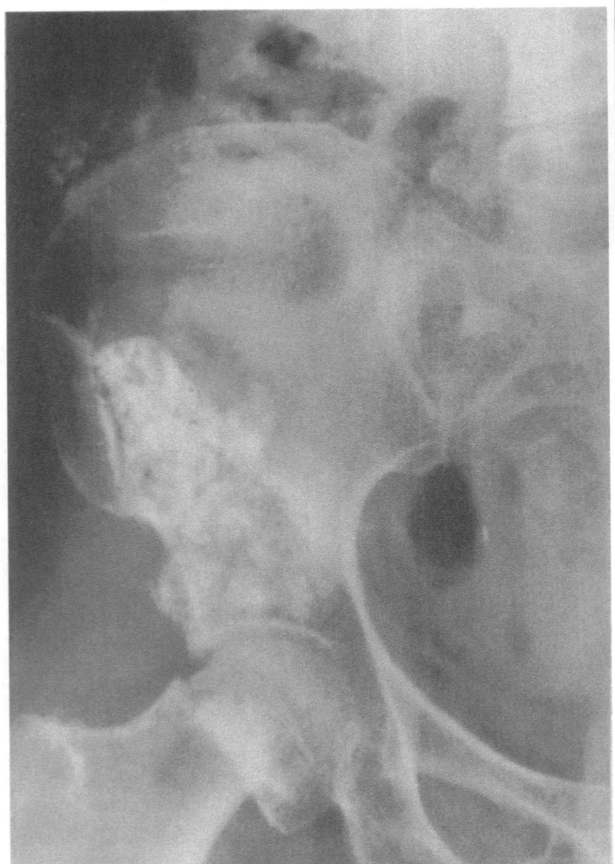

c

Fig. 99 a–d. Calcifications of the abdominal wall that can mimic intra-abdominal calcifications. **a** Old, calcified, abdominal wall hematoma. **b** Corresponding *sonogram* shows only a wide area of acoustic shadowing. **c** Malignant mesenchymoma of the abdominal wall with calcifications projected over the right iliac wing and crest. Associated finding: osteoradionecrosis of the neck of the right femur. **d** Corresponding *CT slice* demonstrates calcifications in the abdominal soft tissues. These have no relation to the bone

Tumors of the Bowel Wall
Calcifying adenocarcinoma, sarcomas, hemangioma

Hematoma
Intraperitoneal, extraperitoneal: see Sects. 3.3 and 3.4

Retroperitoneal tumors
Scattered Calcifications
Peritoneal Carcinomatosis (Fig. 100 c)

Peritoneal Tuberculosis
Same pattern with multiple calcifications, some granular or psammomatous, some plaquelike (see Lesser Pelvis)

Oil Granulomas
These occur after the instillation of oil for prevention of adhesions (a technique now obsolete).

Note: Scattered calcifications, like any other lesions, need to be identified as intra- or extraperitoneal (see Sect. 3.4).

7. Shadows That Can Mimic Abdominal Calcifications

Intraluminal: medications (pills, suppositories) (Fig. 111 b), residual contrast medium, dye ingestion (lead, zinc), mercury, metal (coins, needles) (Fig. 103 a), swallowed bones, IUD, vaginal tampon (Fig. 111 a)
Paraluminal and intramural: suture material, packing, surgical sponge (Fig. 102), metal clips, tubes and catheters (pacemaker, intraspinal electrode for over-stimulation of pain conditions, nasogastric tube, drain, catheter fragment), postsurgical foreign body (Fig. 102), gunshot or war injury, free calculus of the abdominal cavity (Fig. 98)
Skeletal system: residual contrast medium after myelography (oily), intraspinal electrode, gunshot or war injury, previous fracture, abscess, previous bone graft
Abdominal wall and back lesions (see Sect. 4.7, Fig. 99): hematomas, calcified scar, cutaneous appendages, parasitisms, myositis ossificans, foreign bodies (Fig. 110 a, b), suture material
External material (see Fig. 110): ointments, dressings, buttons, skin folds, tattoos, calcified injection abscess, bismuth injection (gluteal), mercury (thermometer), suture material, dried liquid contrast medium, stoma
Differential diagnoses: intramammary calcifications, rib calcifications, basal pulmonary lesions (atelectasis, tumor, metastasis, adhesion, pleuritis calcarea), pericardial calcifications, thorotrastosis
Radiographic artifacts: film/screen defects, faulty development, fingerprints

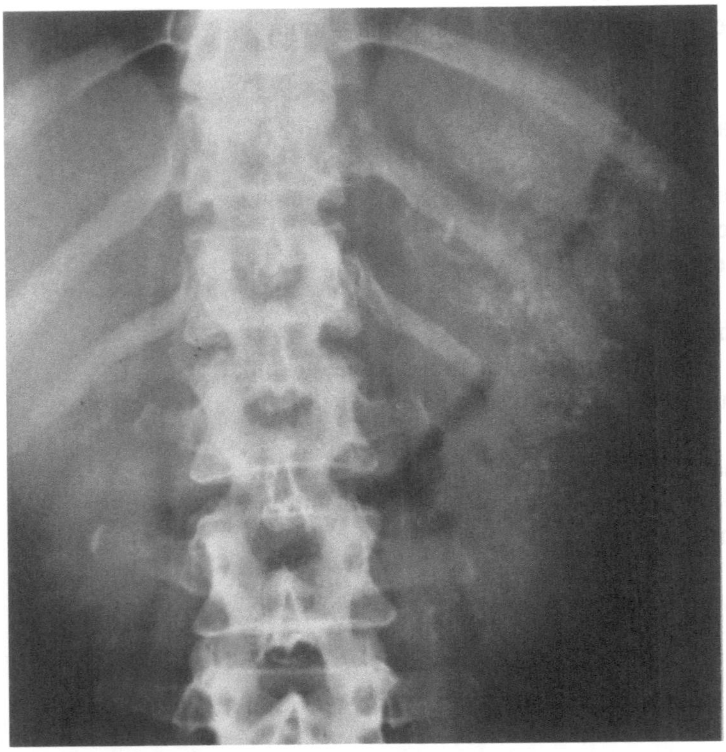
a

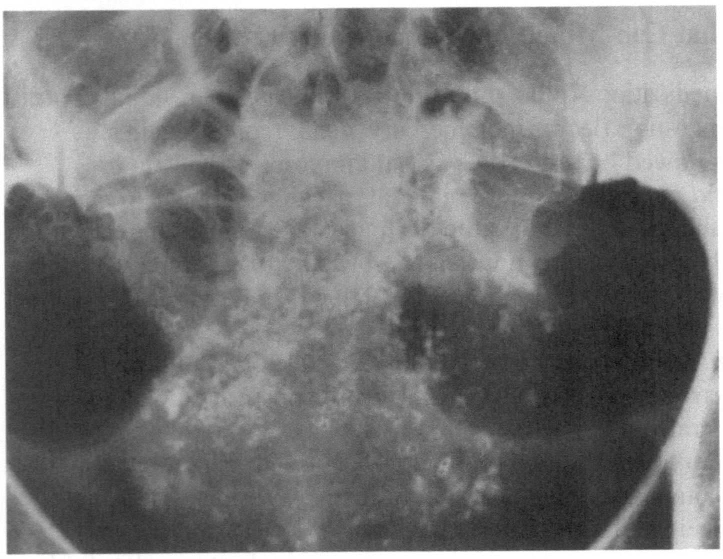
b

Fig. 100a–c. Tumor calcifications. **a** Calcifying mucinous adenocarcinoma of the stomach with multiple speckled calcifications. **b** Calcified recurrence of a rectal carcinoma. Multiple clips are visible following an end-to-end anastomosis of the bowel.

Fig. 100 (continued)
c Calcifying peritoneal carcinomatosis associated with ovarian carcinoma. Differentiation is needed from calcifying tuberculosis and also from calcifying peritoneal echinococciasis (both are rare)

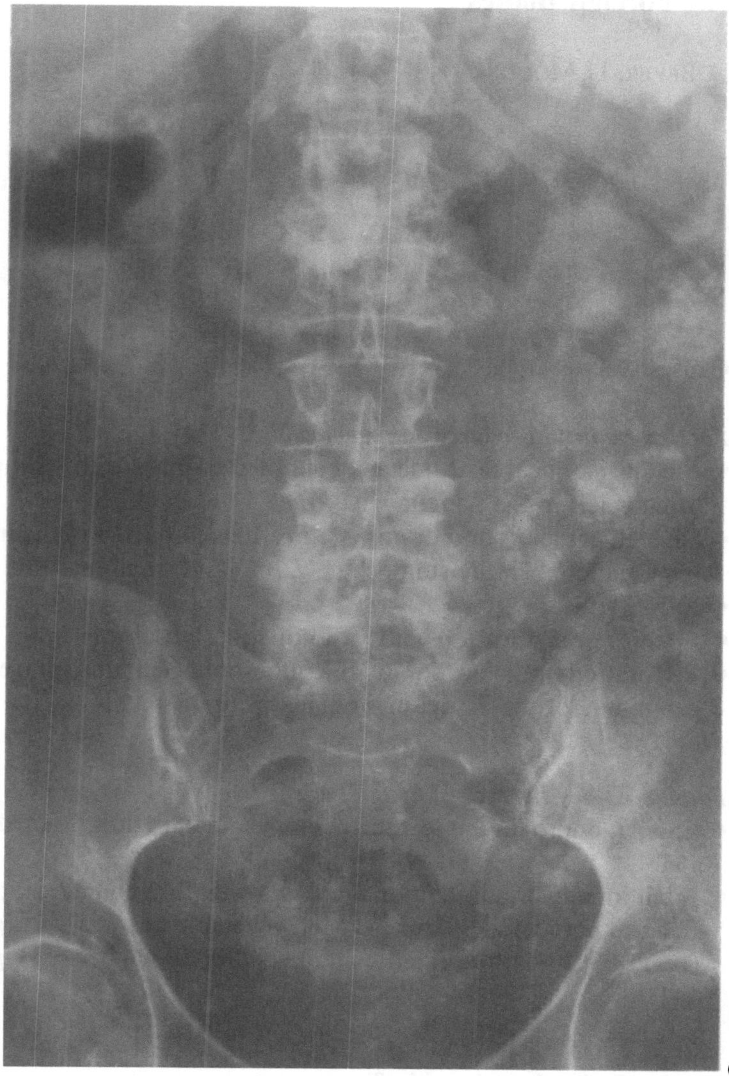

c

References

Baker SR, Elkin M (1983) Plain film approach to abdominal calcifications. Saunders, Philadelphia

Christ F, Rühr D (1985) Das freie Bauchhöhlenkonkrement. ROFO 142/4: 470–472

McAfee JG, Donner MW (1962) Differential diagnosis of calcifications encountered in abdominal radiographs. Am J Med Sci 234: 609

Meschan I (1973) Analysis of roentgen signs, vol 3. Saunders, Philadelphia

3.8 Foreign Bodies

D. Beyer, U. Mödder

Note: Foreign bodies can produce highly acute abdominal symptoms. The majority of foreign bodies are detected incidentally on plain abdominal radiographs. They may become lodged at characteristic sites (Fig. 101).

Causes

Foreign Bodies Introduced Iatrogenically

- Metallic surgical instruments or surgical sponges with radiopaque threads left in the patient (Fig. 102)
- Severed catheters and drains, medications impacted in the intestinal tract, balloons in the stomach (Fig. 105) and small intestine (Fig. 152)
- Intrauterine devices
- Enemas or medication with radio-opaque substances
- Perforation or dislocation of an endoesophageal tube (placed for carcinoma of the cardia or stomach) (Fig. 151)

Foreign Bodies Introduced by the Patient

- Foreign bodies in the rectum, colon, vagina, urethra, or bladder (Fig. 106, 111)
- Intentionally or unintentionally swallowed foreign bodies: coins, toys, denture parts, bones, hair bezoars, vegetable bezoars, dirt (geophagy) (Figs. 103, 104), drug-filled containers ("body packers") (Figs. 107, 108, 111)

Foreign Bodies Introduced by Trauma

- Projectiles, explosive fragments (Fig. 109)
- Broken-off pieces of metal in sharp trauma (Fig. 109)

Caution: Some apparently intra-abdominal "foreign bodies" are actually located behind or below the patient (e.g., fever thermometer; Fig. 110) or in the soft tissues of the abdomen or back (drains, needles, suture material, dressing material, fluid-filled colostomy bag, urine bag). External inspection of the patient is imperative.

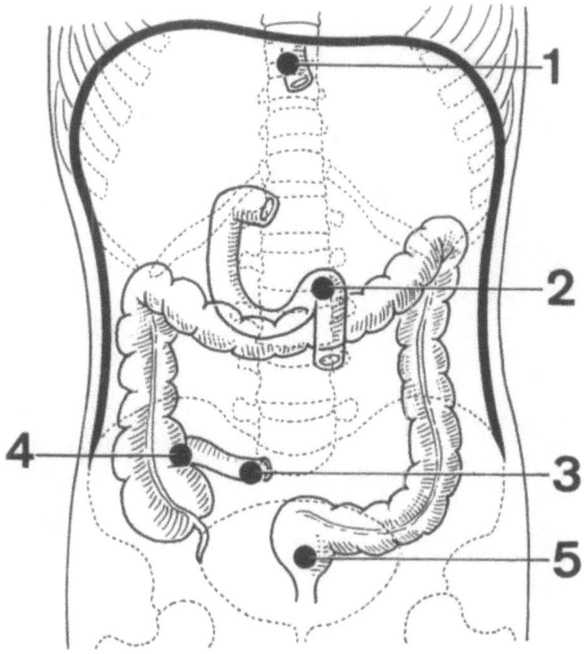

Fig. 101. Typical sites at which swallowed **foreign bodies** are likely to become lodged, producing acute abdominal symptoms. *1*, Esophagogastric junction; *2*, duodenojejunal flexure at the ligament of Treitz; *3*, proximal to a small-bowel adhesion; *4*, ileocecal valve; *5*, rectum (modified from Botsford and Wilson 1981)

Radiologic Signs

Plain Radiographs

Foreign bodies usually present as objects of metallic or calcium density on plain radiographs.
Additional radiographic signs that indicate a foreign body as the cause of acute abdomen are:

- bowel distension oral to the foreign body (Fig. 102, 151, 152)
- a soft-tissue density, possibly with air inclusions (abscess, drug-filled containers (Fig. 107, 108, 111) (Fig. 102b–d)
- free air (perforation)
- inflammatory reaction to an extraintestinal foreign body with adhesions and mechanical bowel obstruction (Fig. 102a)
- late sequelae: peripheral calcification around an extraintestinal foreign body

The location of a foreign body can be difficult to establish with accuracy. With an object in the colon, careful rectal insufflation of air is indicated, although this often causes orad movement of the foreign body. Beware of perforation (Fig. 106c, d)!
If fistulization has occurred, the fistulous tract should be opacified with a water-soluble contrast agent.

Sonography

Sonograms demonstrate the consequences of abscess formation or perforation (free fluid, free air) and may show fluid-filled bowel loops if a mechanical obstruction exists (Fig. 102c).

Computed Tomography

A foreign body of metallic density can create massive artifacts, depending on its size. Like sonography, CT demonstrates the effects of the foreign body, which may involve abscess formation, free air, or bowel obstruction (Fig. 102d, g, 108e, 109c).

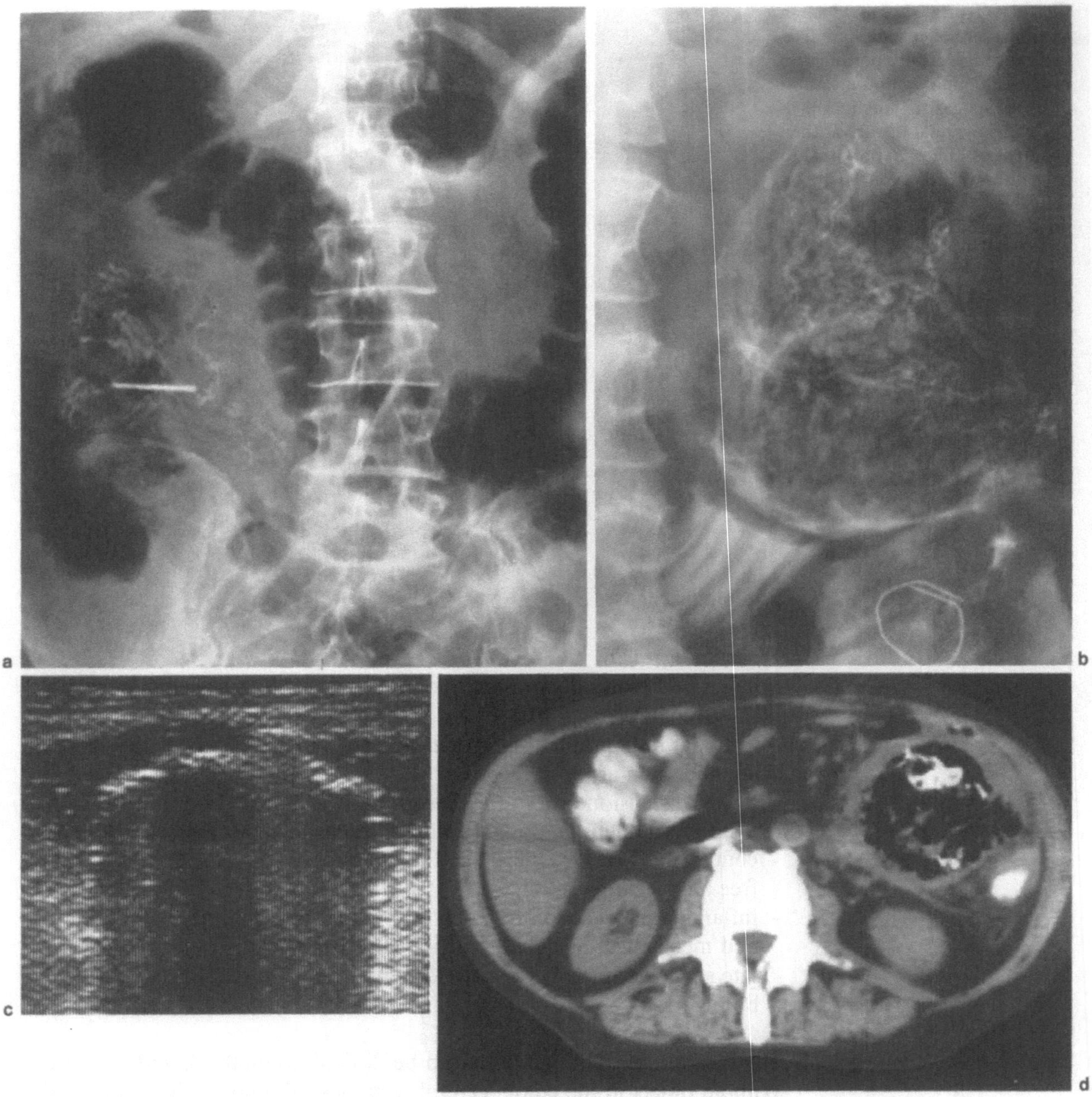

Fig. 102 a–h. Foreign bodies introduced iatrogenically.
a Oversewing of a gastric ulcer in this patient was followed by right lower quadrant pain with tenderness and fever. *Supine film* shows a soft-tissue-dense mass in the right lower quadrant with radiopaque fibers and an element of metallic density occupying the space between the ascending colon, right colic flexure, and transverse colon. *Operation* disclosed a retained surgical sponge. **b** Man, 45 years old, who had undergone splenectomy elsewhere experienced constant epigastric pain and fever, with subsequent drainage of pus through a fistulous opening in the anterior abdominal wall. *Fistulogram* shows that the fistulous opening is marked with a wire loop. The contrast film reveals a space filled partly with air and partly with a mass of soft-tissue density that contains radiopaque fibers. **c** *Sonogram,* left paramedian longitudinal scan, shows an echogenic mass with a wide acoustic shadow surrounded by liquid structures. **d** *CT slice* at the level of the kidneys shows a large, intraperitoneal, gas-containing mass with a thick margin containing radiopaque elements. *Reoperation* disclosed a retained surgical sponge with associated abscess formation.

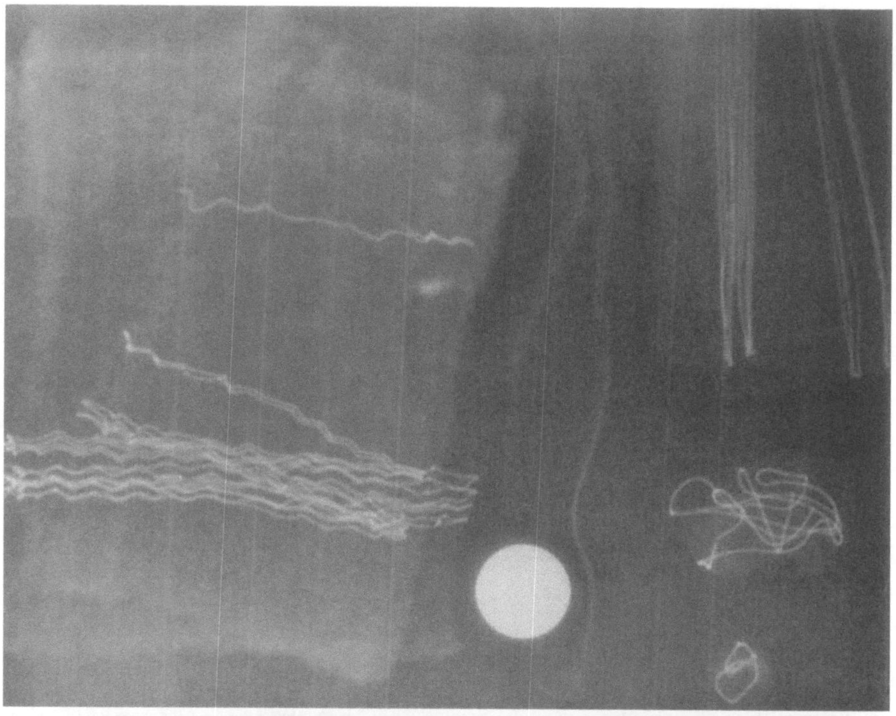

e

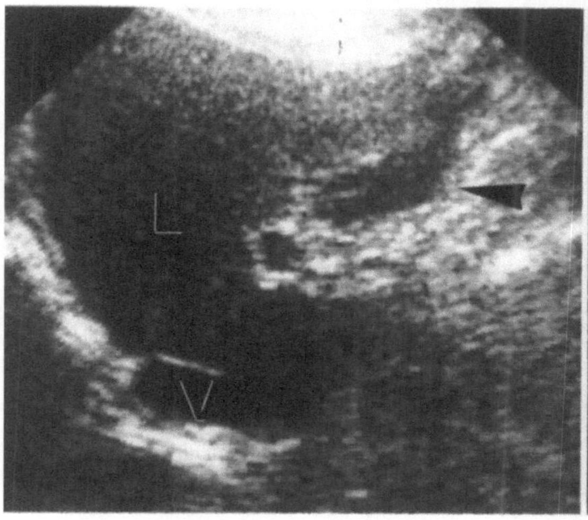

f

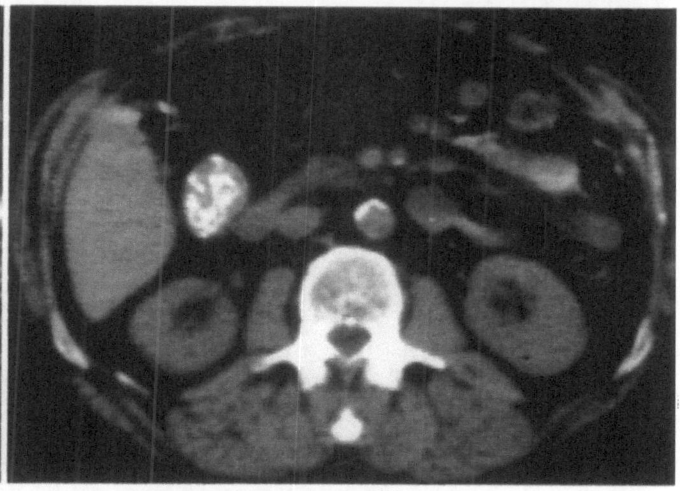

g

Fig. 102 (continued)
e Soft-tissue film of surgical materials: (radiopaque fibers, surgical sponge and swab). **f–h** Postoperative foreign body in the gallbladder bed. Man, 68 years old, with right upper quadrant pain had undergone cholecystectomy 3 months earlier and now was experiencing tenderness below the surgical scar. Laboratory values were normal. **f** *Sonogram* of the upper abdomen (longitudinal scan through the bed of the gallbladder) shows a hypoechoic feature in the area of the cholecystectomy that resembles the gallbladder in shape. No acoustic shadowing. **g** *CT scan* shows a round lesion with high-density, corkscrewlike internal structures in the gallbladder bed. **h** At operation a gauze sponge incorporating radiodense fibers was discovered in the former gallbladder bed
(Dr. H.G. Zilch, Department of Radiology, Passau Municipal Hospital)

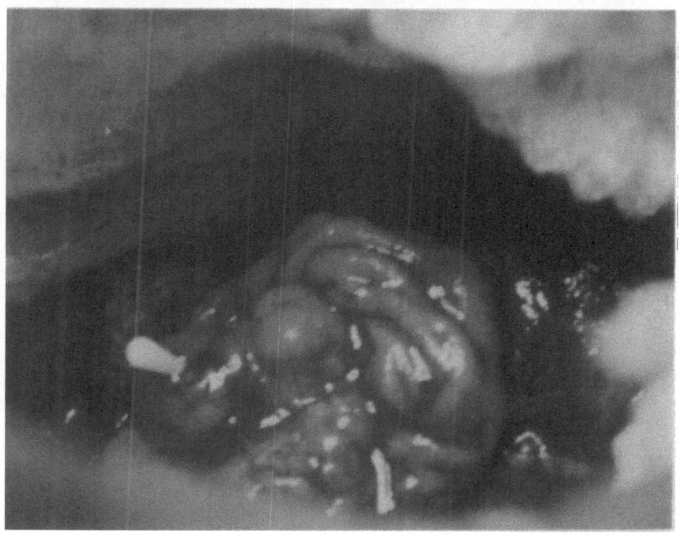

h

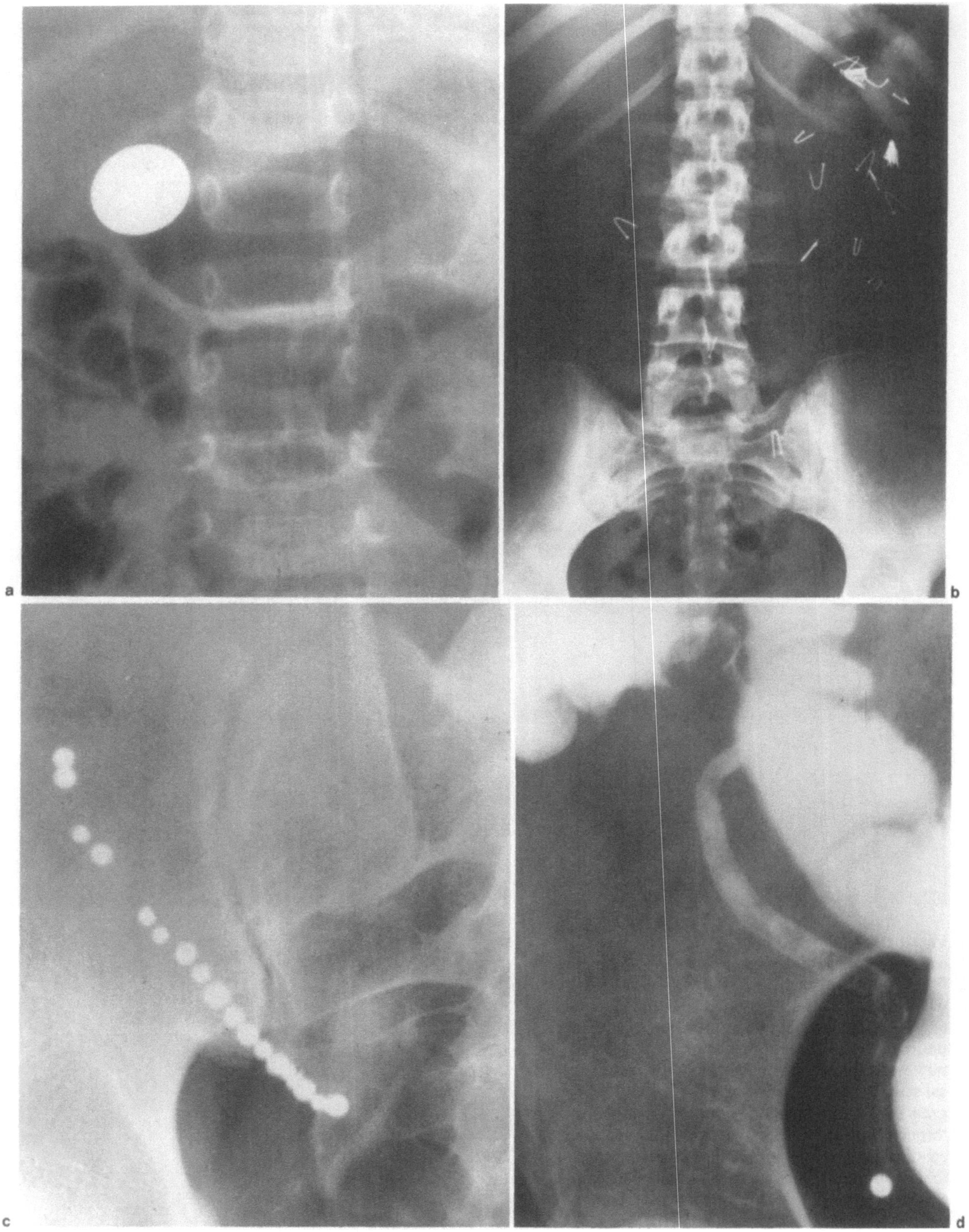

Fig. 103a–d (Legend see page 183)

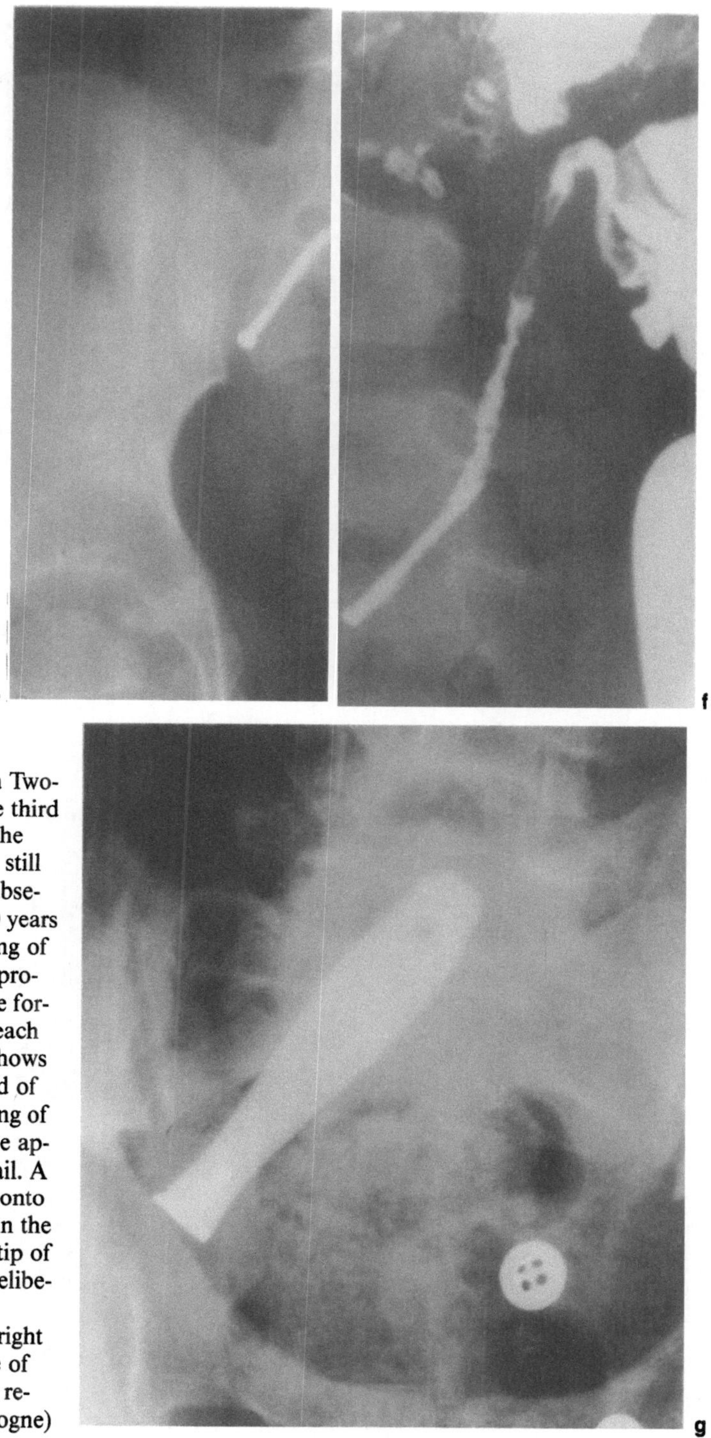

e f g

Fig. 103 a–g. Foreign bodies ingested by the patient. **a** Two-year-old child who swallowed a coin. *Supine film,* the third follow-up radiograph taken after 6 days, shows that the coin still has not traversed the pyloric channel and is still projected over the gas-filled antrum. The coin was subsequently removed endoscopically. **b** Prison inmate, 40 years of age, who came to operation for repeated swallowing of foreign bodies. *Supine film* shows multiple bent pins projected over the mid- and left upper abdomen. After the foreign bodies were passed naturally, it was found that each was wrapped in adhesive tape. **c** *Supine film* (detail) shows multiple shot pellets in the appendix of a patient fond of consuming wild game. **d** *UGI series* shows partial filling of the appendix with a shot pellet visible in the tip of the appendix. **e** *Supine film* of a child after swallowing a nail. A foreign body of metallic density is seen in projection onto the right iliosacral joint. **f** *UGI series* shows the nail in the lumen of the appendix, its point directed toward the tip of the appendix. **g** Supine film of a prison inmate who deliberately swallowed a knife handle. The metal handle, wrapped in adhesive tape, is seen projected onto the right lower quadrant of the abdomen. There is no evidence of bowel obstruction. At operation the knife handle was recovered from the terminal ileum (Dr. H. Modder, Cologne)

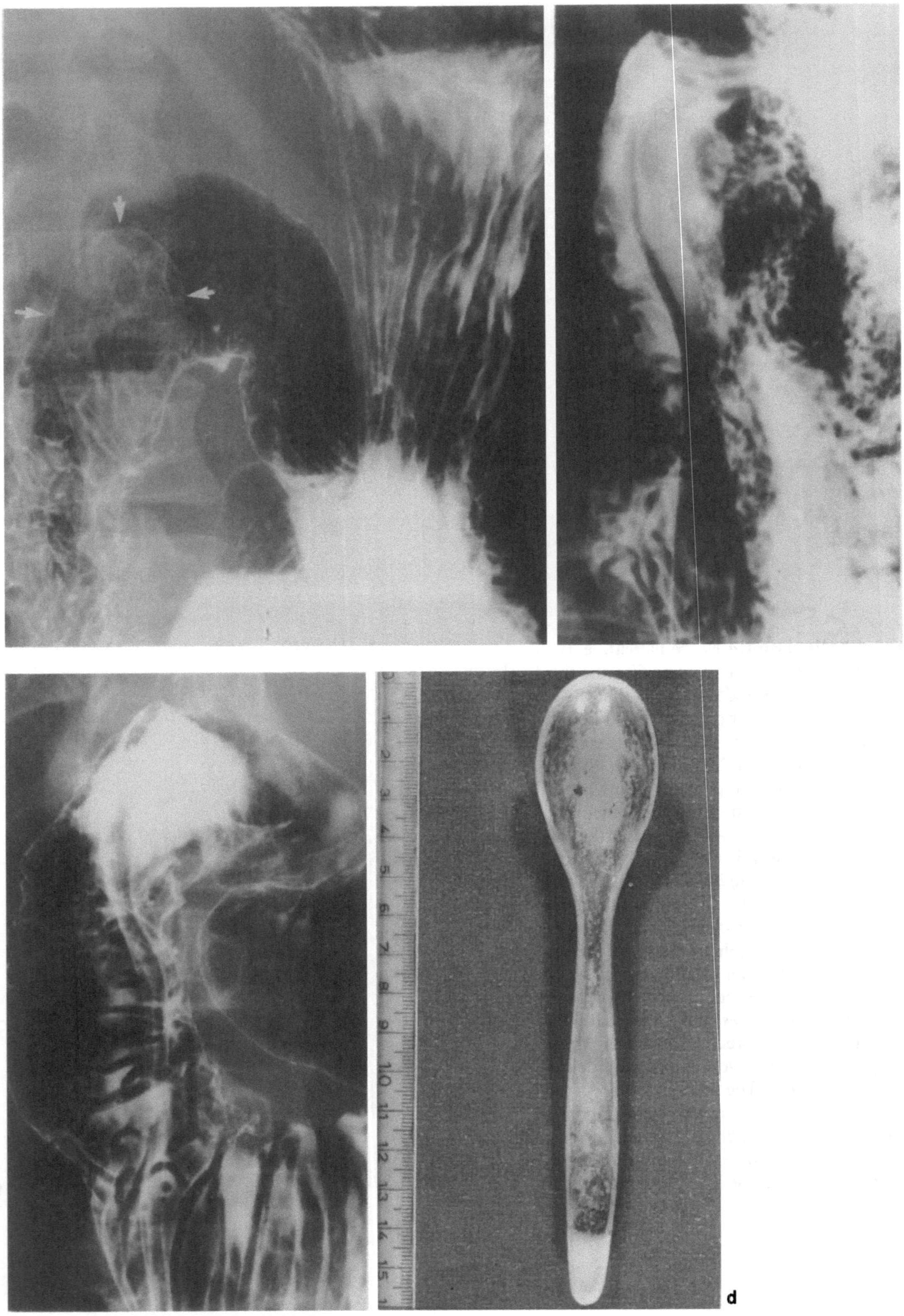

Fig. 104a–d. Intraduodenal foreign body (swallowed 24 years previously). The patient, a 43-year-old woman with a psychological disturbance, had swallowed a plastic spoon while in college with the intention of reducing her weight. She presented with acute gastric pain resembling gastritis. Gastroscopy was not performed. **a** *UGI series* (erect) shows a spoon-shaped foreign body (→) lodged in the atonic duodenum. **b** Film rotated to the left shows the spoon outlined as a filling defect in the duodenum. **c** Hypotonic duodenography shows the spoon standing upright within the duodenum. **d** Status following duodenotomy and removal of the foreign body (Drs. M. Lefke and K. Schmucker, joint radiology practice, Cologne-Weiden)

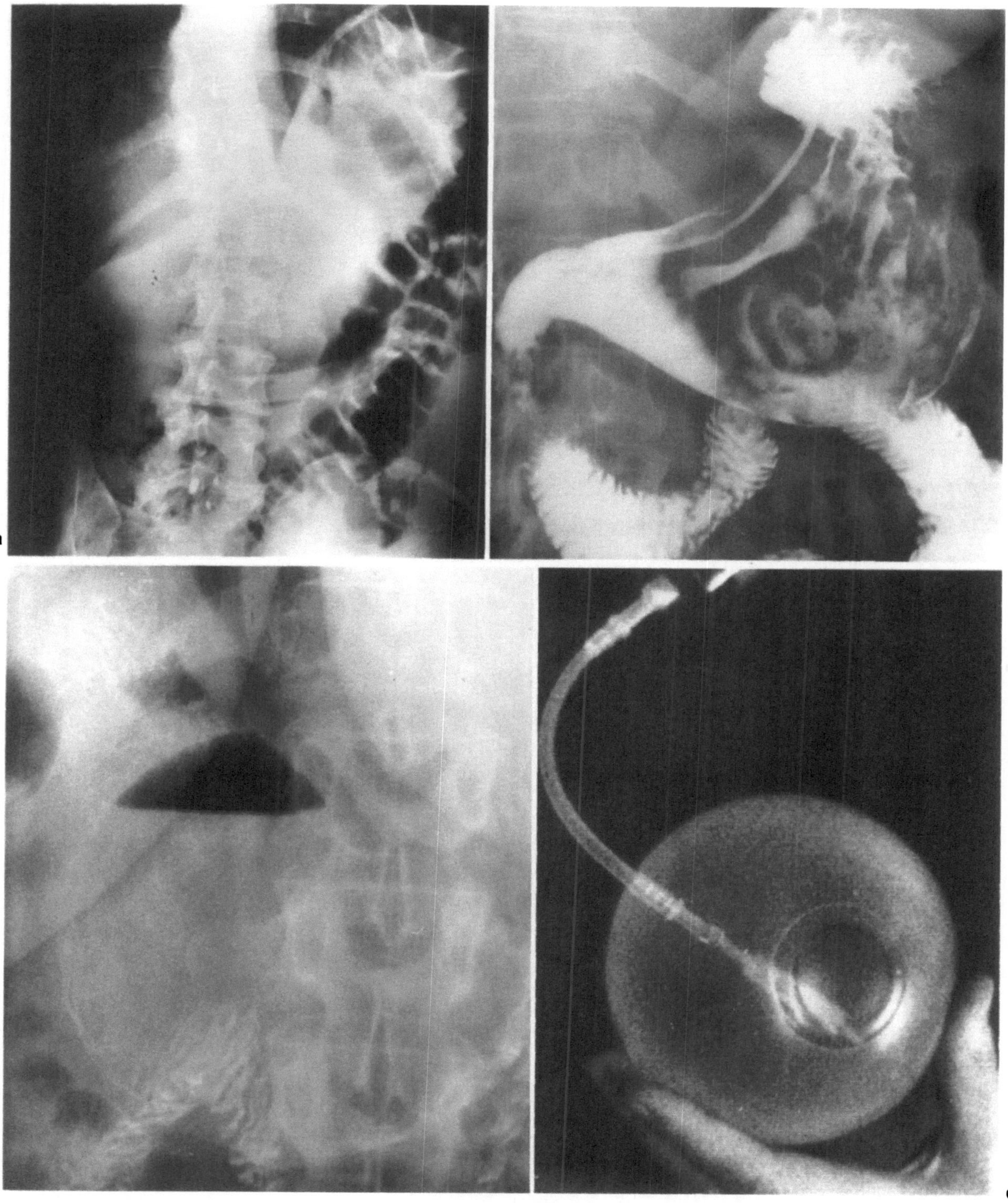

a b c d

Fig. 105 a–d. Intragastric foreign bodies.
a Homemade "gastric tube" deliberately swallowed by a 43-year-old psychiatric patient, who sought to relieve his swallowing difficulties with an esophageal dilator made from the line of a urine bag. He was admitted with acute gastric pain. Supine film shows a thick plastic tube in projection onto the stomach. Surgical removal was required. Residual droplets of an oily myelographic dye projected onto the vertebral canal are present as an incidental finding. **b–d** Intragastric foreign body, a Willmen balloon, introduced iatrogenically for control of extreme obesity. **b** *UGI series* shows an intragastric filling defect about 5 cm in diameter that appears to have irregular margins. The feature, which resembles an ulcer crater, is a cellulose-filled silicone balloon with a reinforced, valve-bearing plate about 5 cm large on its surface. **c** *UGI follow-through* (erect late film) shows an air-fluid level in the gastric balloon caused by the diffusion of gas-forming bacteria into the balloon. **d** Willmen gastric balloon in the filled state prior to implantation

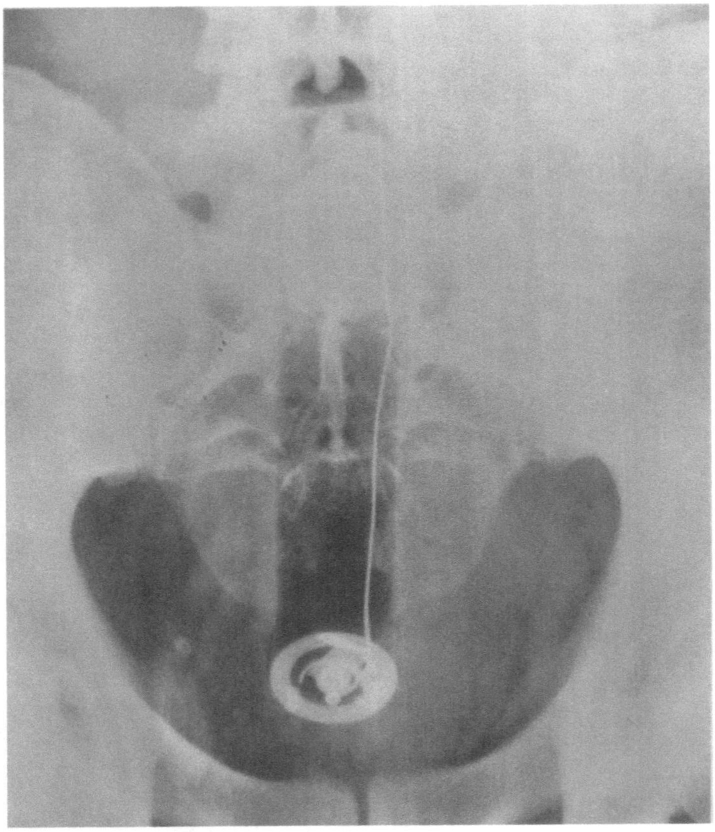

a

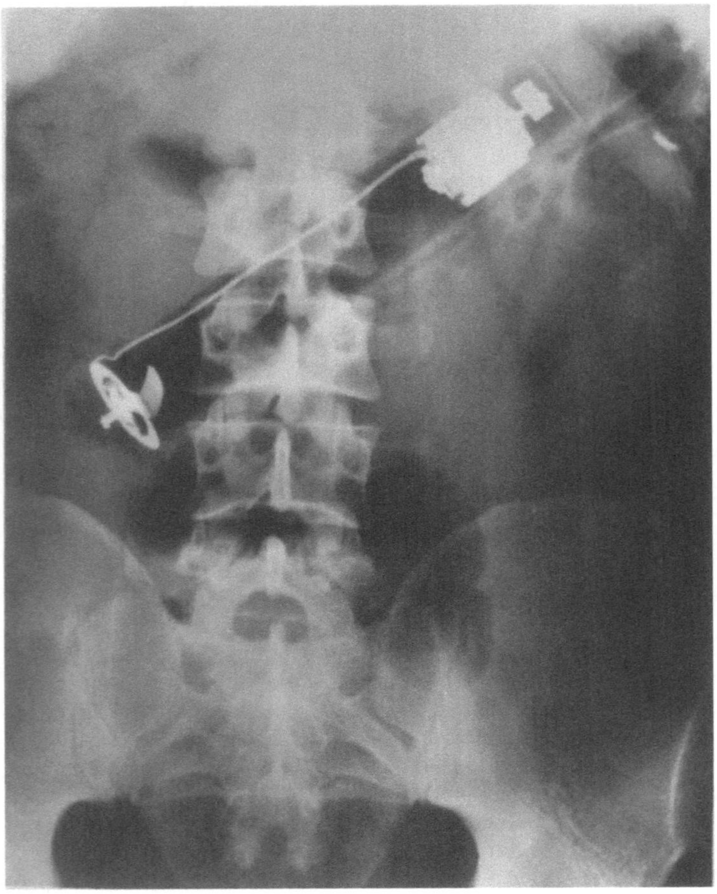

b

Fig. 106 a, b (Legend see page 187)

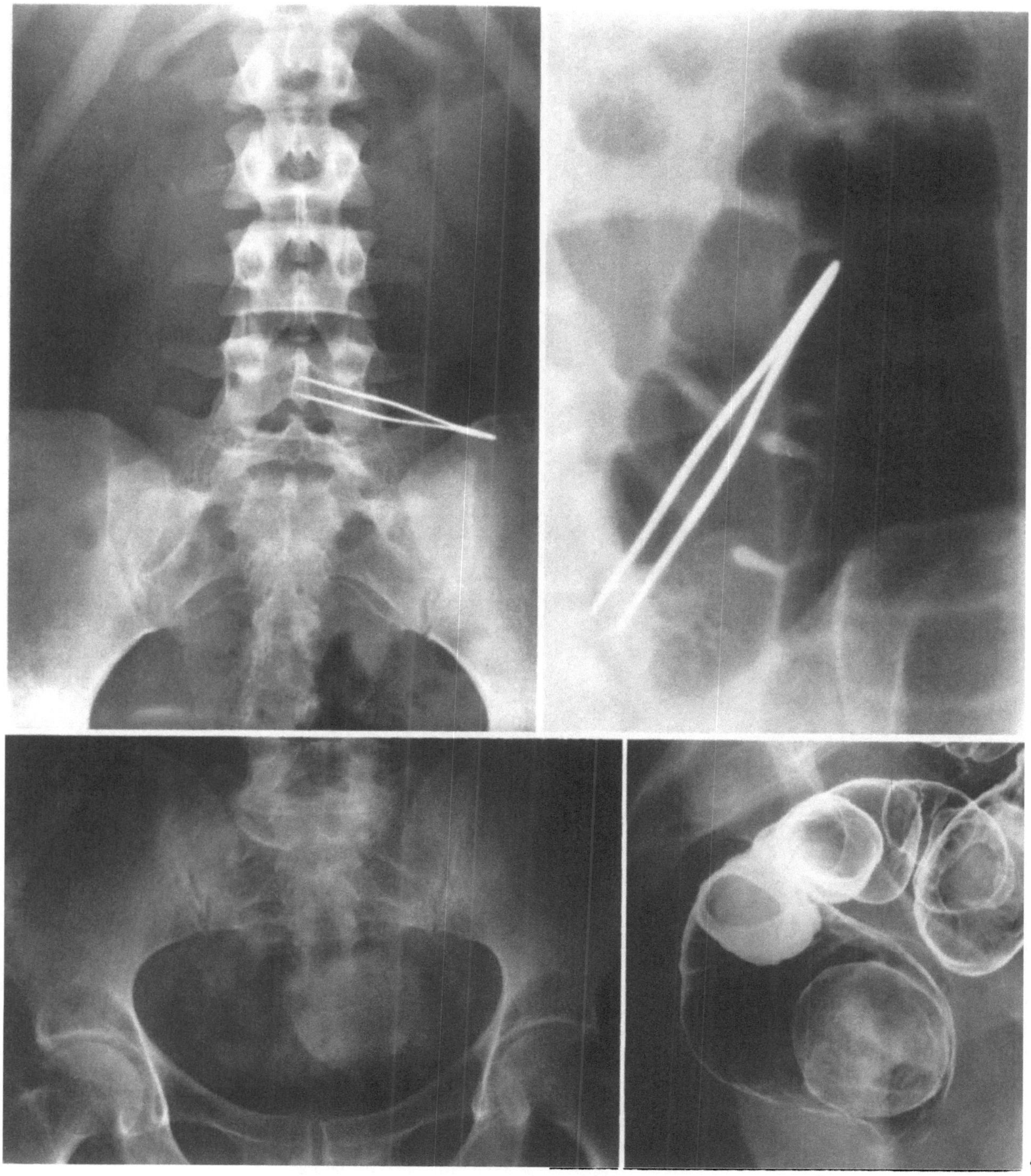

c d e f

Fig. 106a–f. Foreign bodies introduced rectally.
a, b Radiograph taken 6 h after a 25-year-old man inserted a vibrator into the rectum. The cylinder migrated into the sigmoid colon, where it became lodged and could not be mobilized rectoscopically. It had to be removed through a laparotomy. **c** Woman, 20 years of age, who "accidentally sat on a pair of tweezers, which disappeared in the rectum." *Supine film* shows a metal forceps projected over the left lower quadrant and midabdomen, which cannot be localized to a specific segment of the bowel. **d** The colon was carefully dilated with insufflated air, but the forceps migrated further orad into the splenic flexure. Next day the object was passed naturally, and surgery was not required. **e** Rectal coprolith. Woman, 78 years old, with a palpable rectal mass. Proctoscopic examination was normal! Supine film shows a radiopaque mass of unknown origin projected onto the lesser pelvis. **f** *Contrast enema* shows a freely mobile, smoothly marginated coprolith with an elliptical shape

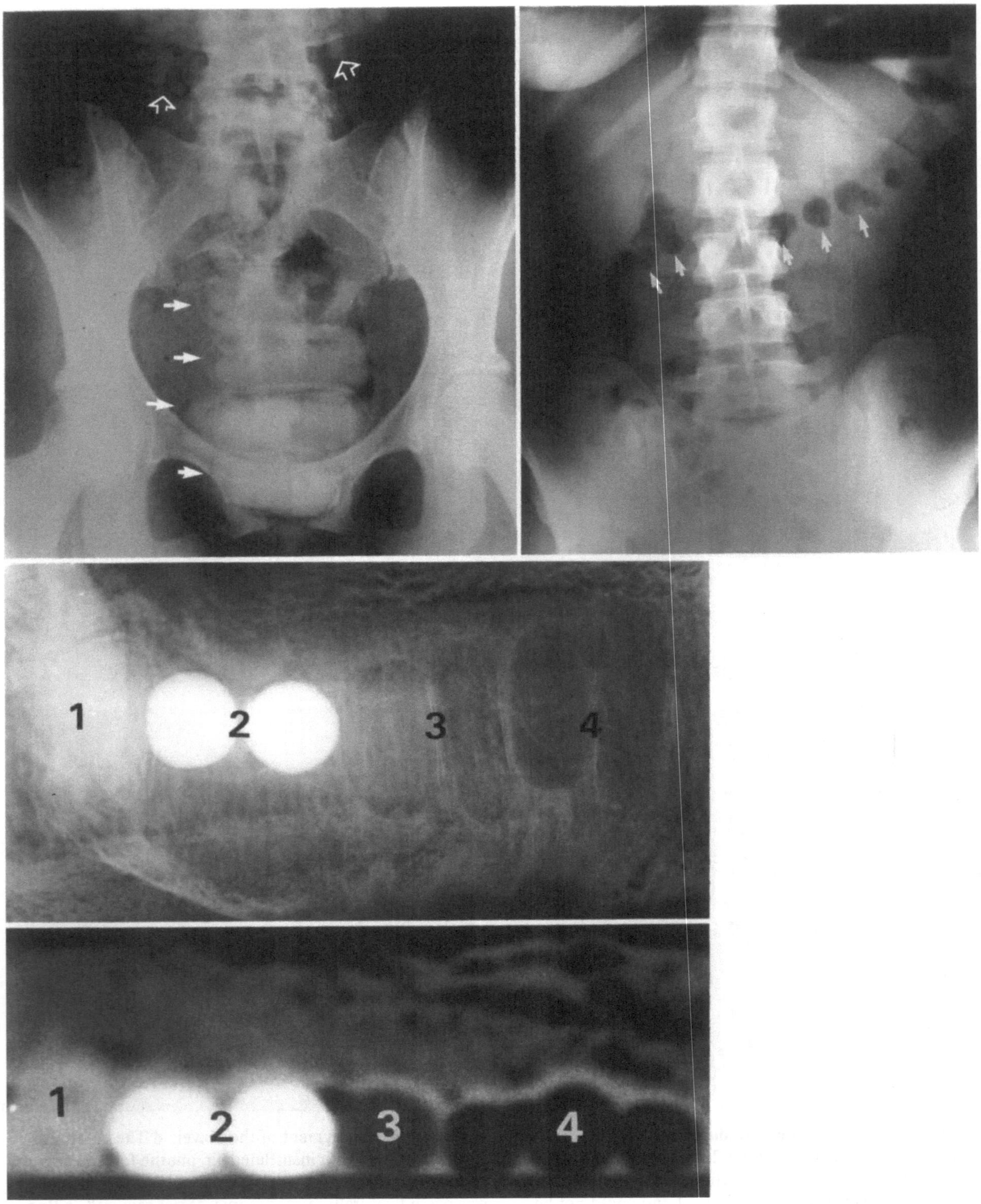

a b c d

Fig. 107 a-d. Intraintestinal foreign bodies in drug smugglers (body packing).
a Woman, 31 years old, referred by police on suspicion of drug ingestion. Supine film reveals four foreign bodies measuring about 7 × 3 cm in the rectum (→) and multiple, small, oval foreign bodies of near-osseous density about 3 × 1 cm in size within the transverse colon (⇒), representing hashish-filled condoms. All the foreign bodies are surrounded by a thin air film, representing the air trapped between the layers of the multiply wrapped drug items. There were no signs of intoxication or bowel obstruction. While the patient was hospitalized, 4 large packets weighing 30 g each and 20 smaller packets weighing 7 g each were passed per rectum. **b** Woman, 24 years old, drew attention to herself by frequent trips to the Middle East and was arrested by border police on suspicion of drug smug-

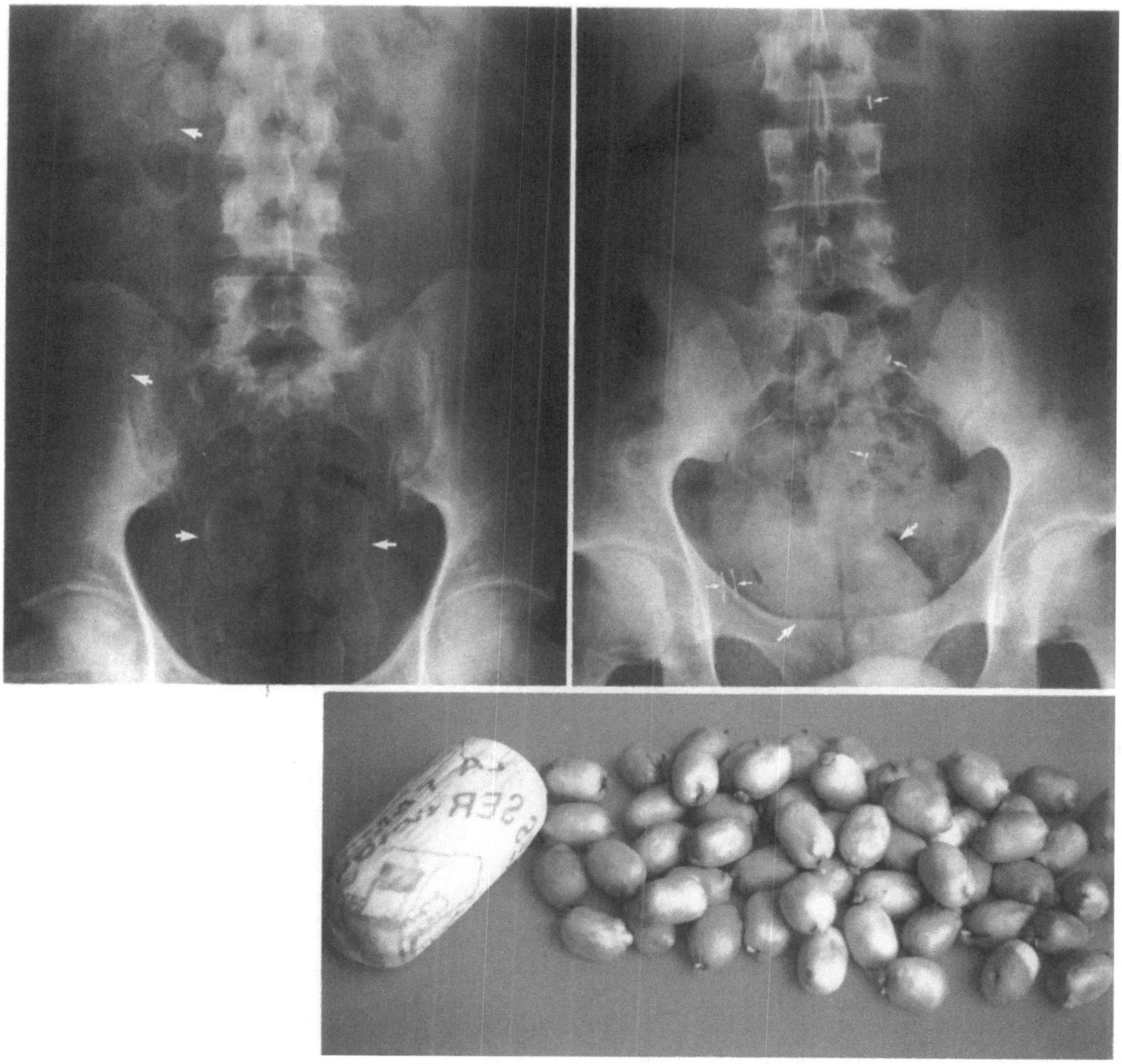

a b c

Fig. 108 a–e. Intraintestinal foreign bodies in drug smugglers (body packing).
a *Supine film* in a 33-year-old man shows multiple, round foreign bodies surrounded by a thin border occupying the colon and rectum (→). Within 2 days the patient passed 86 balloons, each containing 4 g of cocaine. When the balloons were opened, it was found that the cocaine had been wrapped in two layers of plastic separated by a thin sheet of aluminum foil; this created the border effect seen on the X-ray. **b** *Supine film* in a 24-year-old man reveals a sharply marginated foreign body projected onto the rectum, (→) and multiple clips of metallic density projected onto the lower and midabdomen (→). The patient had no history of previous surgery. **c** The larger foreign body in the rectum, measuring 10 × 5 cm, contained 150 g of cocaine. The metallic clips were attached to 55 balloons, each containing 4 g of cocaine. The balloons themselves were not visualized on the plain radiograph.

Fig. 107 (continued)
gling. *Supine film* shows numerous, rounded, airlike structures about 2 cm in diameter within the transverse colon (→), later identified as heroin-filled condoms. The objects were identified solely by their multiplicity and uniform shape, since heroin, unless mixed with other substances, has the same appearance as bowel gas on abdomen plain films. **c** In vitro roentgen appearance of specimens embedded in a watery cellulose paste (*1,* stool; *2,* hashish; *3,* cocaine; *4,* heroin). **d** *CT scans* of the four specimens

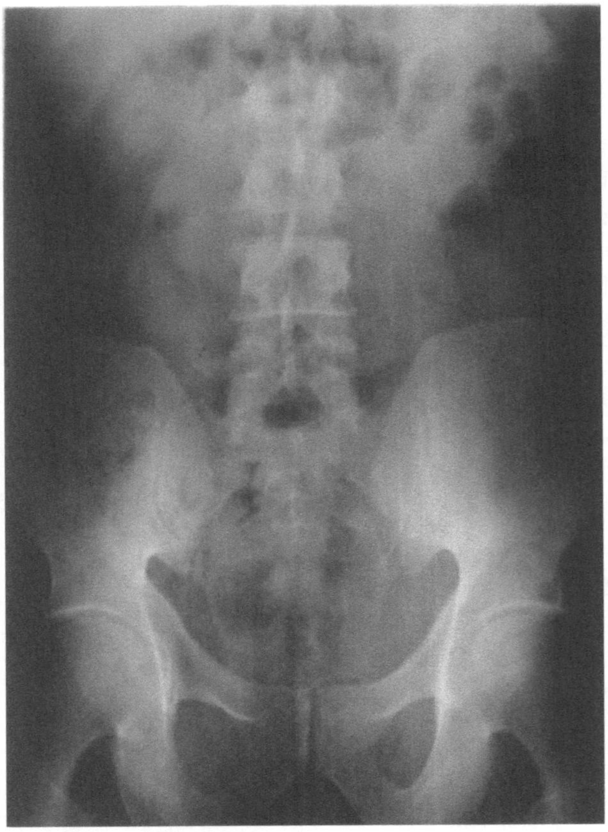

d

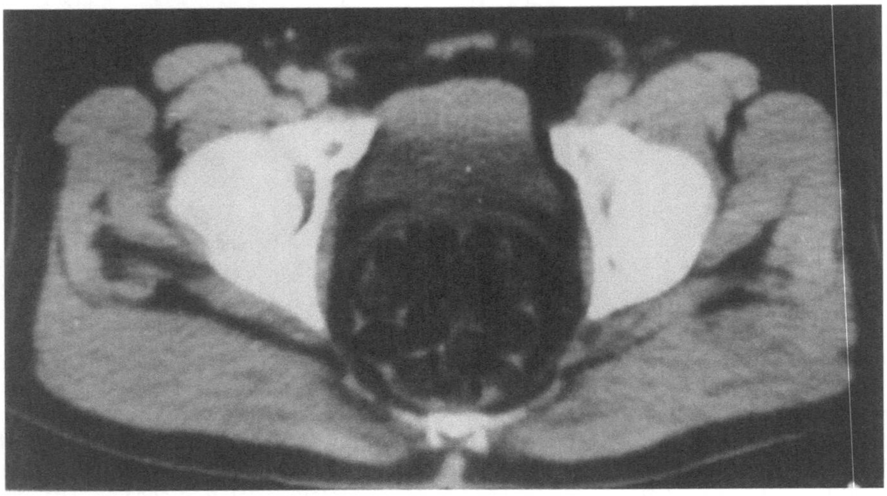

e

Fig. 108 (continued)
d *Supine film* of a 46-year-old man suspected of body packing shows no evidence of intraintestinal foreign bodies. **e** Abdominal *CT scan* reveals multiple, rounded foreign bodies of low density in the markedly distended rectum. Later the suspect passed 106 balloons per rectum, each filled with 5 g of cocaine (Dr. A. J. Kerschot, Department of Radiology, Akademisch Ziekenhuis Antwerpen, Belgium)

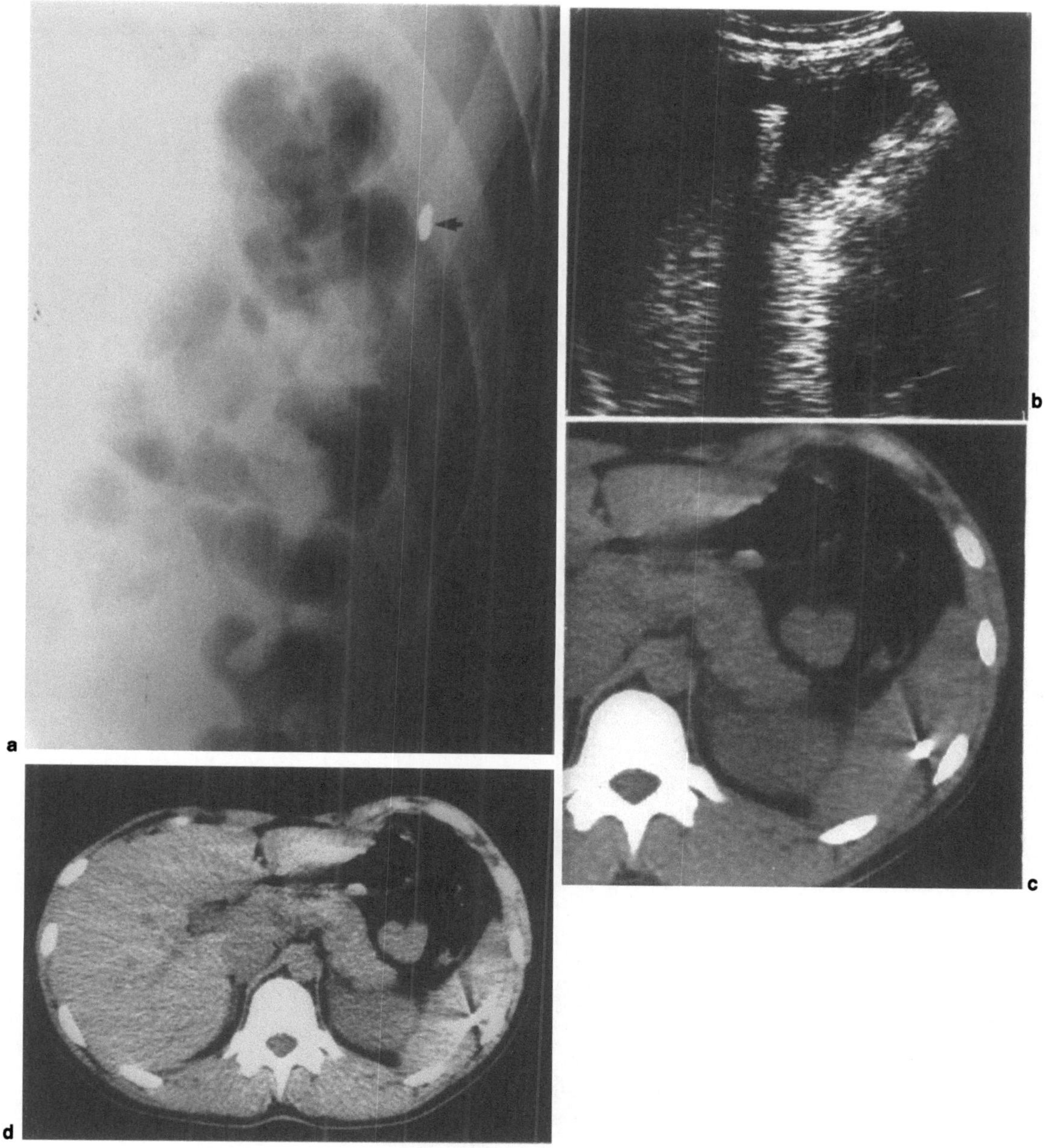

Fig. 109a-d. Indriven metal fragment in the spleen. Man, 26 years old, felt a sudden, stabbing pain in the left side while working with a hammer. The pain was intensified by forced inspiration. **a** *Spot film* of the left upper quadrant shows a metal fragment in position of the spleen that moves with respirations (→). **b** Left lateral *ultrasound scan* of the upper left quadrant shows a small intrasplenic lesion with reverberation echoes and a parasplenic fluid collection. **c, d** *CT scans* show a metallic foreign body lodged in the parenchyma of the spleen. Parasplenic fluid is not visualized

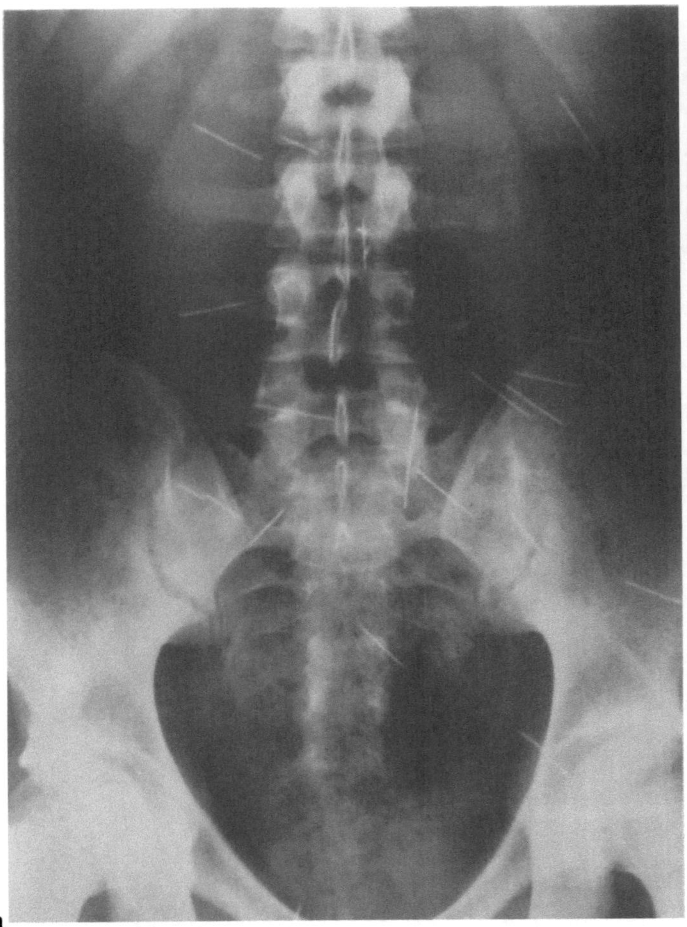

a

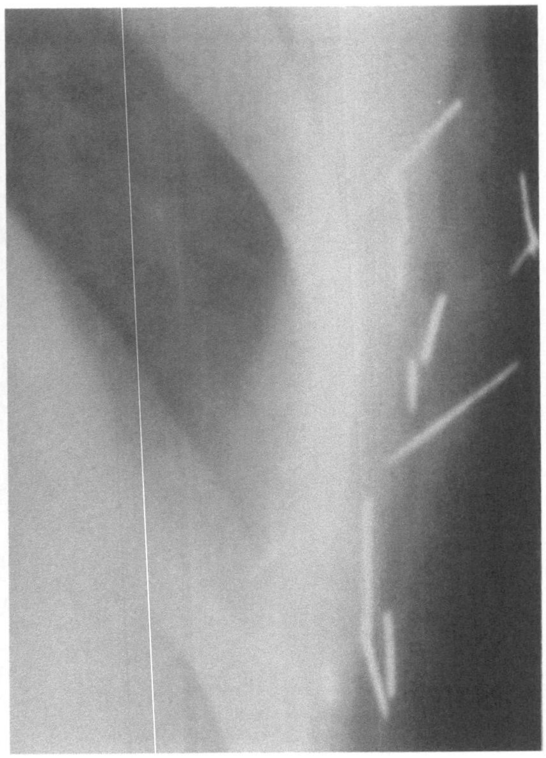

b

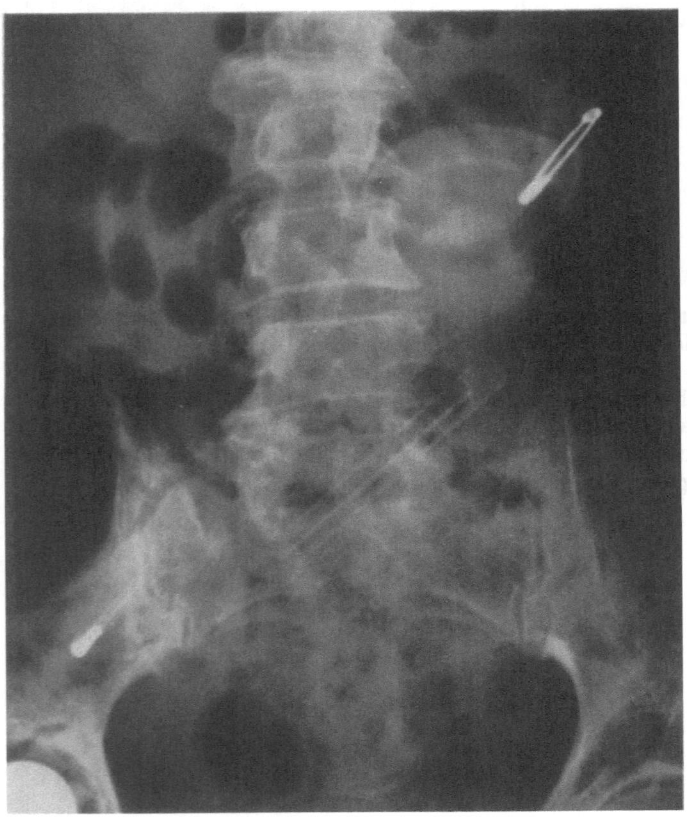

c

Fig. 110 a–c. Apparently intra-abdominal foreign bodies.
a Multiple straight pins in the abdominal skin of a 30-year-old female psychiatric patient. The patient also admits to having swallowed straight pins. *Supine film* shows multiple needles of metallic density, some broken, projected over the abdomen.
b *Spot films* show that all the metallic foreign bodies are embedded in subcutaneous fat. Some are already broken. **c** Woman, 72 years old, who underwent abdominosacral rectal amputation. *Supine film* shows a broken fever thermometer, a safety pin, and a ringlike structure of soft-tissue density projected over the mid-to lower abdomen. All the foreign bodies are *external to* the patient. The ringlike feature is a colostomy bag with a safety pin. The broken fever thermometer lay between the patient and the sheet used to lift the patient

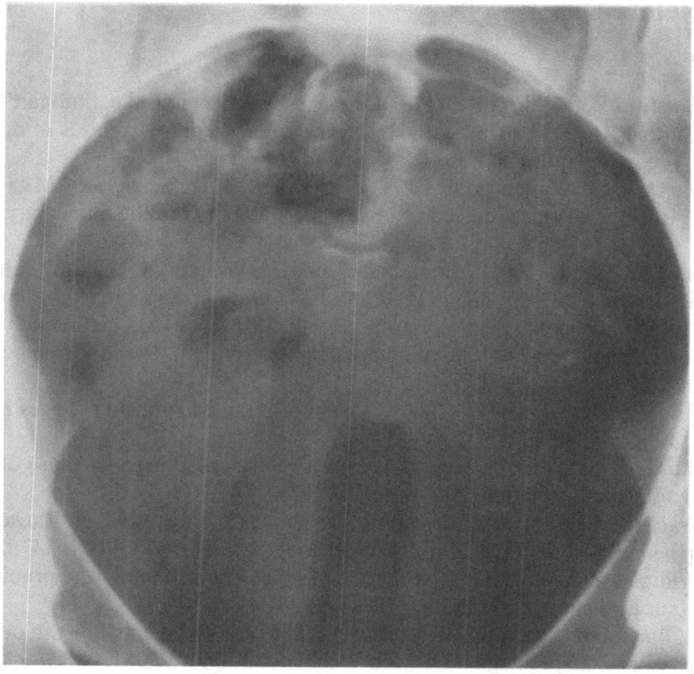

a

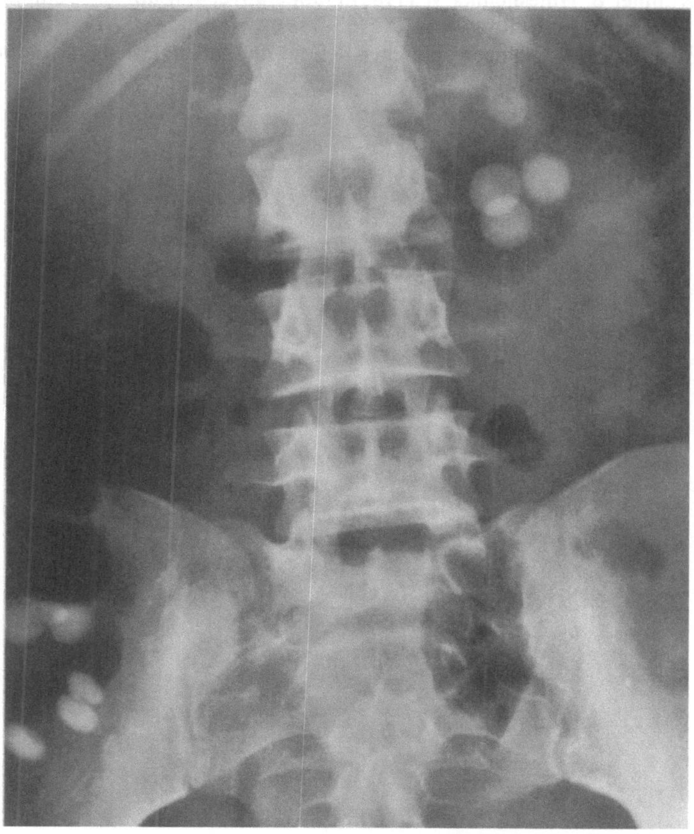

b

Fig. 111 a, b. Foreign bodies without pathologic significance introduced by the patient.
a Woman, 21 years of age, with an intravaginal tampon, which presents as a gas-containing structure projected over the lesser pelvis.
b Radiopaque tablets in the gas-filled stomach and ascending colon

References

Botsford WT, Wilson RE (1981) The acute abdomen. Enke, Stuttgart

Gardner JE, Tevetogla F (1957) The roentgenographic diagnosis of dirt eating (geophagia) in children. J Pediatr 51: 667-72

Kersschot EAJ, Beaucourt LEA, Degryse HRM, De Schepper AMAP (1985) Roentgenological detection of cocaine smuggling in the alimentary tract. ROFO 142/3: 295-298

McCort JJ (ed) (1981) Abdominal radiology. Williams & Wilkins, Baltimore

Meyers MA, Ghahremani GG, Gold BM (1984) Postoperative abdominal abscesses - Retention of surgical foreign bodies. In: Meyers MA, Ghahremani GG (eds) Iatrogenic gastrointestinal complications. Springer, Berlin Heidelberg New York Tokyo

Robinson KB, Levin EJ (1966) Erosion of retained surgical sponges into the intestine. AJR 96: 339-43

Sturdy JH, Baird RM, Gerein AN (1967) Surgical sponges: a cause of granuloma and adhesion formation. Ann Surg 165: 128-134

Wackerle B, Rupp N, Clarmann M, et al. (1986) Nachweis von Rauschgiftpäckchen beim "Body-Packer" durch bildgebende Verfahren. ROFO 145/3: 274-277

Williams RG, Bragg DG, Nelson JA (1978) Gossypiboma - the problem of the retained surgical sponge. Radiology 129: 323-26

Willmen HR, Schneider W, Löffler A (1984) Der "Magenballon" in der Behandlung der Adipositas permagna. Dt Med Wochenschr 109: 1200-1202

Wimmer B, Hillesheimer W (1985) Präoperativer Einsatz der Computertomographie bei Fremdkörpern. Radiologe 25: 135-138

Zilch HG (1985) Ungewöhnlicher Befund im Gallenblasenbett. Radiologe 25: 139-140

4 Major Diseases Associated with Acute Abdomen and Their Accessibility to Diagnostic Imaging

4.1 Acute Inflammatory Abdominal Diseases

4.1.1 Acute Cholecystitis

D. BEYER, R. LORENZ

Etiology and Pathogenesis
The cause of acute cholecystitis in more than 90% of cases is obstruction of the cystic duct by a stone (primary abacterial chemical inflammation with high internal pressure).
Primary infectious "acalculous" cholecystitis caused by stasis of bile flow is rare, with an incidence of less than 10% (severely ill patients on parenteral nutrition with stagnation and inspissation of bile fluid).

Note: Of the 20 million persons with gallstones in the United States of America, 50% are asymptomatic or have only mild, usually nonspecific complaints. Of these, 30% develop an acute cholecystitis *after* several episodes of colic; only 7% are asymptomatic *before* acute cholecystitis supervenes. This underscores the importance of *history taking* in these patients.

Clinical Symptoms
Nausea, vomiting, fever, leukocytosis, possibly mild jaundice. Local tenderness below the right costal arch. Abdomen is nonrigid, bowel sounds are normal or decreased. A palpable resistance is noted with empyema und hydrops.

Note: Biliary colic in the right upper quadrant due to an obstruction of the cystic duct usually subsides after a few hours (and spasmolytic treatment) (Fig. 112a). In *acute cholecystitis* the pain *increases* due to distension of the gallbladder, inflammation of the wall, and ischemia.

Complications
Gallbladder empyema, perforation with diffuse peritonitis, cholangitis, pancreatitis, septicemia, perforation of a stone into the bowel with gallstone ileus, pericholecystitic, intra- und subhepatic abscess

Radiologic Signs

Plain Radiographs

Demonstration of a calculus in the right upper quadrant (Figs. 90, 91, 112a)

Caution: Only 15% of all stones are sufficiently calcified to be visible on plain radiographs!

- Porcelain gallbladder
- Limy bile (with fluid level on L Lat film)
- Gas in the wall of the gallbladder } emphysematous cholecystitis
- Gas in the lumen of the gallbladder } (Fig. 114)

Note: Thirty percent of all patients with emphysematous cholecystitis have diabetes. Males predominate by a 5:1 ratio.

- Distension limited to the colon
- Distension limited to the duodenum (usually evidence of accompanying pancreatitis) (see Fig. 119)
- Indentation of the right colic flexure by the enlarged gallbladder (visible as a soft-tissue density) (Figs. 89, 112e)

Contrast Examination

Nowadays oral or infusion cholangiocholecystography has been completely *replaced* by real-time sonography in acute diagnosis.

Sonography

Note: A major symptom of acute cholecystitis (present in more than 90% of cases) is local tenderness to pressure from the ultrasound transducer over the gallbladder (positive sonographic Murphy sign).

- Thickened, echogenic gallbladder wall with a hypoechoic margin (50%-75% of cases) (Figs. 112, 113)
- Indistinct contour of the gallbladder wall (Fig. 112c)
- Small pericholecystitic fluid collections around the gallbladder fundus (approx. 10%) (Figs. 112c, d, 113a, c)
- Stones within the gallbladder that are movable and (if large enough) cast acoustic shadows
- Stone obstructing the cystic duct, producing hydrops of the gallbladder (rounded organ, transverse diameter >4 cm)
- Echogenic sediment in the lumen (inspissated bile or pus) (Fig. 113a-c)
- Rarely, free intraperitoneal fluid signifying a free perforation
- With gas in the gallbladder lumen (emphysematous cholecystitis): acoustic shadowing and reverberations behind the gas bubbles (easily overlooked!) (Fig. 113c)

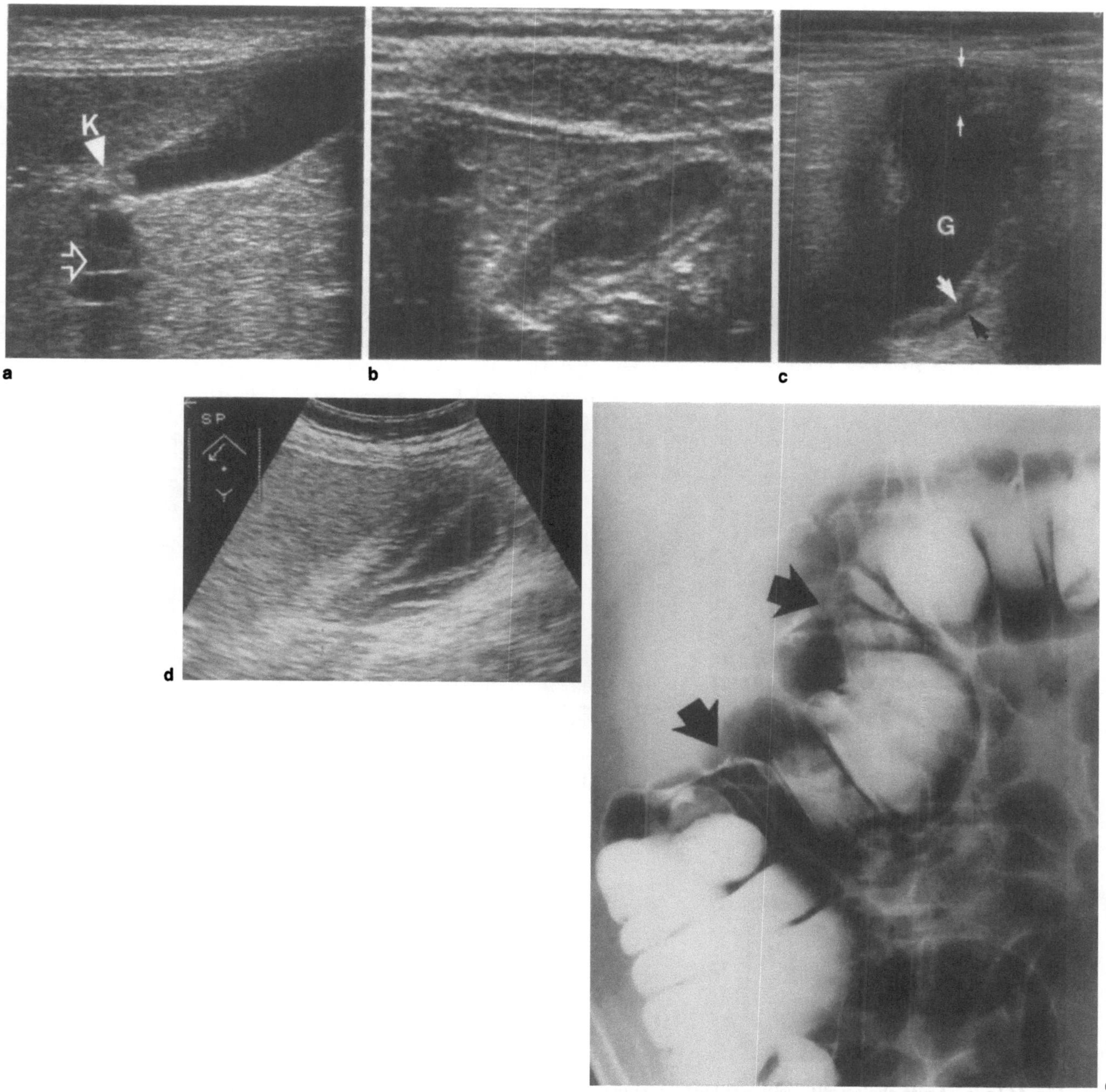

a b c d e

Fig. 112. a Acute cholecystitis.
Acute biliary colic in a 35-year-old women; patient was not febrile. *Sonogram* (longitudinal scan through the right hepatic lobe and gallbladder) shows a calculus (*K*▶) with an accompanying acoustic shadow (⇨) lodged in the infundibulum; the stone is immobile with position changes. There is no evidence of gallbladder hydrops at this time. **b** Woman, 49 years of age, with spontaneous right upper quadrant pain and fever. *Sonogram* (longitudinal scan through the gallbladder and right hepatic lobe) shows a thickened, hypoechoic wall with a partially irregular outer contour and a relatively echogenic inner contour. No calculi are visible. Clinical and sonographic findings indicate cholecystitis. **c** Man, 54 years of age, with increasing epigastric pain, biliary colic 12 h earlier, tenderness in the gallbladder bed, and fever. *Sonogram* (longitudinal scan through the gallbladder) shows a distended, hydropic gallbladder *(G)* with a markedly thickened, hypoechoic wall in the area of the fundus (→←) and the free wall to the abdominal cavity (→←). Part of the wall is not delineated. There also is an obstructing stone in the infundibulum (not shown). *Operation* disclosed gallbladder hydrops by a cystic duct stone with gangrenous cholecystitis. **d** Necrotizing cholecystitis in a 35-year-old man being treated with dacarbazine (DTIC), vincristine, and bleomycin for metastasizing malignant melanoma. Patient had slight tenderness in the gallbladder area. *Sonogram* shows thickening of the gallbladder wall and fluid around the gallbladder. The diagnosis of necrotizing cholecystitis was confirmed at operation. **e** *Supine film* (with contrast enema) shows massive displacement and indentation of the right colic flexure with double contouring (➧) caused by sonographically confirmed gallbladder hydrops (not shown)

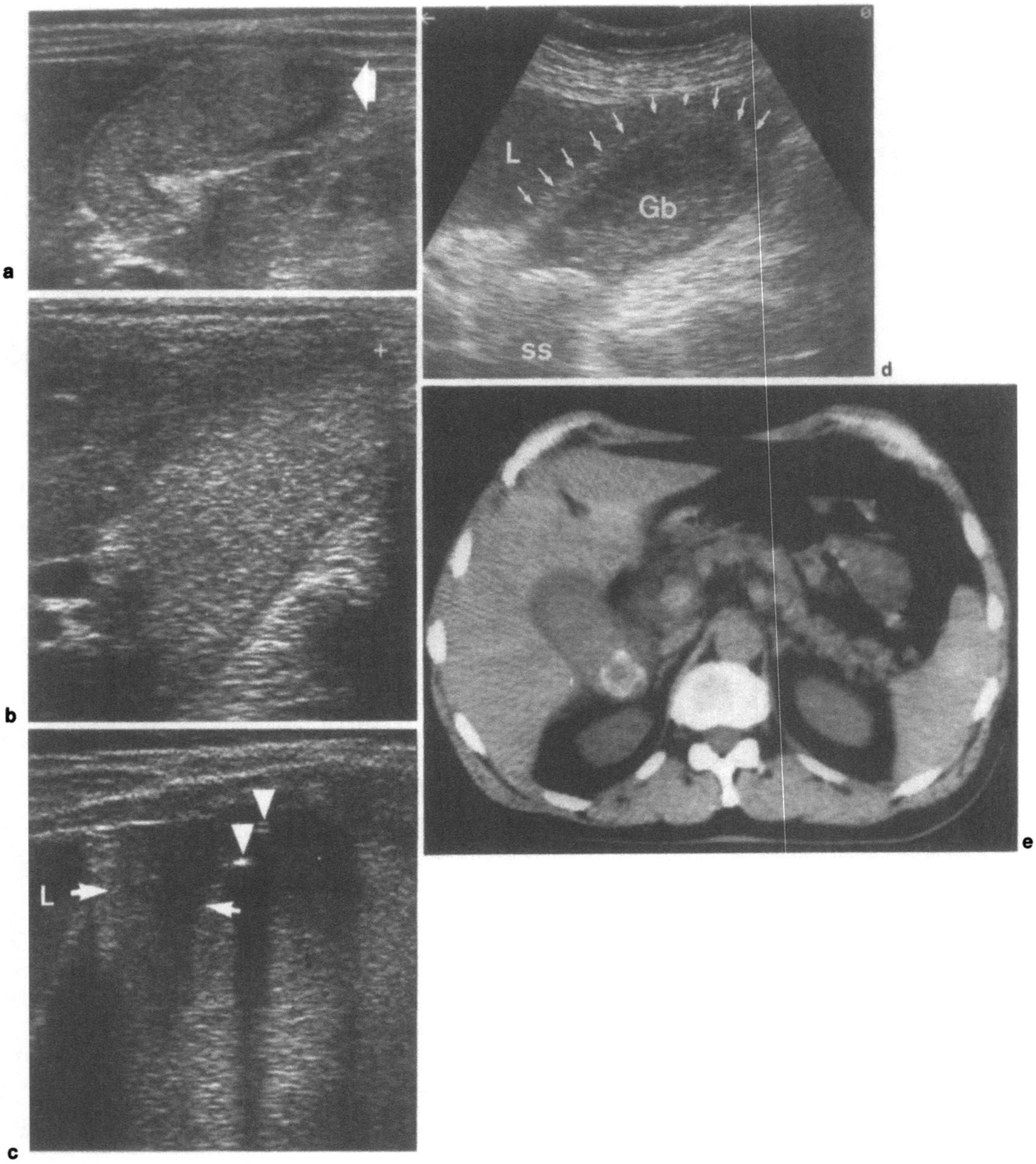

Fig. 113 a–e. Acute cholecystitis with gallbladder empyema. **a** Woman, 49 years old, receiving cytostatic therapy. *Sonogram* (longitudinal scan through the right hepatic lobe and gallbladder) depicts the gallbladder as a solid mass. The hypoechoic area on the fundus (➧) signifies a gangrenous wall swelling and impending perforation. *Operation* disclosed gangrenous cholecystitis and a pus-filled gallbladder. **b** Man, 55 years old, with tenderness in the right upper quadrant, low-grade fever, and hypoperistalsis. *Sonogram* (longitudinal scan through right hepatic lobe and gallbladder) shows a hugely distended, "solid" gallbladder with minimal wall thickening. The cystic duct is obstructed by a stone (not shown). *Operation* disclosed gallbladder hydrops with empyema caused by an obstructing cystic duct stone. **c** Man, 60 years old, with massive tenderness in the epigastrium and local rigidity, fever, shown by *Sonogram* (longitudinal scan through the gallbladder). Sonography performed elsewhere failed to delineate the gallbladder. There is a large "solid" mass in the gallbladder region with anterior gas bubbles (▶) and posterior acoustic shadowing. A semiliquid mass (→) between the right hepatic lobe *(L)* and gallbladder displaces the gallbladder downward. *Operation* disclosed biliary empyema with gas formation and a subhepatic abscess. **d** Acute cholecystitis with empyema secondary to an obstructing stone in the cystic duct. Sonogram shows a moderately thickened gallbladder wall (→) and echogenic material within the gallbladder lumen *(Gb)*. Obstructing cystic duct stone with an acoustic shadow *(ss)*. **e** Woman, 54 years old, with acute epigastric pain, no fever, and sonographically confirmed cholecystolithiasis. *CT scan* reveals a large, calcified, layered calculus in the gallbladder, inspissated biliary fluid, and wall thickening. Gallbladder empyema was found at operation

Caution: In severe cases of acute cholecystitis with empyema, the lumen of the gallbladder may be filled with echogenic material (pus) that does not cast an acoustic shadow and does not form a sediment. The gallbladder then has the appearance of a solid organ. (Fig. 113b)

Radionuclide Imaging
Visualization of the common bile duct and small intestine with [$^{99}Tc^{m}$]IDA compounds within 60 min, with nonfilling of the gallbladder and cystic duct → cystic duct obstruction, giving indirect evidence (together with clinical and sonographic findings) of acute cholecystitis.

Note: The *most reliable* study for the detection of acute cholecystitis is the clinical examination combined with sonography.

Computed Tomography
CT is *not* a prime modality for the diagnosis of acute cholecystitis. However, if complications already exist (abscesses, acute pancreatitis), CT is the method of second choice (see Sects. 4.3 and 4.8) (Figs. 113e, 114a, b).

Emphysematous Cholecystitis

Cause
The major cause is cystic duct obstruction with ischemia and the growth of gas-producing organisms - mostly *Clostridium welchii* - although *E. coli* and *Klebsiella* species can also be causative.

Note: More than 30% of patients have pre-existing diabetes. Males predominate 5 : 1. Some patients do not have stone disease but instead have a primary ischemia with gangrene of the gallbladder and air in the bile ducts. This form has the greatest risk of perforation and a high mortality.

Clinical Symptoms
Nausea, vomiting, fever (one-third of patients are nonfebrile), leukocytosis. Local tenderness below the right costal arch. Nonrigid abdomen, decreased bowel sounds.

Caution: The clinical signs of emphysematous cholecystitis are much less pronounced than those of acute cholecystitis!

Radiologic Signs

Plain Radiographs
Films in both planes show gas in the wall and/or lumen of the gallbladder, which is enlarged. With a patent cystic duct there will also be gas in the bile ducts (Figs. 80a, 81d, 114a, c).

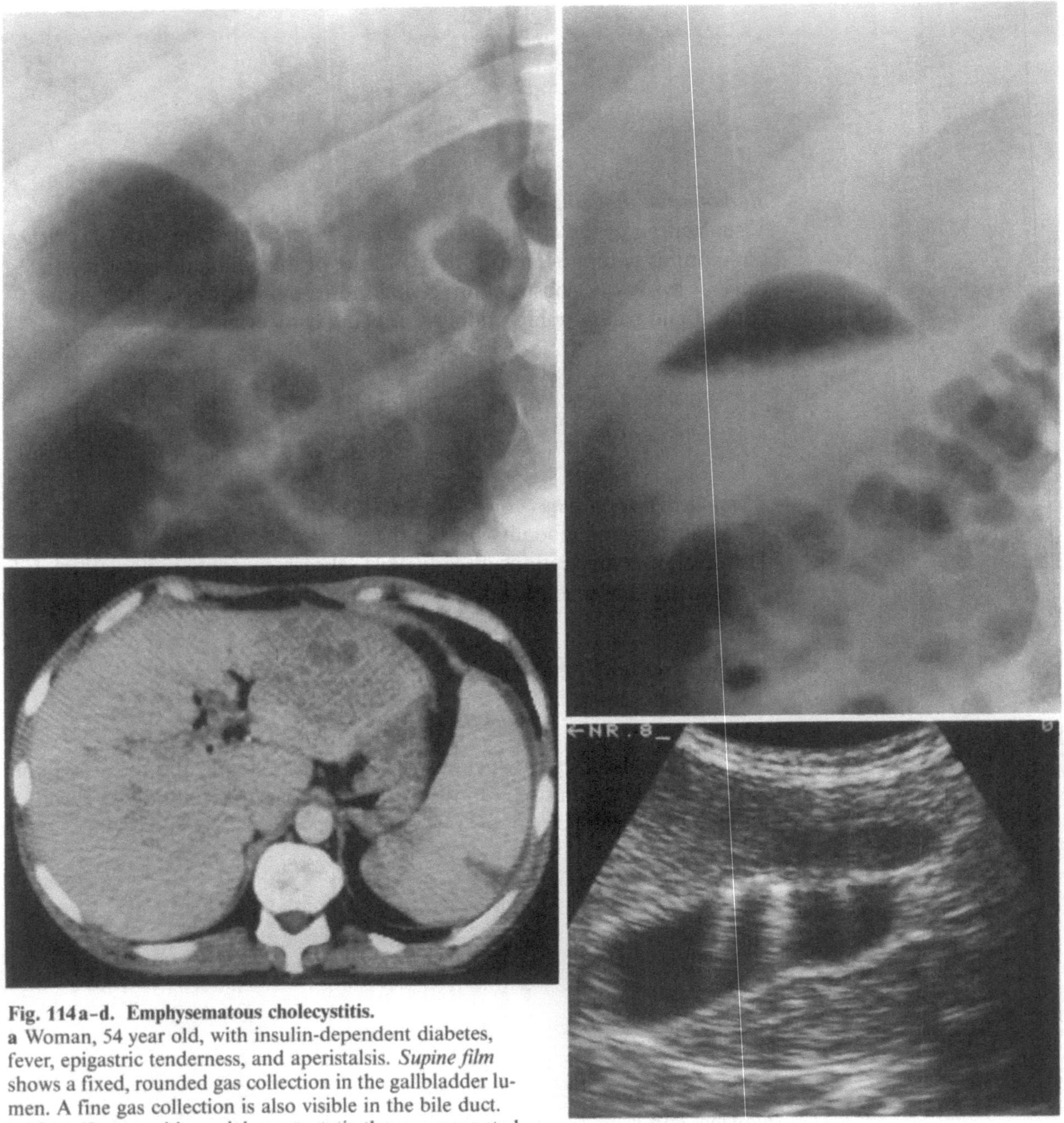

a b c d

Fig. 114a–d. Emphysematous cholecystitis.
a Woman, 54 year old, with insulin-dependent diabetes, fever, epigastric tenderness, and aperistalsis. *Supine film* shows a fixed, rounded gas collection in the gallbladder lumen. A fine gas collection is also visible in the bile duct. **b** Man, 48 years old, receiving cytostatic therapy presented with high fever, a diffusely tender and nonrigid abdomen, and aperistalsis. *CT scan* shows centrally gas-filled bile ducts, an enlarged left hepatic lobe with a low-density mass that appears even less dense centrally, and wedge-shaped, low-density areas in the spleen. *Diagnosis at autopsy:* gas-forming cholangitis with an abscess in the left hepatic lobe and a splenic abscess. Splenic infarction was also apparent. **c** *Erect spot film* demonstrates a fluid level in the gallbladder. *Operation* disclosed emphysematous cholecystitis with gas in the gallbladder lumen and bile ducts; calculi were not present. **d** Woman, 81 years old, with insulin-dependent diabetes. Sonogram shows small gas bubbles in the gallbladder wall with reverberant echoes

Sonography
Scans show a wide echo front in the gallbladder position with acoustic shadows and reverberations (Fig. 114 d). Intramural gas presents a string-of-beads pattern.

Computed Tomography
CT clearly shows the intramural or intracavitary gas collection and enables its assignment to the gallbladder. Air may be present in the bile ducts. CT will disclose even small neighboring abscesses (Figs. 80 c, 114 b).

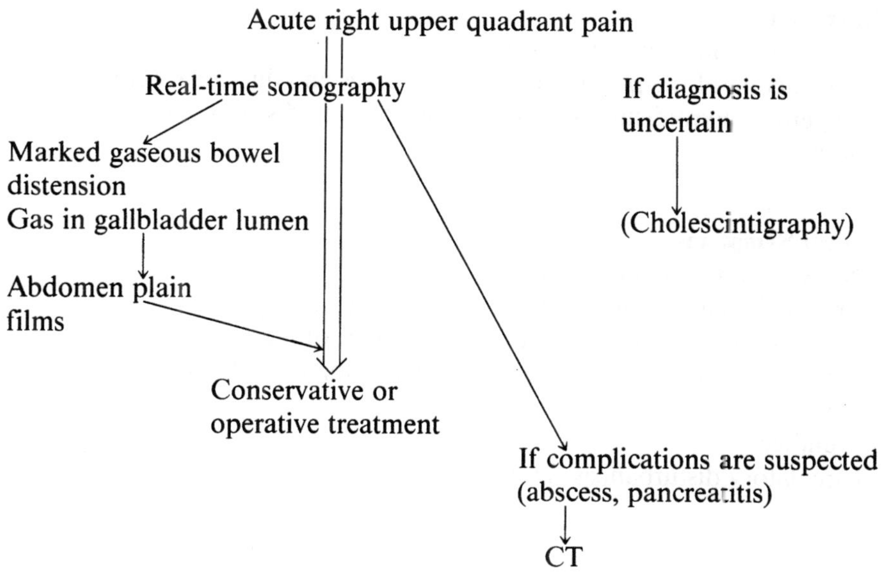

References

Beyer D, Friedmann G, Lorenz R (1983) Ersetzt die Real-time-Sonographie die konventionelle Röntgendiagnostik des biliären Systems? In: Otto RC, Xann FX (eds) Ultraschalldiagnostik 82 - Interventionelle Sonographie. Thieme, Stuttgart

Cohan RH, Mahony BS, Bowie JD, et al. (1987) Striated intramural gallbladder lucencies on US studies: predictors of acute cholecystitis. Radiology 164: 31-35

Frimann-Dahl J (1968) The acute abdomen. In: Strnad F (ed) Röntgendiagnostik des Digestionstraktes und des Abdomens. Springer, Berlin Heidelberg New York (Handbuch der med Radiologie, vol 11/2)

Jeffrey RB, Laing FC, Wong W, Callen PW (1983) Gangrenous cholecystitis: diagnosis by ultrasound. Radiology 148/1: 219-221

Laing FC (1983) Diagnostic evaluation of patients with suspected acute cholecystitis. Radiol Clin North Am 21/3: 477

Largiadèr F, Säuberli H, Wicki O (1983) Checkliste Viscerale Chirurgie. Thieme, Stuttgart

McCort JJ (ed) (1981) Abdominal radiology. Williams & Wilkins, Baltimore

Schulze PJ, Beyer D (1983) Sonographie der Gallenblase und Gallenwege. In: Bücheler E, Friedmann G, Thelen M (eds) Real-time-Sonographie des Körpers. Thieme, Stuttgart

Swart B (1977) Leerbauchdiagnostik des rechten Oberbauches. In: Frommhold W, Gerhardt P (eds) Erkrankungen der Organe des rechten Oberbauches. Thieme, Stuttgart

Way LW, Sleisenger MH (1978) Acute cholecystitis; Cholelithiasis and chronic cholecystitis. In: Sleisinger MH, Fordtran JS (eds) Gastrointestinal disease, 2nd edn. Saunders, Philadelphia, pp 1294-1313

Worthen NJ, Ulzler JM, Funamara JL (1981) Cholecystitis: prospective evaluation of sonography and 99 m-TC-HIDA-cholescintigraphy. AJR 137: 973

4.1.2 Acute Pancreatitis

U. MÖDDER, D. BEYER

Note: Morbidity from acute pancreatitis is on the rise in Western countries. Biliary and alcohol-related forms account for about 80%–90% of cases.

Other Causes
- Abdominal and surgical trauma
- Obstruction of the pancreatic duct by masses and duodenal diverticula
- Hyperparathyroidism, hyperlipidemia, collagen diseases, vascular diseases, etc.

Clinical Symptoms
- Nausea, vomiting, meteorism
- Epigastric pain (approx. 50% radiating to the back)
- Soft abdomen, deep tenderness; with intraperitoneal spread of pancreatic enzymes → diffuse muscular rigidity and hypoperistalsis
- Fever
- Jaundice
- Circulatory disturbances, shock

Note: Pancreatitis can take a *painless* course. A *rise of amylase* in the serum or urine is *not* always present, especially in the severe form of hemorrhagic-necrotizing pancreatitis. The degree of enzyme abnormality bears only a limited relation to the pathoanatomic severity of acute pancreatitis.

Classification by grades of severity: Clinical classification is based on the development of organ complications, response or lack of response to conservative therapy, and the general course of the illness. Attention is also given to the pattern of *laboratory parameters* in assessing severity (leukocyte count over 12000; hyperglycemia over 200 mg%; hypocalcemia less than 4 mmol; PO_2 less than 60 mm Hg). The pathoanatomic status of the organ can be assessed on the basis of these values.
Three grades of severity are recognized:
- Acute edematous form (grade 1)
- Partial necrotizing form (grade 2)
- Total or subtotal necrotizing form (grade 3)

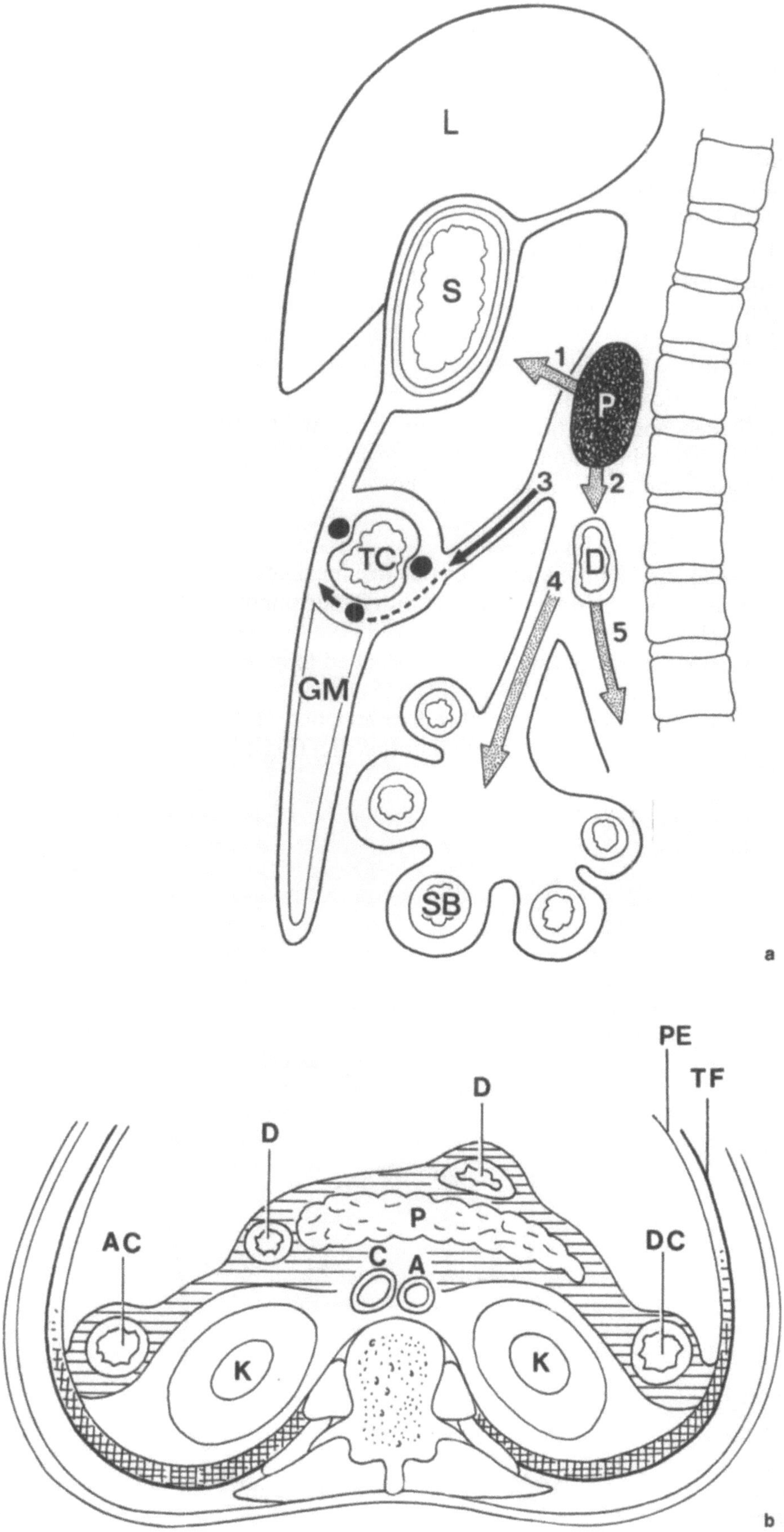

Fig. 115. a Pathways of spread of acute pancreatitis: 1, omental bursa→foramen of Winslow→peritoneal cavity; *2,* duodenum; *3,* transverse mesocolon; *4,* mesenteric root; *5,* retroperitoneal space; *P,* pancreas; *L,* liver; *S,* stomach; *TC,* transverse colon; *GM,* greater omentum; *SB,* small bowel. **b Principal details of the cross-sectional anatomy of the three extraperitoneal compartments that direct the spread of acute pancreatitis.** *Horizontal lines,* anterior pararenal space; *white area,* perirenal space; *cross-hatched area,* posterior pararenal space; *A,* aorta; *C,* inferior vena cava; *AC,* ascending colon; *CD,* descending colon; *D,* duodenum; *TF,* transverse fascia; *K,* kidneys; *P,* pancreas; *PE,* peritoneum

Radiologic Signs

Note: Findings from *ERCP* and *angiography* do *not* contribute to the diagnosis of acute pancreatitis.

Plain Radiographs

Important diagnostic signs relate to abnormal gas patterns and unusual fluid collections.
The *cardinal sign* of acute pancreatitis on the L Lat film is *duodenal atony.* There may be double contouring of the medial aspect of the duodenum caused by protrusion of the enlarged head of the pancreas (Fig. 10a, 116, 119a).

Nonspecific changes:
- Gasless abdomen (duodenal atony is apparent after giving gas-producing granules, e.g., Gastrovison)
- Distension of the small or large bowel

Additional signs (Fig. 117):
- "Halo sign" of the kidneys or positive renal corona, i.e., the adipose capsule of the kidneys contrasts with its surroundings (mostly left-sided; Fig. 118)
- Sentinel loop sign: an isolated, distended loop of small bowel in the left upper quadrant (unreliable) (Fig. 117)
- Colon cutoff sign, i.e., an abrupt termination of the air column in the colon at the left colic flexure (nonspecific) (Fig. 117)

Note: Plain film signs furnish *indirect* evidence of acute pancreatitis. The pancreas itself is not visible on plain radiographs and cannot be directly evaluated.

a

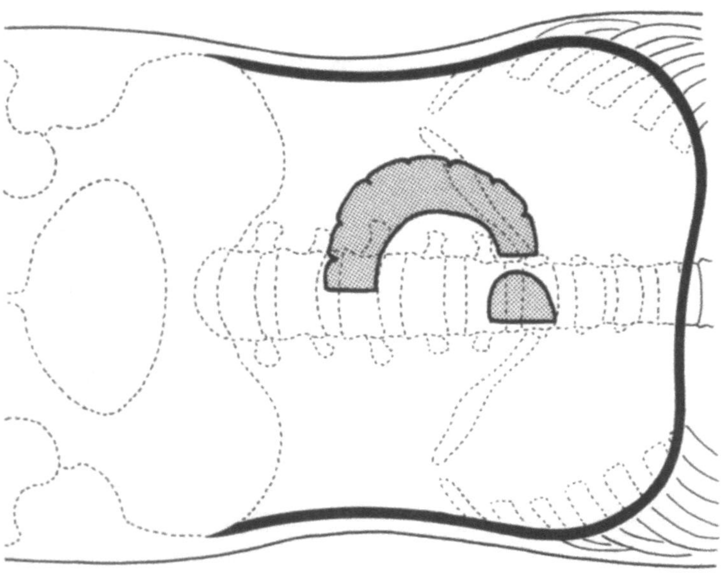

Fig. 116a-d (Legend see page 205)

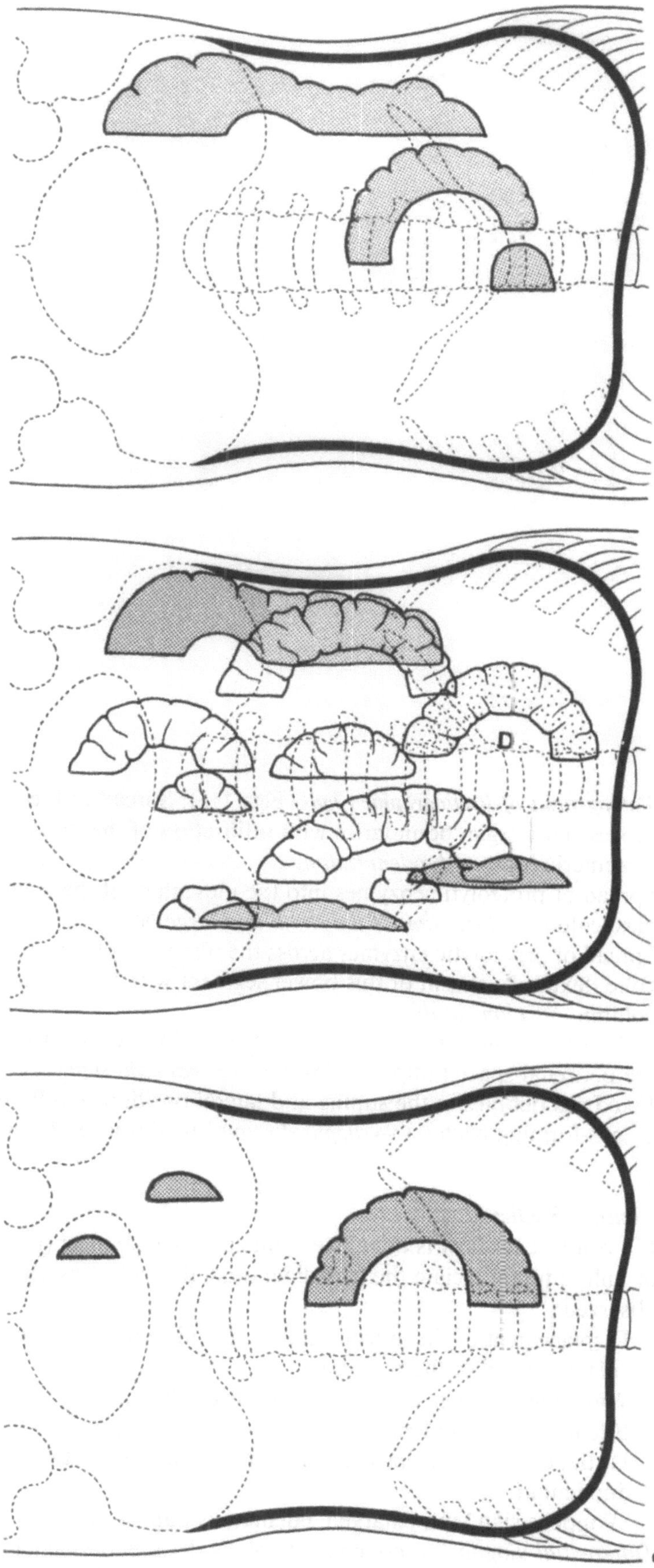

Fig. 116a-d. Left lateral plain film signs of acute pancreatitis.
a Distension limited to the duodenum with fluid levels in the lower duodenal flexure and gastric antrum. There may be enlargement of the pancreatic head with double contouring. **b** Duodenal distension combined with colonic distension and a fluid level in the ascending cecum as evidence of enzyme spread to the retroperitoneum and mesocolon. **c** Duodenal atony combined with small- and large-bowel distension as evidence of acute pancreatitis with spread of enzymes into the retroperitoneum, mesocolon, and small-bowel mesentery, or as a sign of intraperitoneal enzyme spread. **d** Duodenal atony with shorter fluid levels in the terminal ileum as evidence of mesenteric lymphadenitis

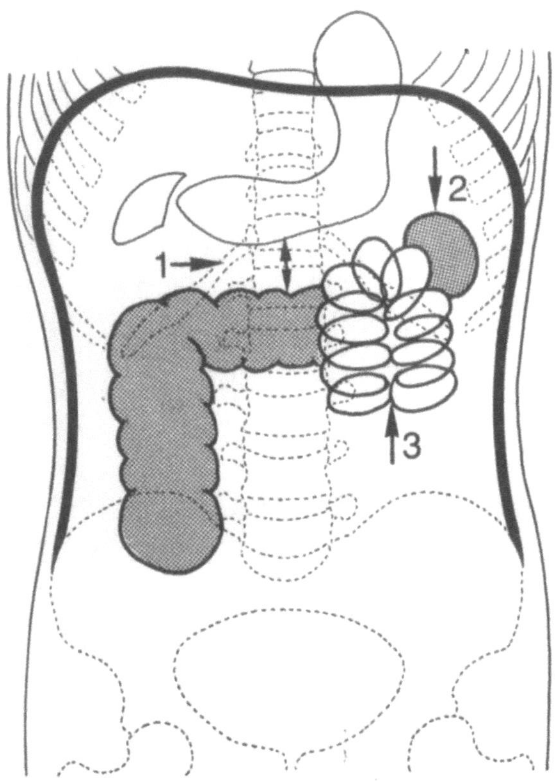

Fig. 117. Dubious radiological signs of acute pancreatitis. Generally these signs are *not* useful diagnostically. *1,* Increased gastrocolic distance; *2,* colon cutoff sign (abrupt termination of the air column at the left colic flexure); *3,* sentinel loop sign (localized, distended loop of small bowel in the left upper quadrant)

Pathogenesis of Radiographic Signs (Figs. 115): Spread of the inflammatory process past organ boundaries with infiltration of the duodenal wall and mesenteric root → *duodenal atony*
Spread of proteolytic enzymes into the mesentery of the small bowel and mesocolon → *distension of the small and large bowel*
Spread of proteolytic enzymes across the phrenicocolic ligament to the left colic flexure → spasm of this bowel segment with termination of the air column → *colon cutoff sign*
Collection of fluid in the anterior and posterior pararenal space, sparing the perirenal space (adipose capsule) → *renal halo sign*
Fixed gas bubbles in the supine and lateral position signify inflammation by gas-forming bacteria →*suppurative pancreatitis with abscess formation*

Contrast Studies

If a contrast swallow is done to exclude a duodenal ulcer (possibly because of failure to appreciate the true diagnosis), the following changes may be observed:

- Displacement of the antrum, stomach, and duodenal loop by the enlarged head of the pancreas
- Widening of the gastric mucosal folds on the greater curvature
- Edema of the duodenal mucosa
- Partial or complete obstruction of the horizontal portion of the duodenum
- "Poppel's sign" (an enlarged, edematous papilla of Vater)

Differential diagnosis: duodenitis, Crohn's disease, duodenal neoplasm, and intramural duodenal diverticula should be considered.

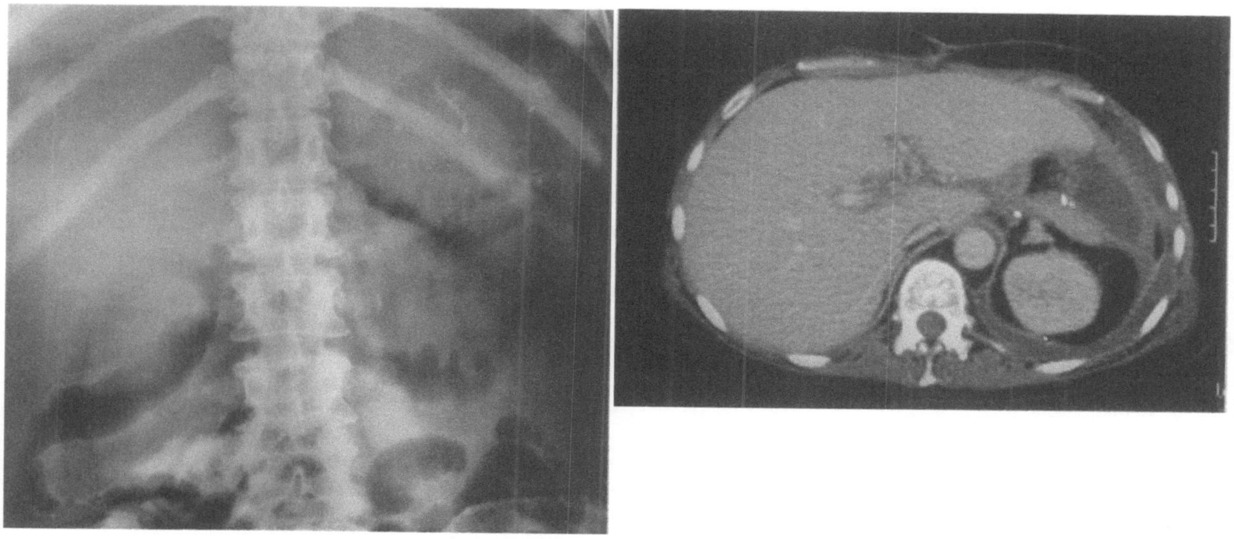

a b

Fig. 118a, b. Halo sign (positive renal corona) in pancreatic fistula.
Woman, 51 years old, who had undergone gastrectomy with esophagojejunostomy.
a *Supine film* shows the left kidney surrounded by a lucent border representing the fat capsule. **b** *CT scan* (with bolus injection) demonstrates the halo sign. The perirenal fat is accentuated by the presence of fluid in the anterior and posterior pararenal spaces due to a pancreatic fistula (confirmed at operation)

Sonography

Note: While the pancreas can be directly imaged with ultrasound, the full length of the organ *cannot* be visualized in all patients (obesity, overlying air). Nevertheless, the use of sonography is justified when there is suspicion of pancreatitis, because a negative study will obviate the need for further investigations, while a positive study will enable an initial assessment of disease severity.

Diagnostic criteria for evaluating the pancreas:
1. Size
2. Contour
3. Echogenicity

Acute edematous pancreatitis (grade 1) (Fig. 119b, c, d)
- Segmental or complete enlargement of the organ
- Indistinct organ boundaries that contrast poorly with the splenic vein and superior mesenteric vein
- Echogenicity diminished due to edema
- Duodenal atony and wall-thickening (Fig. 10b)

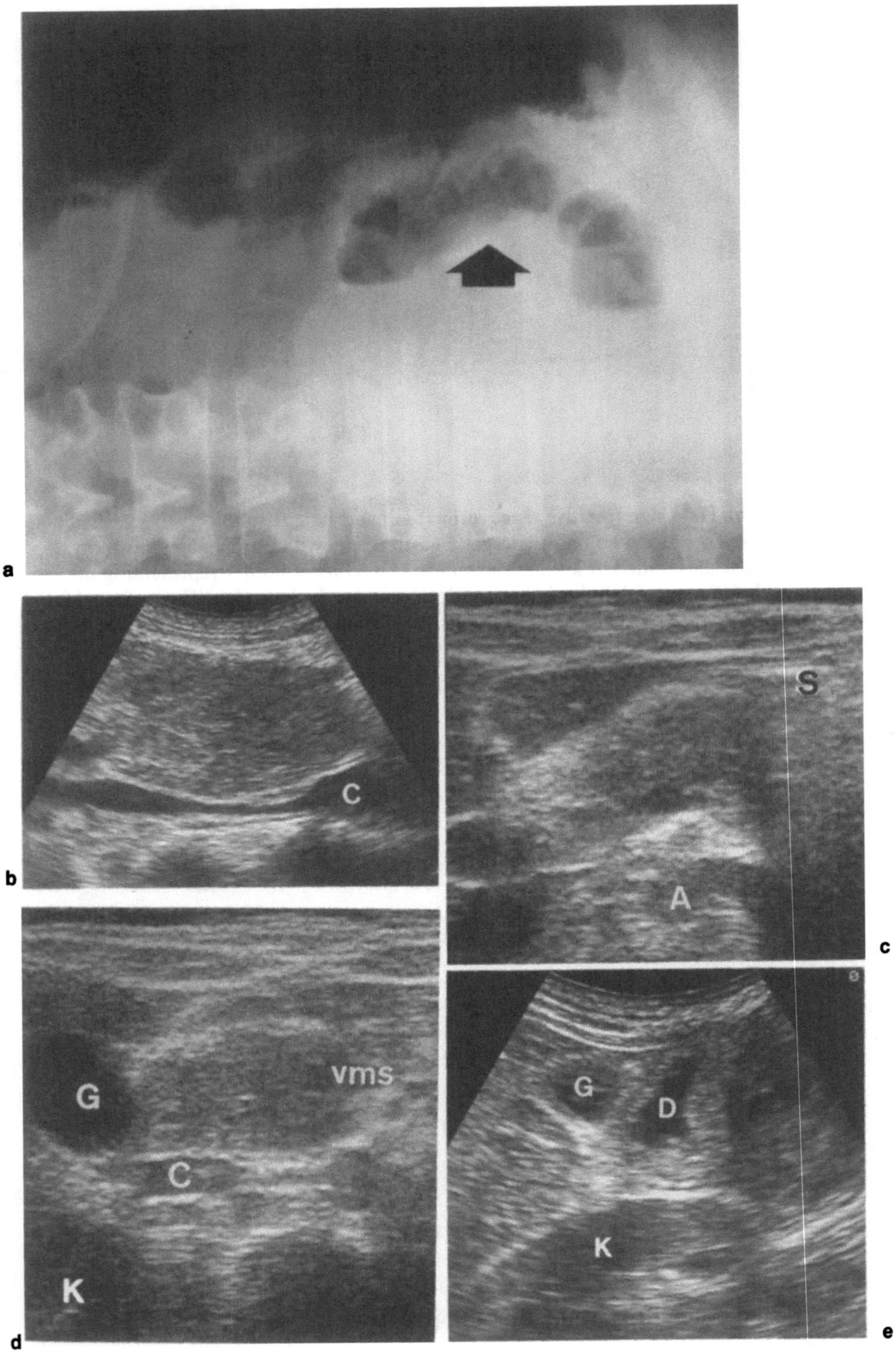

Fig. 119 a–f (Legend see page 209)

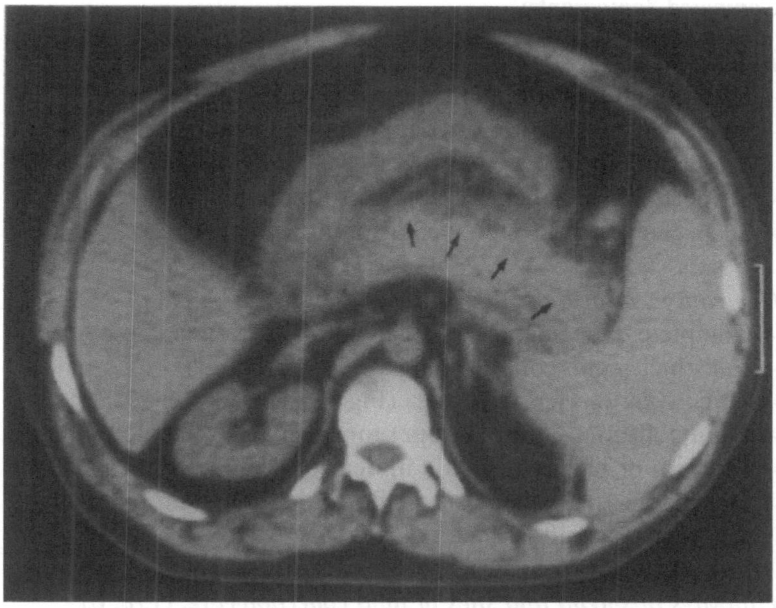

f

Fig. 119 a–f. Acute edematous pancreatitis in a 42-year-old man with nausea, vomiting, and epigastric pain radiating to the back; deep tenderness to pressure. **a** *Left lateral film* shows marked duodenal distension with fluid levels in the lower duodenal flexure and prepyloric antrum. The pancreatic head is markedly enlarged, and a pad sign is noted on the medial duodenal aspect (➡). There is accompanying colonic distension. **b** *Longitudinal sonogram* through the head of the pancreas shows marked distension of the head in the ap and longitudinal dimensions with an attenuated echo pattern. There is moderate compression of the inferior vena cava from anteriorly. **c** *Sonogram* (transverse scan through the body of the pancreas) shows a markedly distended, hypoechoic, and edematous corpus with slight anterior displacement of the stomach, *(S)*; *A*, aorta. **d** *Sonogram* (transverse scan through the head of the pancreas) shows moderate enlargement of the pancreatic head, which occupies the triangle between the gallbladder *(G)*, inferior vena cava *(C)*, and superior mesenteric vein *(vms)*; *K*, right kidney. **e** *Transverse sonogram* through the head of the pancreas shows edematous expansion of the head with reactive wall thickening of the atonic, fluid-filled duodenum *(D)* (*G*, gallbladder; *K*, right kidney). **f** *CT scan* shows a markedly widened pancreas with an indistinct surface contour (→); there is no evidence of high- or low-density areas in the parenchyma

Partial, subtotal, or total necrotizing pancreatitis (grades 2–3) (Fig. 120 a)
Characterized by the coexistence of

- Liquid necrotic, semiliquid, and solid tissue
- Spread beyond organ boundaries with edematous-exudative tissue changes along retroperitoneal planes; the large "tracks" in the anterior pararenal space are preferred; spread may be traced into the lesser pelvis
- Concomitant pleural effusions and ascites may occur
- In pancreatitis with abscess formation, there is superinfection with gas-forming bacteria. Main symptom: echo reverberations behind the gas in the area of inflammatory change

Note: Often the value of sonography in acute pancreatitis is compromised by meteorism, and the study must be supplemented by CT.

Computed Tomography

Indications

- Inability to delineate the pancreas with ultrasound
- Suspected progression of edematous pancreatitis to partial or total necrotizing form
- Suspected hemorrhage or abscess formation
- Suspected spread to the mediastinum

CT features of acute pancreatitis

- Complete or segmental enlargement of the organ (Figs. 119-121)
- Indistinct organ contours (Figs. 119f, 120b, 121)
- Thickening of Gerota's fascia (Fig. 122a)
- Fluid collection in the retroperitoneal space (see below) (Figs. 120-122)
- Uniform or patchy decrease in density (Figs. 120b, 121)
- Diverse picture of necrosis, hemorrhage, and solid parenchyma that accumulates contrast material (Fig. 121)

Pathways of spread and sites of fluid collection (Fig. 115a, b)

- Along the anterior and perhaps the posterior pararenal space, mostly on the left side. Usually fluid does not enter the perirenal space (halo sign on plain abdominal film) (Fig. 118)
- Along the psoas and iliacus muscles into the lesser pelvis, into the inguinal region, into the scrotum
- Into the right retroperitoneal space with involvement of the duodenum and efferent bile ducts
- Through the mesocolon to the transverse colon; into the mesentery of the small bowel along the mesenteric root
- In the direction of the omental bursa, anteriorly or into the subphrenic space; may produce necrotic foci in liver and spleen
- Craniad into the mediastinum, causing widening of the retrocrural space (Fig. 122)

Note: The localization of extrapancreatic fluid collections can be established on CT scans without administration of contrast media. The differentiation of viable from necrotic tissue is most easily accomplished by means of a *bolus injection*.

Caution: CT attenuation values are highly variable in acute pancreatitis due to variations in edema, cellular debris, hemorrhage, and necrosis.

Bolus injection

The i.v. bolus injection of renally excreted contrast material (e.g., amidotrizoate 65%, 40–50 ml) will opacify the organ parenchyma and vessels surrounding the pancreas (aorta, superior mesenteric artery and vein, splenic vein, portal vein) during the arterial and parenchymatous phase.

Larger areas of necrosis can be clearly delineated with i.v. contrast medium (Figs. 120b, 121).

Complete, uniform opacification signifies an acutely edematous, milder form of disease in which the peripancreatic reaction tends to be self-limiting.

Caution: The acute edematous form of pancreatitis (grade 1) may be negative even on CT scans. Necrotizing hemorrhagic pancreatitis (grades 2–3) is *always positive* on CT scans. Often a distinction cannot be made among the exudative, hemorrhagic, and suppurative forms.

Note: The CT features of acute pancreatitis do not always correlate with the clinical presentation! Therapeutic conclusions must be based on an evaluation of *all* clinical, laboratory, and morphologic parameters. It has proved useful to *monitor the course* of the illness with contrast-enhanced CT scans at frequent intervals.

a

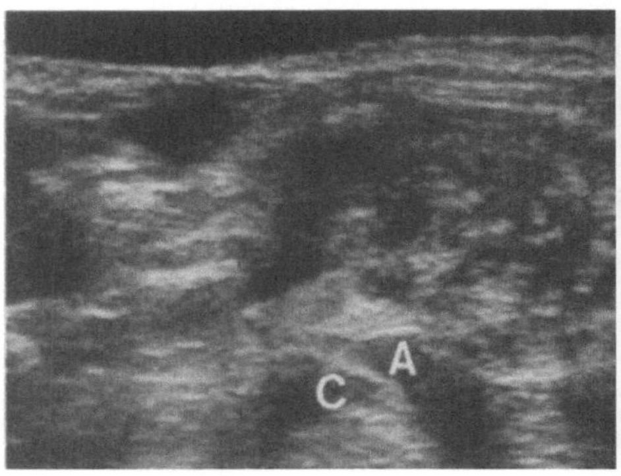

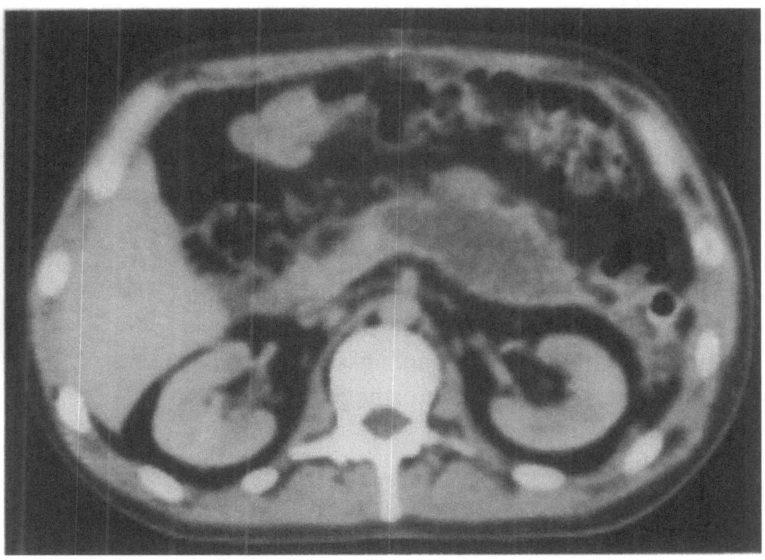

b

Fig. 120a, b. Grade 2 necrotizing pancreatitis.
a *Sonogram* (transverse scan through the body of the pancreas) shows a markedly widened and nonhomogeneous pancreas with displacement of the stomach and spread of fluid into the left anterior pararenal space; *C*, vena cava; *A*, aorta. **b** *CT scan* shows a marked, low-density expansion of the body and tail of the pancreas

a 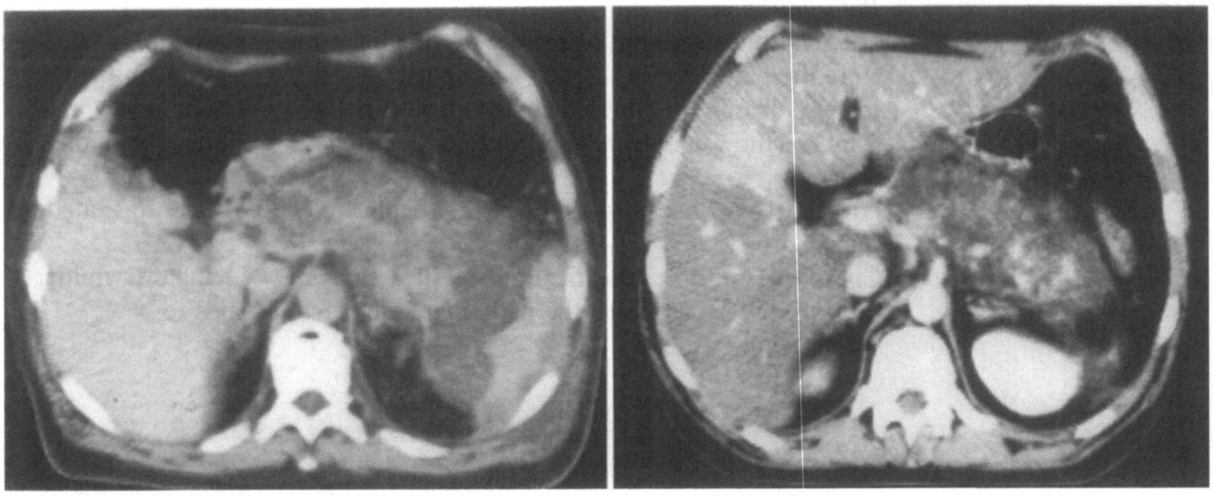 b

Fig. 121. a Grade 3 necrotizing hemorrhagic pancreatitis, characterized by marked fluid accumulation in the pancreatic bed with enlargement of the organ. Only "shreds" of the original parenchyma remain. The nonhomogeneity of the parenchyma is caused by hemorrhage. **b** *CT scan after bolus injection* shows nonhomogeneous contrast accumulation in the necrotic parenchyma of the pancreas

Complications of Acute Pancreatitis
- Shock
- Cardiovascular disturbances
- Pulmonary insufficiency
- Acute renal failure
- Gastrointestinal hemorrhage
- Encephalopathies
- Pseudocysts
- Ascites, pleural effusion
- Abscesses, infections, sepsis
- Hematemesis, melena

Pancreatic pseudocysts (Fig. 122)
These most commonly develop after an acute flare-up of chronic pancreatitis. If the pseudocyst does not resolve spontaneously, *complications* can arise:
- Obstruction or compression of the common bile duct
- Thrombosis of the portal vein and/or splenic vein
- Duodenal stenosis or gastric compression
- Rupture with pancreatogenic ascites
- Vascular erosion and hemorrhage
- Metastatic fat necrosis
- Superinfection

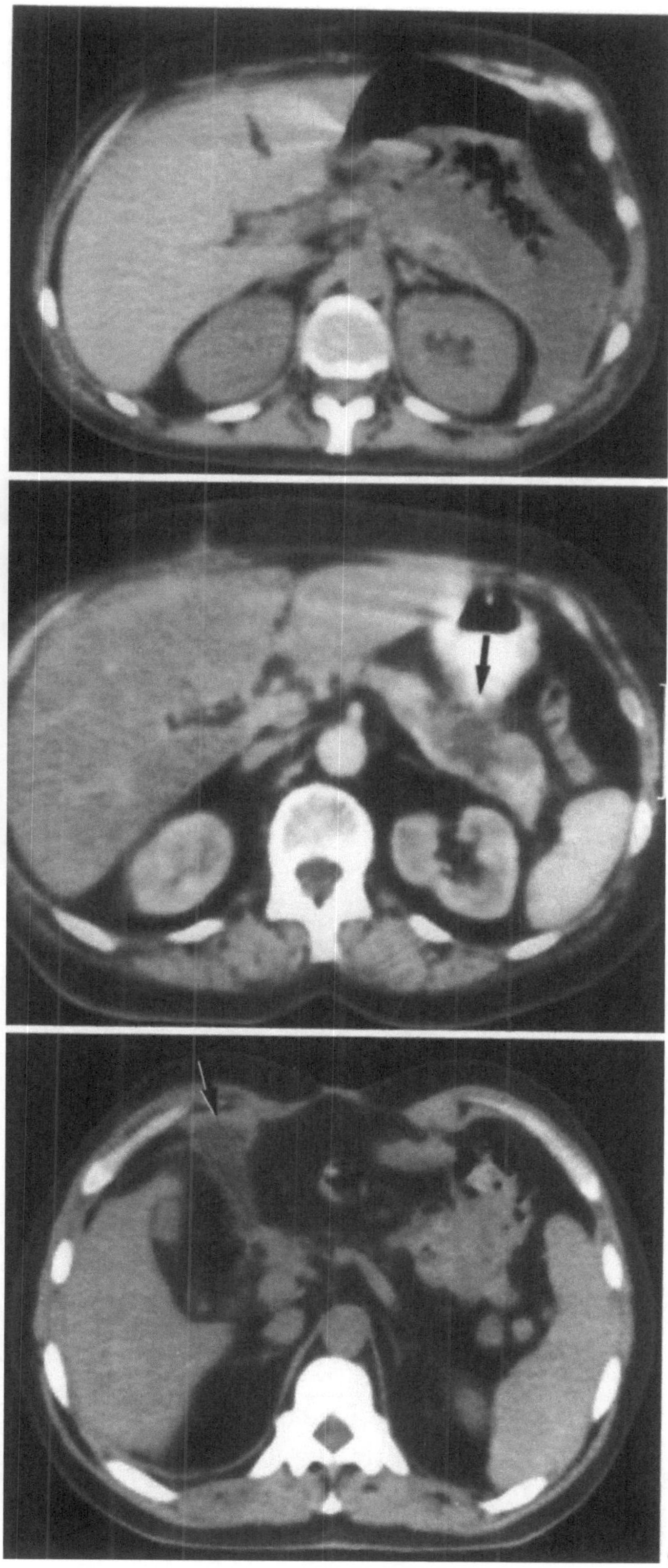
a
b

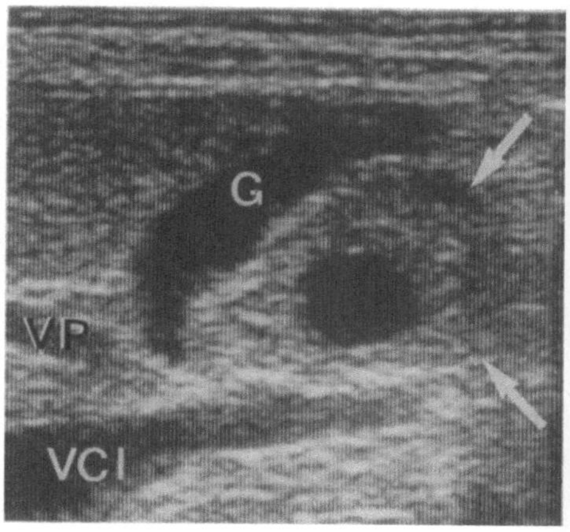

c

d

Fig. 122a–g. Complications of acute pancreatitis. a Necrotizing pancreatitis with abscess formation. *CT scan* documents widening of the anterior pararenal space by protein-rich fluid. It contains numerous gas bubbles as evidence of secondary infection. **b** *CT scan with bolus injection* demonstrates an **abscess** in the tail of the pancreas. There is expansion of the tail with a lack of enhancement (→). Differentiation from pancreatic carcinoma is required. **c Pancreatic pseudocyst.** *Sonogram* (longitudinal scan through the inferior vene cava, *VC*) shows an echo-free liquid focus in the head of the pancreas, which is generally enlarged (→); (*G*, gallbladder; *VP*, portal vein). **d Pancreatic fistula.** *CT scan* shows an abdominal wall abscess caused by a postoperative pancreatic fistula. The fistulous tract extends from the abdominal wall (→) to the head of the pancreas.

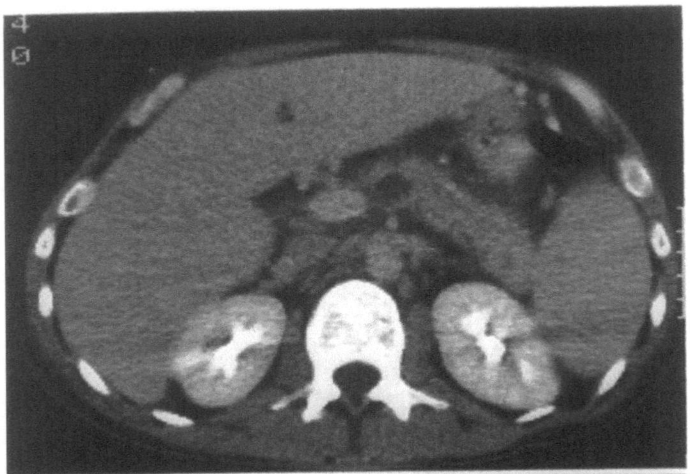

e

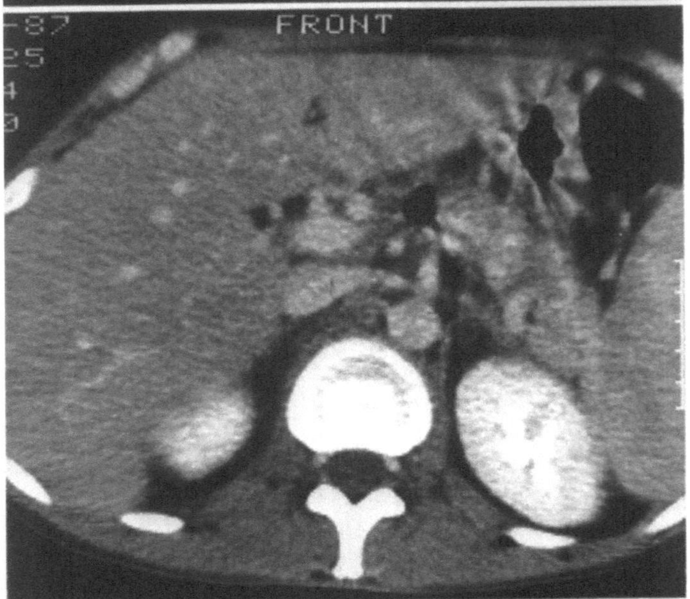

f

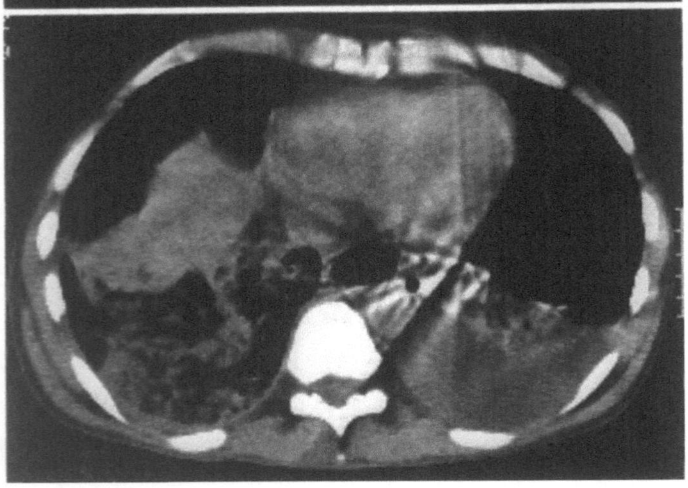

g

Fig. 122 (continued)
e Necrotizing pancreatitis with a necrotic track to the mediastinum and pulmonary necroses. 37-year-old patient with a 6-month history of recurring bouts of pancreatitis. *CT scan* after bolus injection shows edematous pancreatitis with a small pseudocyst at the junction of the body and head of the pancreas. **f** Ten days later fever, leukocytosis, tachycardia, and hypotension. *CT scan* after bolus injection now shows a small gas collection in the area of the former cyst. **g** *CT scan* of the thorax shows extensive periesophageal gas in the left mediastinum with bilateral pleural effusions and pulmonary infiltration on the right side. Autopsy the following day revealed necrosis of the pancreatic head with a broad necrotic track extending toward the mediastinum, esophageal erosion, and pulmonary necroses

Pancreatogenic abscess (Fig. 118)
Causes:
- Infected bile
- Hematogenous spread
- Lymphatic spread from the gallbladder or colon
- Direct transmural infection from the transverse colon

Note: Imaging procedures assist in the primary diagnosis of acute pancreatitis, the monitoring of its course, the assessment of its severity and of the extent of pancreatic and peripancreatic necrosis, and the diagnosis of complications and sequelae after acute manifestations have subsided.

References

Beyer D, Köster R (1980) Diagnostischer Wert der Abdomenübersichtsaufnahmen bei akuter Pankreatitis. Fortschr Röntgenstr 131/1: 9-15

Dürr HK, Bode JC (1976) Klinik und Therapie der akuten Pankreatitis. Leber Magen Darm 6: 282-293

Freeny PC, Lawson TL (1982) Radiology of the pancreas. Springer Berlin Heidelberg New York

Friedmann G, Mödder U (1980) Stadieneinteilung und Verlaufsbeobachtung der akuten Pankreatitis durch Angio-Computertomographie. Leber Magen Darm 10: 303-308

Haertel H, Tillmann U, Fuchs WA (1979) Die akute Pankreatitis im Computertomogramm. Fortschr Röntgenstr 130: 525-530

Hill MC, Barkin J, Isikoff MB, Silverstein W, Kalser M (1982) Acute pankreatitis: Clinical vs CT findings. AJR 139: 263-269

Marks IN, Bank S, Barbezat GO (1976) Alkoholpankreatitis - Ätiologie, klinische Formen, Komplikationen. Leber Magen Darm 6: 257-270

Mendez G, Isikoff MB, Hill MC (1980) CT of acute pankreatitis: Interim assessment. AJR 135: 463-469

Mödder U, Friedmann G, Rosenberger J (1981) Wert der Angio-CT für die Stadieneinteilung, Verlaufsbeobachtung und Therapie bei akuter Pankreatitis. Fortschr Röntgenstr 134: 22-27

Schmidt H, Creutzfeld W (1973) Akute chronische Pankreatitis: In: Demling L (Hrsg) Klinische Gastroenterologie. Thieme, Stuttgart

Schönborn H, Kümmerle F (1978) Die akute Pankreatitis und ihre Intensivtherapie. Intensivmedizin 15: 39-44

Siegelmann SS, Copeland BE, Saba GP, Cameron JL, Sanders RC, Zerhounim EA (1980) CT of fluid collections associated with pancreatitis. AJR 134: 1121-1132

Silverstein W, Isikoff MB, Hill MC, Barkin J (1981) Diagnostic imaging of acute pancreatitis: Prospective study using CT and sonography. AJR 137: 497-502

White ME, Wittenberg J, Müller PR, Simeone JF, et al. (1986) Pancreatic necrosis: CT manifestations. Radiology 158: 343-346

4.1.3 Diffuse Peritonitis

D. BEYER, W. STEINBRICH

Causes

Bacterial transmigration or perforation secondary to:
- Acute appendicitis
- Perforated ulcer or diverticulum
- Purulent salpingitis
- Gallbladder empyema
- Acute pancreatitis
- Bowel ischemia with gangrene
- Suture line leakage

Chemical irritation by the influx of
- Bile
- Urine
- Chemotherapeutic agents (Fig. 124)

Clinical Symptoms
- Diffuse muscular rigidity ("boardlike" abdomen)
- Absence of peristalsis (silent abdomen)
- Shock symptoms

Radiologic Signs (time-dependent)

Plain Radiographs
- L Lat film may show free air if a perforation has occurred (Fig. 123b; see Sect. 3.5.1).
- Combined small- and large-bowel distension with fluid levels (Figs. 123, 124) (see Sect. 3.1.5)
- May show paraintestinal gas (abscess) or intramural/intravascular gas (resulting from gangrene) (see Sects. 3.5.4, 4.1.5.1)

Sonography

Large amounts of free air and massive gaseous bowel distension interfere with ultrasound imaging, so scans should be performed from the flank.
The scans may show:
- Fluid-filled bowel loops
- Free fluid in the paracolic, perihepatic, or perisplenic spaces or lesser pelvis
- Encapsulated fluid collections between bowel loops or in the subphrenic or subhepatic spaces, possibly with gas bubbles (localized intraperitoneal abscess) (see Sect. 4.1.5.1)

Computed Tomography

CT is usually not used in diffuse peritonitis. It has proved useful in grades 2–3 acute pancreatitis (see Sect. 4.1.2) in searching for abscesses (see Sect. 4.1.5.1), detecting and localizing small gas bubbles, and detecting fluid (urine, bile).

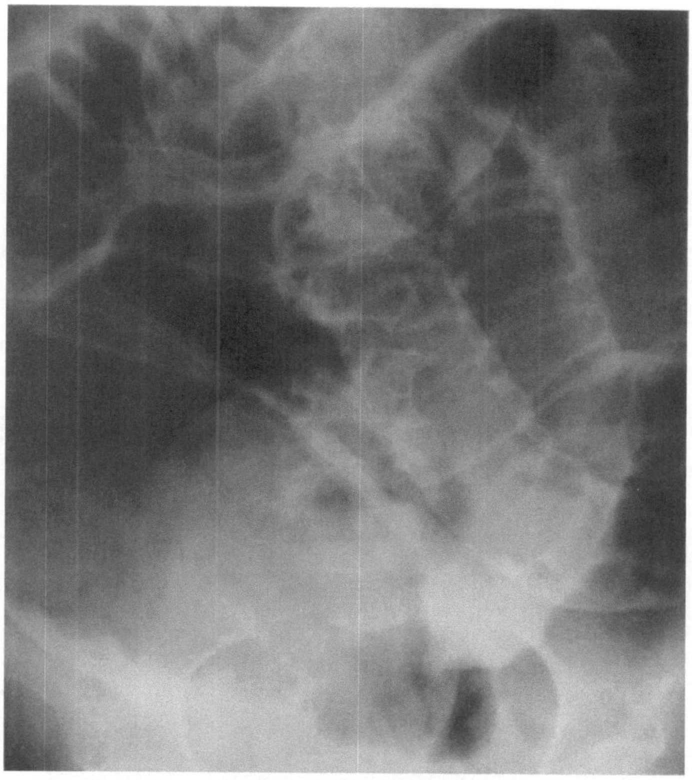

a

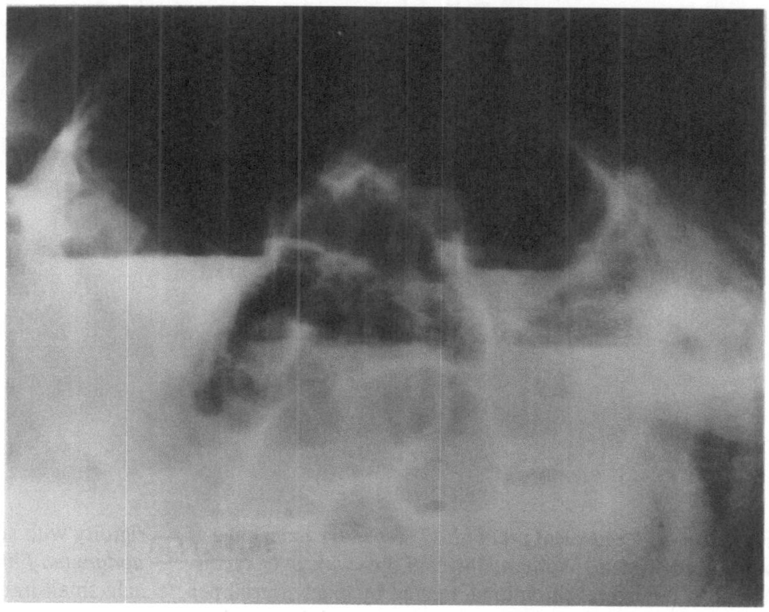

b

Fig. 123 a, b. Diffuse peritonitis after perforation of the cecum secondary to stenosing sigmoid carcinoma. Woman, 73 years old, with abdominal distension, weight loss, and obstipation presented with a rigid abdomen and silent bowel. **a** *Supine film* shows combined distension of the small and large intestine. The visible walls of the small bowel (Rigler's sign) are evidence of the perforation. The cecum is massively distended. **b** *Left lateral film* shows combined small- and large-bowel distension with fluid levels in the ascending colon and small bowel. There is free air below the lateral abdominal wall. Operation disclosed a stenosing sigmoid carcinoma with mechanical colon obstruction and cecal perforation. *Diagnosis:* diffuse peritonitis

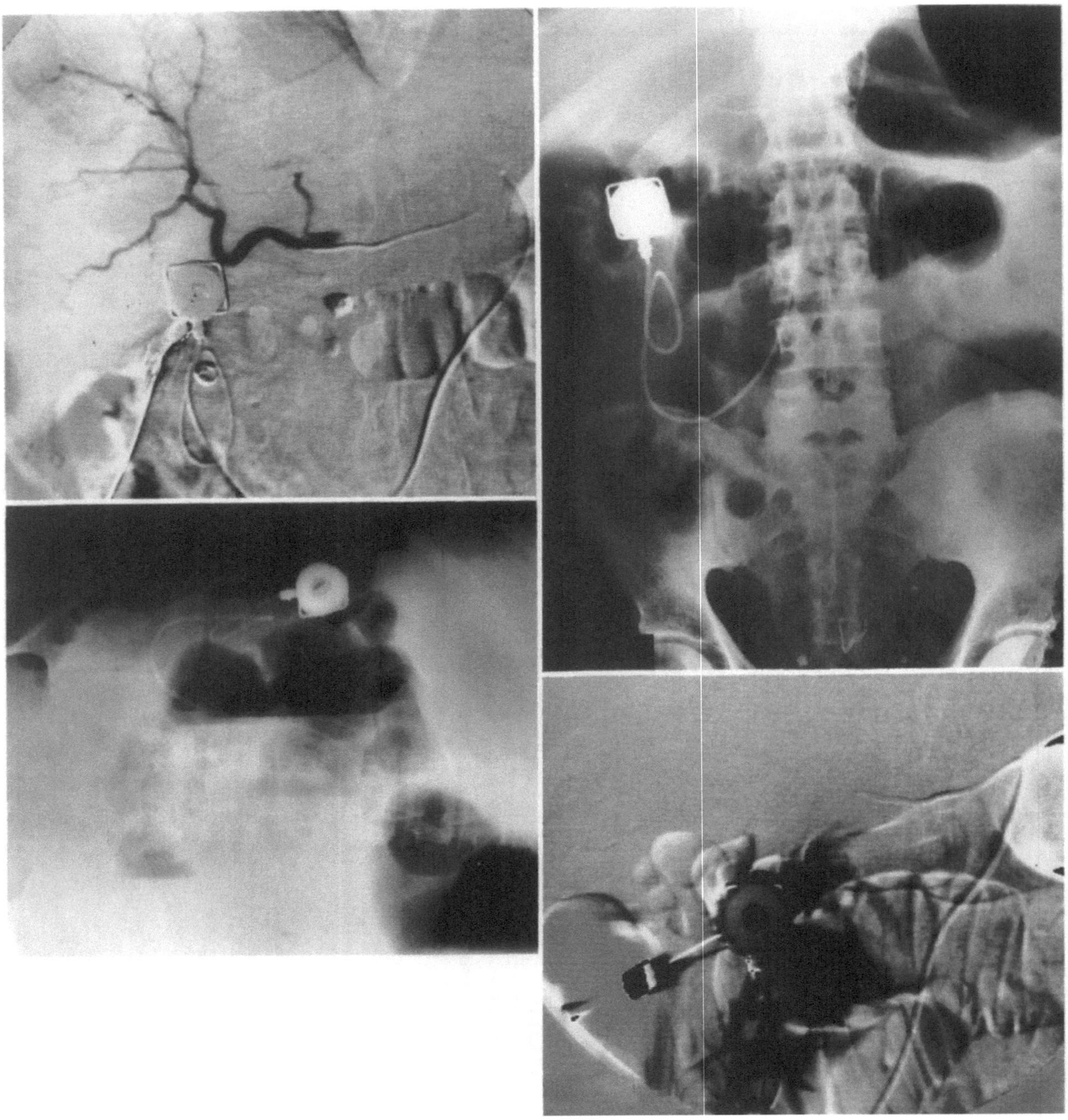

Fig. 124 a–d. "Chemical peritonitis" secondary to leakage of a portacath system. Woman, 36 years old, with liver metastases of a colorectal carcinoma, treated by local arterial perfusion with 5-fluorouracil. **a** Visualization of the port by digital subtraction angiography. The catheter tip has been inserted into the hepatic artery; normal perfusion of the liver. The patient manifested an acute increase in abdominal rigidity with sonographically confirmed ascites. **b** *Supine abdominal film* shows generalized distension of the stomach, small intestine, and colon. **c** *Left lateral film* shows generalized bowel distension with fluid levels. There is no evidence of free air. **d** DSA demonstrates leakage of contrast medium from the catheter chamber into the subcutaneous and peritoneal spaces

4.1.4 Acute Appendicitis

D. Beyer, G. P. Krestin

This is the most common disease requiring surgery in the abdomen.

Caution: The clinical course and findings in acute appendicitis are highly variable. It is difficult to diagnose in children, in the elderly, and during pregnancy.

Causes
Combined action of multiple noxious agents.
The dominant factor is an enterogenic process originating in the lumen of the appendix: coprostasis (fecaliths and foreign bodies), abnormal proliferation of pathogenic intestinal flora.
Rarely, metastatic appendicitis develops in association with angina, osteomyelitis, furuncles, and other pyogenic infections.

Note: The shape and anatomic location of the appendix are extremely variable. Published data on the position of the appendix vary considerably. *A retrocecal position* is reported in up to 65% of cases. An appendix in that position may or may not have a peritoneal investment (Fig. 125).
With an *extraperitoneal* retrocecal appendix, the posterior wall of the ascending colon between the tenia mesocolica and tenia omentalis and also the right pararenal space are primarily affected.
With an *intraperitoneal* appendix, the right paracolic space and lateral colon wall between the tenia omentalis and tenia libera are involved.

Clinical Symptoms
The immediate history is from 12 to 48 h in duration. Pain usually starts in the epigastrium or umbilical area, accompanied by nausea. Later the pain localizes in the right lower quadrant.
Palpation discloses tenderness to pressure and percussion, direct and referred rebound tenderness, and local muscular resistance in the right lower quadrant. Rectal examination elicits pain in the cul-de-sac. In *children* the right leg is held slightly flexed at the hip. Passive extension elicits psoas muscle pain. Additional signs are low-grade fever and leukocytosis.

Differential diagnosis (see Sects. 1, 4.8)
Mesenteric lymphadenitis (see Fig. 134), pseudoappendicitis from *Yersinia* infection, Crohn's disease, right-sided ureteral stone, ovulation, ovarian cyst with a twisted pedicle, ectopic pregnancy, adnexitis, acute cholecystitis, Meckel's diverticulitis, bacterial diarrhea
In children: right basal pneumonia

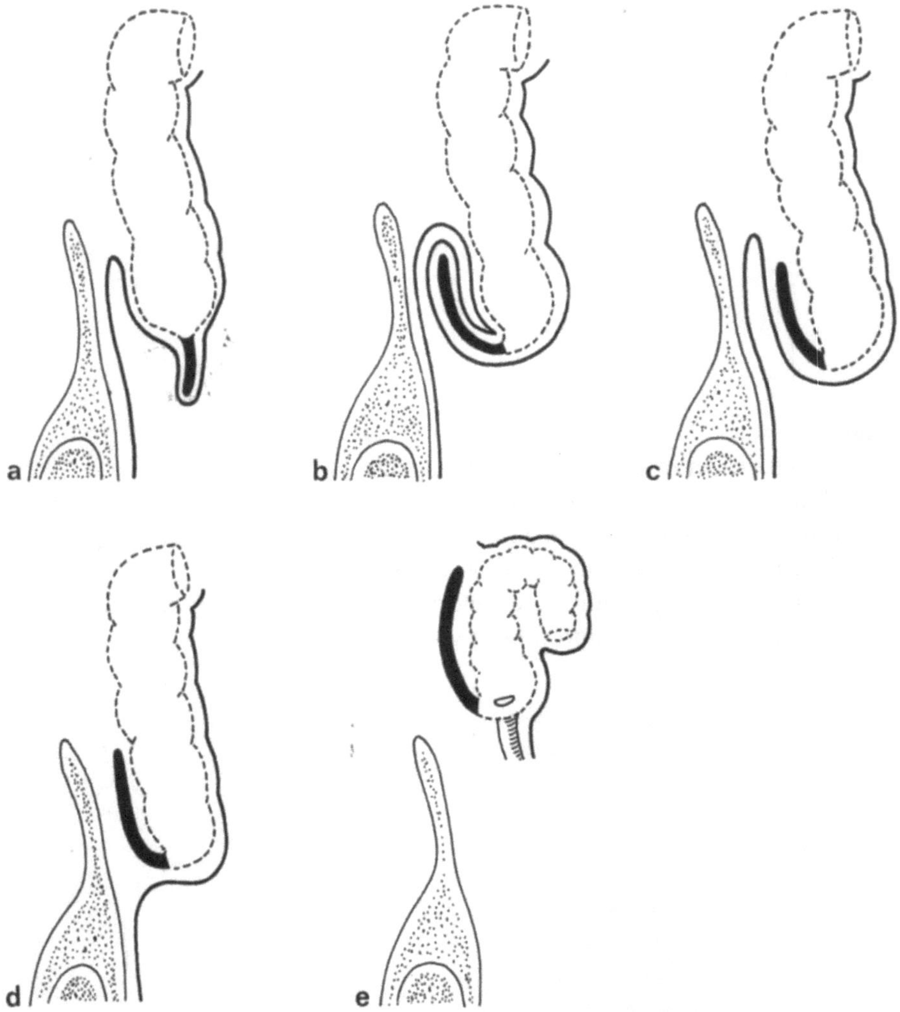

Fig. 125a–e. Normal variations in the position and peritoneal fixation of the appendix. **a** Intraperitoneal appendix hanging downward anterior to the right iliac wing. **b** Intraperitoneal retrocecal appendix. **c** Retrocecal appendix partially contained in a paracecal sac of peritoneum. **d** Extraperitoneal retrocecal appendix. **e** Extraperitoneal retrocecal appendix lying anterior to the right kidney, with associated elevation of the cecum. The terminal ileum, also extraperitoneal, enters the cecum from the posterior aspect. (Modified from Meyers 1982)

Radiologic Signs

Note: Acute appendicitis is usually diagnosed from clinical symptoms and does *not* require a roentgen examination.
Imaging procedures become important only if symptoms are equivocal or complications have occurred. In these cases diagnostic imaging can be important in directing the further course of treatment.

Imaging procedures can differentiate among acute cholecystitis, free perforation, diverticulitis, acute pancreatitis, right-sided ureteral stone, cul-de-sac abscess, salpingo-oopheritis, and right basal pleuropneumonia (in children).

Plain Radiographs (Fig. 127)

Primary Signs
- Appendicolith (fecalith = coprolith) (Figs. 130, 133)
- Gaseous distension of the terminal ileum, cecum, and ascending colon with fluid levels on the L Lat film ("cecal ileus") (Fig. 127)
- Gaseous distension of the appendix (Fig. 128)
- Intraperitoneal abscess with soft-tissue density, possibly displacing the cecum and ascending colon from the flank stripe. Gas formation is unusual (Figs. 130-133)
- Extraperitoneal abscess with a retrocecal, retroperitoneal appendix. Gas formation is possible (see Fig. 145)
- Perforation with free air between the chest wall and liver or in the right lower quadrant under the flank stripe on the L Lat film (see Fig. 140)

Secondary Signs
- Nonvisualization of the lower third of the right flank stripe (Fig. 126a)
- Nonvisualization of the lower third of the right psoas margin (Figs. 126a, 130, 131)
- Mechanical small-bowel obstruction by inflammatory adhesions (Fig. 127)
- Reactive paralytic ileus of the small bowel and colon in diffuse peritonitis due to perforation (see Fig. 145)
- Scoliosis of the lumbar spine convex to the left caused by contraction of the right flank muscles (Fig. 126a)
- Abscess following a perforation (Fig. 126b, 130-133)

Note: Contrast studies are usually *not indicated* in acute appendicitis.

Sonography
- Direct visualisation fo a distended, hypoechoic appendix with thickened wall (target lesion) (Fig. 129)
- Abscess in the right lower quadrant with liquid contents and a thick, irregular wall (Fig. 132)
- With retroperitoneal perforation: displacement of the right kidney with a retroperitoneal abscess that may contain gas (see Fig. 145c)
- Increased fluid content in small-bowel loops
- Possible increase in intra-abdominal fluid volume
- Free air

Note: Sonograms show changes in many patients with acute appendicitis.

Computed Tomography

This modality is very rarely used. CT can demonstrate a right paranephritic abscess, which may contain gas, following the retroperitoneal perforation of a retrocecal appendix. Renal displacement is also apparent (Figs. 132d, 133).

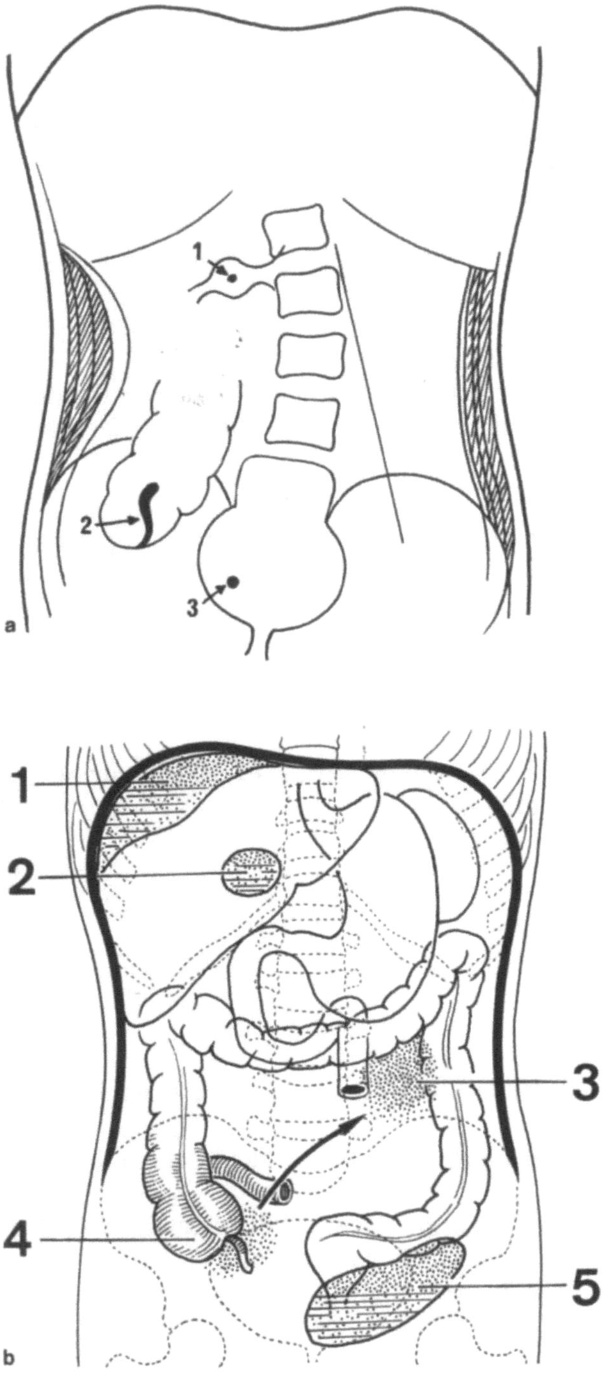

Fig. 126. a Contraction of the right flank stripe with left convex scoliosis of the lumbar spine and obliteration of the right psoas shadow caused by: *1*, perforated duodenal ulcer; *2*, acute appendicitis; *3*, a prevesical ureteral stone. (Modified from Frimann-Dahl 1968). **b Sites of abscess formation after perforation of the appendix with acute appendicitis:** *1*, right subphrenic abscess; *2*, subhepatic abscess; *3*, interloop abscess; *4*, perityphlitic abscess; *5*, cul-de-sac abscess. (Modified from Botsford and Wilson 1981)

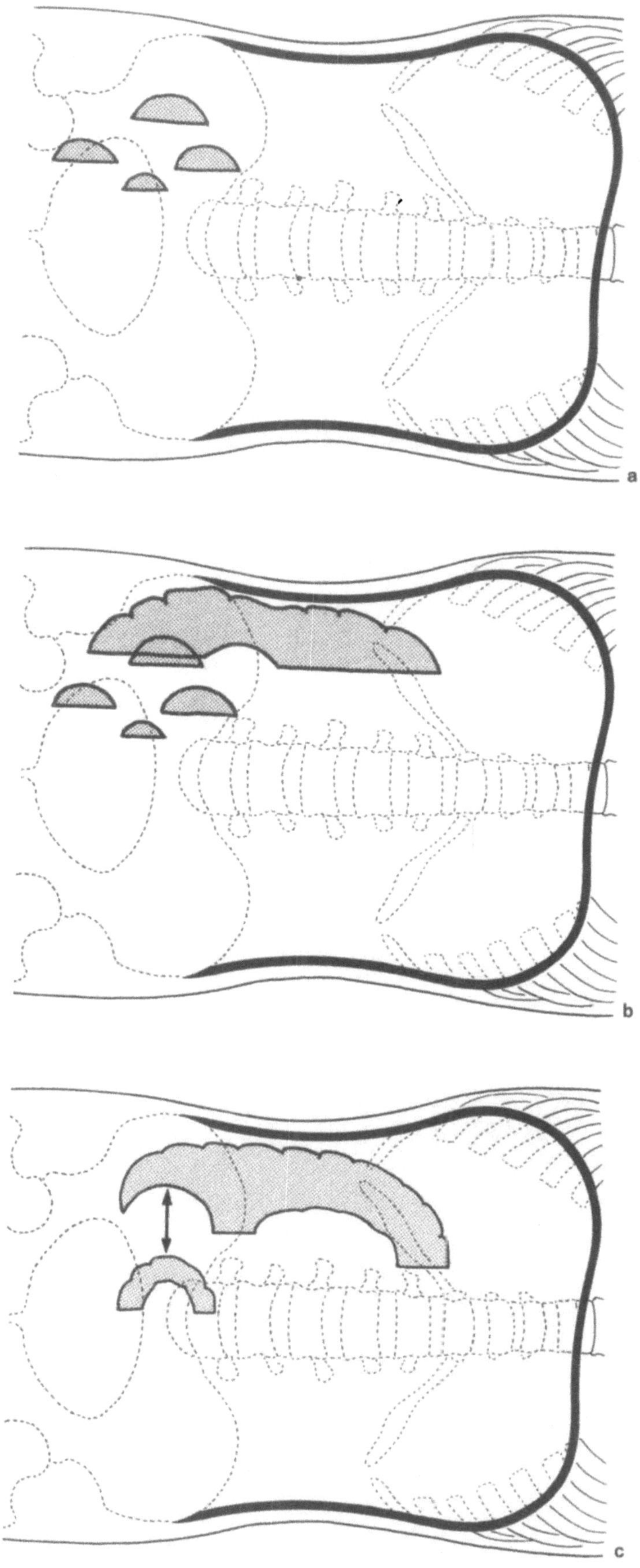

Fig. 127 a–e. Various signs of acute appendicitis on the left lateral plain film.
a Short fluid levels in the area of the terminal ileum. **b** Short fluid levels in the terminal ileum and a long fluid level in the cecum and ascending colon. **c** Distended loop with a fluid level in the terminal ileum. Perityphlitic abscess separates the bowel loop from the gas-filled cecum with a long fluid level.

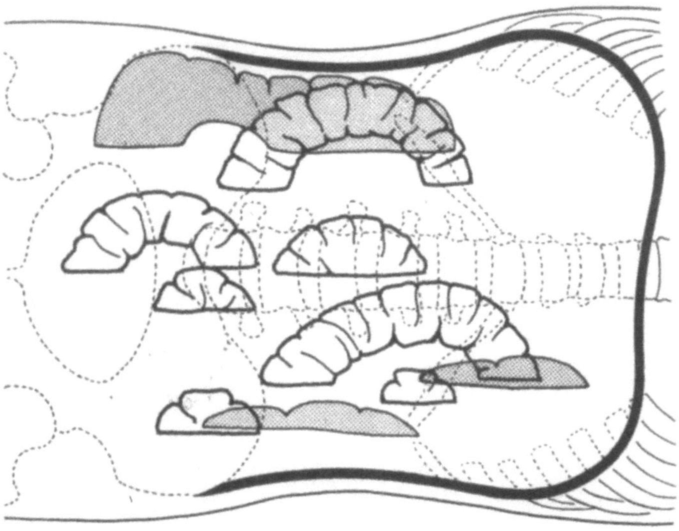
d

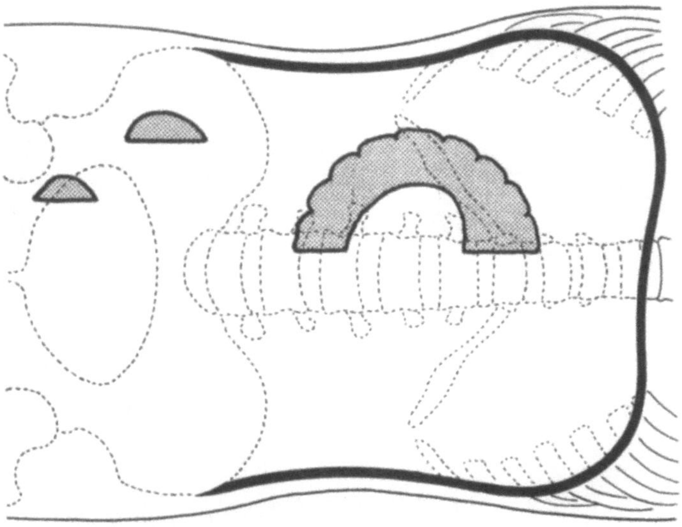
e

Fig. 127 (continued)
d Combined small-bowel and colonic distension with multiple fluid levels and possibly free air signifying perforation of an acute appendicitis with diffuse peritonitis. **e Differential diagnosis: mesenteric lymphadenitis** with short fluid levels in the terminal ileum and duodenal distension

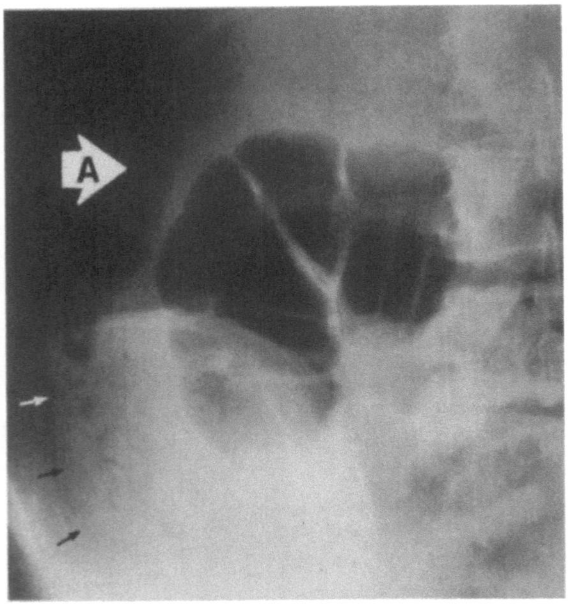

Fig. 128. Retrocecal appendicitis. Woman, 52 years old, with suspected acute cholecystitis. *Erect abdomen plain film* (taken elsewhere) shows colonic distension with no fluid levels. There is an elevated paracolic cecum (→) and fingerlike, air-filled appendix (*A*➡), directed craniad. *Operation* disclosed acute appendicitis of a retrocecal appendix with a mobile cecum

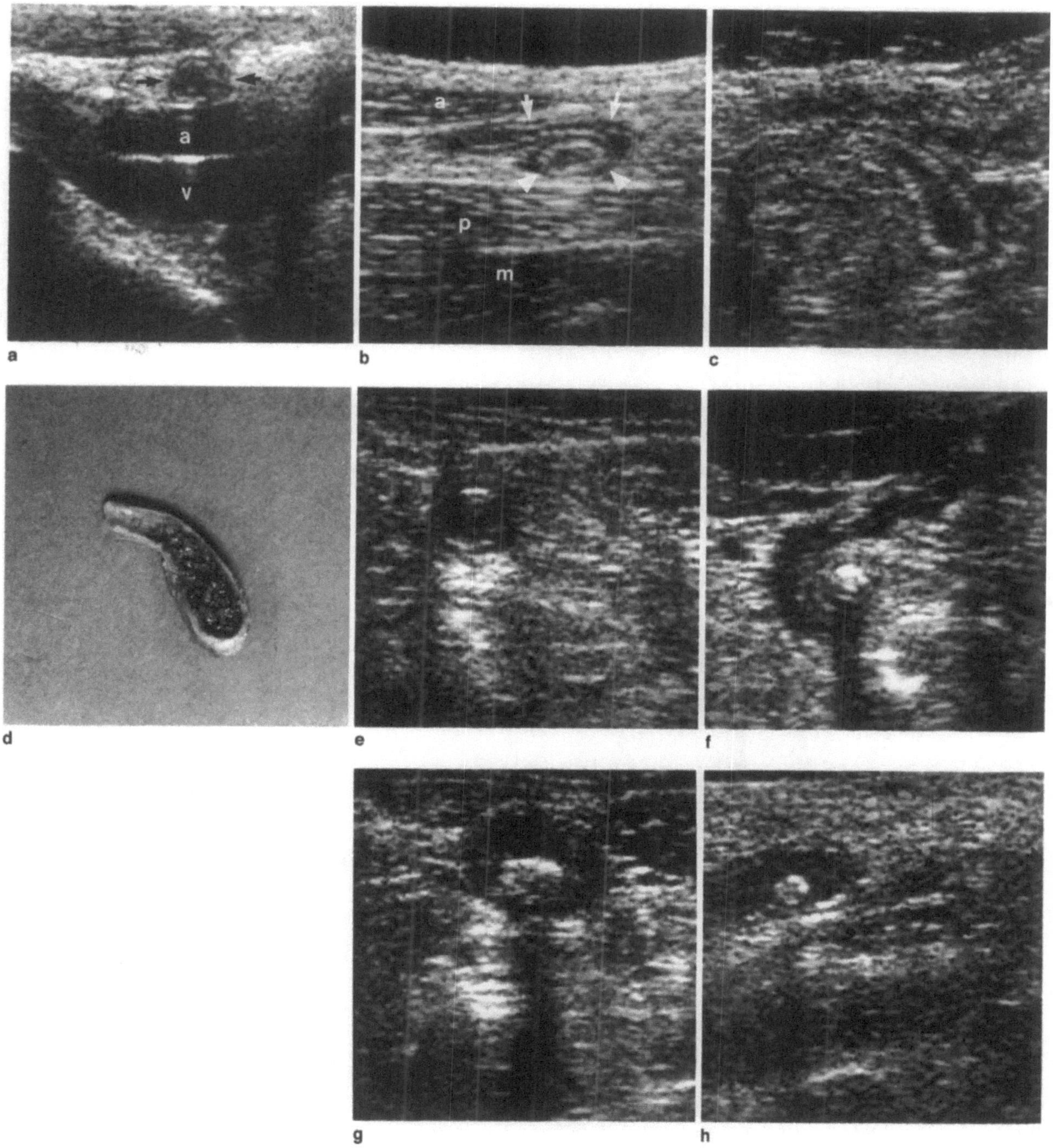

Fig. 129 a–h. Acute appendicitis: various ultrasonographic images using graded compression. **a** Transversely oriented appendix seen as a target phenomenon (→←) above the iliac artery *(a)* and vein *(v)* (longitudinal plane). **b** The appendix (▷) is visualized through the compressed cecum (➧); *a,* abdominal wall; *pm,* psoas muscle (longitudinal plane). **c** Inflamed appendix visualized in toto with correlating gross specimen (**d**) (longitudinal plane). **e** Inflamed appendix appearing as a round structure. Reflecting areas caused by gas (transverse plane). **f, g, h** Inflamed appendices with appendicoliths causing acoustic shadows (**f, g** transverse plane; **h** longitudinal plane). (**a–h** with kind permission of *Radiology,* Puylaert 1986)

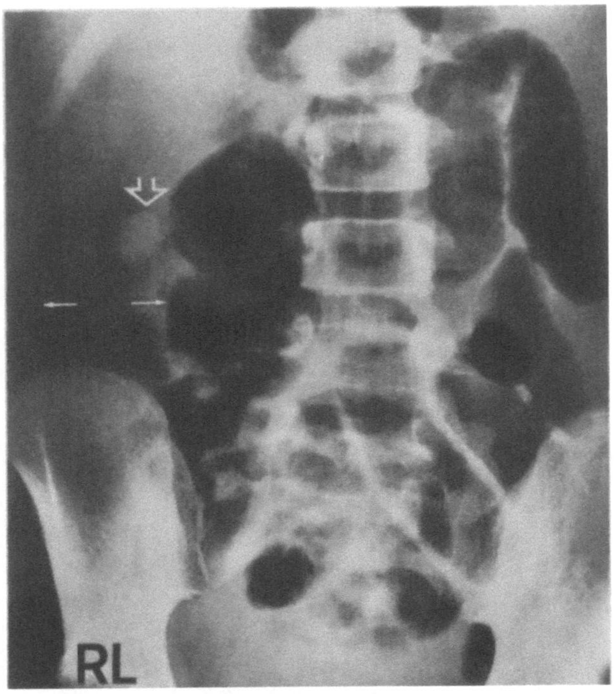

a

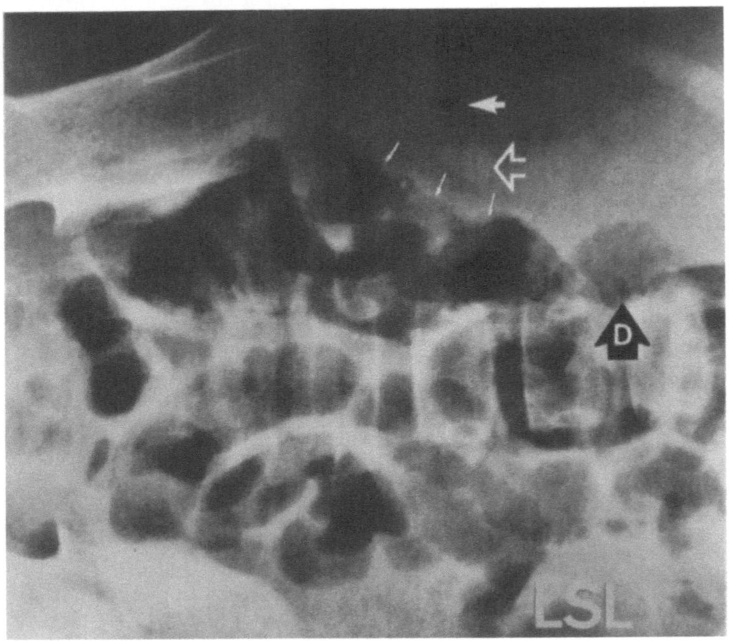

b

Fig. 130 a, b. Retrocecal appendicitis with subhepatic abscess.
Boy, 13 years old, experienced increasing pains below the right costal arch with fever and leukocytosis. **a** *Supine film* shows moderate, combined small-bowel and colonic distension. The ascending colon is separated from the right lateral flank stripe by 3 cm (↔). In this area can be seen 1.5 × 1-cm appendicolith (⇨) surmounted by a small triangular gas pocket. **b** *Left lateral film* shows no evidence of perforation and no displacement of the appendicolith (⇨) and surrounding gas bubble (→). Indentation of the ascending colon is much more apparent than on the supine film (→). There are scattered fluid levels in the small bowel, and the duodenum is dilated (*D*➡). *Operation* disclosed a retrocecal, intraperitoneal appendicitis with an appendicolith and gas-containing subhepatic abscess

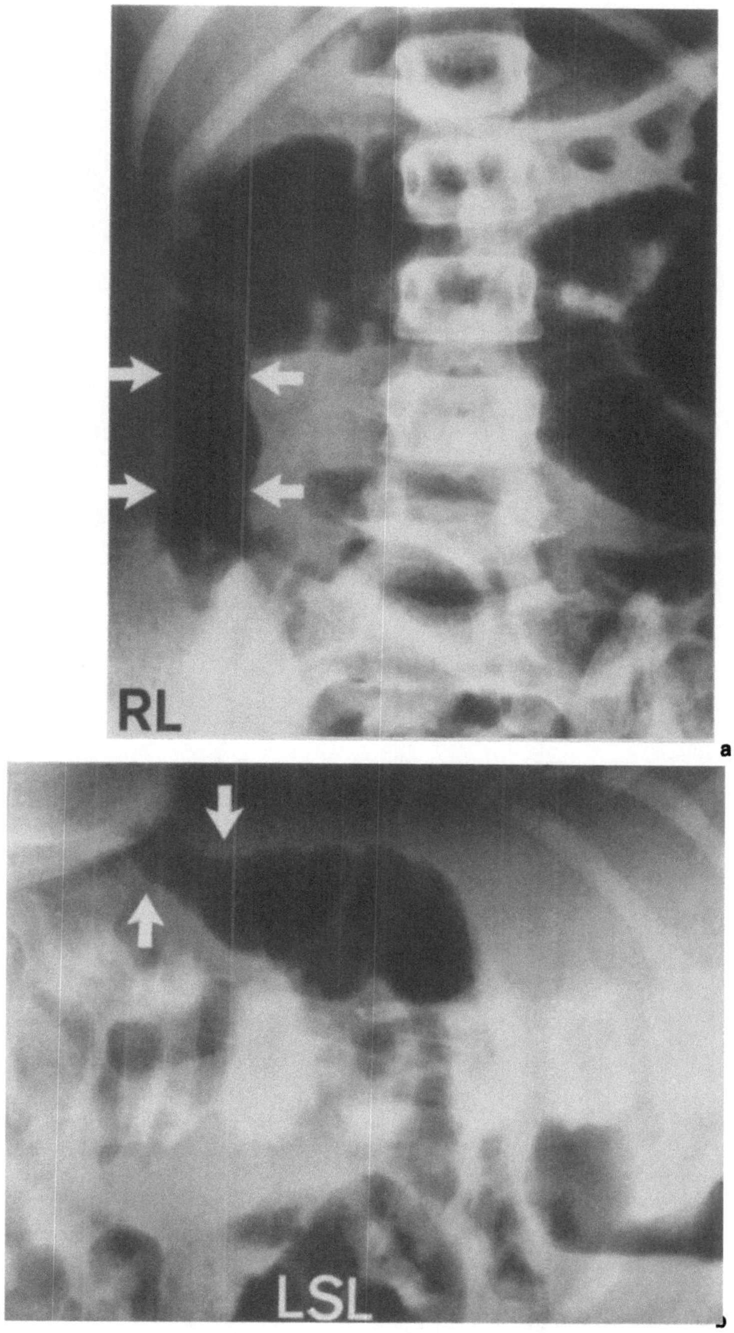

Fig. 131 a, b. Perforation of intraperitoneal appendicitis with perityphlitic abscess. Girl, 11 years old, had for 4 days experienced increasing pain and tenderness in the mid- and right lower abdomen and umbilical area with fever, nausea, vomiting, and diminished bowel sounds. **a** *Supine film* shows combined gaseous distension of the stomach, small bowel, and colon. The cecum and ascending colon are narrow and show loss of haustrations; the ascending colon is separated from the right flank stripe (➧). There is slight scoliosis of the lumbar spine convex to the left from contraction of the right flank muscles. **b** *Left lateral film* shows no evidence of perforation and a few fluid levels in the small bowel. The right colic flexure is distended with gas; the cecum and ascending colon are not distended (➧). *Operation* disclosed the confined perforation of an intraperitoneal appendicitis with a large perityphlitic abscess between the right abdominal wall and cecum

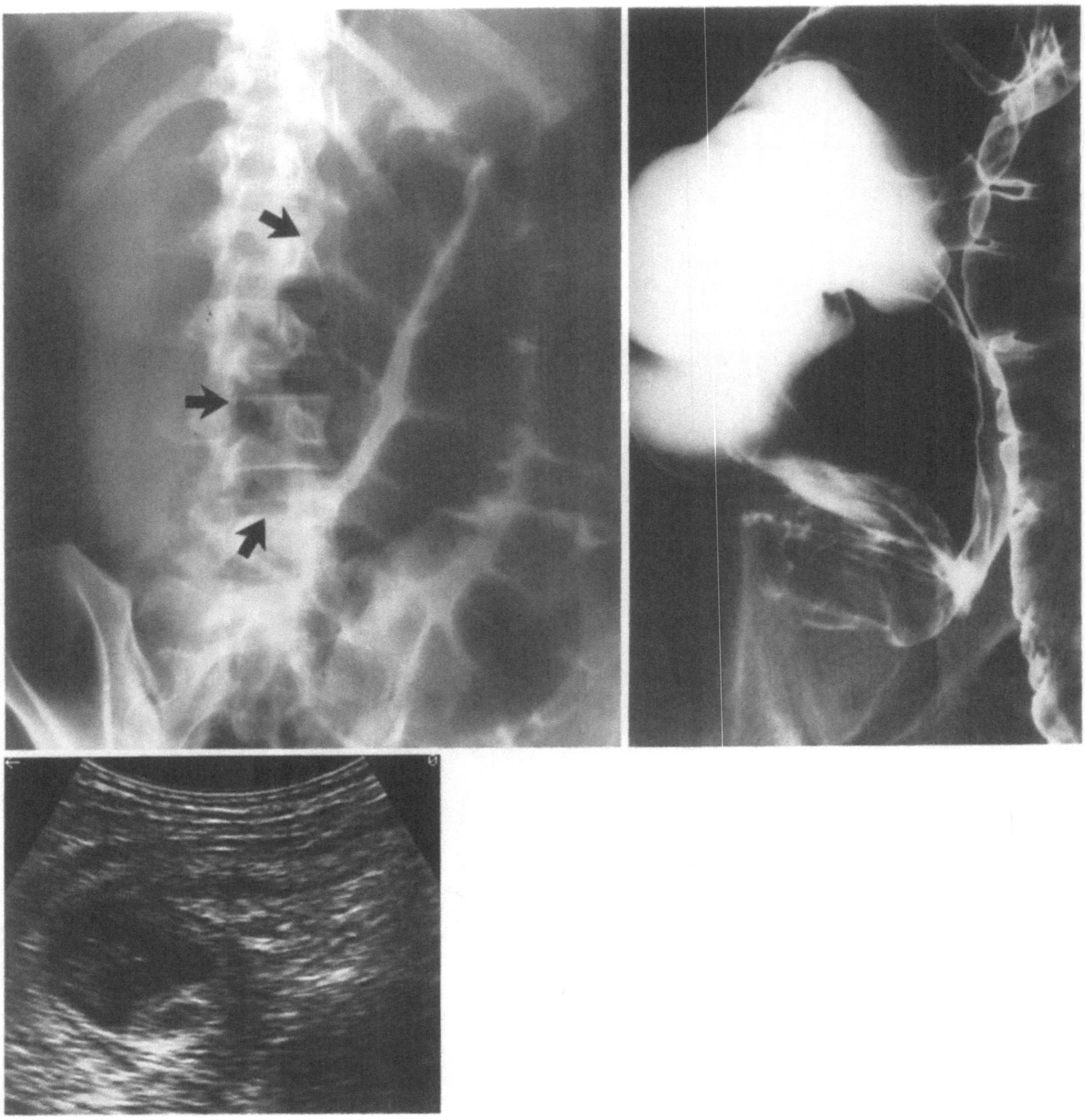

a b c

Fig. 132 a–f. Perityphlitic and paracolic abscesses complicating appendicitis.
a Man, 24 years old, presented with fever and a palpable mass in the right lower quadrant with marked abdominal distension and aperistalsis. *Supine film* shows distension limited to the colon with a soft-tissue mass displacing the ascending colon and right flexure (➡); the psoas shadow is obscured. *Operation* disclosed a huge, retrocolic, retroperitoneal abscess resulting from the retroperitoneal perforation of a retrocecal appendicitis. **b** Woman, 28 years old, who for 6 weeks experienced increasing pain in the right lower quadrant with fever. She received gynecologic treatment for salpingo-oophoritis. *Sonogram,* transverse scan through the right lower quadrant, shows a liquid mass with irregular borders in the cecal area. **c** *Contrast enema* shows a large, rounded indentation of the posterolateral aspect of the cecum with crimping of the cecal wall. *Operation* uncovered a large intraperitoneal, perityphlitic abscess with compression of the cecal pole. **d** Man, 24 years old, who had undergone appendectomy elsewhere presented with fever and tenderness in the right lower quadrant. *CT scan* shows thickened abdominal skin (appendectomy scar) and a soft-tissue mass in the right lower quadrant impressing upon the contrast-filled cecum. There are conspicuous patchy and streaky markings in the mesentery. *Reoperation* disclosed an abscess in the area of the former appendix with compression of the cecum. **e** Boy, 14 years old, who for 3 weeks experienced increasing pain during sports activities and stair climbing. He was referred for orthopedic management. Patient was nonfebrile; radionuclide imaging and radiographs of the hip were normal. A soft bulge in the right groin area was noted on admission to the orthopedic clinic. *Sonogram* (longitudinal scan through the right lower quadrant) shows an extensive, echo-free mass with a thick

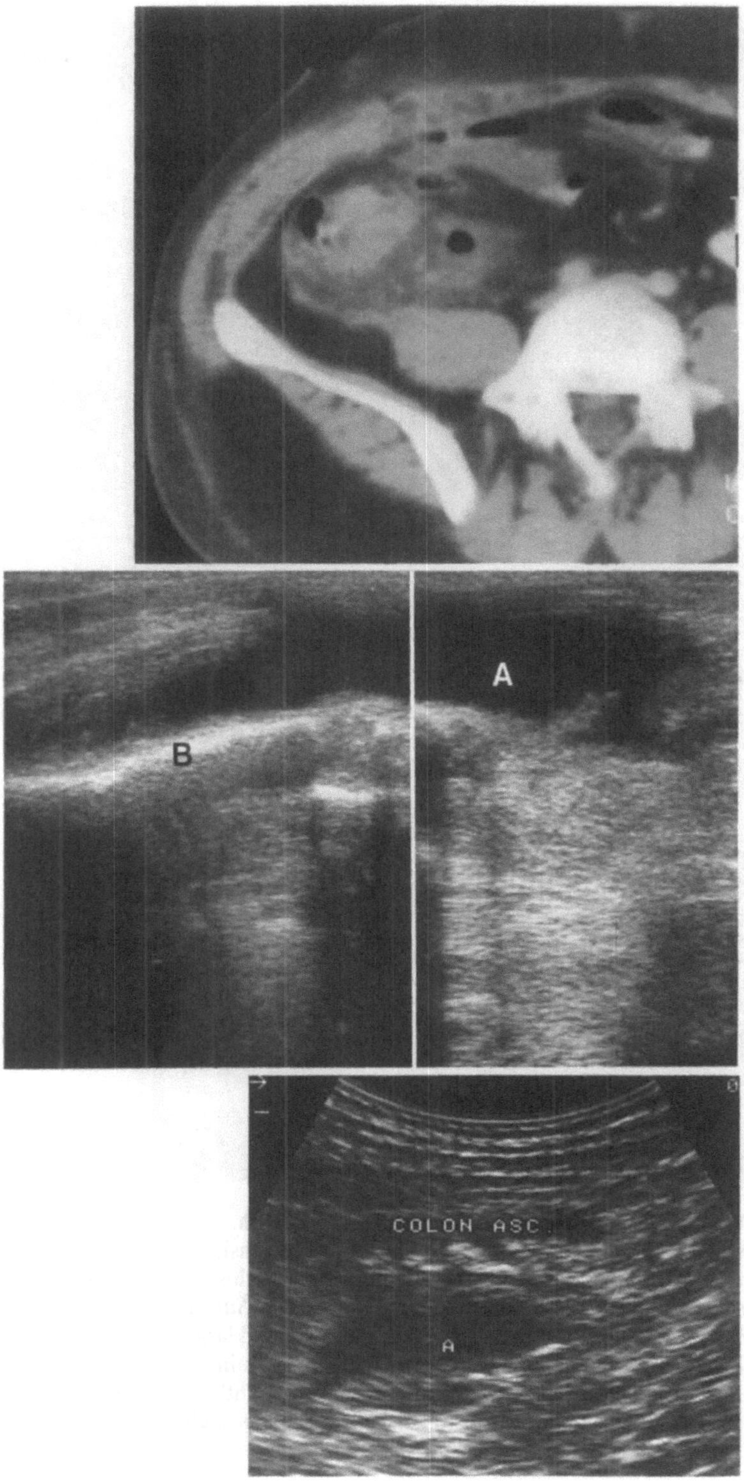

d

e

f

Fig. 132 (continued)
wall *(A)* anterior to the right iliac wing *(B)*; the mass is most extensive below the inguinal ligament. *Operation* disclosed the retroperitoneal perforation of an appendicitis with a large gravitation abscess. **f** Perityphlitic abscess with a retrocecal appendix. Girl, 12 years old, experienced increasing right midabdominal pain and fever for several days; leukocytosis. *Sonogram* shows an elliptical, hypoechoic mass with a thick, irregular wall posterior to the ascending colon, whose wall is slightly thickened

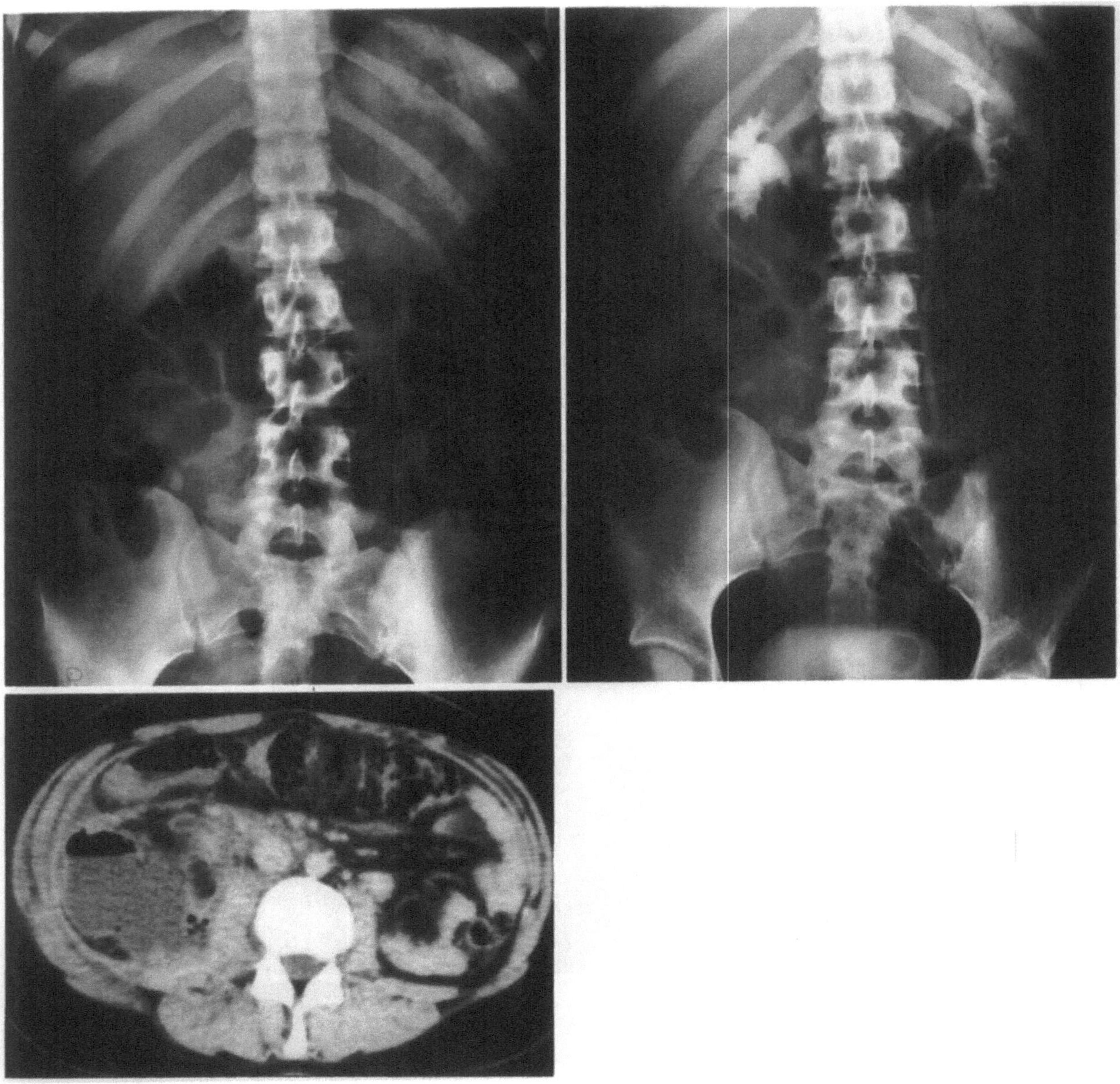

Fig. 133 a–c. Perityphlitic abscess with appendicolith. Woman, 19 years old, with 2-week history of increasing lower abdominal pain and fever. Examination disclosed microhematuria and diminished bowel sounds. **a** *Supine film* shows a nonspecific distension of the small and large bowel. A soft-tissue mass with a calcified coprolith impresses on the medial aspect of the cecum. The right psoas shadow is no longer distinguishable. There is slight bowing of the lumbar spine toward the left side due to pain. **b** *Urogram* shows slight medial displacement of the right ureter with moderate ectasia of the right renal collecting system. The coprolith is clearly visible. **c** *CT scan* shows a large retroperitoneal abscess with an air-fluid level and gas bubbles. Operation disclosed a large retroperitoneal abscess caused by the perforation of a retrocecal appendicitis

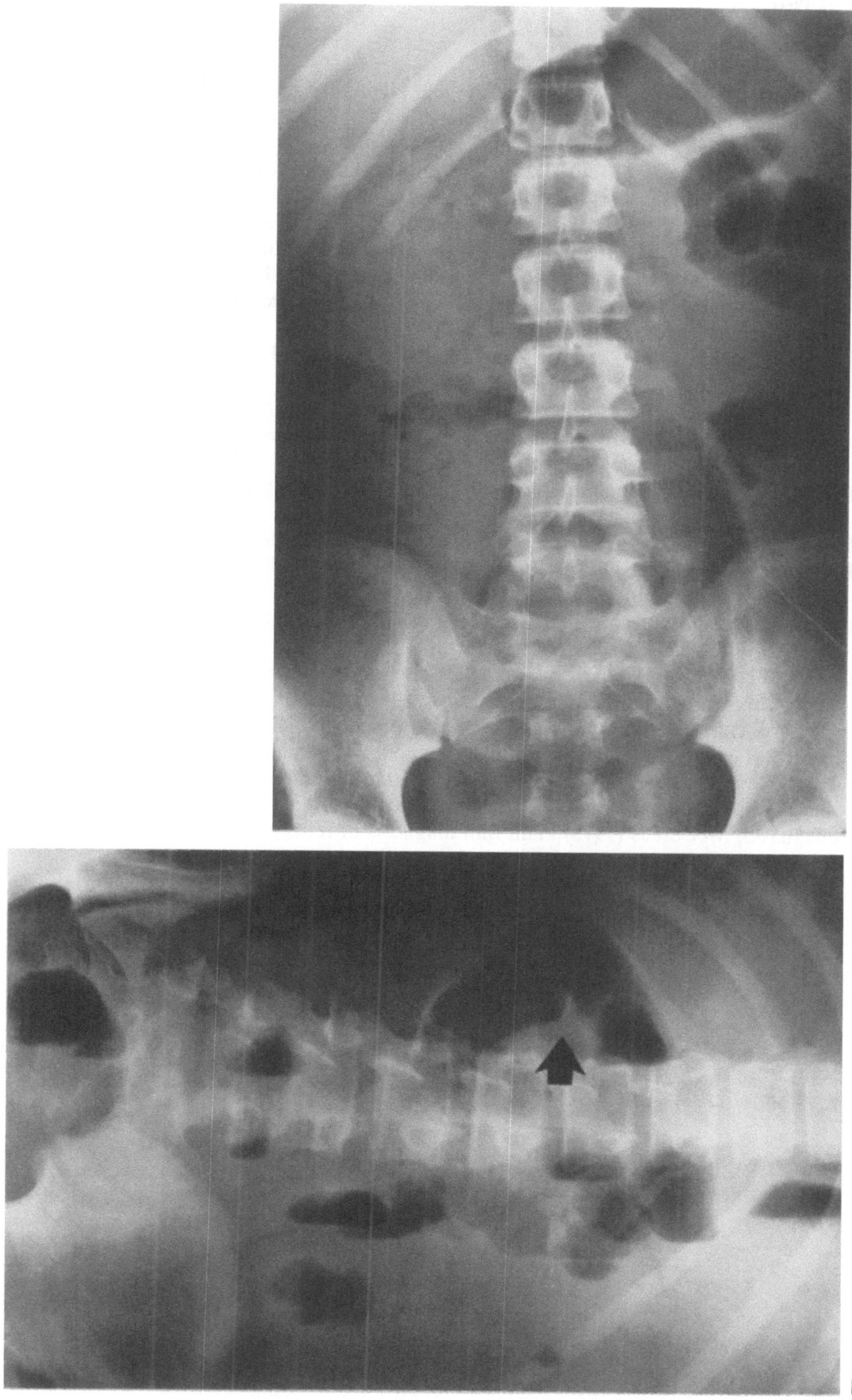

a

b

Fig. 134 a, b. Mesenteric lymphadenitis - its differentiation from acute appendicitis. A 14-year-old boy had complaints suggestive of acute appendicitis. **a** *Supine film* shows a nonspecific bowel gas pattern. **b** *Left lateral film* shows marked isolated duodenal distension (➡) with multiple fluid levels in the small intestine. The cecum is not distended. *Operation* disclosed mesenteric lymphadenitis

References

Baier R, Puppel H, Zelder O, Heiming E (1982) Häufigkeit und Bedeutung von Yersinia-enterocolitica-Infektionen bei akuter Appendizitis. Z Gastroenterol 20: 78-83
Beyer D, Schultze PJ (1983) Sonographie des Magen-Darm-Traktes. In: Bücheler E, Friedmann G, Thelen M (eds) Real-time-Sonographie des Körpers. Thieme, Stuttgart
Beyer D, Friedmann G, Krestin GP (1984) Sinnvoller Einsatz bildgebender Verfahren bei akuter Appendizitis. Fortschr Röntgenstr 140/3: 269-275
Botsford WT, Wilson RE (1981) The acute abdomen. Enke, Stuttgart
Frimann-Dahl J (1968) The acute abdomen. In: Strnad F (ed) Röntgendiagnostik des Digestionstraktes und des Abdomens. Springer, Berlin Heidelberg New York (Handbuch der med. Radiologie, vol 11/2)
Govoni AF, Whalen JP (1981) The acute abdomen. In: Teplick GJ, Haskin ME (eds) Surgical radiology, vol 1. Saunders, Philadelphia
Knothe W (1968) Die Röntgendiagnostik des Appendix. In: Strnad F (ed) Röntgendiagnostik des Digestionstraktes und des Abdomens. Springer, Berlin Heidelberg New York (Handbuch der med. Radiologie, vol 11/2)
Meyers MA (1982) Dynamic radiology of the abdomen. Springer, Berlin Heidelberg New York
Meyers MA, Oliphant M (1974) Ascending retrocecal appendicitis. Radiology 110: 295
Mindelzun RE, McCort JJ (1983) Acute abdomen. In: Margulis AR, Burhenne HJ (eds) Alimentary tract radiology, vol 1. Mosby, St. Louis
Puylaert JBCM (1986) Acute appendicitis: US evaluation using graded compression. Radiology 158: 355-360
Schwerk WB, Wittrup B, Maroske D (1987) Sonographie bei akuter Appendizitis - eine prospektive und kontrollierte Studie Ultraschalldiagnostik 87, Drei-Länder-Treffen Salzburg, Ultraschall in Klinik und Praxis, Supplement 1
Shimkin PM (1978) Radiology of acute appendicitis - commentary. AJR 130: 1001
Swart B, Meyer G (1971) Die Diagnostik des akuten Abdomens beim Erwachsenen - ein neues klinisch-röntgenologisches Konzept. Radiologe 14: 1
Vaudagna JS, McCort JJ (1975) Plain film diagnosis of retrocecal appendicitis. Radiology 117: 533

4.1.5 Abscesses

4.1.5.1 Intraperitoneal Abscesses

G. P. Krestin, D. Beyer, W. Steinbrich

Etiology

Primary Abscesses

- Usually the cause is outside the abdominal cavity (chest, bones, etc.)
- Causative pathogen agent gains access to the peritoneal cavity via blood, lymph, or female genital organs

Secondary Abscesses

Secondary to perforation (nontraumatic)

- Gastric perforation (ulcer, tumor)
  - Into the free abdominal cavity
  - Posteriorly into the lesser sac
- Free duodenal ulcer perforation anteriorly
- Perforated diverticulum (Meckel's diverticulum or colonic diverticulum)
- Perforated appendix (acute appendicitis)

Secondary to an inflammatory process

- Gangrenous cholecystitis
- Appendicitis
- Regional enteritis
- Ulcerative colitis
- Septic abortion
- Salpingitis
- Puerperal infection

Postoperative abscesses

- Perforation or suture line leak in a hollow viscus
- Intra- or postoperative contamination by the surgical wound
- Perforation of a stress ulcer
- Intestinal gangrene after vascular occlusion with ischemia and infarction
- Foreign bodies

Secondary to abdominal trauma (which may or may not breach the peritoneal cavity)

- Rupture of the liver
- Rupture of the gallbladder
- Rupture of the spleen
- Gastrointestinal perforation (also by swallowed foreign bodies)
- Penetrating injury of the bowel
- Rupture of a retroperitoneal abscess into the peritoneal cavity
- Rupture of the urinary bladder

Secondary to circumscribed gangrene of the small or large bowel

Note: The mortality from intraperitoneal abscesses approaches 30% even with intensive care. Unrecognized and untreated abscesses have a mortality rate of almost 100%.

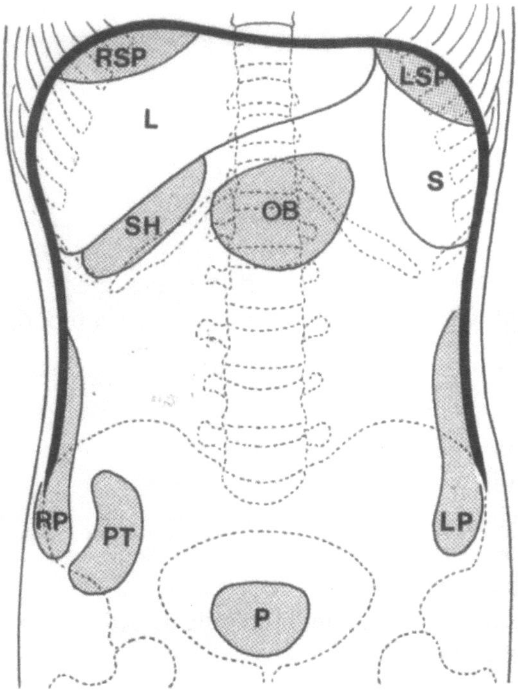

Fig. 135. Major sites of occurrence of intraperitoneal abscesses. *RSP*, right subphrenic; *LSP*, left subphrenic; *SH*, subhepatic; *RP*, right paracolic; *LP*, left paracolic; *PT*, perityphlitic; *OB*, omental bursa; *P*, pelvic abscess; *L*, liver; *S*, spleen

Localization, Cause, and Typical Spread of Intraperitoneal Abscesses
Localization and cause (Figs. 135–137)

Organ Abscesses
- Hepatic abscess (Figs. 141, 142b)
  - Hematogenous infection (bacterial, amebic, etc.)
  - Hepatic rupture
  - Biliary tract disease
  - Postoperative
- Splenic abscess (Fig. 142d)
  - Hematogenous infection
  - Splenic rupture
  - Postoperative

Spread (Fig. 137)
- From rupture of abscess
- To left and right subphrenic space
- To subhepatic space
- To paracolic spaces

Right Subphrenic abscesses (Fig. 138, 140)
- Hepatic rupture
- Perforated ulcer
- Perforated appendicitis
- Biliary tract infection
- Postoperative

Spread
- To subhepatic space
- To right paracolic space
- Into lesser pelvis

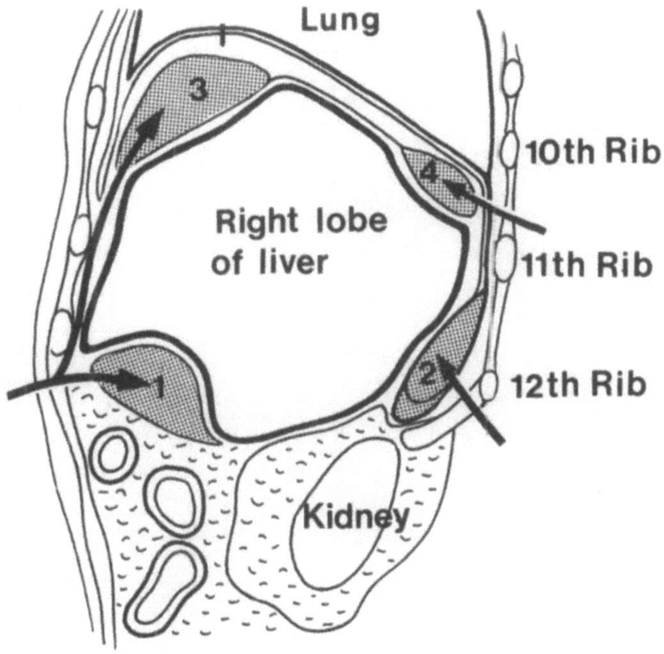

Fig. 136. Sites of occurrence of abscesses in the right upper quadrant and their relation to the right lobe of the liver: *1*, anterior subhepatic; *2*, posterior subhepatic (Morison's pouch); *3*, anterior subphrenic; *4*, posterior subphrenic. The *arrows* indicate the routes of surgical access. (After Meyers, 1982)

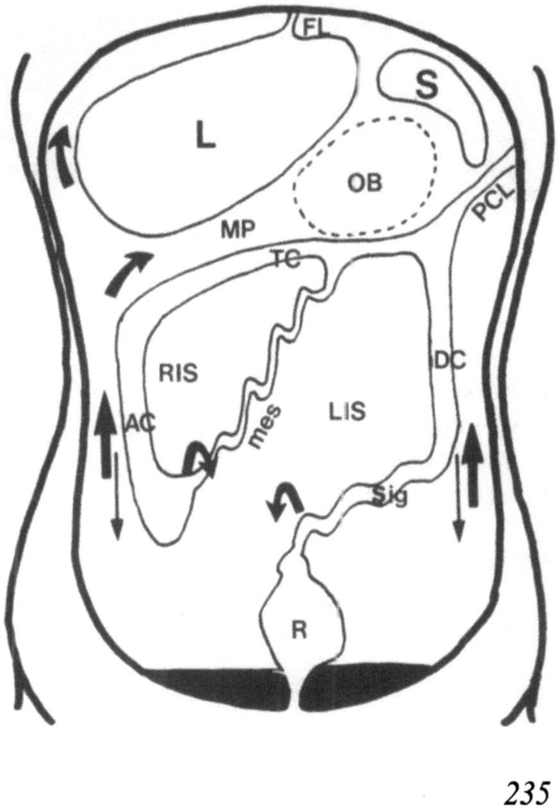

Fig. 137. Pathways of intraperitoneal spread of inflammation. *L*, liver; *S*, spleen; *AC*, ascending colon; *TC*, transverse colon; *DC*, descending colon; *Sig*, sigmoid; *R*, rectum; *OB*, omental bursa; *MP*, Morison's pouch; *FL*, falciform ligament of the liver; *PCL*, phrenicocolic ligament; *mes*, mesentery of small bowel; *LIS*, left inframesocolic space; *RIS*, right inframesocolic space

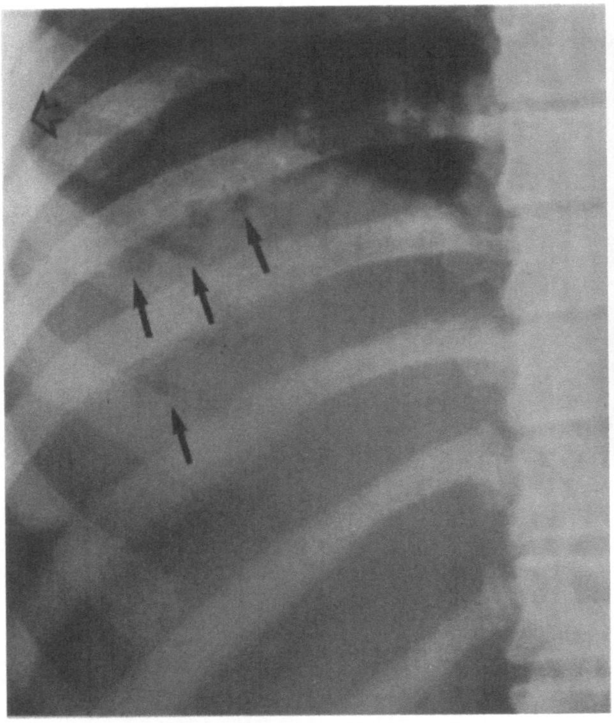

a

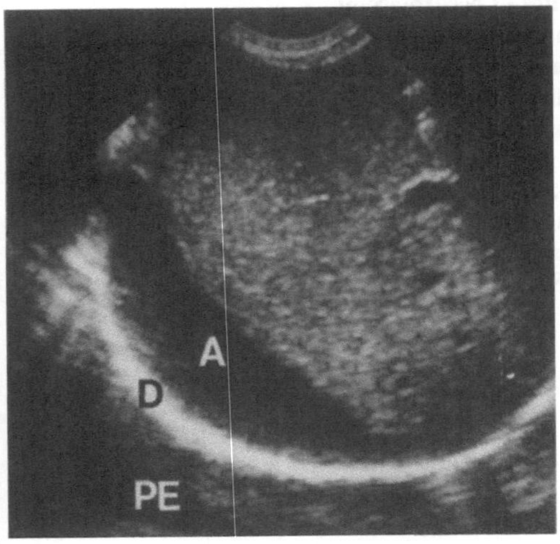

b

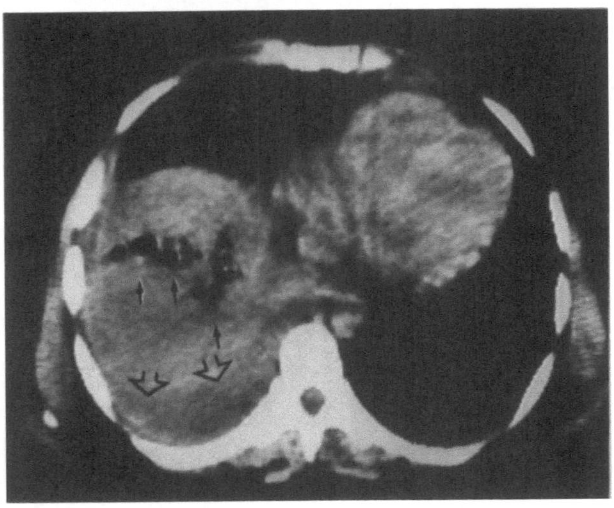

c

Fig. 138 a–c. Right subphrenic abscess. Man, 42 years old, with echinococciasis of the liver confirmed by ultrasound and CT. On day 7 after operative removal the patient developed subfebrile temperatures and right lower quadrant pain; there was no evidence of scar irritation. **a** *Supine film* shows right subphrenic gas bubbles (→), elevation of the right hemidiaphragm, and right angular effusion (⇒). **b** *Sonogram* from the right subcostal space shows a hypoechoic subphrenic area consistent with an abscess *(A)*. The fluid appears gas-free. There is accompanying pleural effusion *(PE); D*, diaphragm. **c** *CT scan* demonstrates a right subphrenic abscess with gas bubbles (→) and pleural effusion (⇒). *Operation* confirmed a postoperative right subphrenic abscess

Left Subphrenic Abscess (Fig. 139)

- Splenic rupture
- Gastric perforation
- Postoperative

Spread

- To left subhepatic space
- Spread caudad is hindered by the phrenicocolic ligament

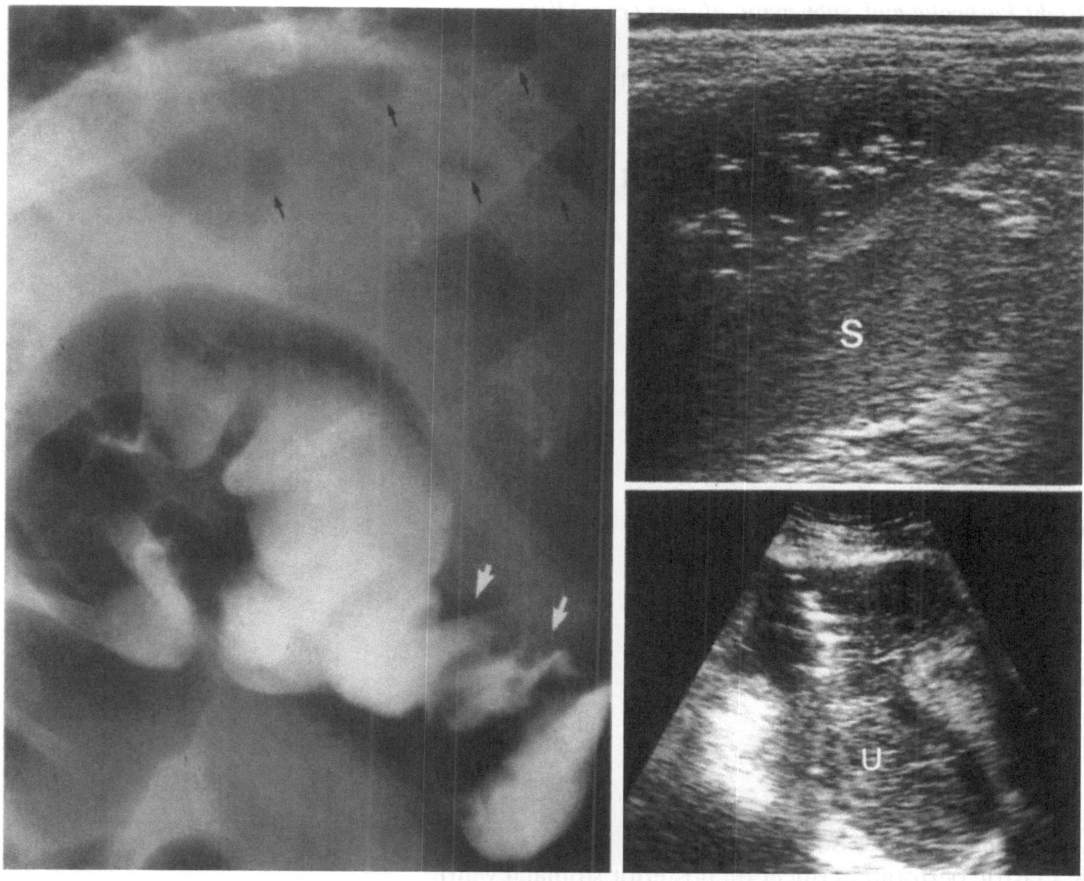

a b c

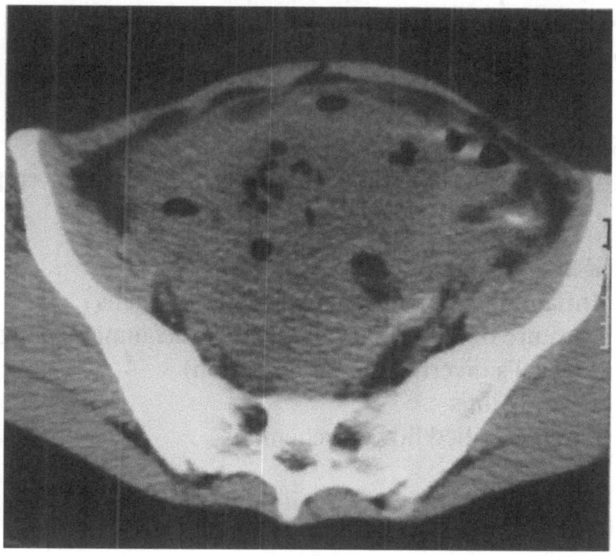

d

Fig. 139 a–d. Left subphrenic abscess. Man, 52 years old, with known retroperitoneal fibrosis. After undergoing ureterolysis with peritonealization, the patient developed fever, leukocytosis, and left upper quadrant tenderness. **a** *Supine film after enema* with water-soluble contrast (detail) shows fixed gas bubbles in the left upper quadrant (→) above the left colic flexure. The "jagged" cranial margin of the colon (➡) signifies secondary inflammatory infiltration. **b** *Sonogram* of the left upper quadrant (longitudinal scan) shows a hypoechoic mass with mobile internal echoes adjacent to the spleen *(S)* representing left subphrenic abscess. *Operation* disclosed a left subphrenic abscess with secondary infiltration of the left colic flexure. **c, d Infected hematoma of the abdominal cavity.** Woman, 22 years old, developed ileus following laparoscopy with fluid aspiration and puncture of the left ovary. Operation disclosed serosal defects, blood in the mesocolon, and a left-sided benign ovarian cyst. A small defect in the ileum was oversewn. Pulmonary embolism ensued on the 6th postoperative day. On day 8 the patient had leukocytosis with severe lower abdominal pain. The abdomen was distended but not tender. **c** *Sonogram* (longitudinal scan) shows a large, loculated fluid collection with gas inclusions and reverberation echoes (*U,* uterus). **d** *CT scan* at the same level shows a fluid collection with gas, displacing the bowel loops laterally. At reoperation an infected, intraperitoneal hematoma was found in the lower abdomen

Right Paracolic and Subhepatic Abscess (Fig. 140)
- Appendicitis with perforation
- Biliary tract and gallbladder infection
- Pelvic abscess
- Inflammations of the bowel
- Circumscribed gangrene of the bowel
- Postoperative

Spread
- To subphrenic space
- Into lesser pelvis

Left Paracolic abscess (see Fig. 146)
- Perforated diverticulum
- Pelvic abscess
- Inflammation of the bowel
- Postoperative

Spread
- To left subphrenic space
- Into lesser pelvis

Abscess in the Lesser Sac (Fig. 141 a–c)
- Gastric perforation (ulcer on posterior stomach wall)
- Pancreatic rupture (after acute pancreatitis)
- Postoperative

Spread
- Into free abdominal cavity (only with a patent epiploic foramen)

Cul-de-sac (Fig. 139 c, d)
- Inflammations of the female genital organs
- Rupture of the urinary bladder (posttraumatic, iatrogenic)
- Meckel's diverticulum (perforation)
- Diverticulitis
- Circumscribed bowel ischemia
- Postoperative

Spread
- Into left and right paracolic spaces
- To left and right inframesocolic space
- To subhepatic space
- To right subphrenic space

Fig. 140 a, b. Perforated appendicitis with subphrenic and subhepatic abscess. Man, 19 years old, with nausea, severe right flank pain, fever, and diffuse abdominal rigidity. **a, b** *Supine and left lateral films* show combined small and large bowel distension with fluid levels. There are gas bubbles in the right subphrenic space and above the right colic flexure (→). The left lateral film additionally shows free intraperitoneal air between the liver and abdominal wall (⇒). *Diagnosis:* perforated appendicitis with subphrenic and subhepatic abscess

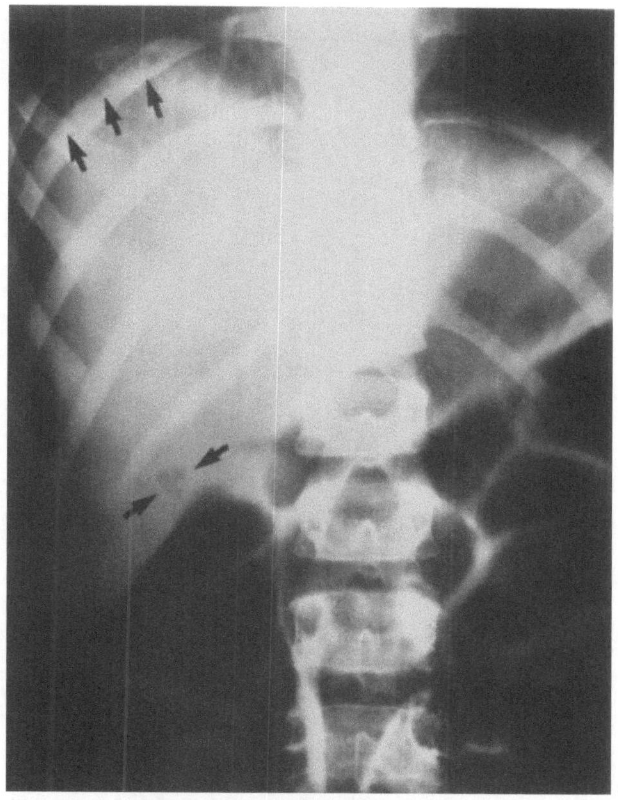

a

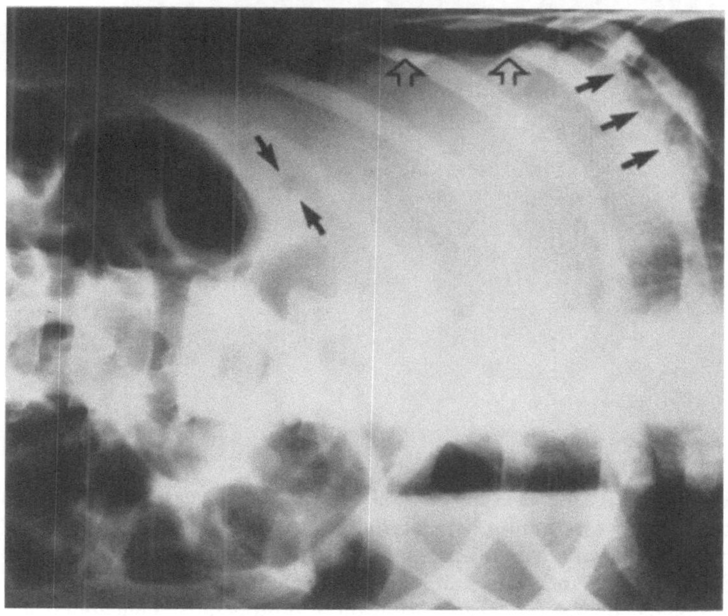

b

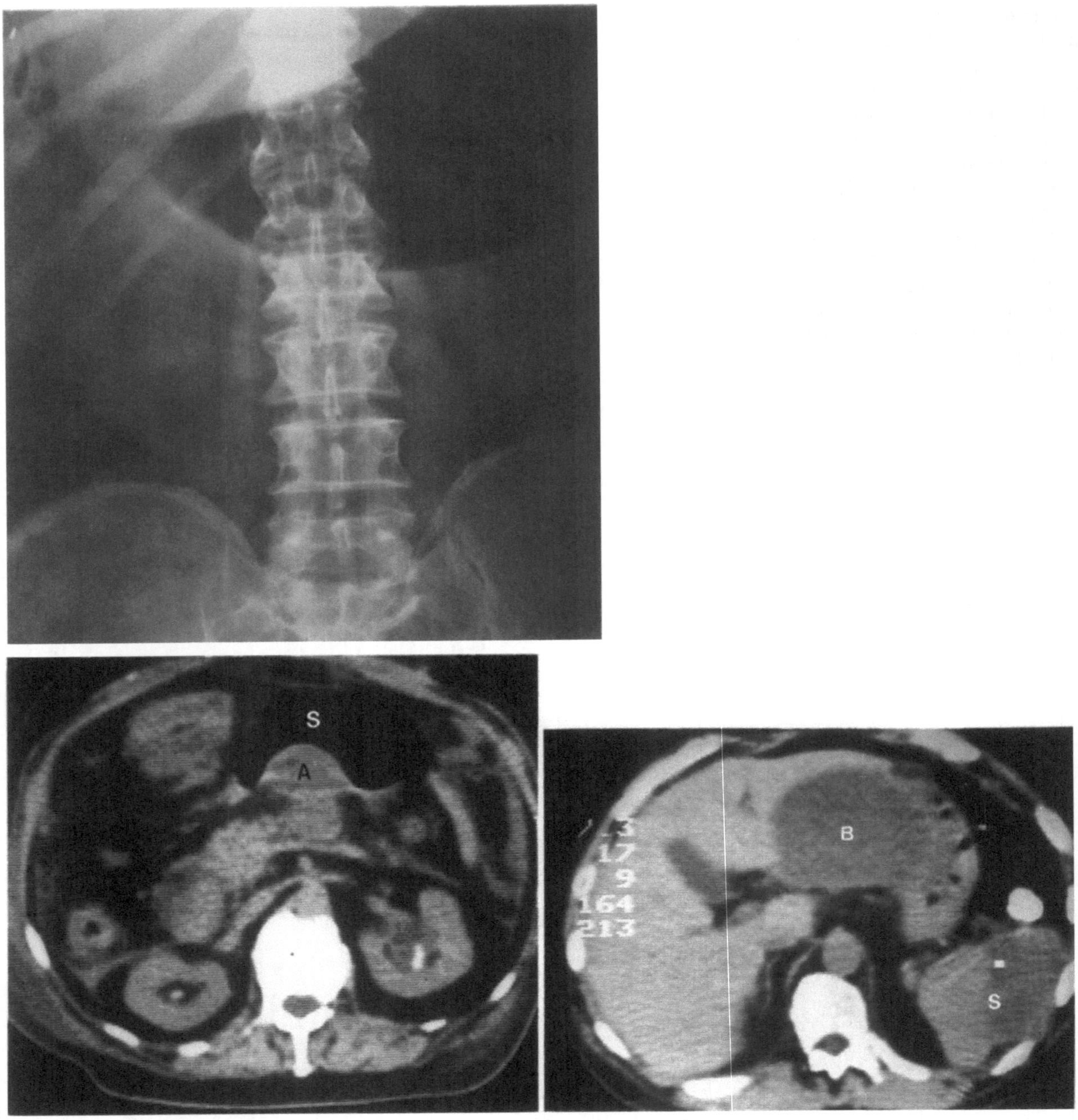

Fig. 141 a–c. Abscess in the omental bursa. Man, 67 years old, who had undergone partial hepatic resection for hepatocellular carcinoma. Five days postoperatively he developed mesogastric pain unaccompanied by fever. **a** *Supine film* shows an atonic, gas-filled stomach and gasless abdomen. Sonograms (not shown) revealed a liquid mass in the pancreatic region, raising suspicion of postoperative hematoma. **b** *CT scan* shows a soft-tissue mass *(A)* between the pancreas and stomach *(S)* in the omental bursa impressing on the posterior stomach wall. There are increased streaky and reticular markings in the right midabdomen and thickening of the retroperitoneal fascial layers following the partial hepatectomy. *Operation* uncovered a postoperative abscess in the omental bursa. **c** Abscess in the omental bursa *(B)* with displacement of the compressed stomach following ulcer-perforation of the posterior gastric wall (*S*, spleen)

Clinical Symptoms

Abdominal symptoms
- Localized tenderness with muscular rigidity (local peritonitis)
- Normal or decreased peristalsis
- Disturbed wound healing, fistula formation
- Nausea, vomiting

Extra-abdominal symptoms
- Inflammatory symptoms (fever, elevated ESR, leukocytosis)
- Sympathetic pleuropneumonia, pleural effusion

Caution: Antibiotics mask symptoms and make them appear clinically less severe.

Radiologic Signs

Plain Radiographs

Primary signs of abscess
- Pathologic, extraluminal, fixed gas collection (Figs. 138–140, 142)
  String-of-beads pattern
  Large gas-containing cavity with or without a fluid level
- Soft-tissue density with organ displacement (Fig. 139)
  Displacement of the colon (paracolic abscess)
  Displacement of the bladder (cul-de-sac abscess)
  Displacement of the stomach (abscess in the lesser sac) (see Fig. 7)
- Obscuring of normally visible contours (e.g., right lower margin of liver)
- Possible fixation of a normally mobile organ

Secondary signs of abscess
- Elevation of restricted motion of hemidiaphragm with a subphrenic abscess (Figs. 138, 139)
- Changes in the basal lung or pleura
- Localized or generalized bowel atony with fluid levels (Fig. 140)
- Scoliosis of the lumbar spine (e.g., with perityphlitic abscess)

Note: A plain chest radiograph is an indispensable part of the diagnostic work-up of intra-abdominal abscesses.

Fistulography (if a fistulous tract is present) (see Fig. 102)
- Permits accurate localization of the abscess
- Extent of the abscess cannot always be evaluated
- The origin of the inflammation can be established in some cases

Sonography (Figs. 138b, 139b, c, 142c)
- Demonstrates a hypoechoic to echo-free mass, possibly with floating echoes ("snowstorm")
- Irregular, echogenic walls
- If gas is present: internal echoes with acoustic shadows or reverberations
- Displacement of adjacent organs
- Usually permits the abscess to be localized with reasonable accuracy

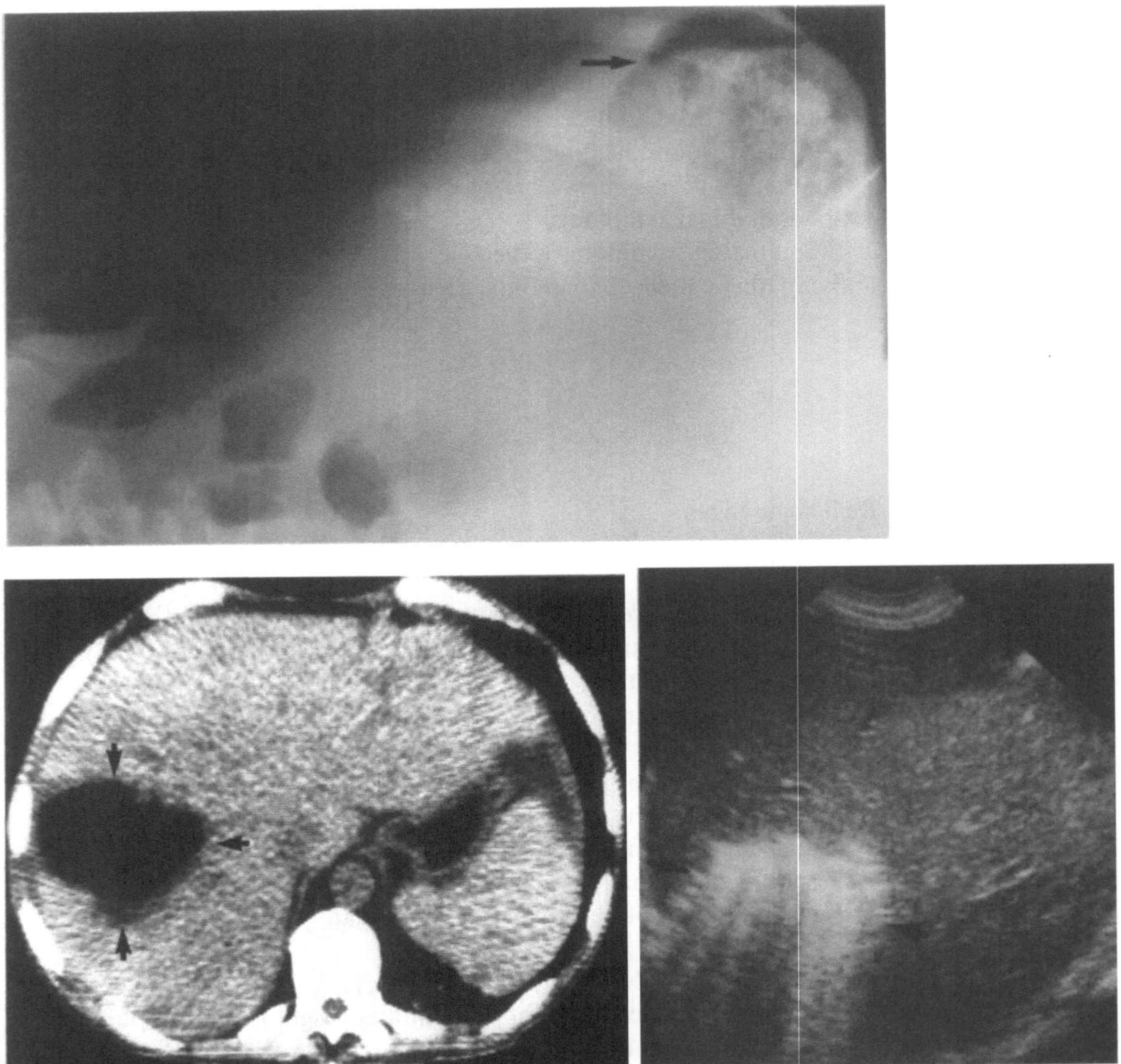

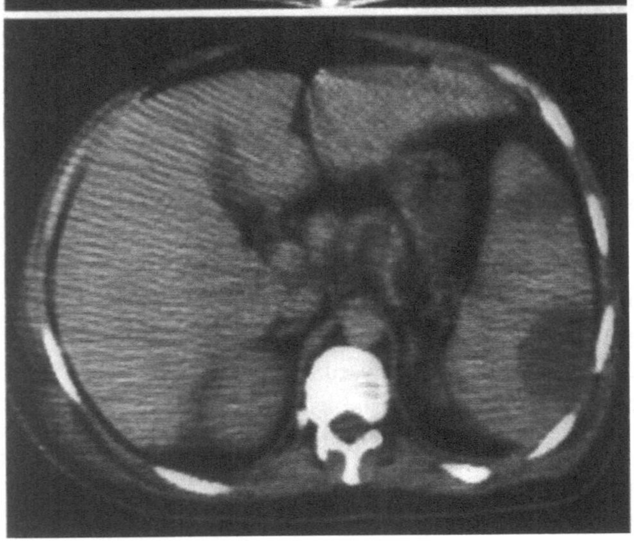

Fig. 142a–d. Hepatic abscess. Following Whipple's operation a 62-year-old man developed right upper quadrant pain, fever, and leukocytosis. **a** *Left lateral film* shows relatively small, fixed gas bubbles with irregular margins over the right upper quadrant and a large gas-fluid level (→). **b** *CT scan* shows a large, gas-containing hepatic abscess in the right lobe of the liver (→). *Operation* disclosed a hepatic abscess. **c** *Sonogram* shows marked acoustic shadowing in the hepatic region produced by a large air-containing mass (→). **d Splenic abscess.** Male, 45 years old, with endocarditis experienced bouts of septic fever for several days accompanied by left upper quadrant pain. *CT scan* shows several low-density areas in the spleen produced by multiple splenic abscesses

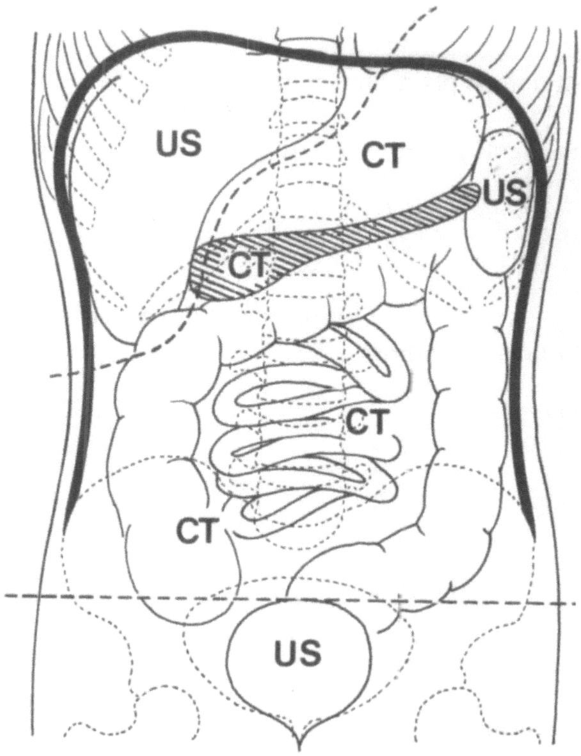

Fig. 143. Regions of the abdomen for which either *sonography (US)* or *CT* have the greatest diagnostic value

Note: Abscesses are demonstrable on plain films in only about 50% of cases. Plain radiography combined with sonography is diagnostic in almost 90% of cases!

Caution: A definitive sonographic diagnosis is possible *only if the scan is positive.* Technical constraints limit the usefulness of the method (dressing material, drains, bowel gas).

Computed Tomography (Figs. 138 c, 139 d, 141 c, b, 142 b, d)
- Pathologic mass with an attenuation value of 15-35 HU
- Gas in an abscess is *always* visible on CT
- Ring enhancement after i.v. contrast is characteristic
- Localization and extent can be accurately established
- Excellent for therapeutic planning

Note: CT is diagnostic in over 90% of abscess cases. Thus, when an abscess is suspected and plain films and sonograms are negative, one should *always* perform CT scans - or operate (Fig. 143)!

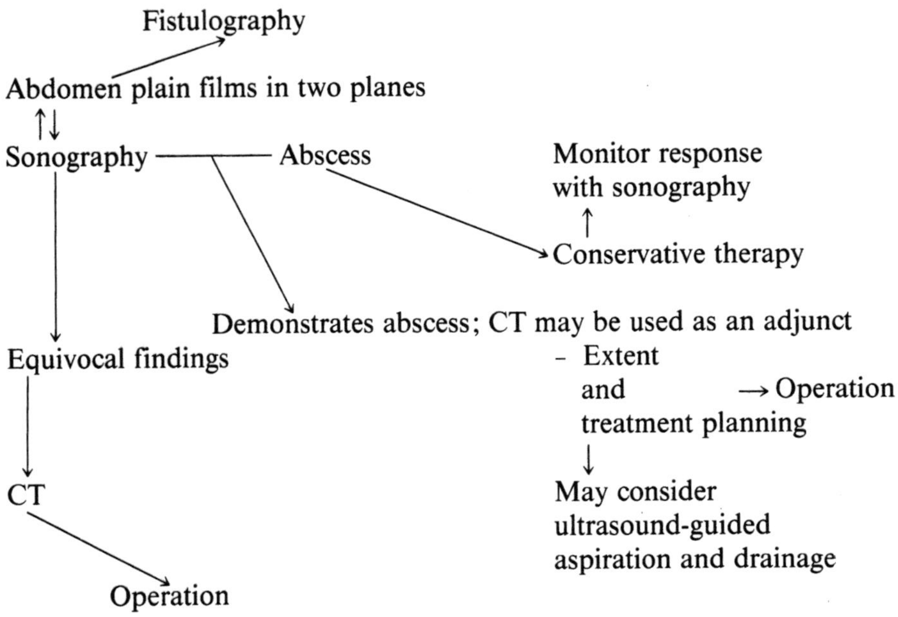

References

Ariel IM, Kazarian KK (1971) Diagnosis and treatment of abdominal abscesses. Williams & Wilkins, Baltimore

Callen PW (1979) Computed tomographic evaluation of abdominal and pelvic abscesses. Radiology 131: 171

Connell TR, Stephens DH, Carlson HC et al. (1980) Upper abdominal abscess: continuing and deadly problem. AJR 134: 759

Doust BD, Quiroz F, Stewart JM (1977) Ultrasonic distinction of abscesses from other intra-abdominal fluid collections. Radiology 125: 213

Halber MD, Daffner RH, Morgan CL, Trought WS, Thompson WM, Rice RP, Korobkin M (1979) Intraabdominal abscess: current concepts in radiologic evaluation. AJR 133: 9

Kressel HY, Filly RA (1978) Ultrasonographic appearance of gas-containing abscesses in the abdomen. AJR 130: 276

Krestin GP, Beyer D, Steinbrich W (1984) Radiologische Diagnostik intraabdomineller Abszesse durch gestuften Einsatz bildgebender Verfahren. Röntgenblätter 37: 295

Kumpan W (1987) Computertomographische Analyse postoperativer abdomineller Kompartments. Eine Vergleichsstudie an 100 Patienten mit abdominellen Abszessen. Radiologe 27: 203-215

Meyers MA (1970) The spread and localization of acute intraperitoneal effusions. Radiology 95: 547

Mintz MC, Arger PH, Kressel HY (1983) Algorithmic approach to the radiologic evaluation of a suspected abdominal abscess. Semin Ultrasound 4: 80

Mueller PR, Simeone JF (1983) Intraabdominal abscesses: diagnosis by sonography and computed tomography. Radiol Clin North Am 21: 425

Rice RP, Masters SJ (1973) Intraabdominal abscess. Semin Roentgenol 8: 365

Wittich GR, van Sonnenberg E, Karnel F, Casola G et al. (1987) Perkutane Drainage komplizierter Abszesse und Flüssigkeitsansammlungen. Radiologe 27: 216-220

4.1.5.2 Extraperitoneal Abscesses

G. P. Krestin, D. Beyer, W. Steinbrich

Etiology

Primary Abscesses
- Cause is outside the retroperitoneal space
- Causative pathogenic agents gain entry to the retroperitoneum through blood or lymph

Secondary Abscesses
Resulting from open or blunt abdominal trauma
- Rupture of kidney
- Rupture of duodenum
- Rupture of colon
- Rupture of bladder
- Avulsion of ureter
- Rupture of pancreas
- Penetrating injury (with or without perforation of the duodenum or colon)

Resulting from retroperitoneal perforation of a hollow viscus
- Perforated duodenal ulcer
- Perforated appendicitis
- Rectal perforation (iatrogenic or by foreign body)

Resulting from an inflammatory process
- Pyelonephritis with abscess formation
- Pancreatitis
- Appendicitis
- Regional enteritis (retroperitoneal fistula)
- Spondylitis or spondylodiscitis (tuberculous abscess)

Postoperative
- Perforation or suture line leak in a hollow viscus
- Perforation of a stress ulcer
- Infection of a lymphocele
- Contamination by the operative wound
- Infection of a vascular prosthesis
- Gangrene following a vascular lesion

Note: Retroperitoneal abscesses remain confined to a particular space for some time. Spread to adjacent compartments is a late event.

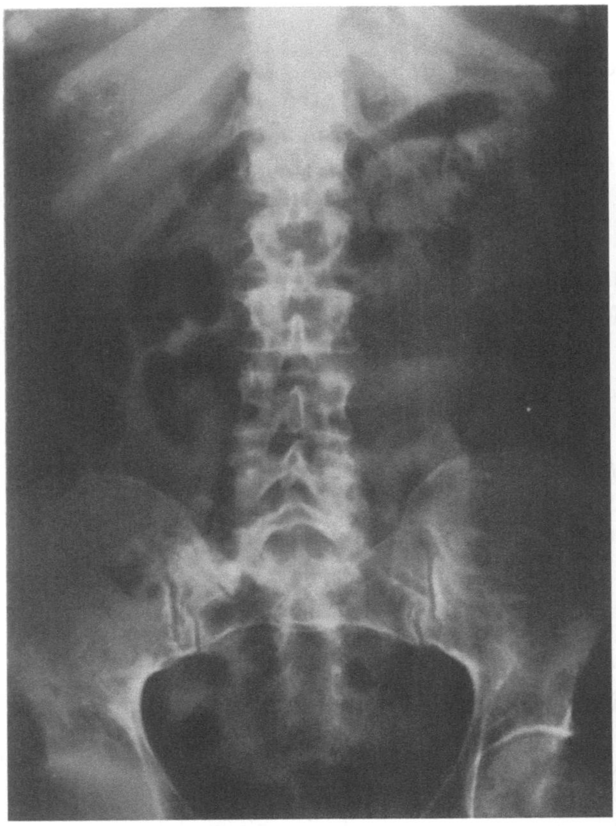

a

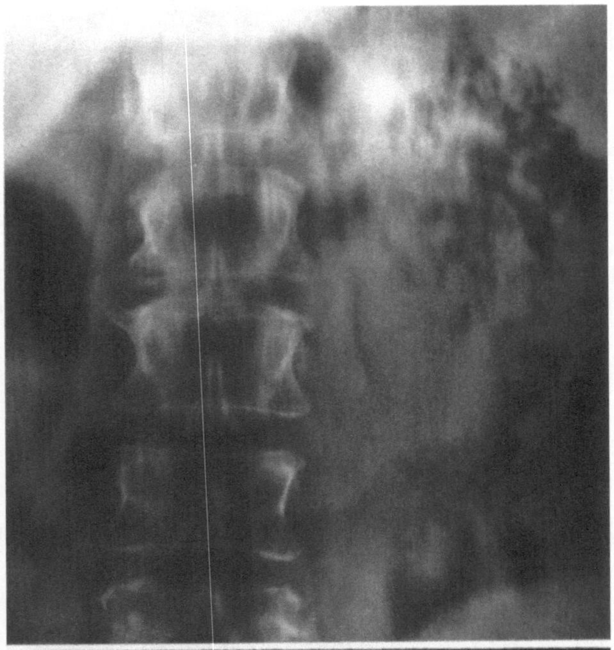

b

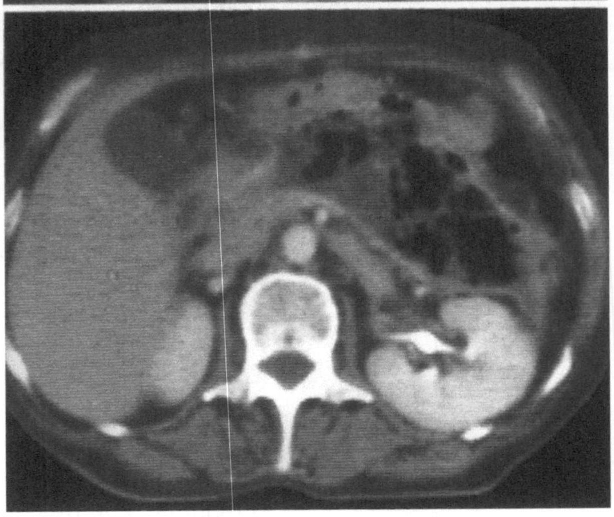

c

Fig. 144a–c. Retroperitoneal abscess secondary to pancreatitis. Woman, 61 years old, with girdling epigastric pain and signs of peritonitis, with elevated amylase and lipase values. *Supine film* (**a**) and *sagittal tomogram* (**b**) show fixed gas bubbles projected over the left kidney and extending past the renal borders. **c** *CT scan* shows a large, gas-forming abscess in the anterior pararenal space as a sequel to pancreatitis

Localization and Cause

Anterior pararenal space
- Pancreatic abscess
- Duodenal rupture or perforation
- Appendiceal perforation
- Colonic rupture or perforation
- Postoperative

Perirenal space
- Renal abscess
- Rupture of kidney
- Postoperative

Posterior pararenal space
- Rectal perforation
- Infection of vascular prosthesis
- Infection of the vertebral column
- Postoperative

Psoas Abscess
- Infection of the vertebral column
- Prosthetic infection

Clinical Symptoms

Systemic symptoms
- Inflammatory signs (fever, elevated ESR)
- Sympathetic pleural effusion (rare)

Abdominal symptoms
- Back pain
- Tenderness to percussion of the renal beds
- Postural guarding (lumbar scoliosis)
- Irritative psoas pain
- Reflex colonic distension
- Nausea, vomiting

Caution: The symptoms of retroperitoneal abscesses may be considerably less pronounced, less acute, and less specific than those of intraperitoneal lesions.

Note: The mortality from retroperitoneal abscesses may be 100% without treatment and may approach 50% even with intensive care.

Radiologic Signs

Plain Radiographs

Primary signs of abscess

Extraluminal fixed gas collection (Figs. 144–147)
- Forms cystlike or streaky patterns along fascial planes
- Fluid levels are rare

Mass producing organ displacement
- Displacement of the colon (e.g., perityphlitic abscess) (see Fig. 132)
- Displacement of the kidney (perirenal abscesses) (Fig. 145)
- Displacement of the ureter (e.g., psoas abscess)
- Anterior displacement of the rectum (retrorectal abscess)

Obscuring of normally visible contours
- Psoas shadow (especially with marked disparity between sides) (Figs. 145, 149)
- Renal contours (increased or decreased density, "corona" from perirenal fluid)
- Flank stripe (with abscess of posterior pararenal space)

Note: The urogram and/or plain tomogram can be very helpful in demonstrating primary signs of retroperitoneal abscess.

Secondary signs of abscess
- Elevation of the diaphragm and basal pleuropneumonia (e.g., with pancreatic abscess)
- Bowel distension (usually colon) (Fig. 145)
- Scoliosis of the lumbar spine (e.g., psoas abscess) (Figs. 145, 149)

Fig. 145a–c. Retroperitoneal abscess, secondary to a retroperitoneal perforation of the appendix. Girl, 16 years old, with pain in the right flank and right lower quadrant. She was febrile and had normal urinary findings. *Supine film* (**a**) and *urogram* (**b**) show fixed gas bubbles over the right flank. There is also mediad displacement of the right kidney (→) and mild scoliosis of the lumbar spine convex to the left. Congenital meningocele of the lumbar spine is additionally present. **c** *Sonogram* shows displacement of the right kidney *(K)* by a pararenal mass that contains gas and produces posterior acoustic shadowing and reverberations (➡)

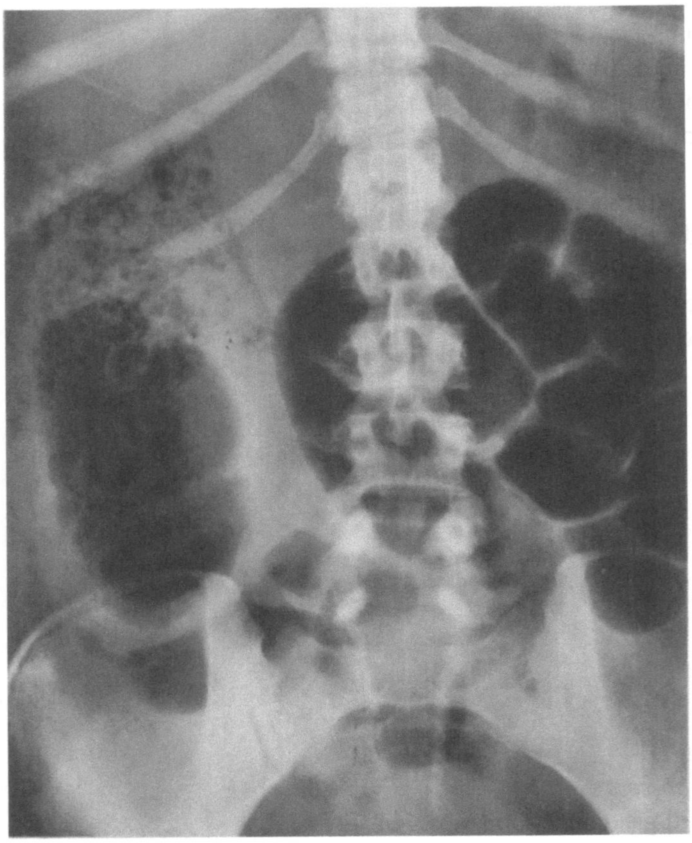

a

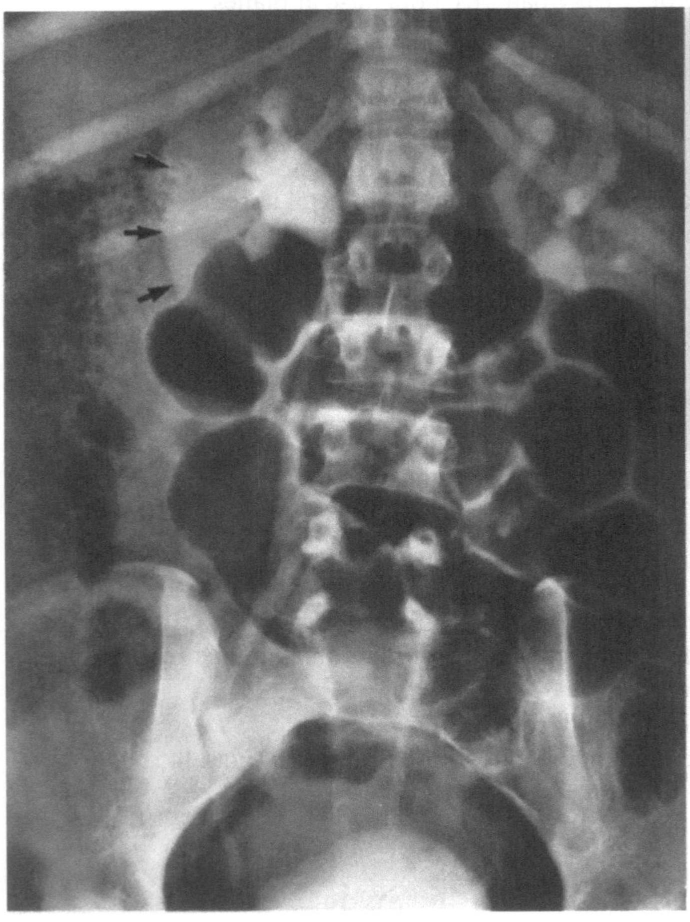

b

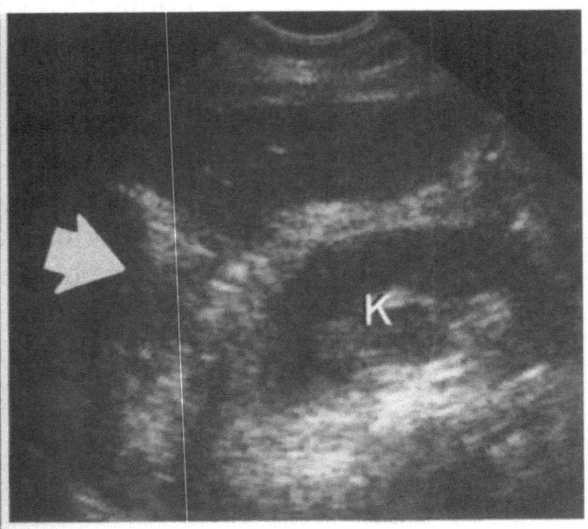

Localizing signs (see Fig. 59)

Anterior pararenal space
- Density or extraluminal gas extends past psoas contours
- Flank stripe is preserved
- Spread to the contralateral side is possible

Perirenal space
- Increased or decreased density of renal contours ("corona")
- Mostly unilateral
- Change in organ position

Posterior pararenal space
- Density or extraluminal gas may spread in the flank stripes
- Psoas contours are preserved
- Mostly unilateral

Note: Plain films show pathologic changes in only about 40% of cases. Localization based on a typical pattern of spread is rarely possible.

Sonography (Figs. 145 c, 146 d, 148 d)
- Hypoechoic to echo-free mass in the retroperitoneal space (a floating, "snowstorm" echo pattern can occur)
- Irregular, echogenic walls
- If gas is present: internal echoes with acoustic shadows or reverberations
- Displacement of the kidneys as evidence of retroperitoneal localization
- Lesions cannot always be definitively assigned to retroperitoneal compartments

Note: Sonography is diagnostic in about 70% of cases; in 30% it is *not* diagnostic because of overlying bowel gas.

Computed Tomography (Figs. 144 c, 146 c, 147 b, 148 e, 149 c, d)
- Mass lesion with attenuation value of 15-35 HU
- Gas within the mass is *always* demonstrable
- Peripheral enhancement after i.v. contrast medium is highly characteristic of an abscess
- Accurate localization (organ assignment, identification of involved compartment) is possible
- Extent can be accurately established
- Excellent for directing treatment planning

Note: CT is diagnostic in more than 90% of retroperitoneal abscesses. When a retroperitoneal abscess is suspected, CT should be incorporated earlier into the diagnostic program than with an intraperitoneal lesion!

Caution: None of the methods presented can consistently differentiate an older, circumscribed (and possibly infected) hematoma from an abscess.

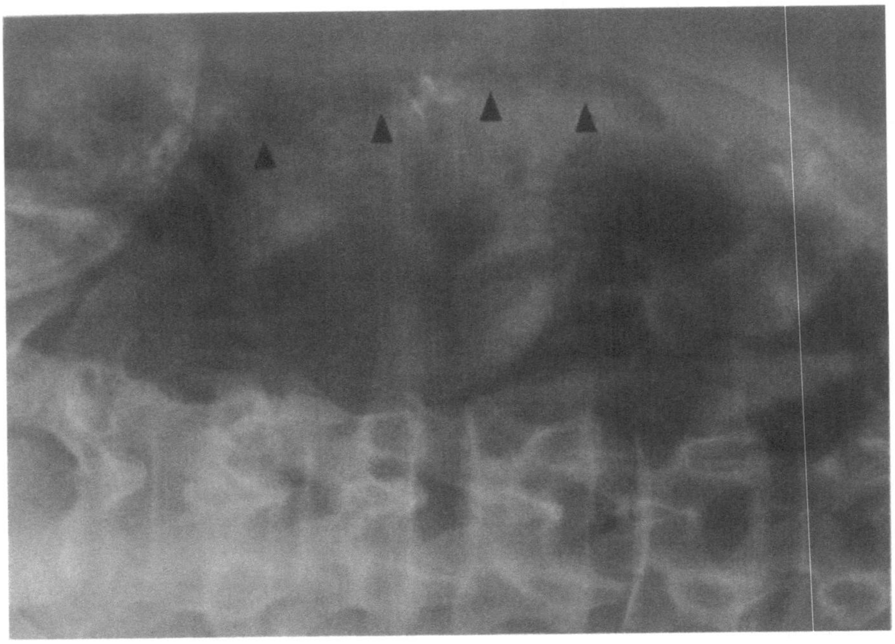

a

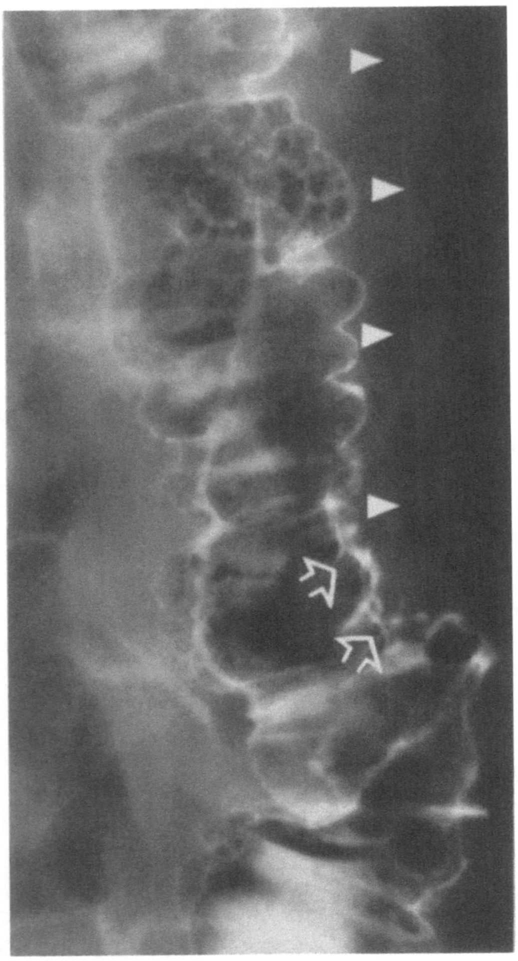

b

Fig. 146a–d. Left paracolic abscess with infiltration of the descending colon following perforation of a sigmoid diverticulum into the retroperitoneum with diverticulitis. Man, 58 years old, with known sigmoid diverticulosis and recurring bouts of diverticulitis. Seven days ago he experienced a new episode of left lower quadrant pain accompanied by fever and an elevated ESR. After a trial of conservative therapy, fever persisted, and the pain became localized to the left mid- and upper abdomen. **a** *Right lateral film* (detail) shows a nonspecific bowel gas pattern with no fluid levels. Extraluminal gas, presumably paracolic, is projected over the left flank lateral to the large bowel (►). **b** *Enema* with water-soluble contrast for bloody stool shows gas bubbles in the left paracolic space (►) with apparent infiltration of the descending colon (⇒).

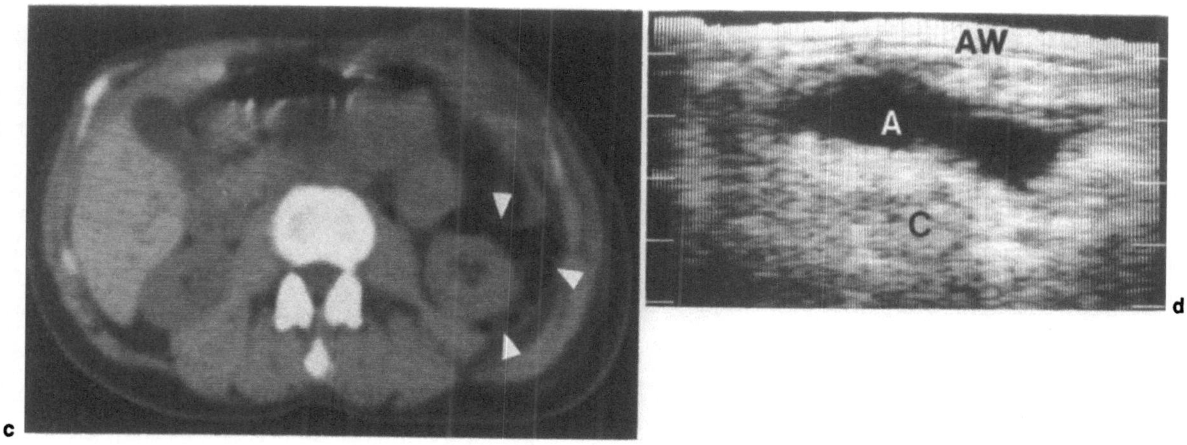

Fig. 146 (continued)
c *CT scan* shows a sizable gas collection in the anterior pararenal space and a lesser collection posteriorly (▶), indicative of an abscess. **d** *Sonogram* shows a fluid-containing abscess *(A)* between the abdominal wall *(AW)* and colon *(C)*

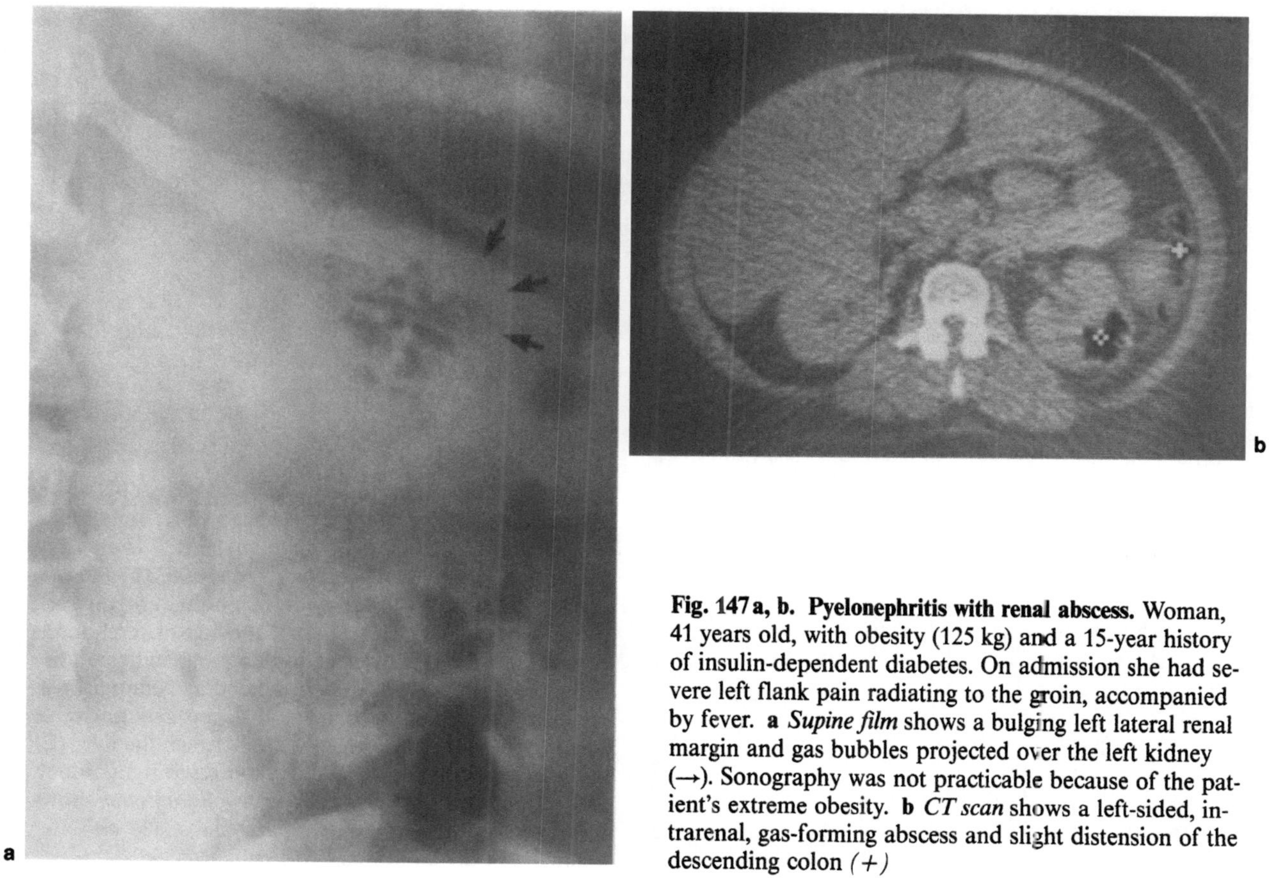

Fig. 147 a, b. Pyelonephritis with renal abscess. Woman, 41 years old, with obesity (125 kg) and a 15-year history of insulin-dependent diabetes. On admission she had severe left flank pain radiating to the groin, accompanied by fever. **a** *Supine film* shows a bulging left lateral renal margin and gas bubbles projected over the left kidney (→). Sonography was not practicable because of the patient's extreme obesity. **b** *CT scan* shows a left-sided, intrarenal, gas-forming abscess and slight distension of the descending colon *(+)*

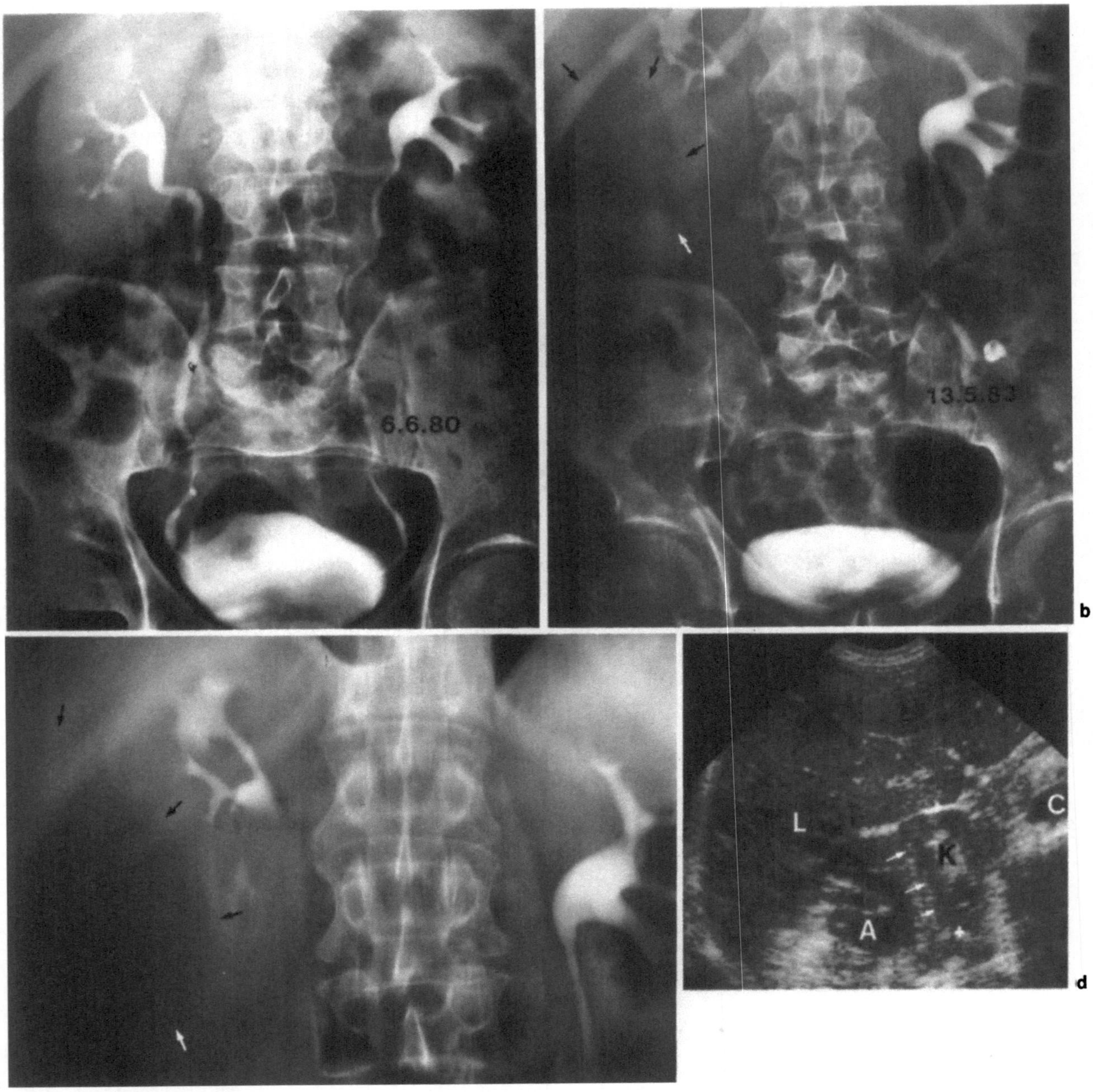

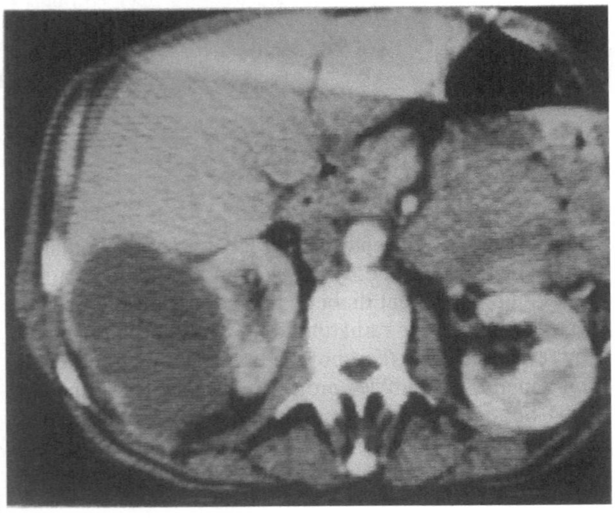

Fig. 148 a–e. Perirenal abscess. Man, 53 years old, with right flank pain, fever, and an elevated ESR; condition was diagnosed and treated as pyelonephritis. *Urograms* taken on 6 June 1980 (**a**) and on 13 May 1983 (**b**) and *film tomogram* (**c**): Comparison with the normal urogram of 6 June 1980 shows obliteration of the inferolateral border of the right kidney with renal displacement and compression of the pyelocaliceal system mediad and craniad (→), raising the suspicion of a tumor. **d** *Sonogram* (transverse scan) shows a hypoechoic mass *(A)* between the liver *(L)* and the medially displaced and compressed right kidney *(K); C,* inferior vena cava. **e** *CT with bolus injection* shows a low-density mass in the right pararenal space with indentation of the kidney and ring enhancement

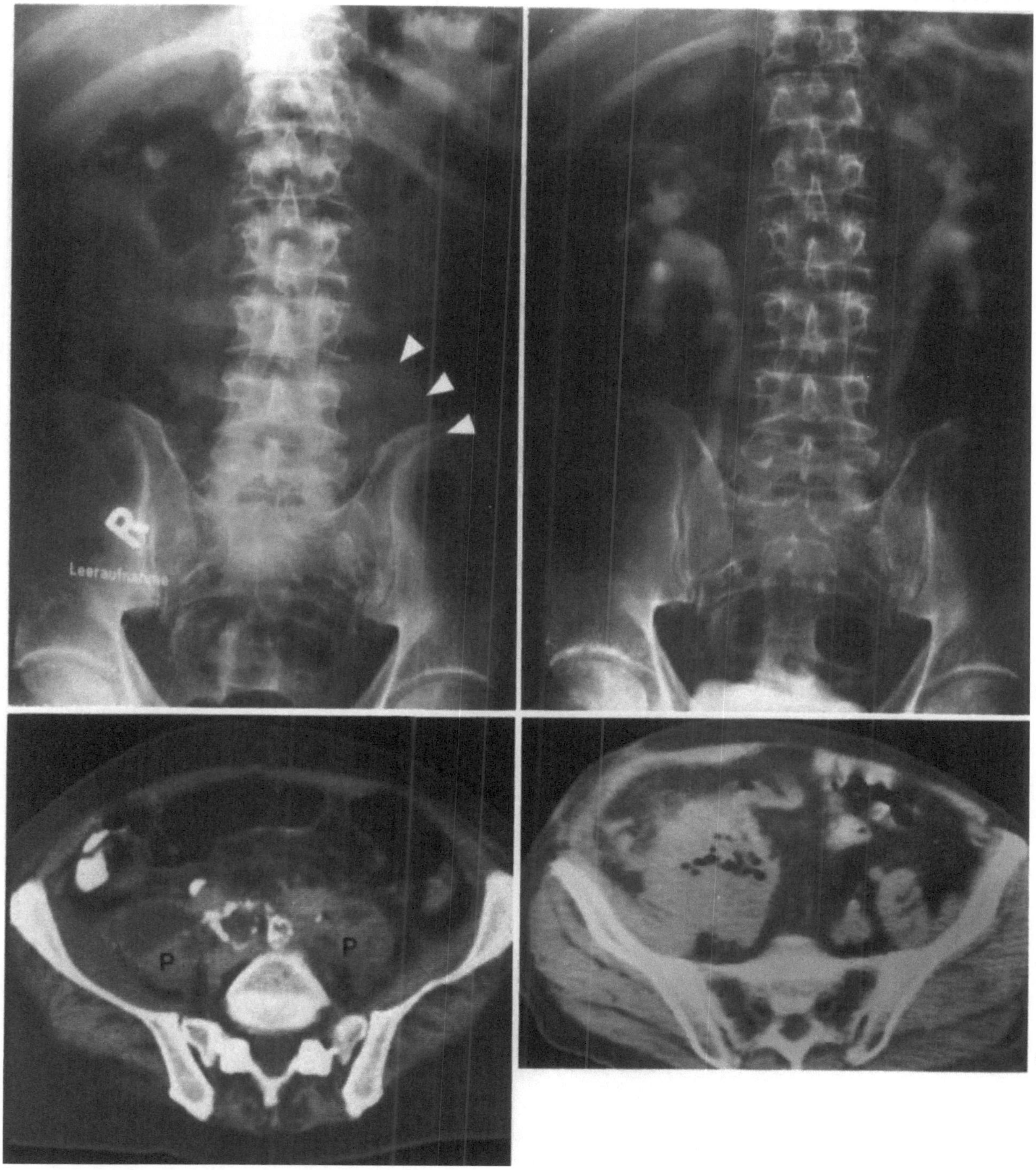

Fig. 149 a–d. Bilateral psoas abscesses leading to bilateral renal and ureteral stasis secondary to infection of a vascular prostheses. Man, 65 years old, with grade 3 bilateral arterial occlusive disease following the insertion of an aortobifemoral bypass. Two months later he developed fever and groin pain. **a** *Supine film* shows a nonspecific bowel gas pattern. The psoas shadows are well-defined superiorly; the right lower psoas contour is indistinct, and the left contour fades away laterally (►). **b** *Urogram* shows bilateral renal and ureteral stasis extending to the level of the L5/S1 junction on the right side and to the L4 level on the left side. **c** *CT scan* shows bilateral, low-density masses with indistinct margins in the region of the psoas muscle *(P)*. The right ureter is dilated, and the left ureter is within the mass. Vascular calcifications are pronounced. **d** *CT scan* shows a **psoas abscess caused by anaerobic bacteria.** The right psoas muscle is expanded and contains gas bubbles. There is concomitant involvement of the mesentery and right abdominal wall

References

Altemeir WA, Culbertson WR, Pullen WD, Shook CD (1973) Intraabdominal abscesses. Am J Surg 125: 70
Friedmann G, Bücheler E, Thurn P (1981) Ganzkörper-Computertomographie. Thieme, Stuttgart
Gerzof SG, Robbins AH, Birkett DH (1978) Computed tomography in the diagnosis and management of abdominal abscesses. Gastrointest Radiol 3: 287
Goldman R, Hunter TB, Haber K (1980) Silent abdominal abscess: role of the radiologist. AJR 134: 759
Hiatt JR, Williams RA, Wilson SE (1983) Intraabdominal abscess: etiology and pathogenesis. Semin Ultrasound 4: 71
Krestin GP, Beyer D, Steinrich W (1984) Radiologische Diagnostik intraabdomineller Abszesse durch gestuften Einsatz bildgebender Verfahren. Röntgenblätter 37: 295
Meyers MA (1974) Radiological features of the spread and localization of extraperitoneal gas and their relationship to its source. Radiology 111: 17
Meyers MA, Whalen JP, Peele K, Berme AS (1972) Radiologic features of extraperitoneal effusions. Radiology 104: 249
Stevenson EOS, Ozeran RS (1979) Retroperitoneal space abscesses. Surg Gynecol 128: 1202
Vermooten V (1933) The mechanism of perinephric and perinephritic abscesses. J Urol 30: 181

4.2 Acute Bowel Diseases

The most common acute disease of the small and large bowel is *intestinal obstruction* - a collective term covering any hindrance to the aboral progression of gastrointestinal contents, including paralytic ileus. Various forms of intestinal obstruction are distinguished clinically according to:

- *Etiology* (mechanical, vascular, functional, intestinal pseudo-obstruction)
- *Time factor* (acute, subacute, chronic, chronic recurring)
- *Localization* (high or low small-bowel obstruction, colon obstruction)
- *Completeness* (partial or incomplete, total or complete)

Note: Rules of thumb for intestinal obstruction

1. The higher the level of the obstruction, the more acute the systemic manifestations.
2. With a low colon obstruction (which usually is incomplete initially), some time is required for the full-blown picture of intestinal obstruction to develop, since the damming back of bowel contents takes more time.
3. Untreated, a primary mechanical obstruction will invariably progress to paralytic ileus.

What does the surgeon need to know from the radiologist when intestinal obstruction is suspected?

- Mechanical obstruction or paralytic ileus?
- In a mechanical obstruction, where is the obstruction located?
- In the small or large bowel?
- Radiologic evidence of a primary or secondary impairment of intestinal blood flow?
- Free air signifying a perforation?
- Evidence of peritonitis?
- Evidence of retro- or extraperitoneal disease?

4.2.1 Mechanical Obstruction of the Small Bowel

D. Beyer

Note: Approximately 20% of patients with acute abdominal conditions admitted to hospital have intestinal obstruction. Of these 80% have small-bowel obstruction.

Causes (Fig. 150)
Luminal obturation (without vascular occlusion)
Bands, adhesions, atresia, meconium ileus, duplications of the small bowel, neoplasms, strictures, stenoses, gallstones, foreign body, worm infestation, bezoars, food material
Strangulated obstruction (with vascular compression)
Strangulated hernias, intussusception, volvulus

Clinical Symptoms

Initial symptoms: abdominal pain, vomiting, inability to pass gas or stool.
Later: abdominal distension
With complete small-bowel obstruction:
- Waves of cramping pains coming at intervals of 4-5 min with hyperperistalsis and intervening quiescent periods
- Soft abdominal wall
- Spontaneous pain at the midline (high small-bowel obstruction → epigastrium; low small-bowel obstruction → umbilical region). Later: subsidence of cramping pain. Hyperperistalsis → bowel paralysis

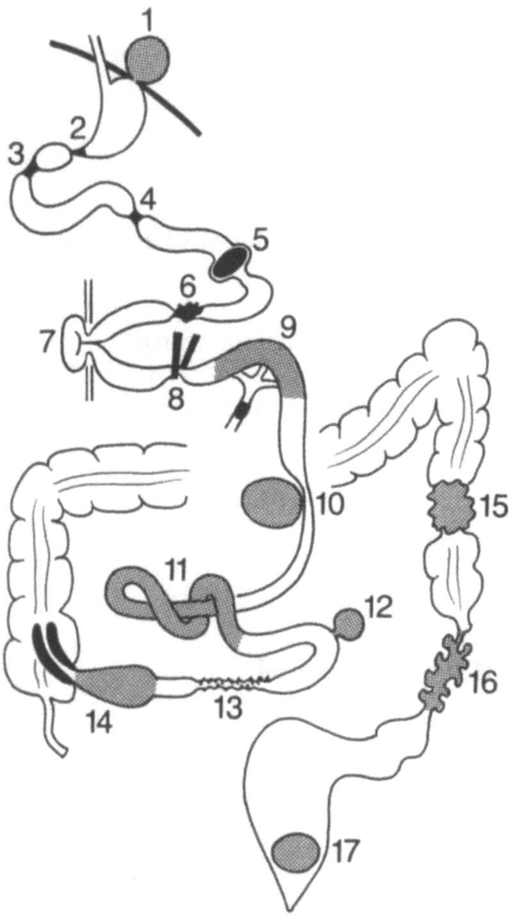

Fig. 150. Principal causes of surgically treatable intestinal obstruction (modified from Zittel 1983). *1,* Incarcerated diaphragmatic hernia; *2,* pyloric stenosis; *3,* duodenal stenosis/atresia; *4,* small-bowel stenosis/atresia; *5,* obturation by gallstone, foreign body, worm bolus; *6,* malignant tumor of the small intestine; *7,* incarcerated external or internal hernia; *8,* obstruction by adhesive band; *9,* bowel ischemia and mesenteric infarction; *10,* compression by bowel duplication, mesenteric cyst, mesenteric tumor; *11,* volvulus; *12,* Meckel's diverticulum; *13,* inflammation of the terminal ileum (Crohn's disease, tuberculosis, actinomycosis); *14,* intussusception; *15,* colonic tumor; *16,* diverticulitis; *17,* meconium ileus, coloanal atresia, congenital coloanal stenosis

Radiologic Signs

Plain Radiographs

Note: Besides the clinical picture and history, plain radiography in two planes is *the* definitive diagnostic procedure!

- Moderate small-bowel distension (supine) with a few, small fluid levels on the L Lat film; ground-glass haziness over the abdomen → largely fluid-filled loops → sonographic evaluation! (Fig. 156)
- Marked small-bowel distension (supine) with extensive fluid levels in uncoiled, hairpinlike small-bowel loops framed by an empty colon (Figs. 151, 154). Concomitant hyperperistalsis *confirms* mechanical small-bowel obstruction!

Caution: The exact site of the obstruction usually cannot be ascertained on plain radiographs.

Contrast Examination (UGI Series with water-soluble amidotrizoate)
(Figs. 153 a, 156 c, 155 e)
Indicated for a suspected high obstruction and for a partial obstruction of unknown cause.
Advantage: laxative effect of the water-soluble contrast medium (e.g., in postoperative ileus)
Disadvantage: Medium is heavily diluted by the copious fluid in the obstructed bowel; the obstructive lesion itself may not be visualized.

Sonography
Sonography is the *main adjunctive study* in the obstructed, fluid-engorged bowel that contains little gas.

Sonographic signs
- Increased fluid content in the dilated small bowel (Figs. 154 c, 155 c, d, 156 b, 157 c, 158 b)
- "Keyboard" appearance of Kerckring's folds on the longitudinal scan (Figs. 154 c, 156 b; Fig. 14 d)
- "Stepladder sign" (Kerckring's folds cut tangentially by the longitudinal scan) (Fig. 14 d)
- The obstructing lesion may be visualized (target sign, intussusception, tumor, gallstone) (Figs. 155 c, d, 158 b)
- The other abdominal organs can be evaluated

Computed Tomography (Figs. 157, 152, 153)
Usually is *not* indicated for mechanical bowel obstruction.
- Demonstrates fluid-filled, dilated small-bowel loops with fluid levels in the supine position
- The obstructive lesion may be visualized

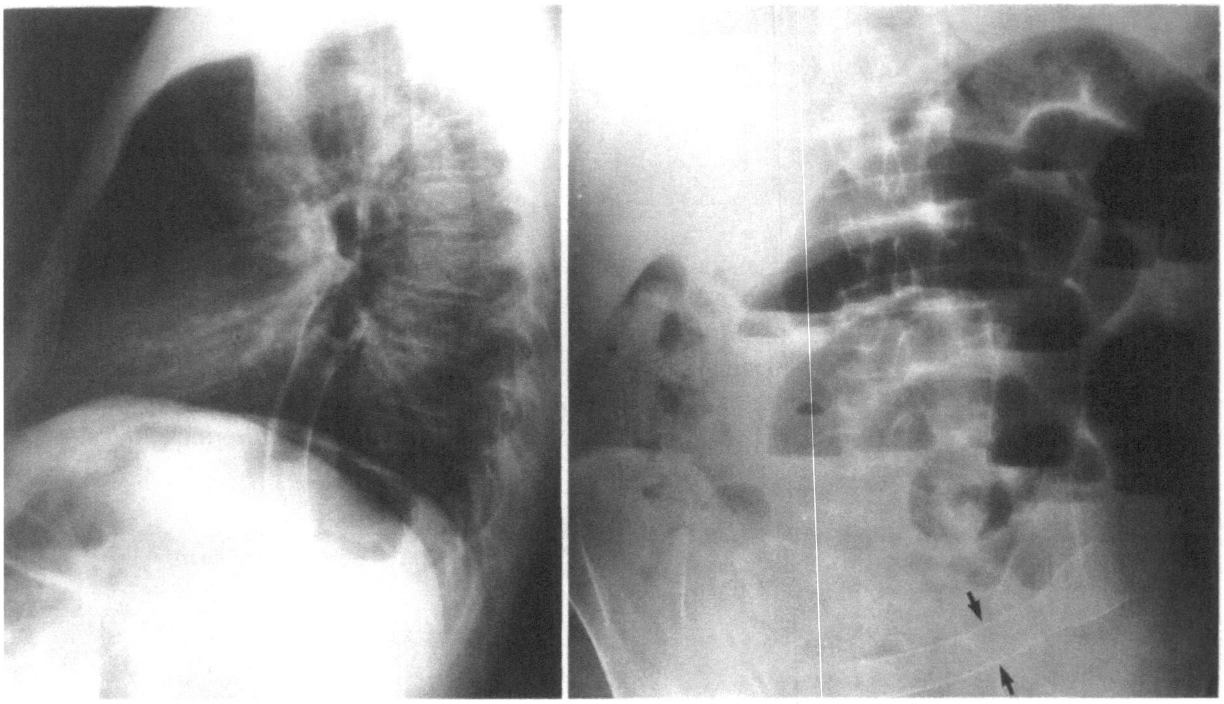

a b

Fig. 151 a, b. Mechanical obturation of the small bowel caused by migration of an endoesophageal tube to the ileocecal junction.
Man, 59 years old, with a 35-cm-long carcinoma of the lower third of the esophagus and hepatic metastases. An endoesophageal tube was placed endoscopically. **a** Lateral chest film shows the tube correctly positioned in the lower third of the esophagus. **b** Twelve days later the patient developed colicky abdominal pains with nausea, vomiting, abdominal distension, and hyperperistalsis. Erect abdominal film shows isolated small-bowel distension with air-fluid levels; the esophageal prosthesis (→) is projected onto the lower abdomen. Operation disclosed a mechanical bowel obstruction caused by the displaced endoesophageal tube, whose oral (not aboral) end was positioned directly in front of the ileocecal valve. The tube was removed by ileotomy (Dr. C. Penschuck and Dr. T. Saul, Department of Surgery, Goslar District Hospital)

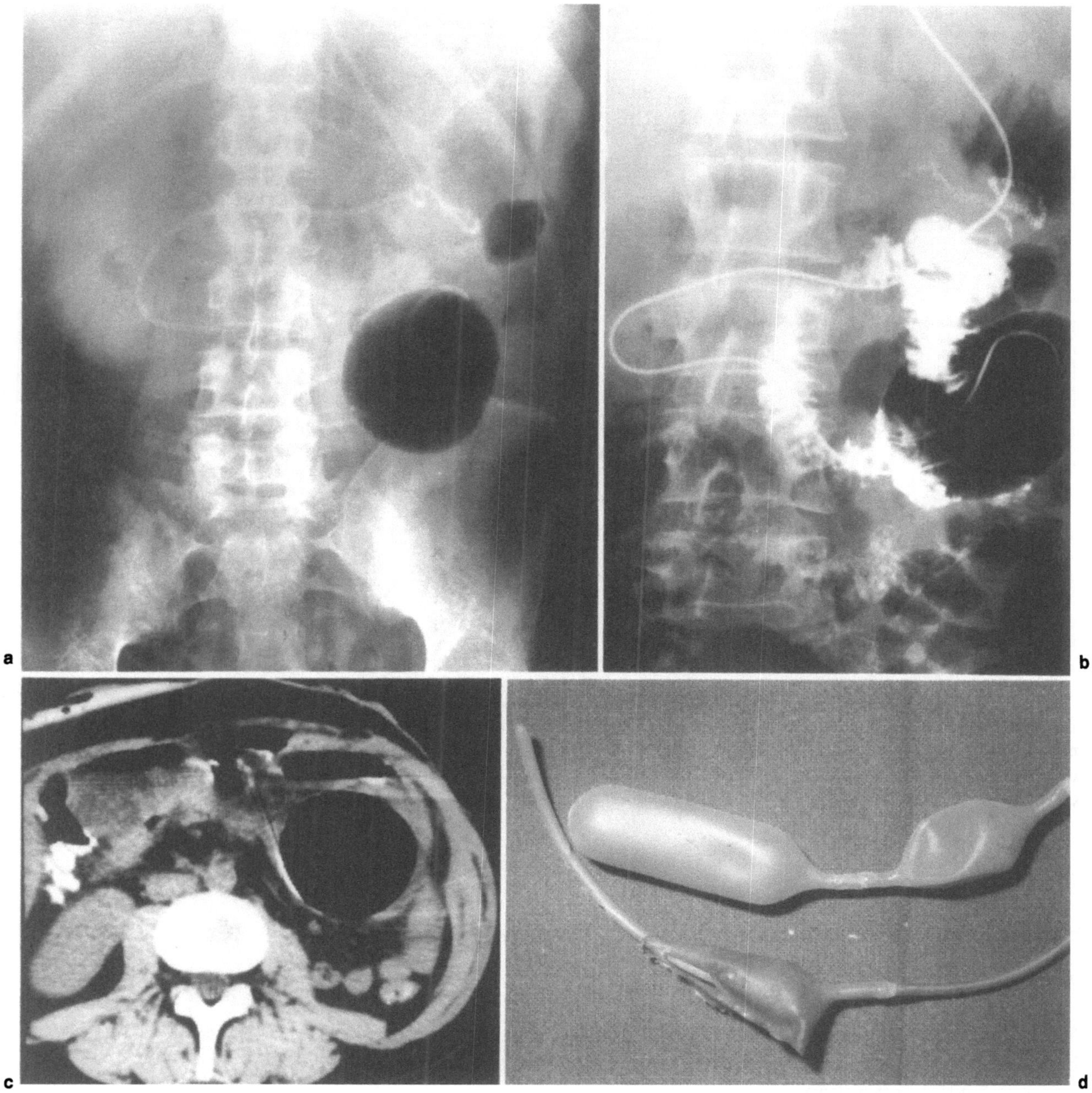

Fig. 152a–d. High mechanical small-bowel obstruction by a feeding catheter.
Man, 42 years old, who had undergone Whipple's operation developed extensive enterocutaneous fistulae with connections to the bile duct, pancreas, and stomach. An indwelling intestinal tube (Solvisond type) was inserted to feed the patient and bypass the fistulous region. This tube consists of a single-lumen catheter with a balloon at the tip, which detaches after a certain period of time. Behind this balloon is a second balloon which carries the tube to the designated site by peristalsis and also secures the tube in the desired position. **a** Three weeks after tube placement the patient developed signs of high mechanical ileus with vomiting and a massive increase in fluid production through the fistulous system. **b** *UGI series* shows an intraintestinal, air-filled, smoothly marginated mass at the end of the feeding tube. Removal of the tube was impossible due to overinflation of the balloon, so a percutaneous fine needle aspiration was planned. **c** *CT scan* shows a large air-filled cavity, which was marked and then aspirated through a thin needle inserted laterally. At that point the tube could be withdrawn without difficulty (**d**). Overinflation of the balloon may have been caused by the diffusion of bowel gas or gas-forming bacteria, but this is uncertain. A second catheter of the same type was inserted, and the obstructive symptoms recurred after 2 weeks, necessitating a second fine needle aspiration of the overinflated balloon under CT guidance

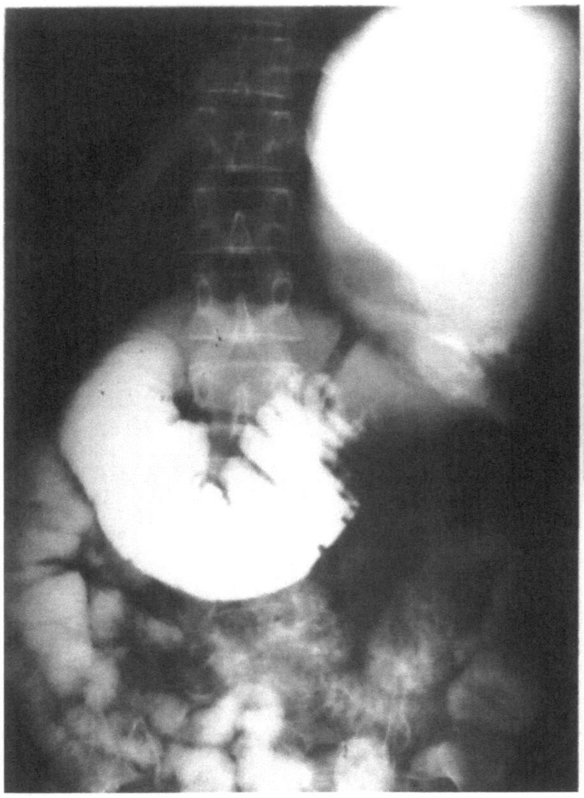

a

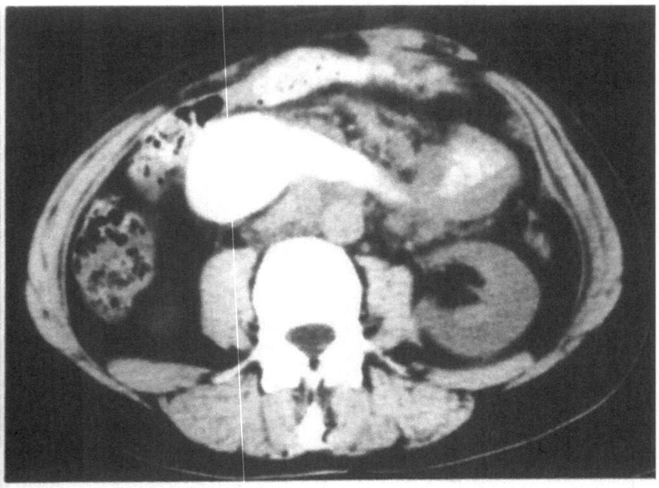

b

Fig. 153 a, b. High mechanical bowel obstruction by retroperitoneal lymphomas and the local recurrence of colon carcinoma. Man, 58 years old, admitted with vomiting and upper abdominal complaints. **a** *UGI series* shows marked dilatation of the stomach and duodenum with a high-grade stenosis at the level of Treitz's ligament. Small-bowel transit is normal aboral to the obstruction. **b** *CT scan* shows massive dilatation of the contrast-filled duodenum. Retroperitoneal lymphomas. Stenosis of the duodenum by locoregional recurrence

Special Forms of Mechanical Small-Bowel Obstruction

*1. **Obstruction by Adhesive Bands*** (see Fig. 154)

Most common after surgery of the lower abdomen (appendectomy scar). Females predominate because they are more frequently candidates for lower abdominal operations.
Characteristic *radiologic features* are absent.
With recurrent intestinal obstruction by adhesions (multiple abdominal scars) and the danger of renewed adhesion formation after further surgery: UGI study with water-soluble amidotrizoate often is sufficient to reestablish transit.

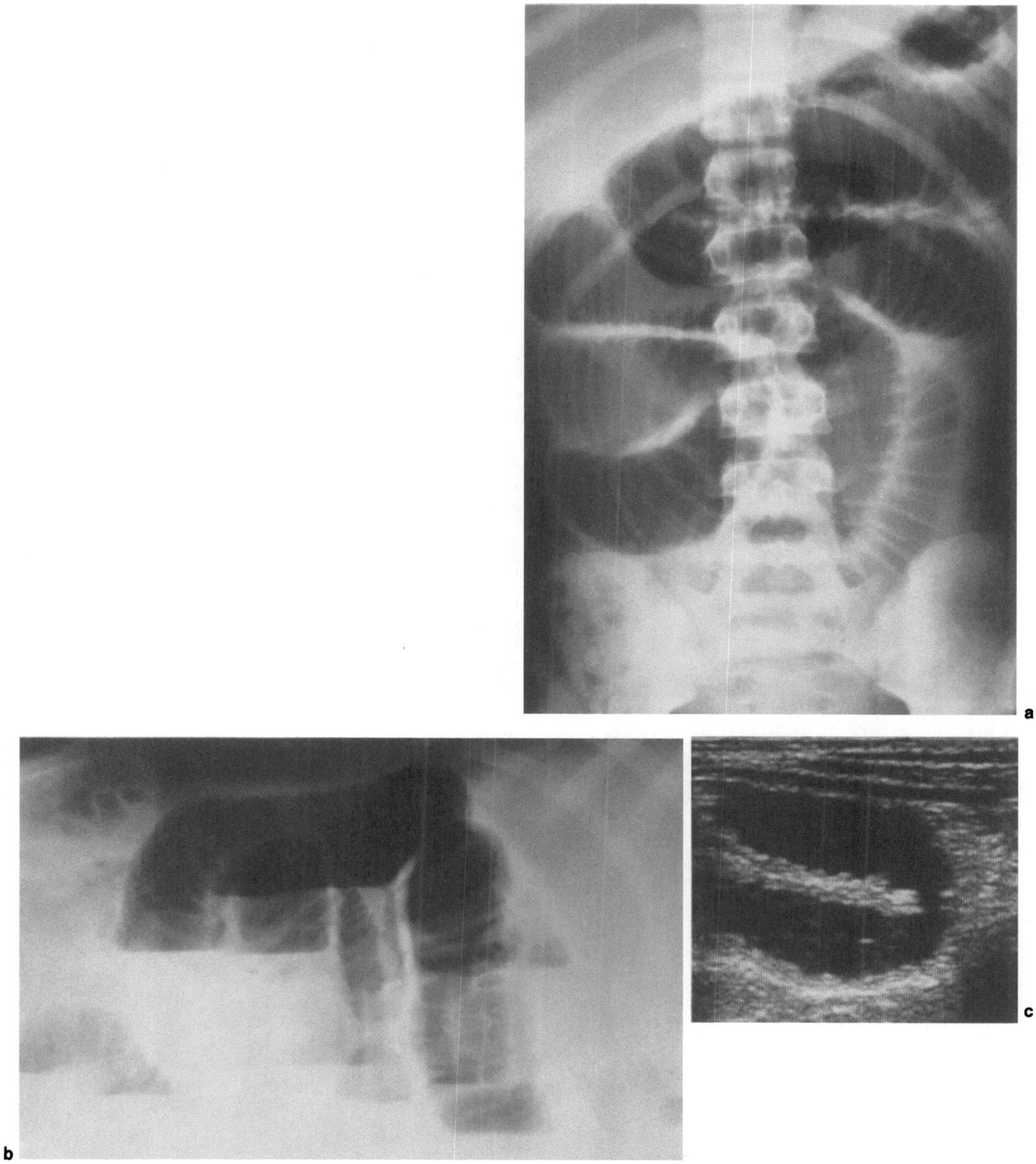

Fig. 154 a–f. Obstruction of the bowel by an adhesive band. Man, 24 years old, with cramping pain at 1-min intervals, hyperperistalsis, and a nonrigid abdomen. He had undergone an appendectomy 3 years previously. **a** *Supine film* shows distension limited to the small bowel and an empty colon. Kerckring's folds are clearly visible. **b** *Left lateral film* shows uncoiled and dilated small-bowel loops with multiple fluid levels; there is no evidence of perforation. **c** *Sonogram* from the flank shows dilated and fluid-filled small-bowel loops with the "keyboard sign."

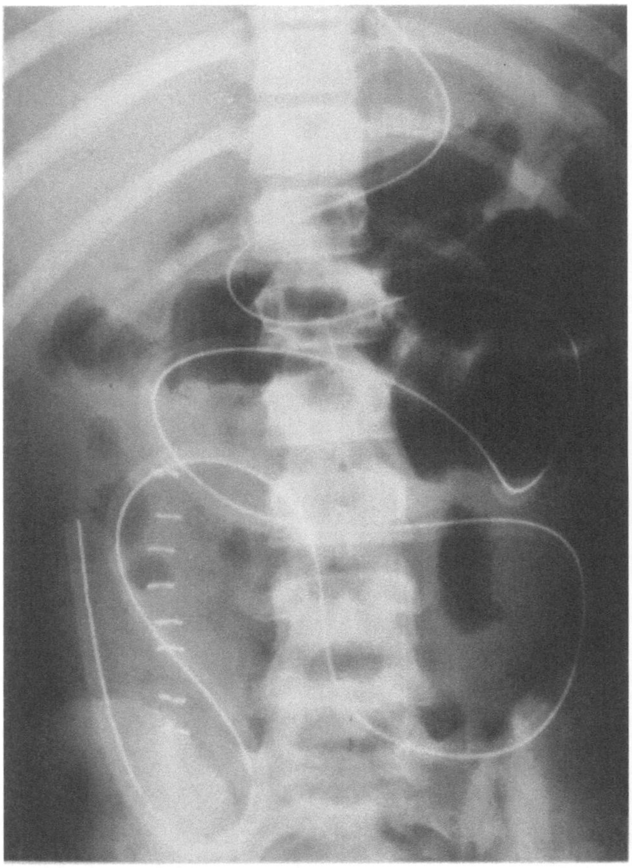

d

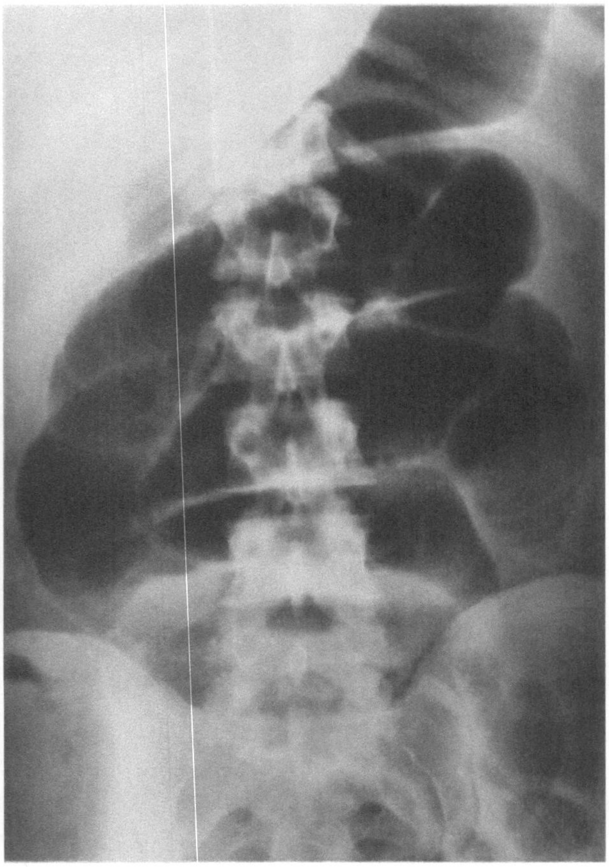

e

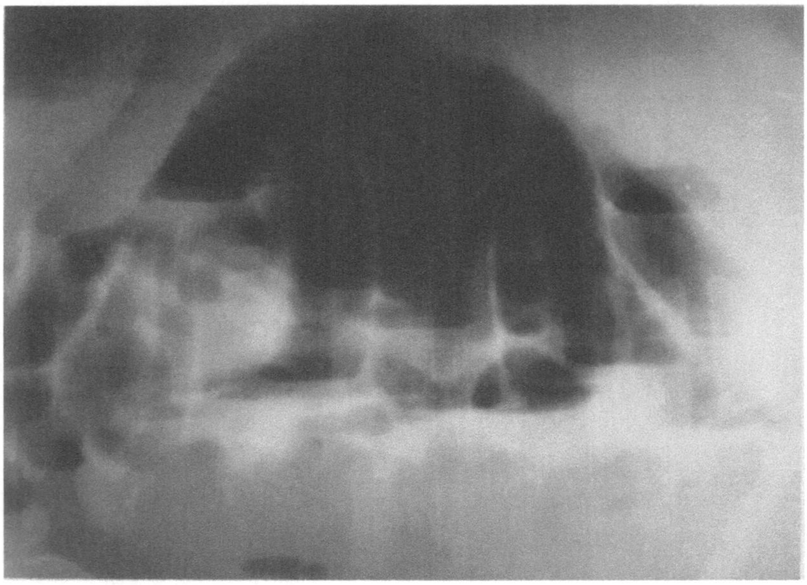

f

Fig. 154 (continued)
d *Postoperative supine film:* Surgery was followed by paralytic ileus. A Miller-Abbot tube was inserted to decompress the small bowel. **e, f Pseudomembranous enteritis secondary to cytostatic and antibiotic therapy; no mechanical obstruction.** Simulation of mechanical small-bowel obstruction in a 35-year-old woman who developed hyperperistalsis, diarrhea, and abdominal cramps while receiving long-term cytostatic and antibiotic therapy for a malignant disease. *Supine film* shows distension limited to the small bowel and an empty colon (**e**). *Left lateral film* shows greatly distended small-bowel loops with a fluid level. UGI series with water-soluble contrast showed swift passage of the contrast medium through the distended small bowel with no sign of stenosis (**f**)

Fig. 155 a–e. Crohn's disease with mechanical obstruction of the small bowel. Woman, 28 years old, who underwent colectomy for granulomatous colitis (of Crohn) and terminal ileostomy. For days she experienced increasing abdominal distension with tenderness and hyperperistalsis. **a** *Supine film* shows distension limited to the small bowel with dilated loops mainly in the epigastric region. **b** *Left lateral film* shows markedly distended small-bowel loops with multiple fluid levels and no free air.

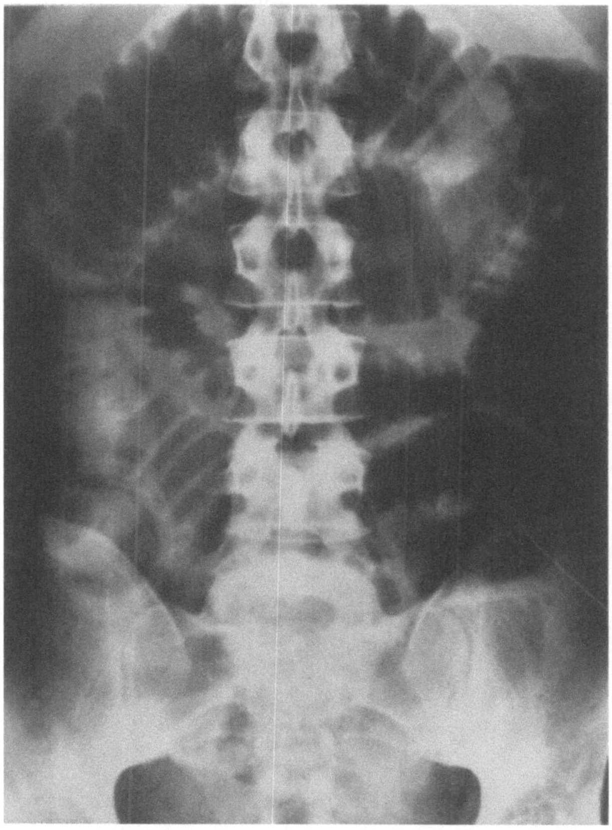

a

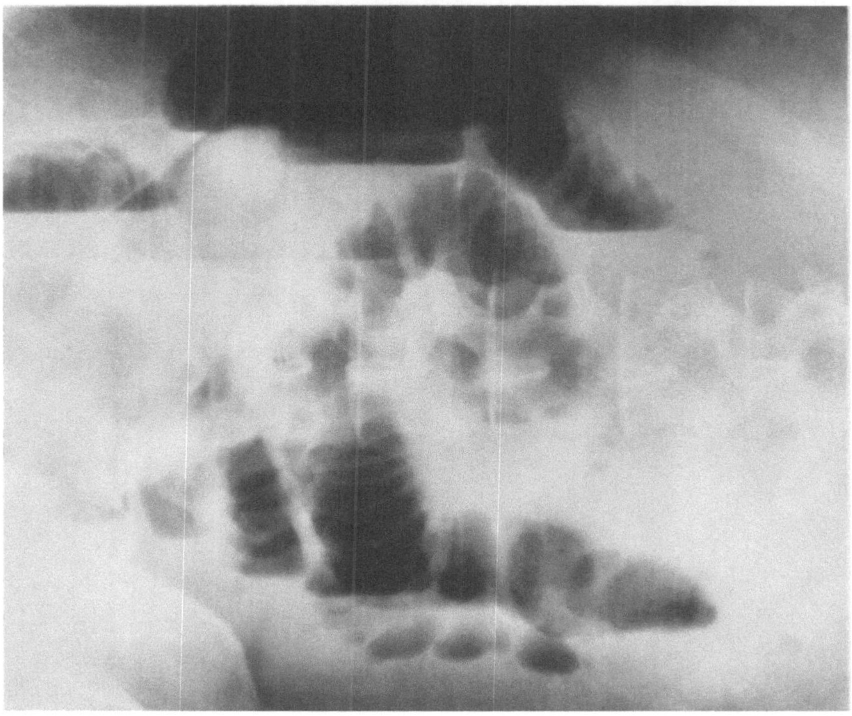

b

c d

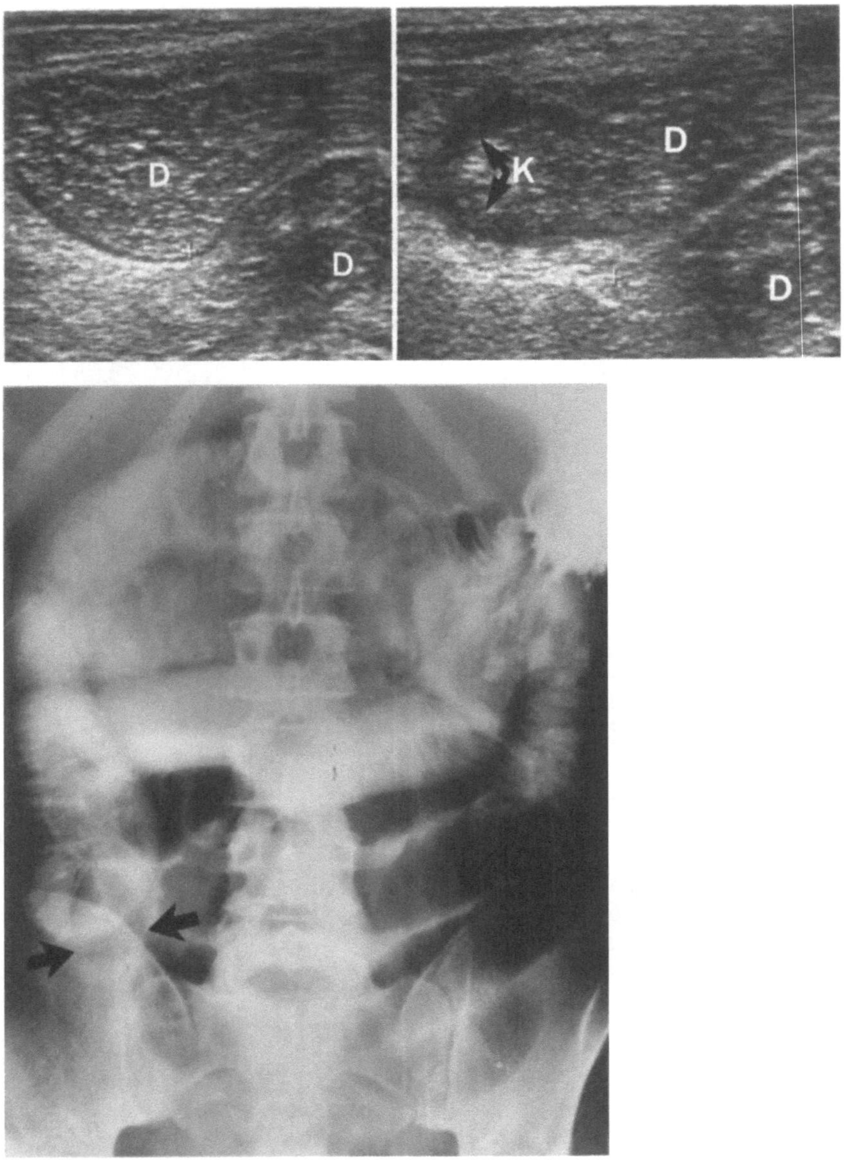

e

Fig. 155 (continued)
c *Sonogram* shows dilated small-bowel loops *(D)* with semiliquid contents and hyperperistalsis.
d *Sonogram* of the right lower quadrant shows a target lesion (*K*➡) just proximal to the terminal ileostomy signifying transmural inflammation with wall thickening. There is dilatation of the small-bowel loops orad. Findings are consistent with Crohn's disease of the small bowel proximal to the ileostomy. **e** *UGI series* with water-soluble contrast shows a markedly dilated small bowel with a failure of drainage through the ileostomy (➡). *Operation* disclosed involvement of a 10-cm segment of the terminal ileum by Crohn's disease with associated mechanical obstruction of the small bowel

2. Intussusception in Adults

Note: Unlike the condition in infants (Chap. 5), intussusception in adults tends to be a subacute, chronically recurrent entity with partial or transient complete intestinal obstruction caused in 90% of cases by pedunculated small bowel polyps, small bowel tumors, Meckel's diverticulum, or prior surgery (see Fig. 156a–c).

Radiologic Signs

Some 90% of intussusceptions are ileocolic, 6% ileoileal, 4% colocolic.

Plain radiographs (Fig. 157)

- Isolated small-bowel distension with fluid levels
- Radiopaque soft-tissue mass (intussusceptum), which is often palpable
- Little or no gas in the midabdomen and right lower quadrant
- With ileocolic intussusception: convex soft-tissue defect in the ascending or transverse colon

Contrast enema is diagnostic.

Sonograms demonstrate the invaginated bowel as a "target within a target" (Figs. 157, 247).

CT also will demonstrate the intussusceptum after the ingestion of dilute amidotrizoate solution (Fig. 157).

Note: Intussusception is most common in children (see Sect. 5.2.2).

3. Gallstone Ileus

Note: This type of obstruction is rare and is mainly a disease of the elderly; 85% of patients are female.
Usually the clinical course with epigastric discomfort and nausea is not very acute; often recurrent episodes alternate with pain-free intervals of varying duration.

Radiologic Signs

Plain radiographs (Fig. 158)

- Gas in the bile ducts or gallbladder (may be absent)
- Large, calcified, intraluminal stone, usually in the right lower quadrant (may be absent with an uncalcified stone!)
- Failure to demonstrate a stone in the gallbladder region despite a past history of cholelithiasis (sonography!) (Fig. 158)
- Distension limited to the small bowel with hyperperistalsis as evidence of the mechanical obstruction

UGI series with water-soluble amidotrizoate can establish the diagnosis by demonstrating the obstructing stone and possibly the biliary-enteric fistula (Fig. 158).

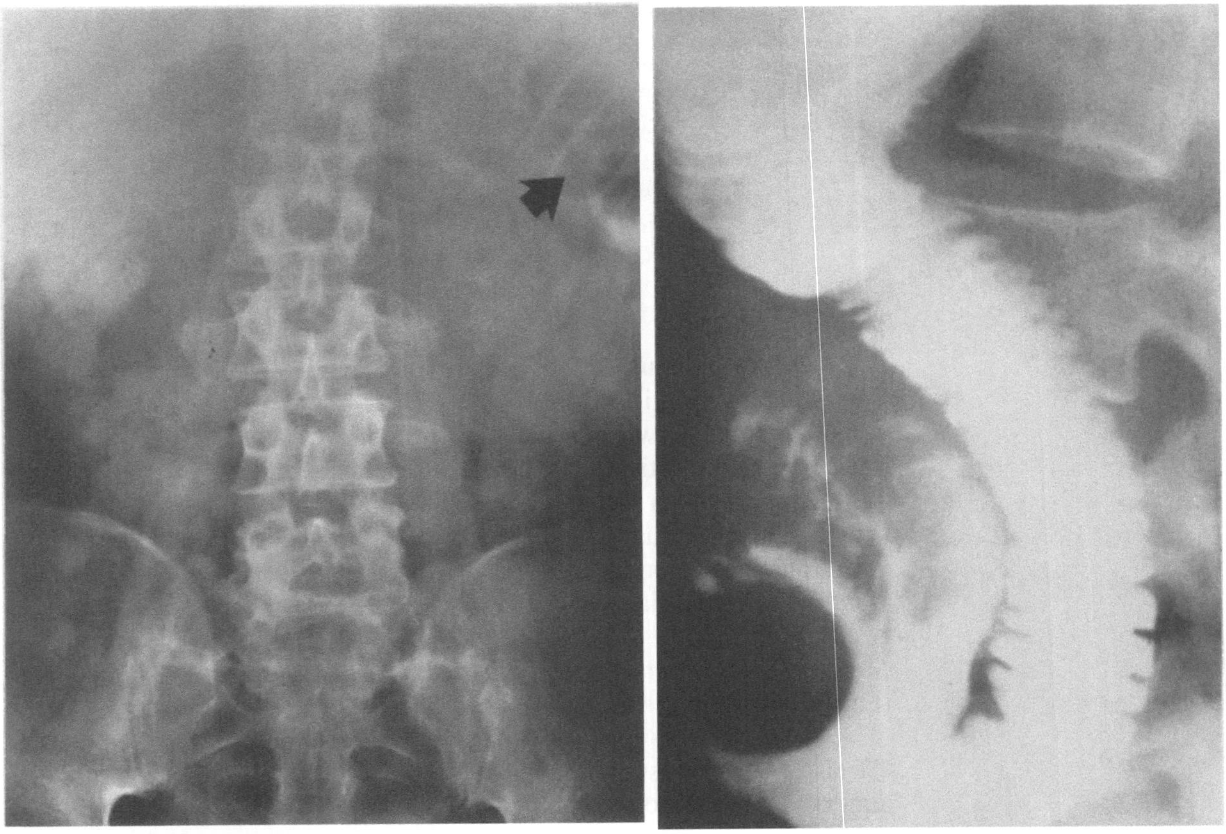

a c

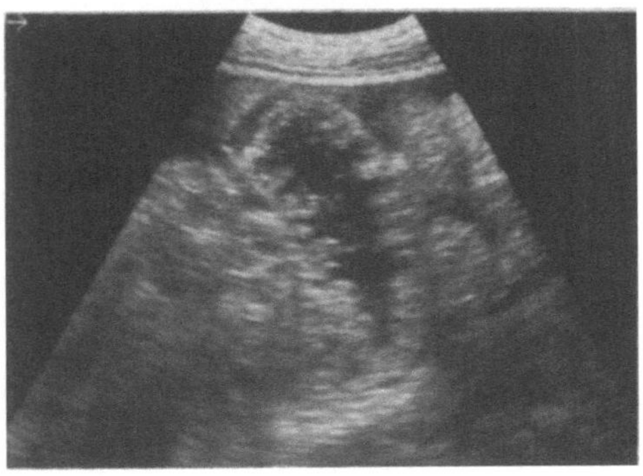

b

Fig. 156 a–c. Jejunojejunal intussusception. Man, 44 years old, who had undergone a Billroth II resection 12 years earlier suffered constant blood-stained vomiting and epigastric pain. **a** *Supine film* shows a single, distended small-bowel loop (➡) in the left upper quadrant with an otherwise gasless abdomen. **b** *Sonogram* of the left upper quadrant shows isolated dilatation of a jejunal loop with the "keyboard sign" and concurrent low-grade ascites. **c** *UGI series* with water-soluble contrast shows dilatation of the efferent loop of the Billroth II anastomosis with signs of jejunojejunal intussusception (confirmed at operation)

Fig. 157 a–g. Mechanical small-bowel obstruction by intussusception of a leiomyoma of the terminal ileum into the ascending colon.
Woman, 67 years old, with increasing abdominal distension and incipient hyperperistalsis. **a** *Contrast enema* shows amputation of the ascending colon by an intraluminal mass. **b** *Contrast enema* with the image plane rotated to the left (detail) clearly displays the tip of the tumor intussusceptum. **c** *Sonogram* shows a hay-fork sign with the double target pattern characteristic of intussusception. **d** *Sonogram* shows multiple concentric rings (double target pattern). **e Mechanical small-bowel obstruction by ileocolic intussusception secondary to Hodgkin's infiltration of the terminal ileum.** *Gastrografin UGI series* clearly demarcates the intussusceptum *(In)* from the contrast-filled cecum and ascending colon *(C. asc.)*. ▷

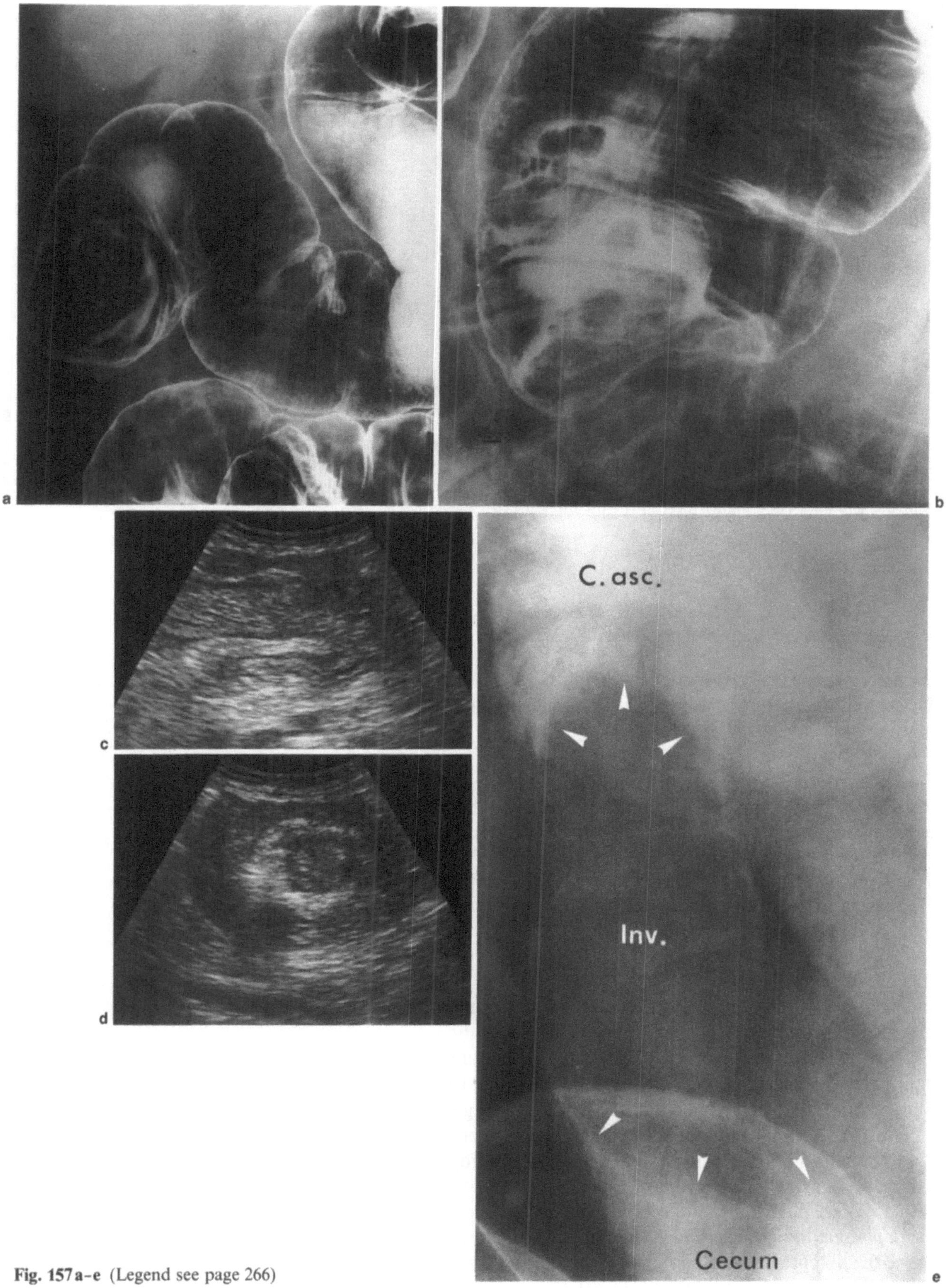

Fig. 157 a–e (Legend see page 266)

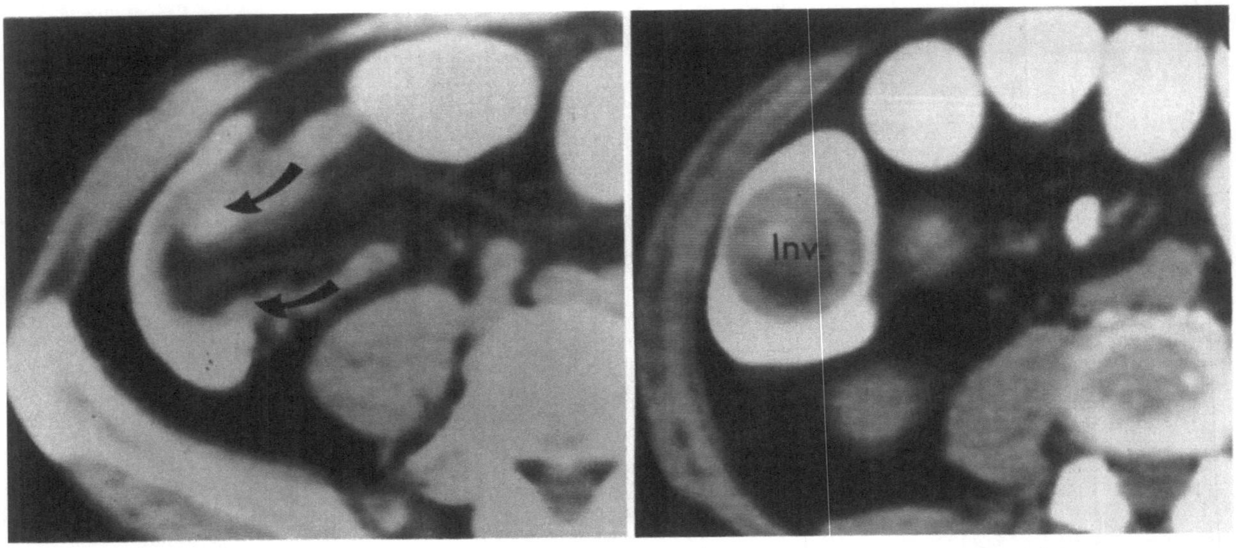

f g

Fig. 157 (continued)
f *CT scan* appearance of the ileocolic intussusception (↗). The mesenteric vessels entering the intussusceptum are visualized. **g** *CT scan* at a higher level shows the intussusceptum *(Inv)* in the Gastrografin-filled ascending colon (**e–g,** courtesy of Prof. Dr. G. Schindler, Department of Diagnostic Radiology, University of Wurzburg)

4. Incarceration of External and Internal Hernias

External hernias (95%) (Figs. 159 b, 163)
Direct and indirect inguinal, femoral, umbilical, obturator (rare), scar hernias

Internal hernias (5%) (Fig. 159)
Paraesophageal (stomach), Bochdalek (through lumbocostal trigone, usually colon), Morgagni (right parasternal) (Fig. 160), Larrey (left parasternal) hernias
Traumatic hernias (see Fig. 216) (with rupture of diaphragm)
Herniation through the foramen of Winslow, paraduodenal hernias, paracecal hernias (Figs. 161, 162)

Radiologic Signs
Incarcerated hernias present the general features of mechanical bowel obstruction (Fig. 163).
External hernias: Most are detectable by inspection and palpation. With inguinal and femoral hernias, care must be taken that the abdomen survery film encompasses the affected area. Extraperitoneal gas projected over the anterior pelvic ring will be noted with this type of hernia.
Large umbilical hernias usually appear on plain radiographs as a soft-tissue density on the standard supine film or on the supine film taken with a cross-table beam.
In *diaphragmatic* hernias, nonspecific gas collections are projected onto or above the diaphragm. The hernia may be demonstrable with an UGI series (water-soluble amidotrizoate) or CT (Fig. 160).
Other types of internal hernia are extremely rare, and very few are diagnosed radiologically. Most are diagnosed at operation.

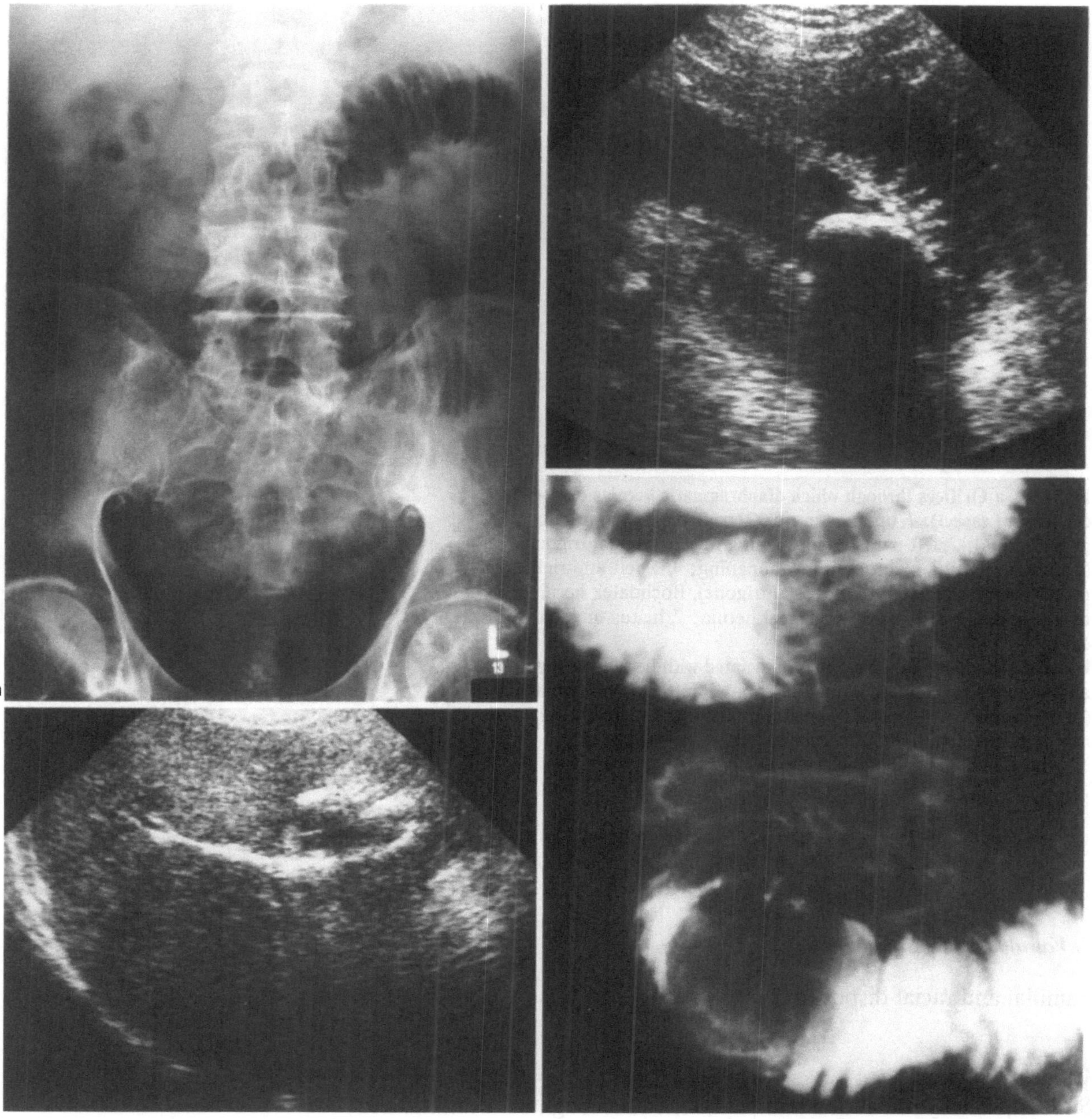

Fig. 158 a–d. Gallstone ileus.
Man, 86 years old, had an episode of acute pain 2 days before admission with signs of mechanical bowel obstruction including hyperperistalsis and abdominal distension. **a** *Supine film* shows isolated small-bowel distension. A fluid level was visible on the left lateral film (not shown). **b** *Sonogram* shows massively dilated and fluid-filled jejunal loops and a hyperechoic area with a broad acoustic shadow. **c** *Sonogram* of the liver shows a significant collection of gas in the bile ducts. The fluid-containing gallbladder is not visualized (Priv. Doz. Dr. Kuhn, Department of Radiology, University of Düsseldorf). **d** Gallstone ileus. *UGI series* shows a large gallstone after perforation into the duodenum in the jejunum outlined by the contrast material. There is no complete obstruction

Sonography (Fig. 163 c, d)
Usually only a direct sonographic examination of the contents of the hernial sac showing edema of the bowel wall as evidence of incarceration contributes to the diagnosis.

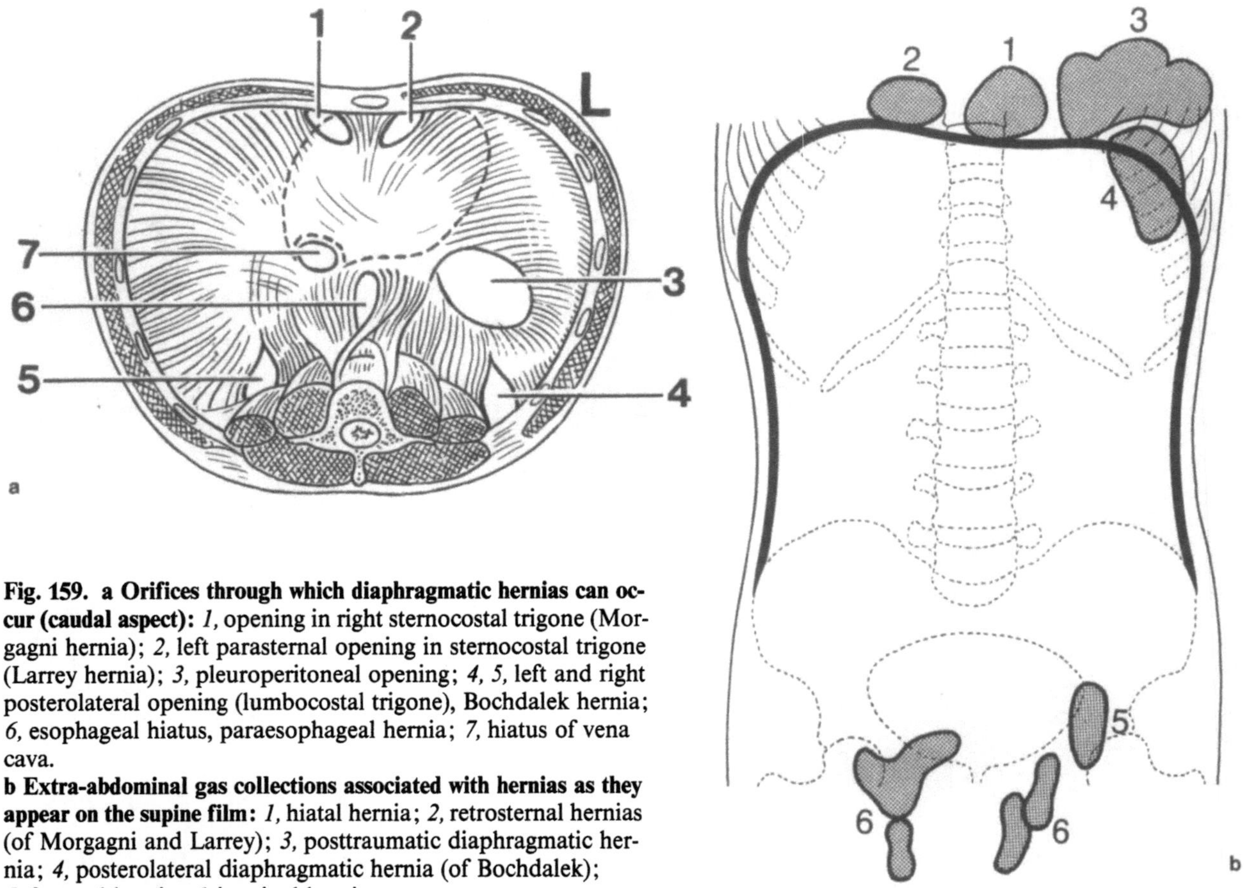

Fig. 159. a Orifices through which diaphragmatic hernias can occur (caudal aspect): *1,* opening in right sternocostal trigone (Morgagni hernia); *2,* left parasternal opening in sternocostal trigone (Larrey hernia); *3,* pleuroperitoneal opening; *4, 5,* left and right posterolateral opening (lumbocostal trigone), Bochdalek hernia; *6,* esophageal hiatus, paraesophageal hernia; *7,* hiatus of vena cava.
b Extra-abdominal gas collections associated with hernias as they appear on the supine film: *1,* hiatal hernia; *2,* retrosternal hernias (of Morgagni and Larrey); *3,* posttraumatic diaphragmatic hernia; *4,* posterolateral diaphragmatic hernia (of Bochdalek); *5,* femoral hernia; *6,* inguinal hernias

5. Volvulus of the Small Intestine

Familial and racial disposition

Clinical Symptoms

Sudden, colicky midabdominal pain, reflex hiccough or vomiting, and shock symptoms. The patient feels extremely ill.

Radiologic Signs

Plain films show gastric and duodenal distension with fluid levels in the L Lat position.
Usually the abdomen is gasless and contains fluid-filled loops of small intestine (sonography) and many smaller fluid levels. *UGI series* with water-soluble amidotrizoate shows a high obstruction of the small bowel with a beaklike termination of the contrast column in the distal duodenum. With incomplete obstruction, loops of jejunum will be seen in the *right* side of the abdomen (Fig. 163 e).

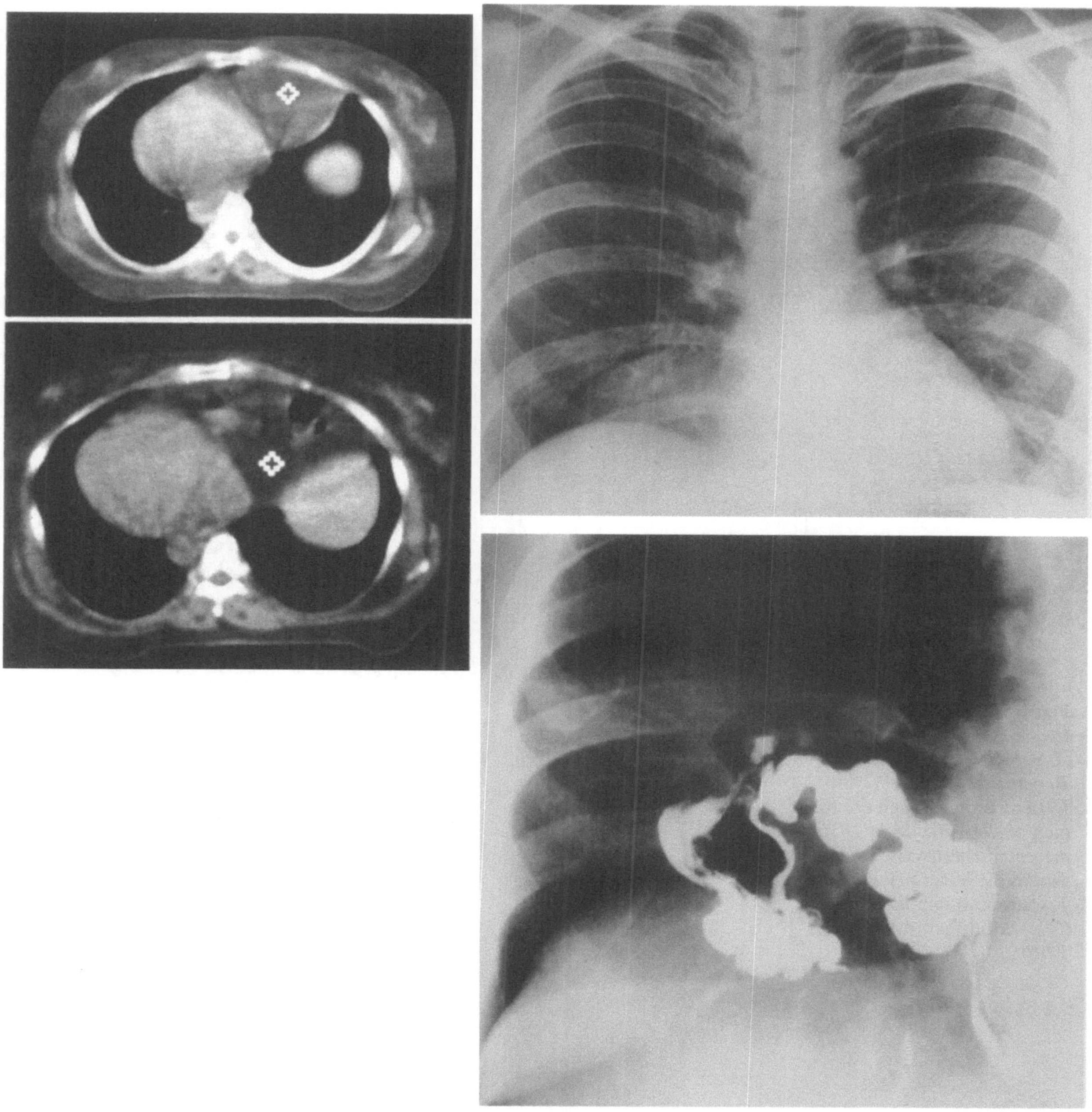

a b c d

Fig. 160 a–d. Morgagni herniation of the colon misdiagnosed as a lipoma.
The patient, an obese woman 55 years old, had a homogeneous, sharply marginated, right paracardial density on her chest X-ray film 11 years earlier, which was interpreted as a diaphragmatic protrusion. Marked enlargement of the density was noted 5 years later. **a** *Thoracic CT scan* shows a homogeneous, lipomatous mass in the right paracardial area, diagnosed as a paracardial lipoma. Increasing complaints 5 years later prompted another chest X-ray examination, which showed further enlargement of the paracardial mass with dystelectasis of the right middle lobe. **b** *Chest film* shows dystelectasis of the right middle lobe. The "right paracardial lipoma" now contains air-filled structures with fluid levels. **c** *Thoracic CT scan* demonstrates marked enlargement of the paracardial mass with gas inclusions. **d** *Contrast enema* displays portions of the colon herniating into the right paracardial area. (Dr. H. Tschakert, Department of Radiology, Knappschafts Hospital, Recklinghausen)

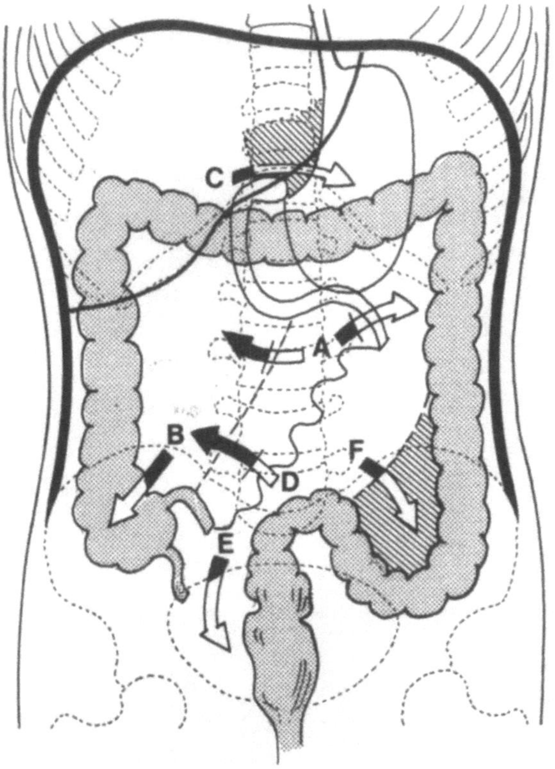

Fig. 161. Location and relative frequency of internal hernias. *A*, Paraduodenal hernias (53%); *B*, pericecal hernias (13%); *C*, herniation through the foramen of Winslow (8%); *D*, transmesenteric hernias (8%); *E*, hernias into the lesser pelvis (7%); *F*, transmesosigmoidal hernias (6%). (Modified from Meyers 1976)

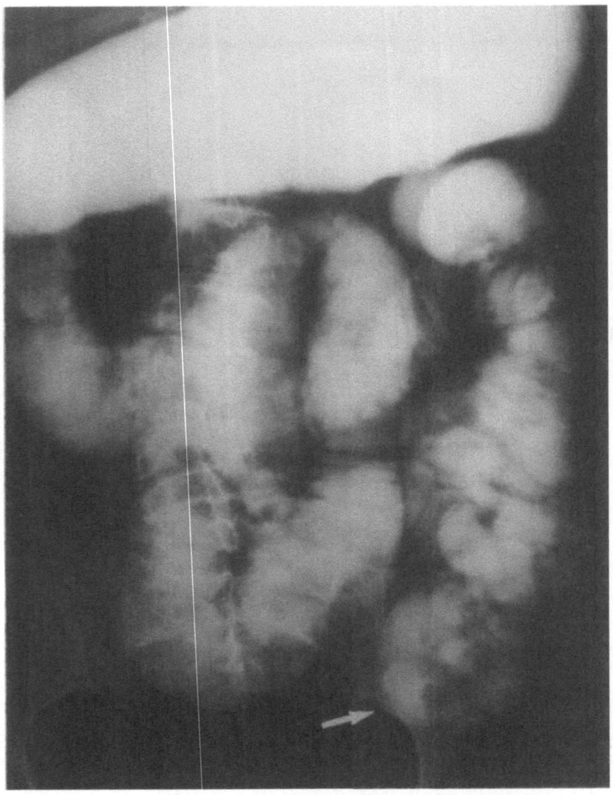

a

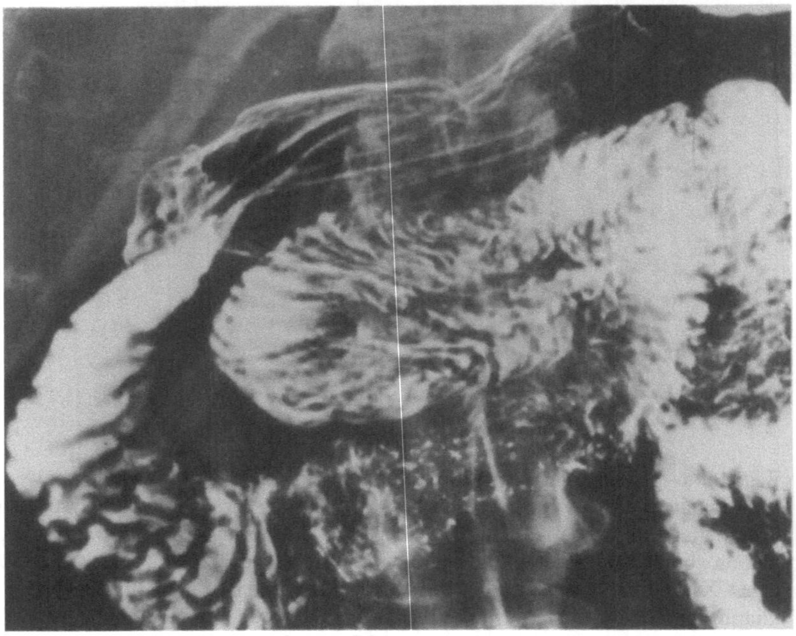

b

Fig. 162a, b. Mechanical bowel obstruction by an internal hernia after hemicolectomy. Woman, 76 years old, who had undergone a left hemicolectomy 8 years earlier developed a mechanical bowel obstruction with vomiting and hyperperistalsis. **a** *Gastrografin UGI series* shows massively dilated loops of small bowel with termination of the contrast column in the midabdomen (→). Operation disclosed mechanical obstruction by an internal hernia below the improperly closed mesocolic incision after hemicolectomy. **b** *UGI series* shows a **paraduodenal internal hernia (Treitz's hernia) (b)** Courtesy of Prof. Dr. W. Wenz, Department of Radiology, Albert-Ludwig University, Freiburg)

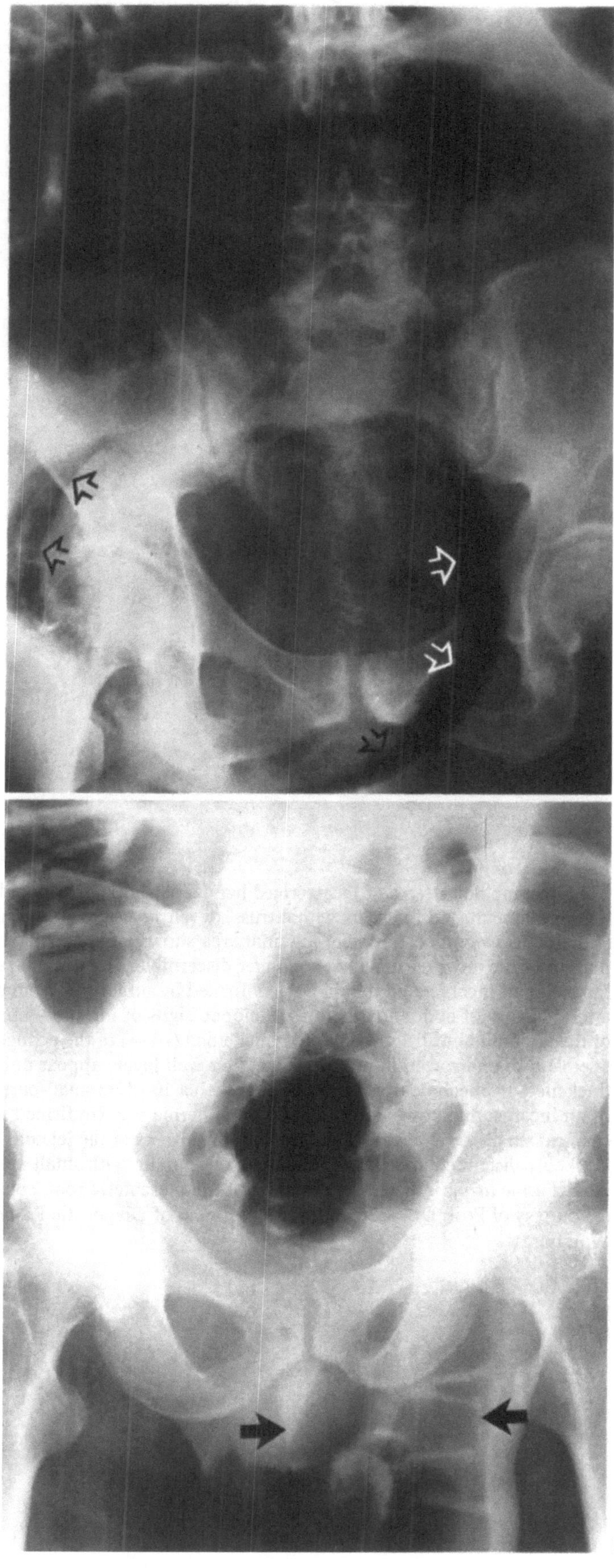

a

b

Fig. 163. a Incarcerated small-bowel hernia with ischemia and perforation in a 64-year-old woman who had a large, neglected inguinal hernia for many years. She presented now with obstipation, retention of flatus, and local tenderness in the hernial sac. *Clinical examination* disclosed a non-rigid abdomen, local tenderness in the hernial sac, and a pulse rate of 120. *Supine film* shows massive small-bowel distension mainly affecting several loops of jejunum. A crescentic, almost circular gas collection (⇒) is visible in the hernial sac. The left lateral film (not shown) excluded free air and showed no symptoms other than a distended small bowel with fluid levels. *Operation* disclosed a large incarcerated hernia of the small bowel, mainly the ileum. A 40-cm segment of ileum was ischemic and had to be resected. There was a small perforation with local gas collection in the hernial sac. **b** Large, left-sided inguinal hernia involving descending and sigmoid colon (➡⬅). Transit is unobstructed.

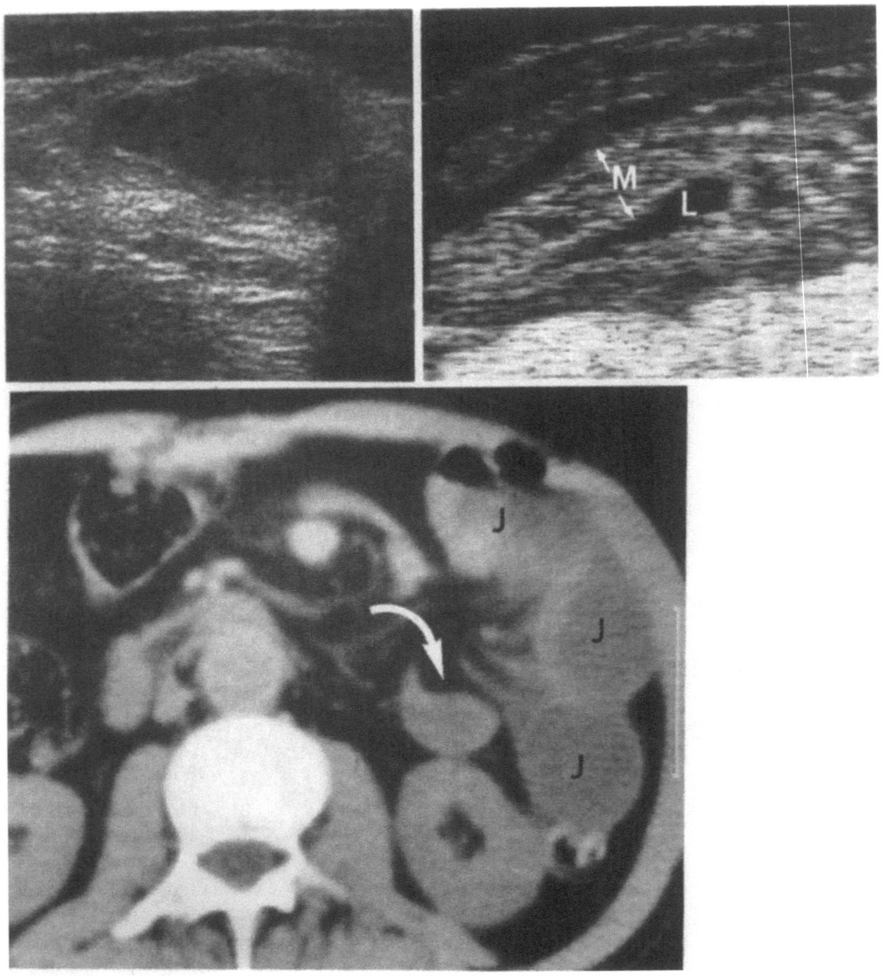

c d e

Fig. 163 (continued)
c, d Sonographic patterns of incarcerated hernia. c Man, 65 years old, with a right inguinal hernia, managed for years with a truss, developed signs of mechanical bowel obstruction. *Sonogram* of the right inguinal area shows a hypoechoic mass with smooth margins. True bowel structure is no longer discernible. There is no transit of gas bubbles. Suspicion of incarcerated hernia was confirmed by surgery. **d** Woman, 68 years old, with a long history of abdominal hernia developed signs of intestinal obstruction. *Sonogram* of the abdominal wall shows marked thickening (←→) of the echogenic mucosa *(M)* by edema and a narrowed lumen *(L)*. The outer wall layers appear only as a minimally thickened, hypoechoic ring. (Examination with a 10-MHz small-part scanner.) Suspicion of an incarcerated bowel loop in abdominal hernia was confirmed at operation. **e Mechanical small-bowel obstruction secondary to volvulus of the jejunum.** *CT scan* shows markedly distended and fluid-filled loops of jejunum with small air-fluid levels. The *curved white arrow* indicates the twisting of the mesenteric root, confirmed at operation (**e** courtesy of Prof. Dr. G. Schindler, Department of Diagnostic Radiology, University of Wurzburg)

4.2.2 Mechanical Obstruction of the Large Bowel

D. BEYER, R. LORENZ

Note: Up to 25% of all forms of intestinal obstruction have their cause in the colon. With the exception of volvulus and intussusception, the clinical symptoms of mechanical colon obstruction tend to be far less dramatic than those of small-bowel obstruction. Circulatory disturbances from strangulation are not so common. Because the absorptive and secretory functions of the colon are minor compared with the small bowel, fluid and electrolyte losses with their associated systemic effects are less significant than in small-bowel obstructions.

Caution: An unrelieved mechanical colon abstruction can lead to cecal perforation with peritonitis and septic shock.

Causes
- Colorectal carcinoma (most frequent cause)
- Tumors of adjacent organs (ovary, uterus, prostate, peritoneal carcinomatosis)
- Diverticulitic abscess
- Hernias involving the colon
- Inflammatory rectal stenosis
- Foreign bodies introduced per rectum
- Coprostasis and decompensated obstipation (fecal impaction) complicated by water-insoluble medications, inspissated barium sulfate or medications inducing bowel hypotonia
- Ischemia of the colon (pseudoileus)

Clinical Symptoms
- Indsidious onset ("digestive difficulties")
- Failure to pass gas or stool despite increasing laxative use
- Increasing abdominal distension
- Normal food intake without nausea or vomiting
- Soft abdominal wall
- Normal or increased bowel sounds

Note: With a tumor obstructing the cecum or right colon, there is a sudden onset of symptoms of mechanical small-bowel obstruction with hyperperistalsis!

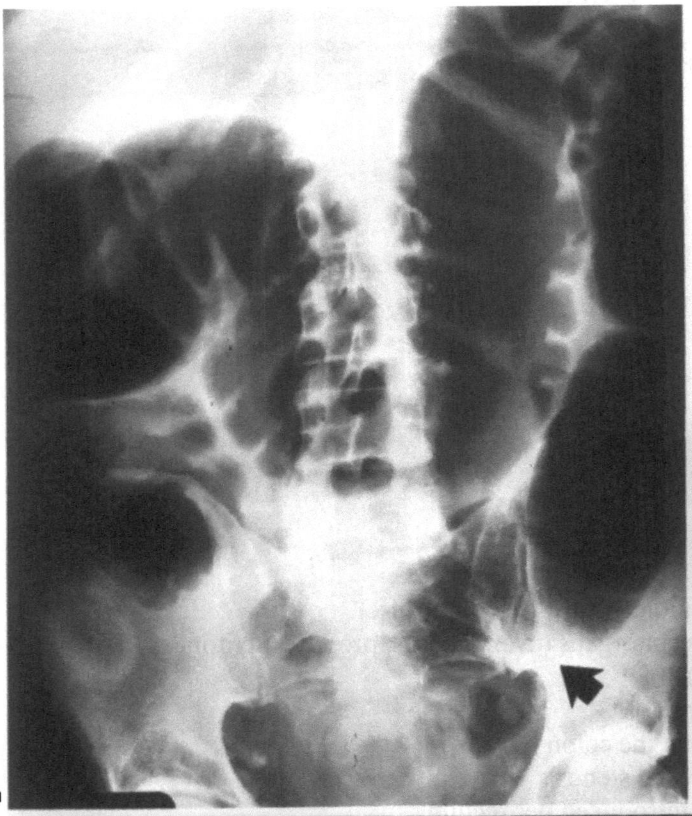

a

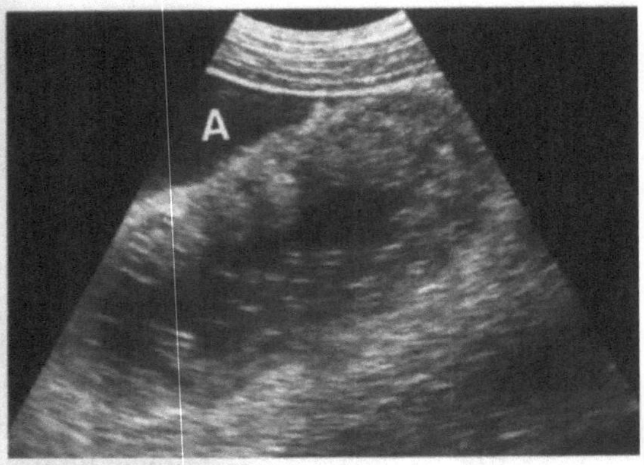

c

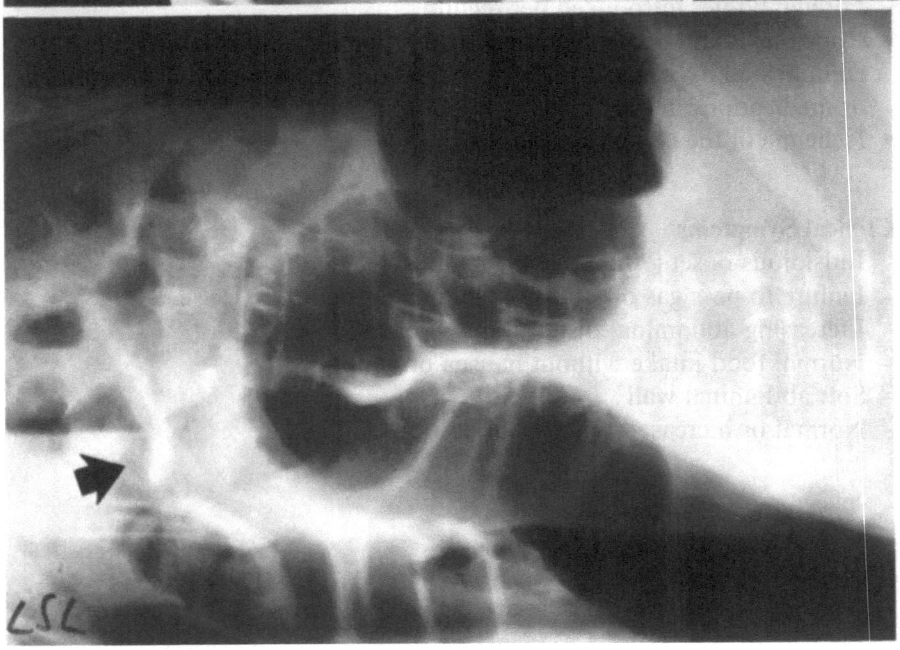

b

Fig. 164a–c. Mechanical colon obstruction secondary to diverticulitis.
Man, 76 years old, did not pass stool for several days and developed increasing abdominal distension with slight hypoperistalsis, fever, and tenderness in the left lower quadrant. **a** *Supine film* shows distension limited to the colon with a hugely dilated colon that shows a cutoff sign at the level of the left iliac wing (➡). **b** *Left lateral film* shows massive generalized distension of the colon with fluid levels mainly in the cecum and transverse colon. As on the supine film, the gas column is strongly constricted at the level of the sigmoid (➡). The small bowel contains scattered fluid levels. **c** *Sonogram* (longitudinal scan through the left lower quadrant) shows a markedly dilated colon with a thickened wall and an adjacent, localized fluid collection *(A)*. Overall findings are consistent with diverticulitic abscess, which was confirmed at operation. The plain film findings by themselves are indistinguishable from sigmoid carcinoma

Radiologic Signs

Plain Radiographs

- Distension limited to the colon (supine). The degree of large-bowel distension depends on the location, duration, and completeness of the obstruction (Figs. 164–167; Fig. 21 a, b)
- Decreased haustral markings (Fig. 21 a, b)
- Sudden termination of the gas column *proximal to* the obstruction by tumor, colitis, diverticulitis, foreign body (Figs. 164 a, b, 165 a, b, 166 a, b, 167 a, b: see Fig. 21 a)
- Aboral colon segments (rectum) are gasless (Figs. 164 a, b, 166 a, b, 167 a, b; Fig. 21 a, b)
- L LAT film shows marked distension of the cecum, ascending and transverse colon with a long fluid level in the cecum and ascending colon (usually there is only little fluid in the colon!) (Figs. 164 b, 165 b, 166 b, 167 b)
- Right colon abstruction, obstruction of the ileocecal valve, or the distal ileum have the radiographic appearance of small-bowel obstruction → water-soluble contrast enema, sonography (mass)

Note: With a *competent* cecal valve mechanism (80%), there will be massive cecal distension with a significant risk of perforation (Laplace's law). An *incompetent* cecal valve (20%) will allow partial decompression of the colon with reflux into the small bowel → combined colon and small-bowel distension (Fig. 165 a, b).

Contrast Examination (see Figs. 21 c, f, 22, 166 c)

Emergency enema with water-soluble contrast medium demonstrates the site of the obstruction and gives information on its cause (tumor, diverticulitis, foreign body). A more detailed diagnosis is unnecessary.

Sonography (Figs. 164 c, 165 c)

Colonic distension is a serious obstacle. Scans may demonstrate a tumor, diverticulitic abscess, or extracolic tumor as the cause of the obstruction. Best imaging modality to detect a cecal carcinoma or an intussusception.

Computed Tomography

Colonic distension has little impact on CT visualization. Scans demonstrate the obstruction clearly and without superimposition and can direct further treatment by confirming local inoperability, lymph node metastases, or hepatic metastases (Fig. 167 c).

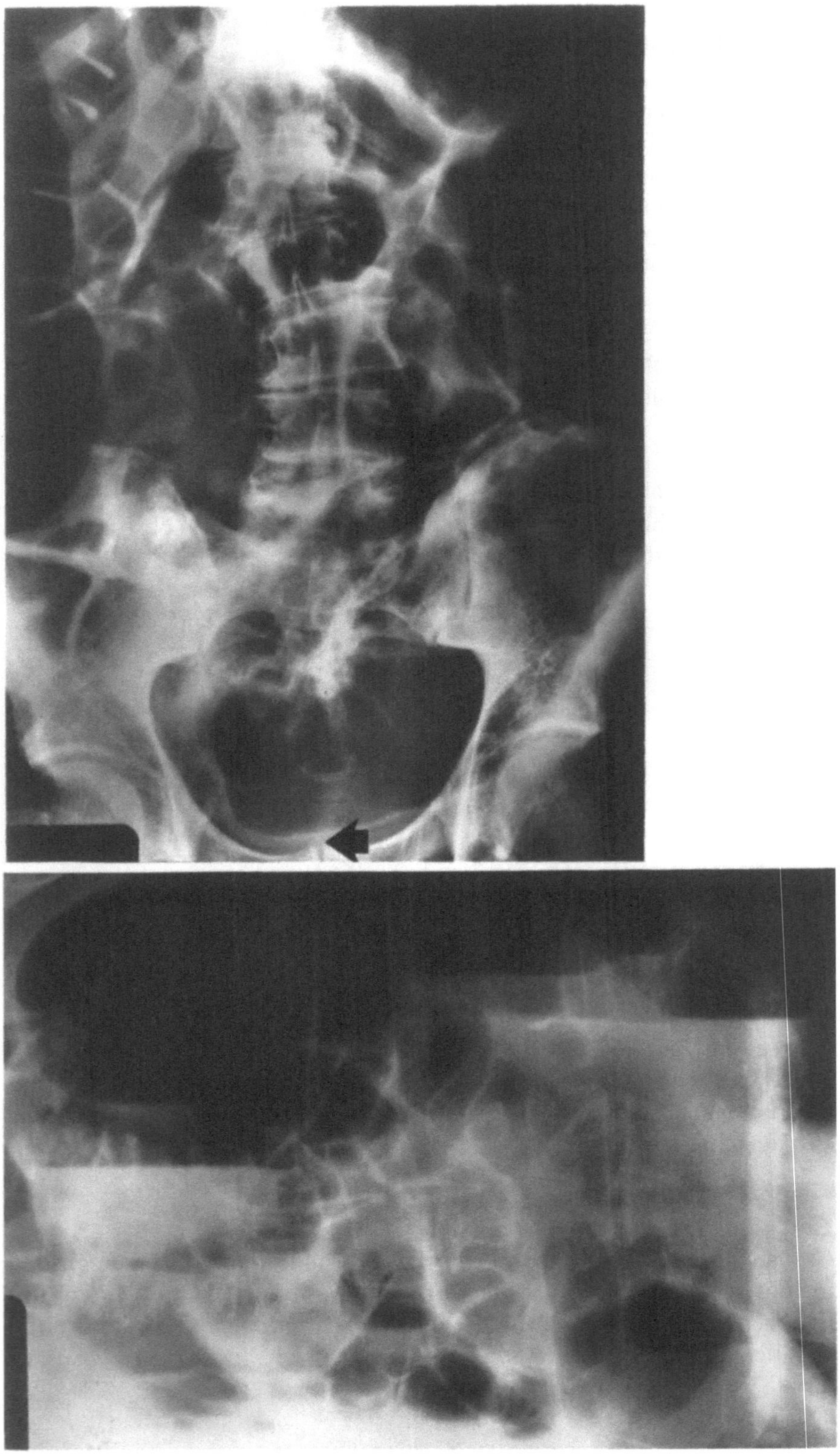

a

b

Fig. 165 a, b. Mechanical colon obstruction due to sphincteric stenosis. Man, 84 years old, did not pass stool for several days and had increasing abdominal distension. He had passed threadlike stools several weeks earlier. Rectal examination was precluded by sphincteric stenosis. **a** *Supine film* shows massive colonic distension combined with moderate small-bowel distension centrally. The gas column terminates above the anus (➨). **b** *Left lateral film* shows massive colonic distension, mainly involving the cecum and transverse colon, with no evidence of perforation. Multiple fluid levels also are seen in the distended small bowel. Findings normalized after instrumental dilatation of the anal sphincter

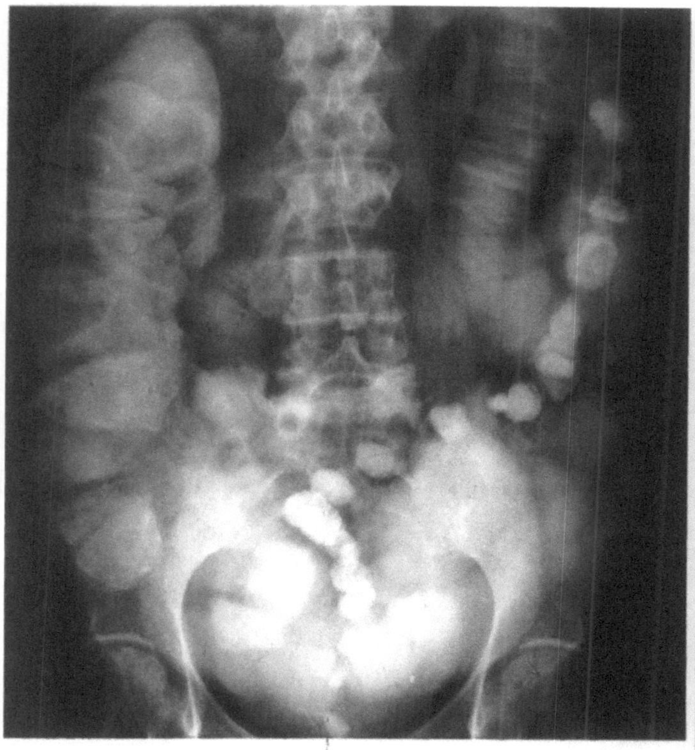

a

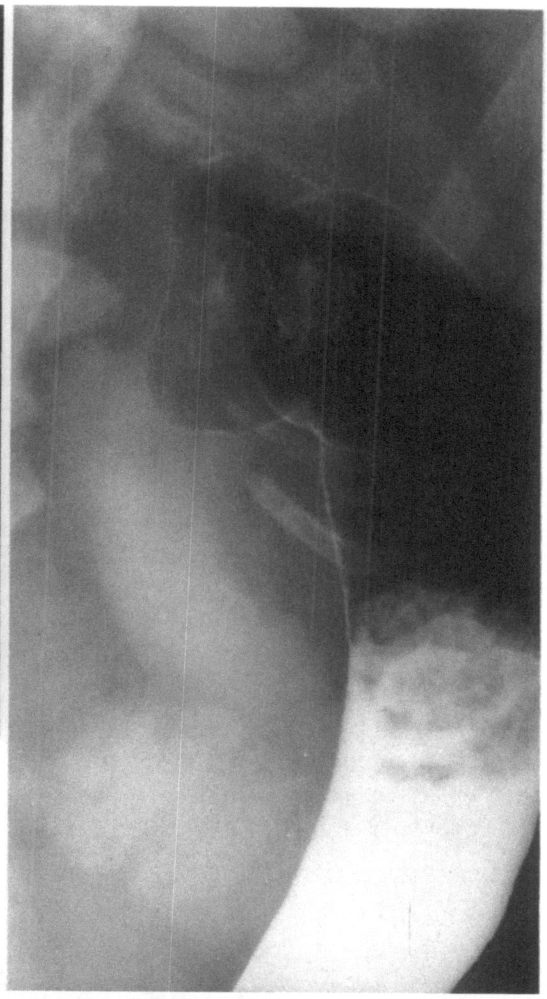

b

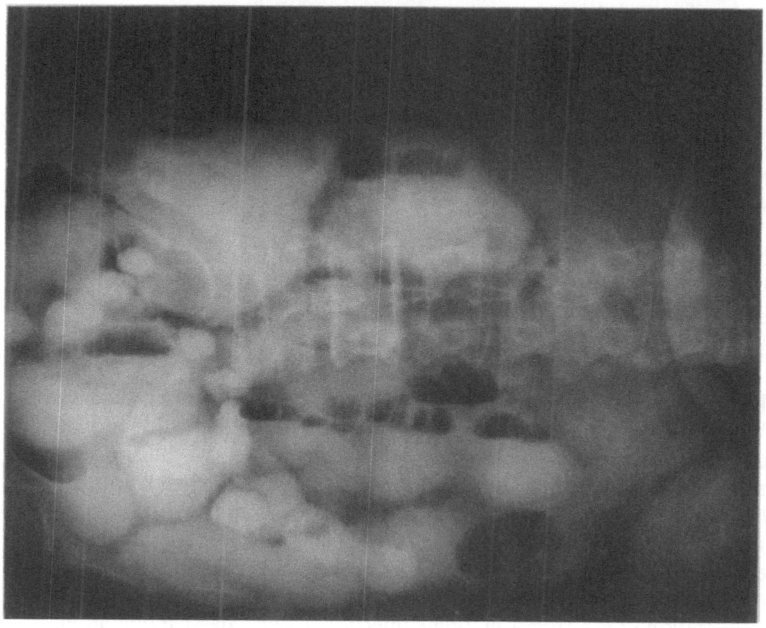

c

Fig. 166 a–c. Mechanical colon obstruction caused by a small carcinoma of the left colic flexure. Woman, 65 years old, with slowly progressive abdominal distension and obstipation. A barium sulfate UGI series had been performed 2 days earlier. **a** *Supine film* shows combined distension of the small and large bowel extending approximately to the midtransverse colon. The descending colon shows a normal caliber with barium feces. **b** *Left lateral film* shows multiple air-fluid levels in the small and large bowel extending to the left colic flexure. **c** *Gastrografin enema* shows termination of the contrast column at the left flexure by a carcinoma with intraluminal extension. A pedicled polyp is adjacent to the obstructing tumor. Operation disclosed mechanical colon obstruction caused by a small carcinoma

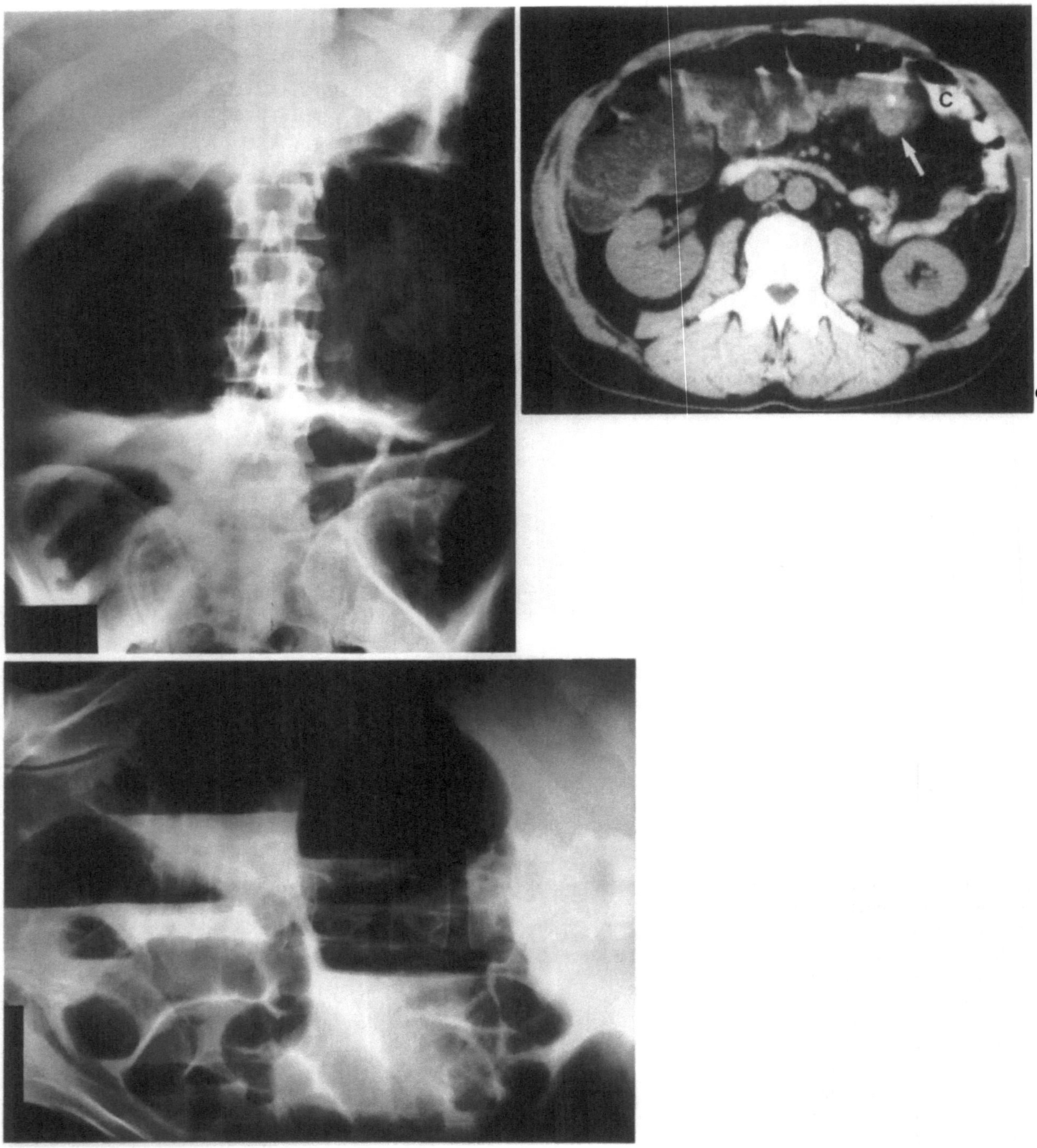

a

b

c

Fig. 167 a–c. Mechanical colon obstruction by peritoneal carcinomatosis. Woman, 54 years old, with ovarian carcinoma presented with abdominal distension and increased bowel sounds. No tenderness of the abdomen. **a** *Supine film* shows massive combined distension of the small and large bowel that is especially marked in the transverse colon. **b** *Left lateral film* shows combined small- and large-bowel distension with multiple fluid levels which are most conspicuous in the ascending colon and transverse colon. There is no evidence of free air. **c** *CT scan* of the abdomen after administration of Gastrografin, bolus injection, shows massive dilatation of the fluid-filled transverse colon with air-fluid levels. There is localized narrowing of the left flexure by a soft-tissue mass (→) external to the transverse colon. The colon *(C)* is narrowed the site of the stenosis. Peritoneal carcinomatosis was confirmed at *operation*

Volvulus of the Colon

Note: Volvulus affects only those portions of the colon that have a long and mobile mesentery. Sigmoid volvulus is most common, followed by volvulus of the cecum and transverse colon. A fault of embryonic fixation is usually causative (Fig. 168). Familial and racial dispositions exist.

Clinical Symptoms

Sudden colicky pain, shock, and subjective feeling of illness.
Later: massive abdominal distension, nausea, vomiting

Caution: Gangrene can develop from vascular occlusion!

Radiologic Signs

Plain Radiographs

All forms of colonic volvulus are characterized by an enormous distended, coffee-bean-shaped large-bowel segment with fluid levels (closed loop obstruction) (Figs. 169 a, 170 a, b, d) and a central "double wall" that points to the twisted mesentery (Figs. 168, 170 a, b). The colon segments proximal to the stenosis become dilated, while distal segments are decompressed and contain little or no gas (Figs. 169, 170).
In cecal volvulus, therefore, one will find concomitant distension of the small intestine

Contrast Examination (Figs. 169 c, 170 d)

Enema by water-soluble contrast medium demonstrates "beaking" of the contrast column at the site of the torsion. An incomplete volvulus will allow small amounts of the contrast medium to pass through.

Note: With massive gaseous distension of a ptotic transverse colon, the radiographs can mimic a "pseudovolvulus" of the transverse colon. The clinical features, however, are inconsistent with a volvulus. The most frequent cause is a left-sided colorectal carcinoma.

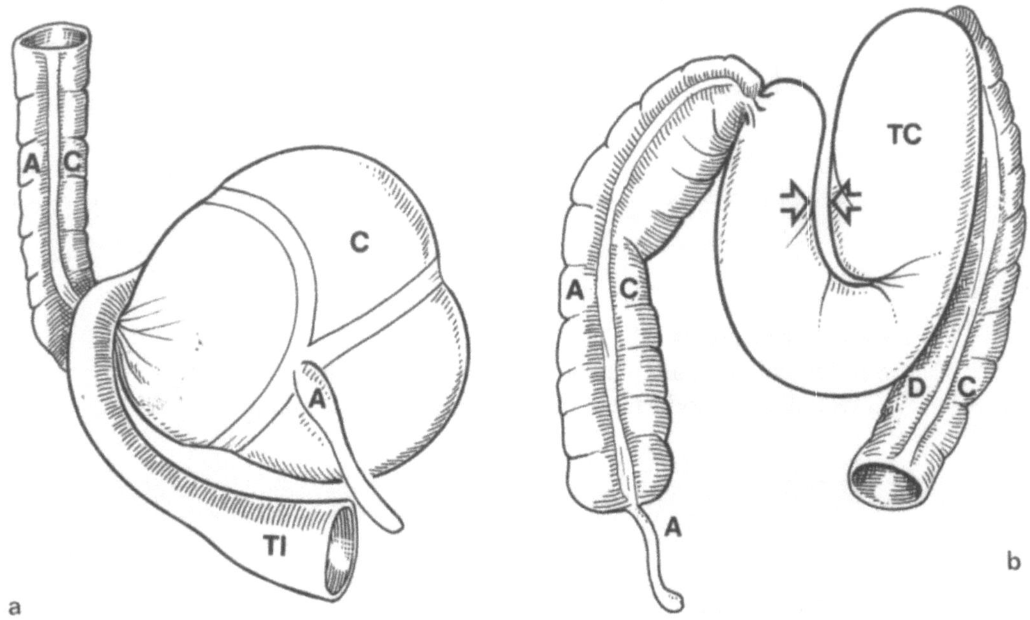

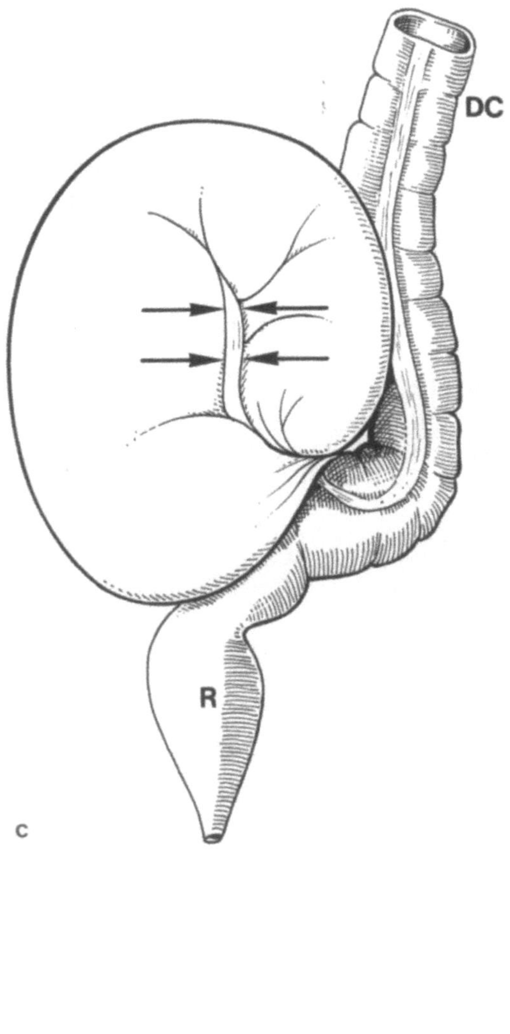

Fig. 168a–c. Various forms of colon volvulus in the supine position.
a *Cecal volvulus.* The greatly dilated cecum *(C)*, identified by the vermiform appendix *(A)*, is twisted clockwise and obstructs transport into the ascending colon *(AC)*. The terminal ileum *(TI)* is looped around the twisted and dilated cecum. **b** *Volvulus of the transverse colon.* The transverse colon that is dilated by volvulus and sags downward frequently simulates a sigmoid volvulus. The caudal border of the colon is rounded. The central, double bowel wall does not extend to the descending colon or sigmoid. *A*, appendix; *AC*, ascending colon; *TC*, transverse colon; *DC*, descending colon. **c** *Sigmoid volvulus* is characterized by a massively distended, coffee-bean-shaped sigmoid colon with a central double wall that points to the torqued sigmoid mesentery (→). *DC*, descending colon; *R*, rectum. (Modified from McCort 1981)

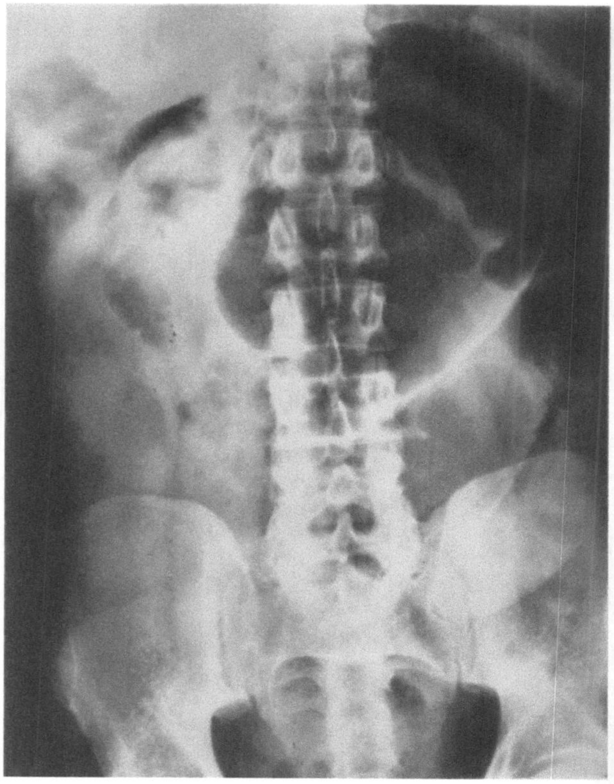

a

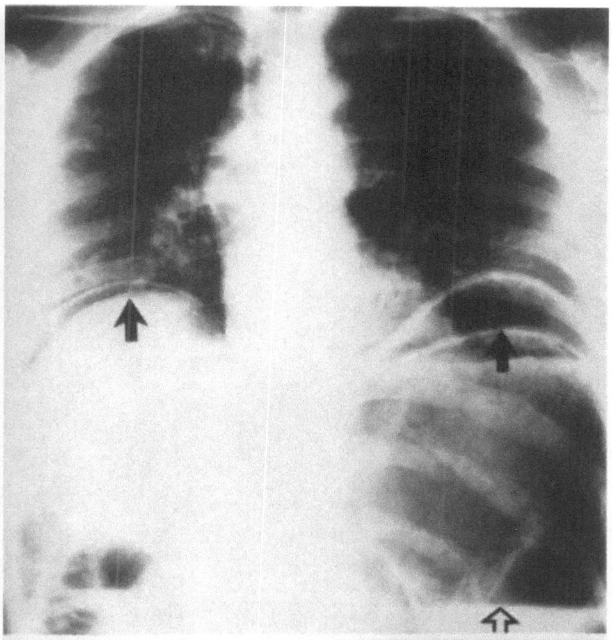

b

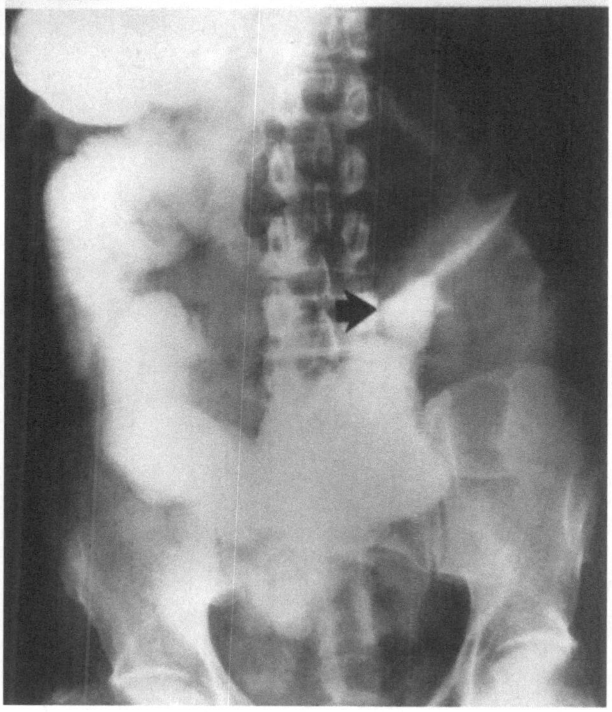

c

Fig. 169 a–c. Cecal volvulus with perforation. South African black man, 38 years old, experienced sudden colicky pains, shock, and severe malaise accompanied by massive abdominal distension and vomiting. **a** *Supine film* shows greatly distended colonic segment in the left upper quadrant and midabdomen. Small-bowel distension is slight. **b** *Erect chest film* shows the massively distended colonic segment with a fluid level projecting into the left upper quadrant (➡). Free intraperitoneal air under both hemidiaphragms signifies a perforation (⬆). **c** *UGI series* with water-soluble contrast shows markedly dilated small-bowel loops with no passage of contrast medium into the air-filled segment of colon (➡). *Operation* disclosed cecal volvulus with perforation and incipient cecal ischemia. (Figs. 169, 170 courtesy of Dr. J. Mirwis, Department of Radiology, Baragwanath Hospital, Soweto, Republic of South Africa)

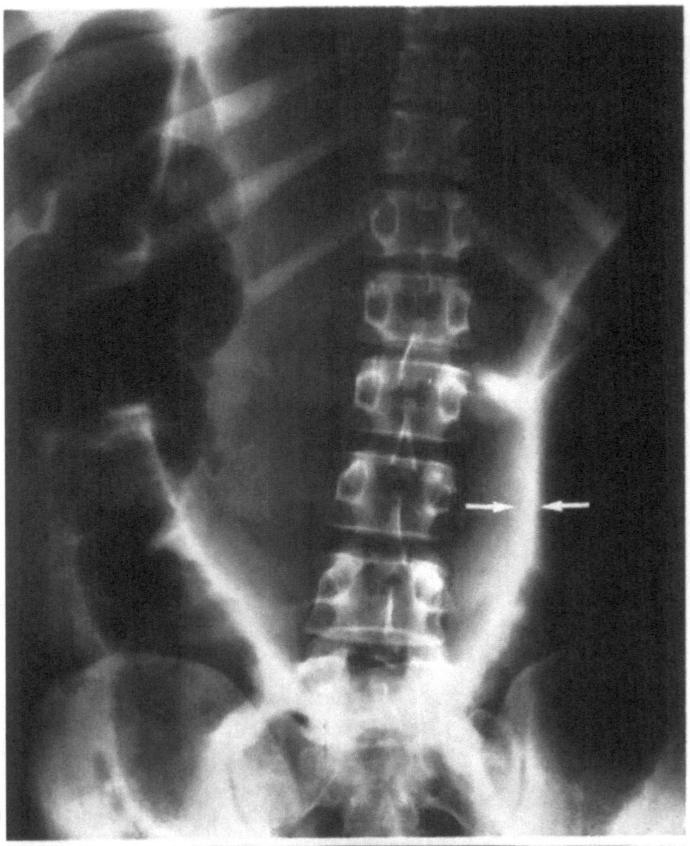

a

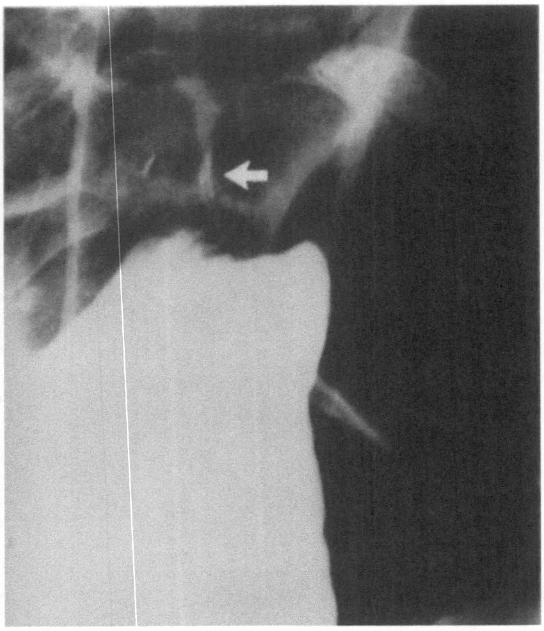

c

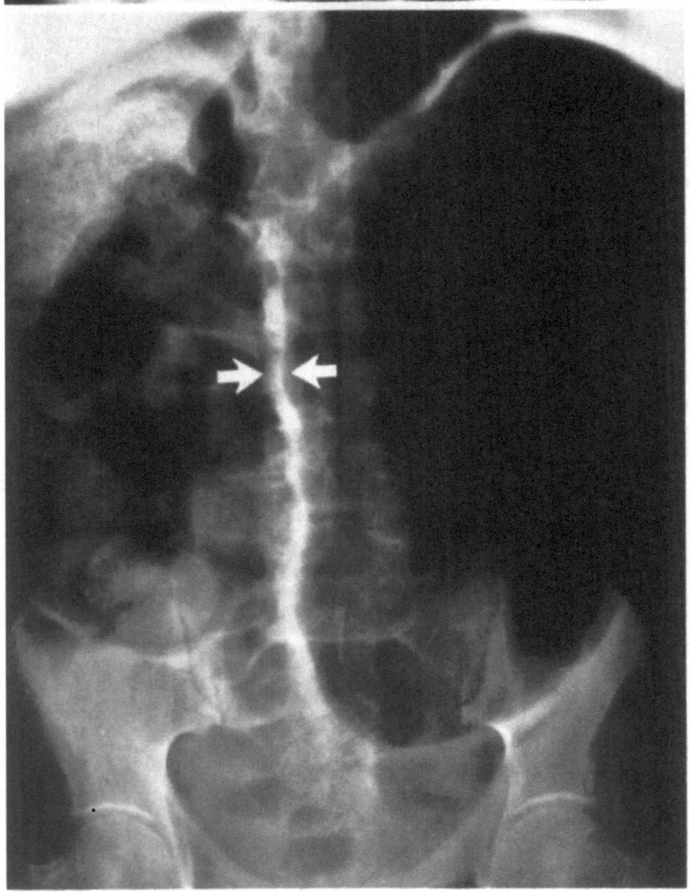

b

Fig. 170 a–d. Sigmoid volvulus. South African black man, 16 years old, experienced sudden acute abdominal pain, nausea, and vomiting accompanied by massive abdominal distension and aperistalsis. **a** *Supine film* shows a colon distended to more than arm-thickness. The thickened double wall (→←) belongs to the twisted sigmoid. **b** Confirmatory *contrast enema* shows a beaklike termination of the contrast column at the torsion site (➧). **c** Another case of sigmoid volvulus in a younger South African black man with massive bowel distension. Again the double wall points to the sigmoid mesentery, indicating sigmoid volvulus (➧).

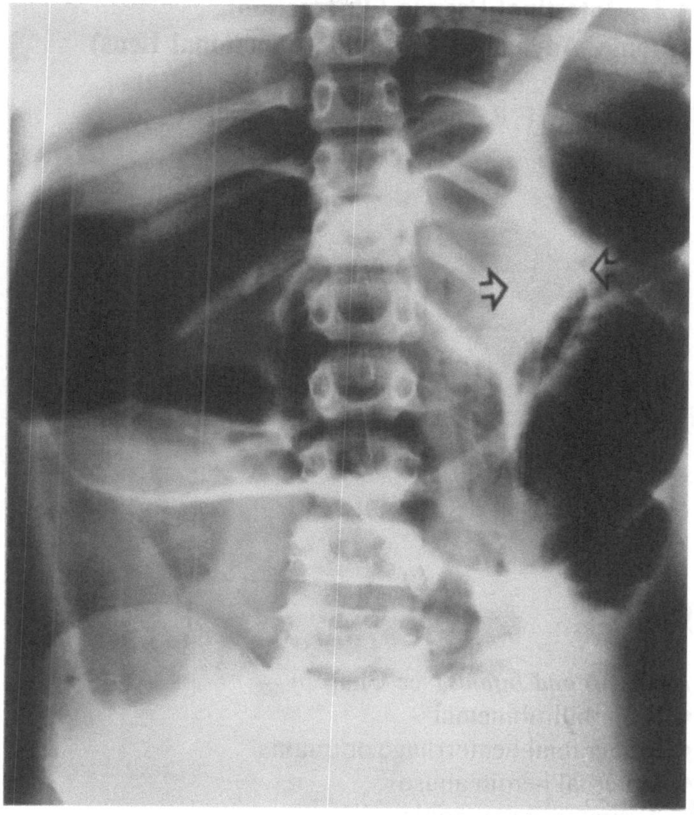

d

Fig. 170 (continued)
d Volvulus of the transverse colon. Black South African, 14 years old, experienced sudden colicky pain and shock with massive abdominal distension and vomiting. *Supine film* shows massive colonic distension mainly affecting the ascending and transverse portions. The central double wall points to the epigastrium and thus to the twisted mesentery of the transverse colon (⇒ ⇐). The descending colon is devoid of gas. *Operation* confirmed volvulus of the transverse colon. (Source quoted in Fig. 169)

4.2.3 Intestinal Pseudo-Obstruction (Atonic, Adynamic, Paralytic, Functional Ileus)

D. BEYER, K. F. R. NEUFANG

Note: Intestinal pseudo-obstruction is a collective term for all acute or subacute disorders of the gastrointestinal tract that are characterized radiologically by isolated or combined gaseous distension of the bowel without an abrupt termination of the gas column. The only radiologic sign distinguishing pseudo-obstruction from mechanical obstruction is the markedly decreased fluid content of the bowel with little tendency to form fluid levels. Differentiation from other syndromes and especially from mechanical obstruction must rely on clinical symptoms and on contrast studies.

Causes

Newborns and Infants (see Chap. 5)
- Hyperbilirubinemia
- Intracranial hemorrhage or trauma
- Maternal heroin abuse
- Aspiration pneumonia
- Necrotizing enterocolitis
- Aganglionosis (Hirschspring's disease)

Children and Adults
- Intestinal ischemia (see Sect. 4.2.4)
- Inflammatory bowel disease
  - Enteritis necroticans (Fig. 30)
  - Pseudomembranous enteritis or enterocolitis caused by antibiotic usage (especially clindamycin) (see Fig. 154e, f), gold therapy for rheumatoid arthritis
  - Ulcerative colitis } toxic megacolon (see Figs. 180, 181)
  - Crohn's disease }
- Inflammatory or infections conditions
  - Peritonitis (see Sect. 4.1.3)
  - Acute pancreatitis, cholecystitis, appendicitis (see Sect. 4.1.2), gastroenteritis
  - Intra-abdominal abscess (see Sect. 4.1.5.1)
- Drugs
  - Ganglion-blocking agents
  - Psychoactive drugs with anticholinergic effects (antiparkinsonian drugs, phenothiazines, tricyclic antidepressants, morphine and its derivatives)

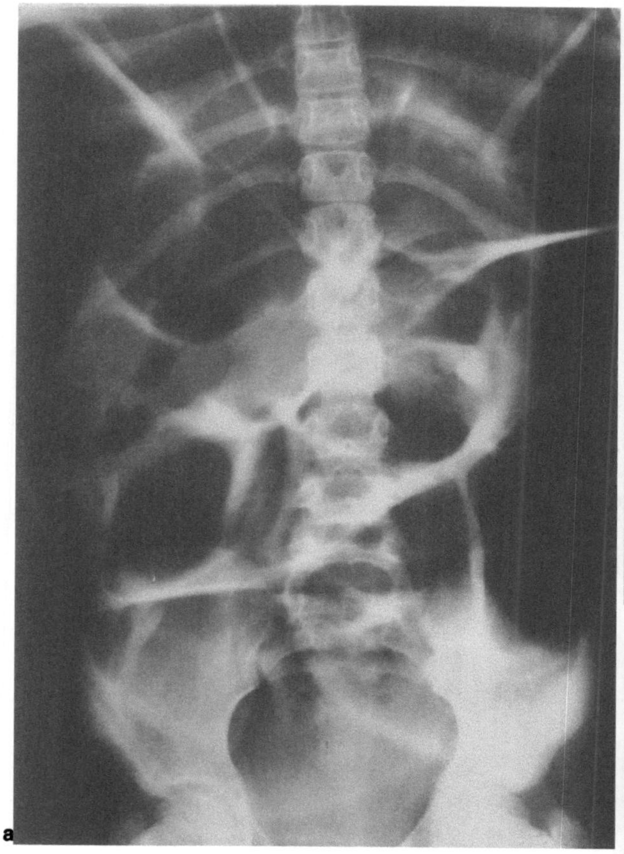
a

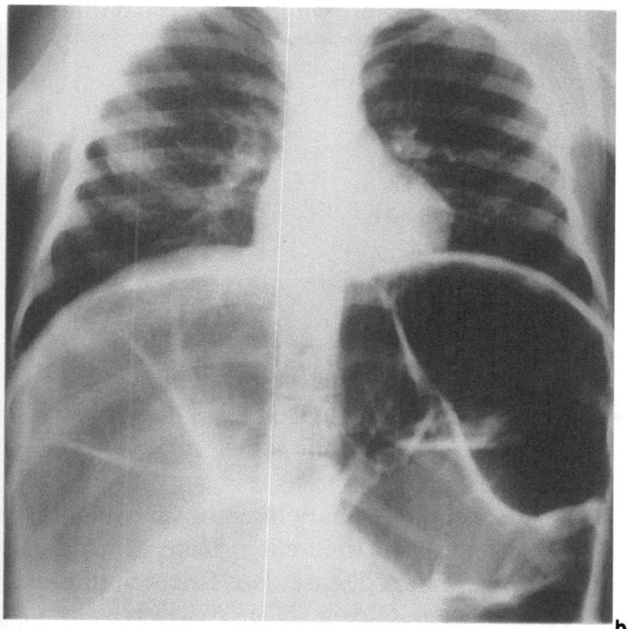
b

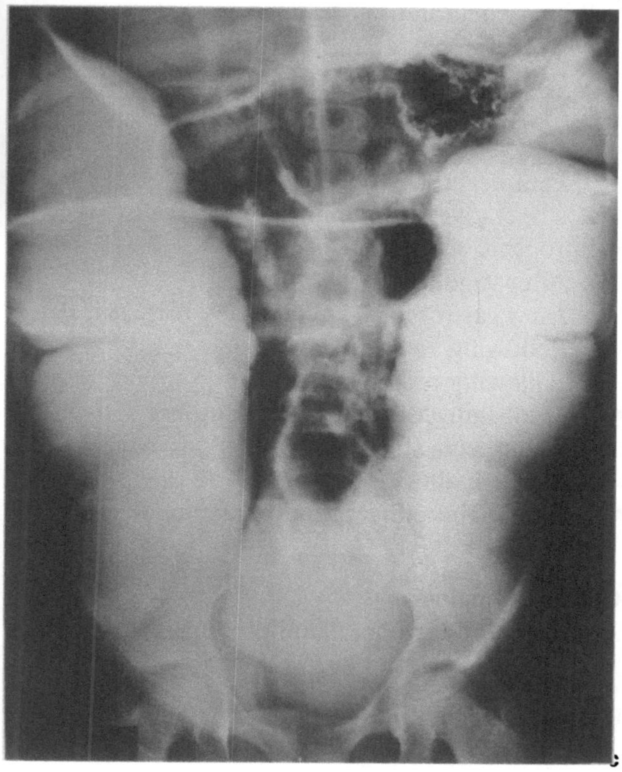
c

Fig. 171 a–c. Pseudo-obstruction of the colon.
Girl, 12 years old, had undergone ileorectostomy for megacolon 2 years earlier in Yugoslavia. Since then she has had abdominal distension and growth retardation. **a** *Supine film* shows massive colonic distension from the cecum to the rectum with no narrowing. There is associated distension of the small bowel. **b** *Erect chest film* shows massive elevation of the diaphragm with distended loops of colon interposed between the liver and anterior abdominal wall. **c** *UGI follow-through* shows massive colonic distension without stenosis. There is no evidence of Hirschspring's disease

- Diseases that interfere with myoneuronal transmission or alter muscular contractility
  - Diabetes (Fig. 8 c, d)
  - Myxedema
  - Porphyria
  - Lead poisoning
  - Uremia (Fig. 8 a)
  - Hypokalemia
  - Amyloidosis (Fig. 35)
  - Scleroderma
  - Sprue
  - Chagas' disease *(Trypanosoma cruzi)*
- Systemic extra-abdominal diseases that impair intestinal transport
  - Septic or hypervolemic shock
  - Hypoxia
  - Pleural and pulmonary diseases (pneumonia, pleurisy) (Fig. 24 a, b)
  - Cardiac diseases (infarction, acute pericarditis)
  - Retroperitoneal diseases (see Sect. 4.5) (trauma, hemorrhage, abscess, renal or ureteral colic) (Fig. 25)
- Primary neuromuscular diseases
  - Amyotrophic lateral sclerosis
  - Poliomyelitis
  - Multiple sclerosis
  - Cauda equina lesions
  - Paraplegia
- Postoperative, adynamic, paralytic ileus (Fig. 31)
- Iatrogenic bowel distension
  - After vagotomy (Fig. 8 c, f)
  - After gastroscopy or coloscopy (Fig. 28 c, d)
  - Following assisted ventilation
  - Following radiotherapy
- Psychogenic gastrointestinal disorders
  - Aerophagia (Fig. 28 a, b)
  - Laxative abuse
- Idiopathic intestinal pseudo-obstruction (Fig. 171)

Clinical Symptoms
Abdominal distension, inability to pass stool or gas, absende of peristalsis

Radiologic Signs

Plain Radiographs
Plain films show combined small- and large-bowel distension with L Lat fluid levels. Mechanical colon obstruction with gaseous reflux into the small bowel can be differentiated from the atonic, paralytic, functional ileus of intestinal pseudo-obstruction only from *clinical manifestations* and on *UGI* study.
If the water-soluble contrast medium is able to traverse the atonic bowel (even slowly) to the anus, a diagnosis of pseudo-obstruction is justified. A complete blockage of the contrast medium signifies a mechanical colon obstruction. Besides its diagnostic value, Gastrografin also has therapeutic efficacy by stimulating intestinal peristalsis.

References for 4.2.1, 4.2.2, 4.2.3

Alessi V, Salerno G (1985) The "hay fork" sign in the ultrasonographic diagnosis of intussusception. Gastrointest Radiol 10: 177-179

Beyer D (1983) Sonographie des Peritonealraumes. In: Bücheler E, Friedmann G, Thelen M (eds) Real-time-Sonographie des Körpers. Thieme, Stuttgart

Beyer D, Friedmann G (1983) Sonographie des Magen-Darm-Traktes. In: Bücheler E, Friedmann G, Thelen M (eds) Real-time-Sonographie des Körpers. Thieme, Stuttgart

Beyer D, Köster R (1984) Bildgebende Diagnostik akuter intestinaler Durchblutungsstörungen. Springer, Berlin Heidelberg New York Tokyo

Beyer D, Horsch S, Bohr M, Schmitz T (1980) Röntgensymptomatik der experimentellen Darmischämie beim Hund nach Ligatur der A. mesenterica superior. Fortschr Röntgenstr 4: 377-385

Beyer D, Köster R, Horsch S (1980) Radiologische Frühdiagnostik der akuten Darmischämie durch Nativaufnahmen des Abdomens und Angiographie. Experimentelle und klinisch-radiologische Ergebnisse. In: Müller-Wiefel H, Barras JP, Ehringer H, Krüger M (eds) Mikrozirkulation und Blutrheologie - Therapie der peripheren arteriellen Verschlußkrankheiten. Witzstrock, Baden-Baden

Beyer D, Heuser L, Krestin GP (1984) Adjuvante sonographische Diagnostik bei Ileusverdacht. In: Lutz (ed) Ultraschalldiagnostik 1983. Thieme, Stuttgart

Fleischer AC, Dowling AD, Weinstein ML, James AE (1979) Sonographic patters of distended, fluid-filled bowel. Radiology 133: 681-685

Friedmann G, Wenz W, Ebel K-D, Bücheler E (1980) Emergency roentgen diagnosis. Thieme, Stuttgart

Frimann-Dahl J (1968) The acute abdomen. In: Strnad F (ed) Röntgendiagnostik des Digestionstraktes und des Abdomens. Springer, Berlin Heidelberg New York (Handbuch der med Radiol, vol 11/2)

Govoni AF, Whalen JP (1981) The acute abdomen. In: Teplick JG, Haskin ME (eds) Surgical radiology. Saunders, Philadelphia

Hentschel M (1984) Praxis der Chirurgie des Ileus. Enke, Stuttgart

Hyson EA, Burell M, Toffler R (1983) Drug-induced gastrointestinal disorders. In: Meyers MA, Ghahremani GG (eds) Iatrogenic gastrointestinal complications. Springer, Berlin Heidelberg New York

Johnson CD, Rice RP, Kelvin FM, Forster WL, Williford ME (1985) The radiological evaluation of gross cecal distension: emphasis on cecal ileus. AJR 145: 1211-1217

McCort JJ (1981) Abdominal radiology. Williams & Wilkins, Baltimore

Meyers MA (1976) Dynamic radiology of the abdomen. Normal and pathologic anatomy. Springer, Berlin Heidelberg New York

Mindelzun RE, McCort JJ (1983) Acute abdomen. In: Margulis AR, Burhenne HJ (eds) Alimentary tract radiology. Mosby, St. Louis

Penschuk C, Saul T (1985) Seltene Dislokation einer Oesophagusprothese vor die Ileocöcalklappe mit tiefem Dünndarmileus. Chirurg 56: 345-346

Preston DM, Lennard-Jones JE, Thomas BM (1985) Towards a radiologic definition of idiopathic megacolon. Gastrointest Radiol 10: 167-169

Schindler G (1984) Stellenwert der Computertomographie in der radiologischen Diagnostik des akuten Abdomens. Röntgenpraxis 37: 48-57

Swart B (1968) Duodenum und Nachbarschaft. In: Strnad F (ed) Röntgendiagnostik des Digestionstraktes und des Abdomens. Springer, Berlin Heidelberg New York (Handbuch der med Radiol, vol 11/2)

Swart B (1977) Leerbauchdiagnostik des rechten Oberbauches. In: Frommhold W, Gerhardt P (eds) Erkrankungen der Organe des rechten Oberbauches - Klinisch-radiologisches Seminar. Thieme, Stuttgart

Swart B, Meyer G (1974) Die Diagnostik des akuten Abdomens bei Erwachsenen - ein neues klinisch-röntgenologisches Konzept. Radiologe 14: 1-57

Tschakert H (1985) Als Lipom fehlgedeutete Morgagni-Hernie Digit. Bilddiagn 5: 16-17

Zittel RX (1983) Akute chirurgische Erkrankungen. Thieme, Stuttgart

4.2.4 Acute Intestinal Ischemia - Mesenteric Infarction

D. Beyer, W. Gross-Fengels

Etiology and Pathogenesis (Fig. 172)

- Arterial embolism } of the superior mesenteric artery
- Arterial thrombosis } of the superior mesenteric artery
- Thrombosis of the superior mesenteric vein/portal vein
- Nonocclusive ischemia (functional occlusion)
- External compression
- Trauma

Arterial Embolism (about 25% of all intestinal ischemias)
Sources of emboli: 90% originate in the left heart (ventricular aneurysm, atrial fibrillation, aortic and mitral valves). The remainder derive from extracardiac sources (paradoxic embolism, parietal thrombi from aneurysms of the aorta, tumor embolism).

Arterial Thrombosis (about 40%)
Some 90% of arterial thrombi arise from arteriosclerotic plaques in the superior mesenteric artery (about two-thirds close to the origin, one-third in the periphery). Infrequent causes are compression by abdominal aortic aneurysms, dissecting aneurysms, and inflammatory diseases of the vessel wall.

Venous Thrombosis (about 15%)
About 80% originate from antecedent disease in the bed supplying the portal vein, previous surgery or trauma, or previous inflammatory processes such as pancreatitis, appendicitis, diverticulitis, and abscesses. Less frequent causes are hemorrhagic diathesis and alterations of blood viscosity, hormonal contraceptives, and portal venous thrombosis associated with hepatic cirrhosis.

Nonocclusive Ischemia (about 15%)
Does *not* involve direct occlusion of the vessel lumen. A multifactorial etiology is the rule.
Causes: prolonged circulatory insufficiency (low cardiac output, result of massive diuretic therapy or digitalis intoxication).

External Compression
By mesenteric tumors or hemorrhage (anticoagulant overdose, hemorrhagic diathesis), volvulus, intussusception, or incarceration.

Trauma
Traumatic (rarely iatrogenic) laceration or avulsion of a blood vessel.

Caution: The gastrointestinal tract can tolerate ischemia for 4-12 h, depending on the site and completeness of vascular obstruction and development of a collateral flow. Surgical decision making and diagnostic imaging must be accomplished swiftly to avoid infarction of the ischemic bowel segments, which carries a 70%-90% mortality rate.

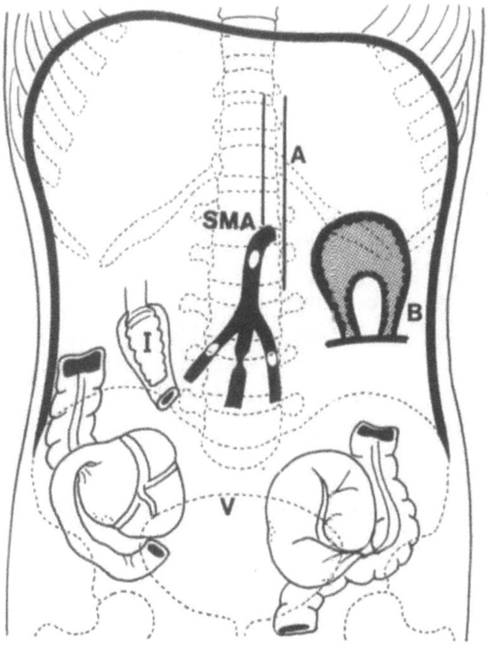

Fig. 172. Causes of primary and secondary bowel ischemia with consequent mesenteric infarction and gangrene. Primary ischemia is caused by occlusion of the superior mesenteric artery *(SMA)* after its origin from the aorta *(A)* or the superior mesenteric vein. Secondary ischemia is caused by adhesive bands *(B)*, intussusception *(I)*, or volvulus *(V)*

Clinical Symptoms

Early stage

Initially the patient experiences colicky or cramping abdominal pain that is poorly localized. Embolism is characterized by a sudden onset, while a gradual onset is typical of arterial or venous thrombosis and nonocclusive ischemia. Additional signs are nausea and vomiting, a nonrigid abdomen, intial hyperperistalsis with diarrhea, and shock symptoms.

Latent stage

Abdominal pain spontaneously subsides about 2-6 h after symptoms begin. There is increasing meteorism, and the abdominal wall remains soft. Peristalsis is absent or diminished (paralytic ileus). Shock symptoms become more pronounced, and bloody diarrhea may be present.

End stage

Diffuse abdominal tenderness supervenes about 12-48 h after onset of symptoms, accompanied by muscular rigidity, aperistalsis (silent abdomen), fever, and shock. Classic picture of diffuse seepage peritonitis.

Laboratory values are nonspecific: leukocytosis (30000-50000 in late cases). Blood studies show metabolic acidosis and hypokalemia.

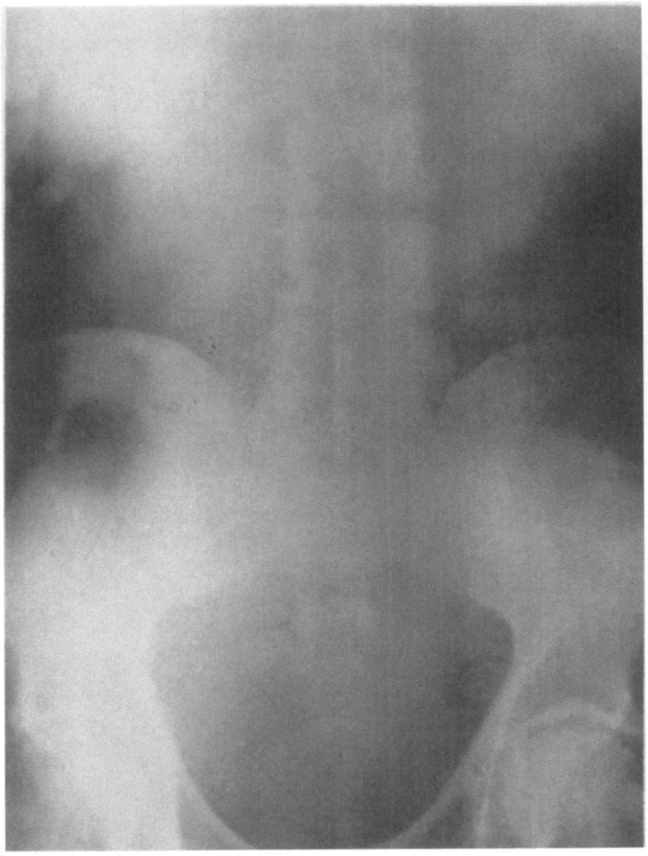

a

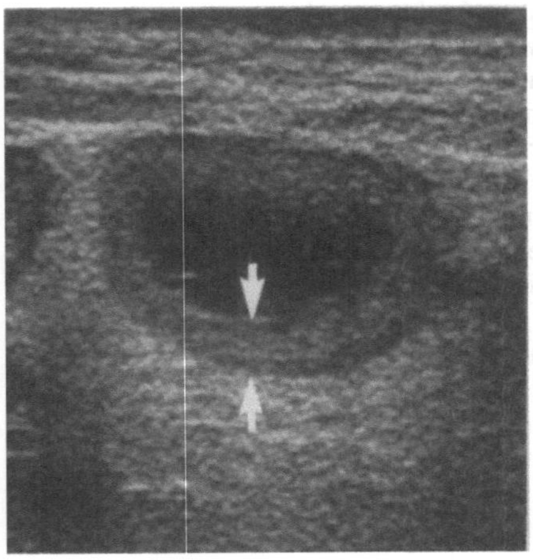

b

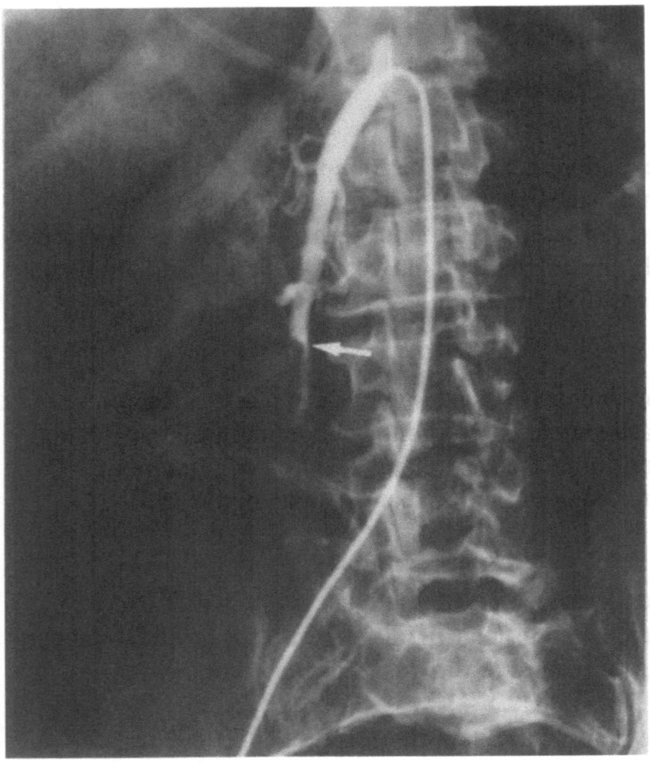

c

Fig. 173a–c. Mesenteric arterial embolism in a 71-year-old man with acute abdominal pain of sudden onset. Patient had been placed in ICU for an absolute arrhythmia and atrial fibrillation and had undergone embolectomy of the left ulnar artery 5 days earlier. *Clinical findings:* diffuse abdominal tenderness, hyperperistalsis, nonbloody diarrhea. **a** *Supine film* (grid cassette, ICU) 60 min after onset of symptoms shows a "gasless abdomen". **b** *Sonogram* about 80 min after symptom onset shows marked thickening of the small-bowel walls (→←), which have fluid contents. Peristalsis is still normal; there is no ascites. **c** Because of the clinical symptoms and "gasless abdomen," immediate *angiography* was performed. Selective mesenteric angiogram 90 min after symptom onset shows complete occlusion of the main trunk of the superior mesenteric artery (⇐) with associated arteriosclerotic wall changes. *Operation* (started 3 h after acute event): Embolectomy was precluded by severe arteriosclerotic changes, and so the entire small bowel and ascending colon had to be resected. Patient died 3 days postoperatively

Radiologic Signs

Plain Radiographs

Early stage

Plain films show a gasless abdomen with increasing ground-glass haziness ("white abdomen" - a nonspecific sign) from hyperperistalsis with diarrhea. This is especially typical of mesenteric embolism (Fig. 173 a).

Caution: The gasless abdomen sign is often misinterpreted by radiologists. A gasless abdomen *does not* exclude mesenteric infarction, especially in the early stage. Diagnosis is aided by careful clinical observation history taking and sonography!

Latent stage

- Isolated distension of the affected loops of small bowel with fluid levels on the L Lat radiograph (Figs. 174, 175 b)
- Decreased mobility of the small-bowel loops when the patient is repositioned ("rigid loop sign") (Fig. 174 b)
- Thickening of the bowel wall by edema and intramural bleeding confined to affected segments (Figs. 174, 175; Fig. 34 a)

End stage

- Combined small- and large-bowel distension in the supine position as evidence of paralytic ileus, with multiple fluid levels in the small and large bowel in the L Lat position (Fig. 32)
- Gas accumulation in the bowel wall (Fig. 32 b, c)
- Gas in the mesenteric and portal veins (Fig. 32 b, c)
- Possibly free air on the L Lat film signifying perforation of gangrenous bowel segments

Sonography

Sonography is the most important adjunctive study to plain films in the early and latent stages. It confirms a beginning bowel-wall edema (Figs. 173 b, 174 c; Fig. 34 b), excludes other causes of separation of small-bowel loops (ascites, pseudomyxoma, fluid engorgement of the intestine) (see Figs. 35 c, 37 c, 38 d, e), and can quickly establish an indication for angiography. Sonography may show a thrombus in the superior mesenteric vein (Fig. 176).

UGI Series with a water-soluble contrast medium

This study is rarely indicated. In unclear cases it may give evidence of ischemia (especially when caused by thrombosis of a mesenteric venous branch) by demonstrating a short segment of edematous mucosa (Fig. 177).

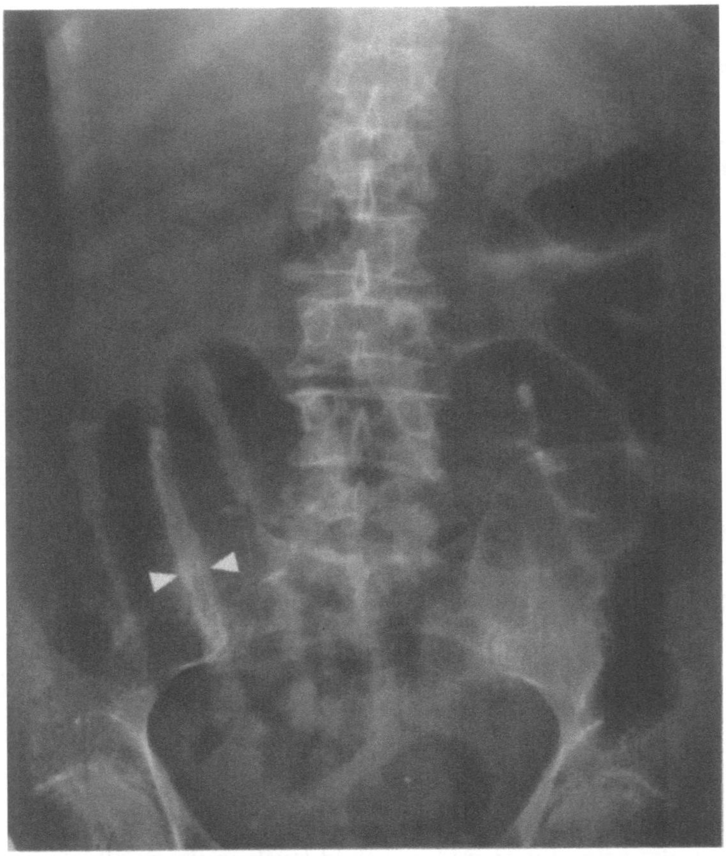
a

Fig. 174a–c. Mesenteric arterial embolism in a 72-year-old woman with violent, rapidly increasing abdominal pain and nonbloody diarrhea. *Clinical findings:* nonrigid abdomen, diffuse abdominal tenderness, silent bowel, tachycardia. **a** *Supine film* 10 h after symptom onset shows isolated small-bowel distension with massive bowel wall thickening mainly affecting the ileum. There is marked loop separation and luminal narrowing (▶ ◀). **b** *Left lateral film* shows isolated small-bowel distension with fluid levels. The rigid, edematous loops of ileum are immobile with position change (rigid loop sign). **c** *Sonogram* shows markedly thickened bowel loops (→←) floating in ascitic fluid *(A)* and a thickened mesentery. *Operation* about 11 h after symptom onset disclosed hemorrhagic infarction of almost the entire small bowel with massive edematous thickening of the loops. Subtotal resection of the small bowel was carried out. Patient died 14 days postoperatively from cerebrovascular accident

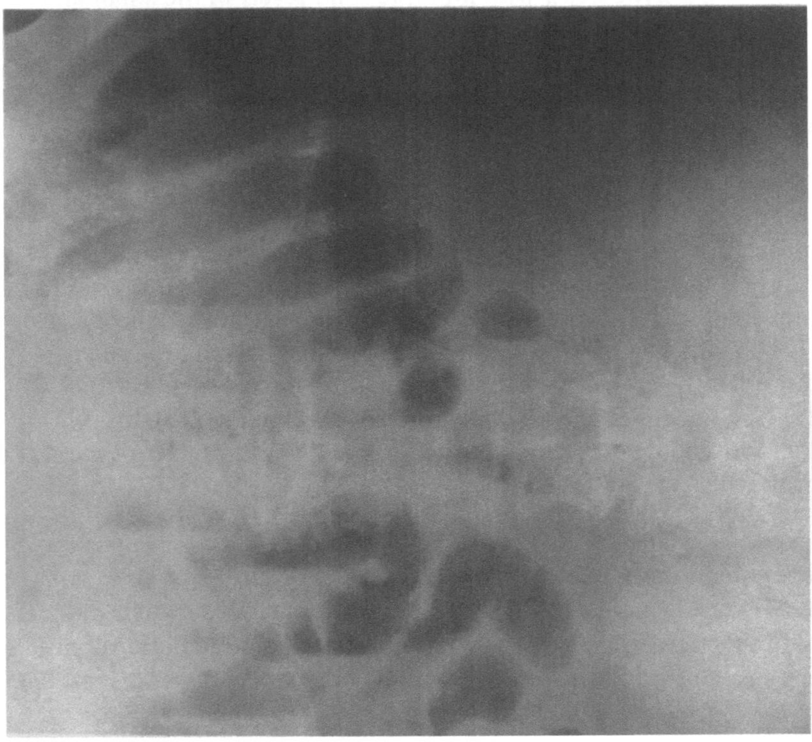
b

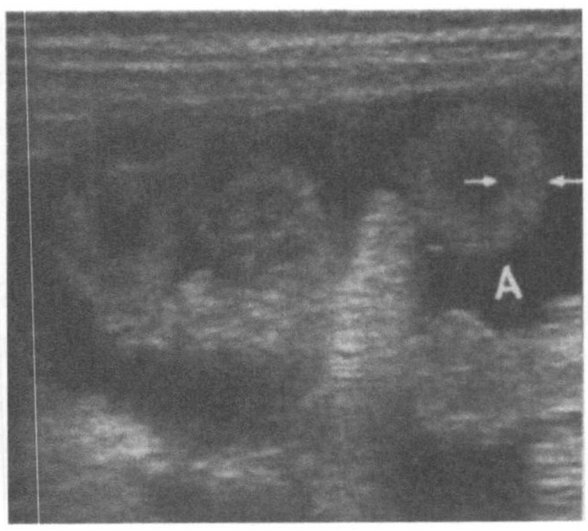

c

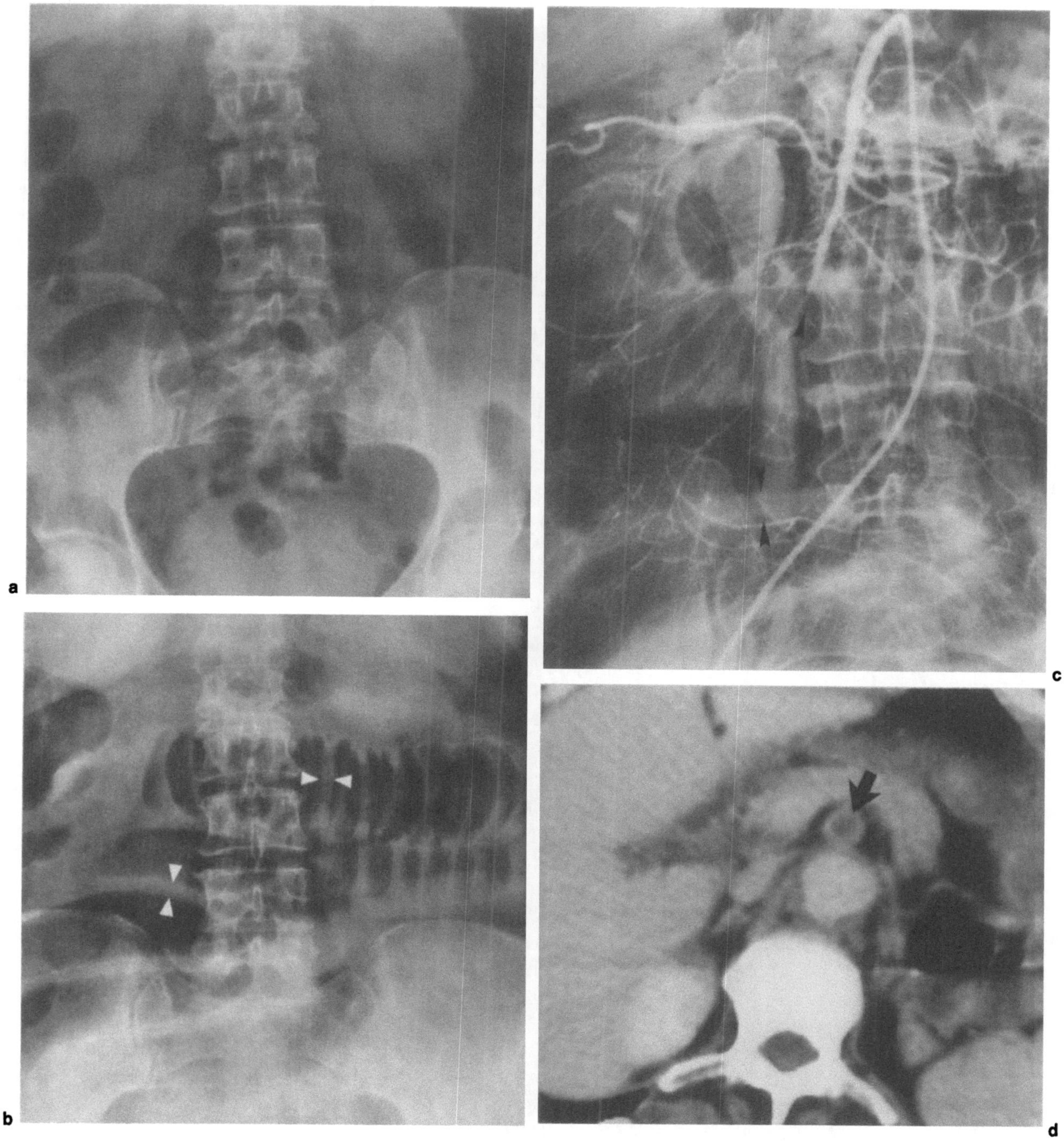

Fig. 175 a–d. Slow development of mesenteric arterial thrombosis over a 7-day period in a 68-year-old woman. Patient had persistent vomiting on 1st day and was hospitalized on 4th day because of bloody diarrhea. *Clinical findings:* nonrigid abdomen with no localized tenderness, pulse 96/min, minimal reduction of peristalsis (!). **a** *Supine film* shows a relatively gasless abdomen and minimal small-bowel distension without wall edema or separation. Left lateral film (not shown) depicted no free air and minimal fluid levels. Films were repeated on 7th day. *Clinical findings:* soft, diffusely tender abdomen, absence of peristalsis, pulse 120/min. **b** *Supine film* at this time shows isolated small-bowel distension with edematous Kerckring's folds in the distended jejunum; marked ileal wall edema with separation of loops (▶ ◀). **c** *Selective mesenteric angiogram* shows a sudden stop of the contrast column in the artery 11 cm distal to its origin from the aorta (▶). There is marked wall edema in the ischemic ileum (▶ ◀). *Operation* disclosed small-bowel ischemia from mesenteric arterial thrombosis mainly affecting the ileum. A 120-cm length of small bowel was resected; the patient survived. **d** Another patient with the same symptoms as in **a**. *CT scan after bolus injection* demonstrates a central, low-density thrombus (➧) in the superior mesenteric artery, which shows marked luminal dilatation

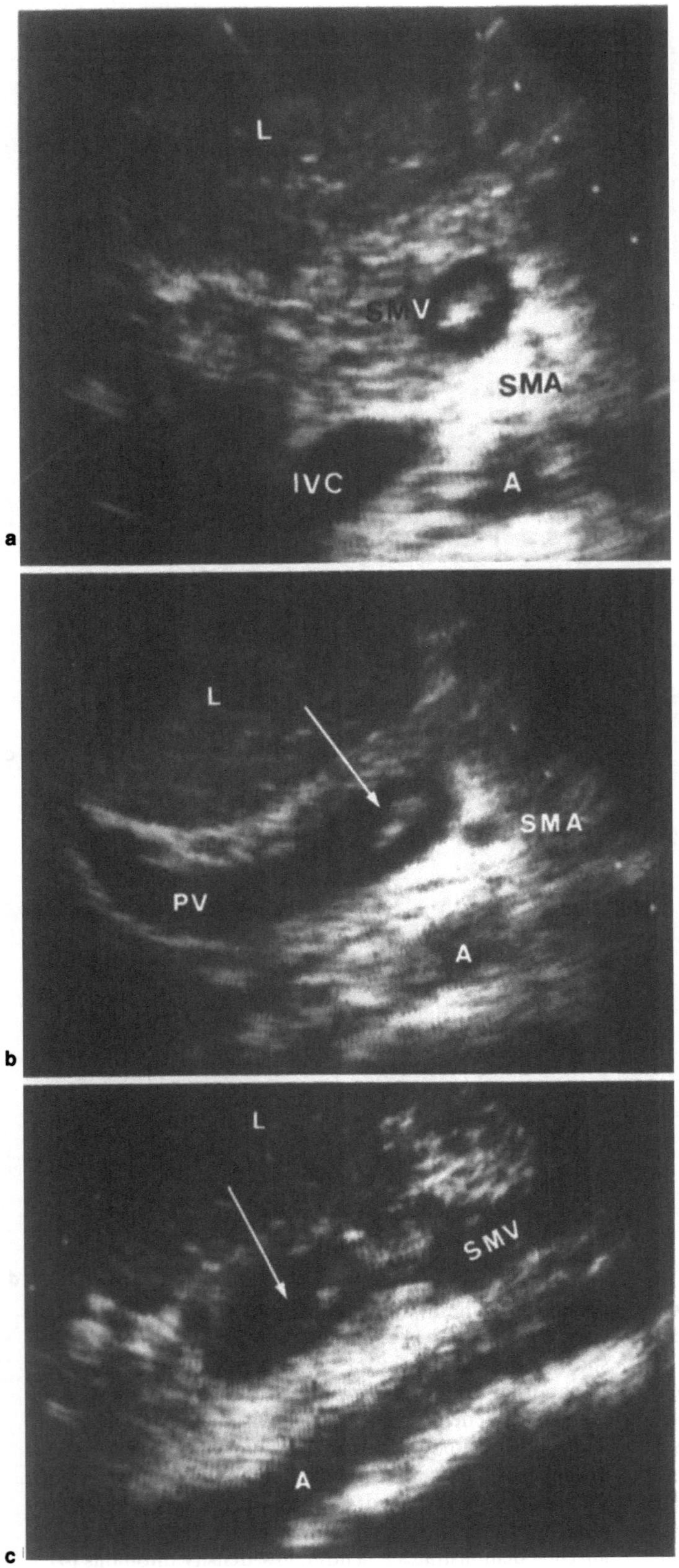

Fig. 176 a–f. Mesenteric venous thrombosis complicating appendicitis in a 39-year-old man who had had right lower quadrant pain for 2 days with fever and vomiting. Appendicitis was found at laparotomy. Appendectomy was uneventful but was followed by recurrence of fever, leukocytosis, and elevated hepatic enzymes. Blood culture was positive for *E. coli.*
a *Sonogram* (transverse scan at the level of the pancreatic head) shows a dilated superior mesenteric vein *(SMV)* with echogenic material at its center. *IVC,* inferior vena cava; *A,* aorta; *L,* liver; *SMA,* superior mesenteric artery.
b *Sonogram* (oblique scan through the porta hepatis) shows a normal-appearing portal vein *(PV)* with no intraluminal thrombotic material. The markedly dilated confluence of the splenic vein and SMV is filled with thrombus. *A,* aorta; *L,* liver; *SMA,* superior mesenteric artery.
c Longitudinal scan through the aorta *(A)* and superior mesenteric vein *(SMV)* shows a large intravenous thrombus whose apex is in the confluence of the SMV and splenic vein; *L,* liver.

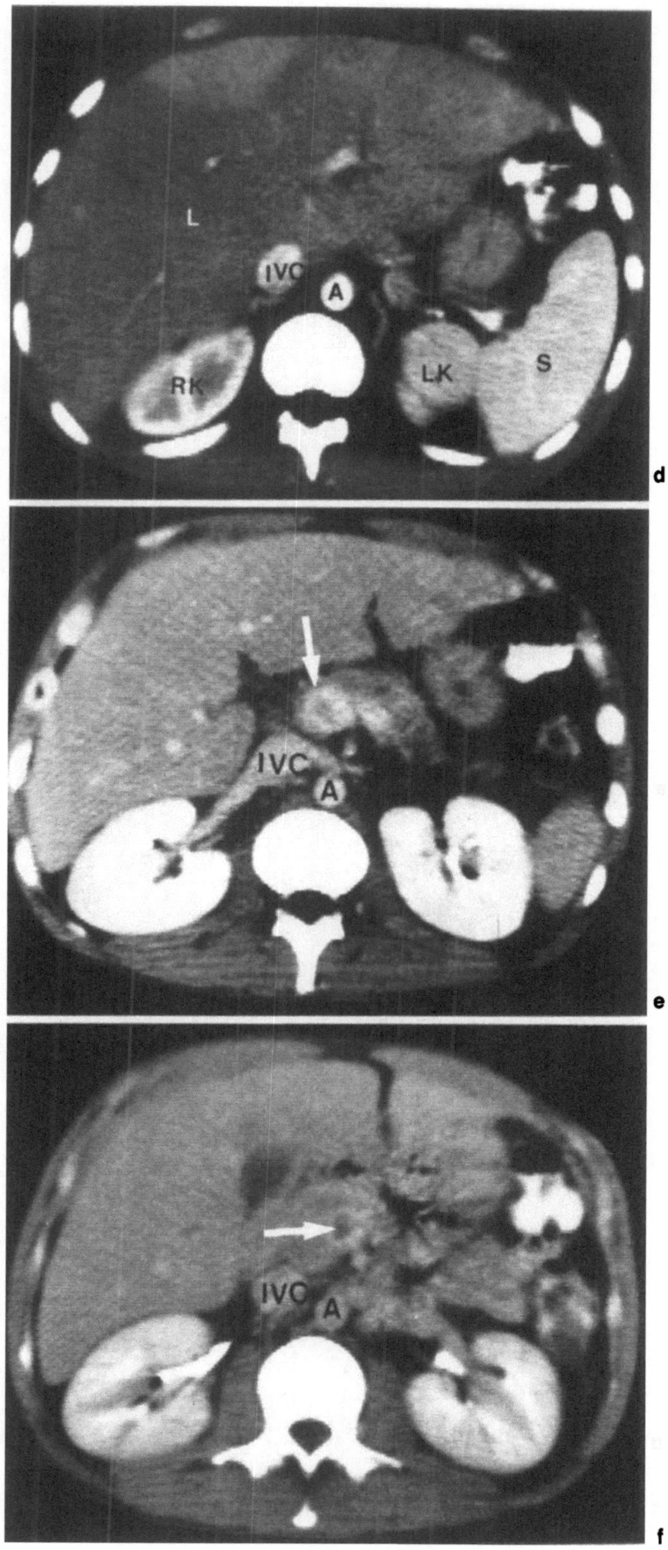

Fig. 176 (continued)
d *CT scan after bolus injection* of the upper abdomen, shows a large perfusion defect in the liver *(L)*. *IVC*, inferior vena cava; *A*, aorta; *RK*, right kidney; *LK*, left kidney; *S*, spleen. **e** *CT scan with bolus injection* shows the cranial part of the SMV to be markedly dilated and that there is a filling defect during bolus injection; *A*, aorta; *IVC*, inferior vena cava. **f** *CT scan after bolus injection* shows total occlusion of the lower part of the SMV with a low-density thrombus at the center of the vessel. *Treatment:* antibiotics and high-dosage heparinization. Reexamination at discharge confirmed absence of thrombus in the SMV. *IVC*, inferior vena cava; *A*, aorta. (Courtesy of Dr. T. K. Oei, Radiology Department of St. Annadal Hospital, University of Limburg, Netherlands)

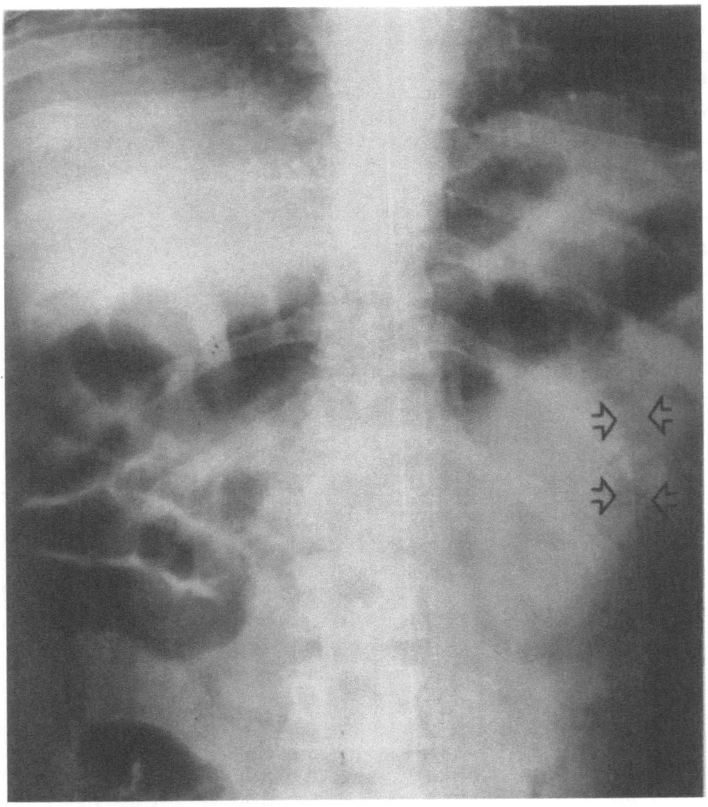

a

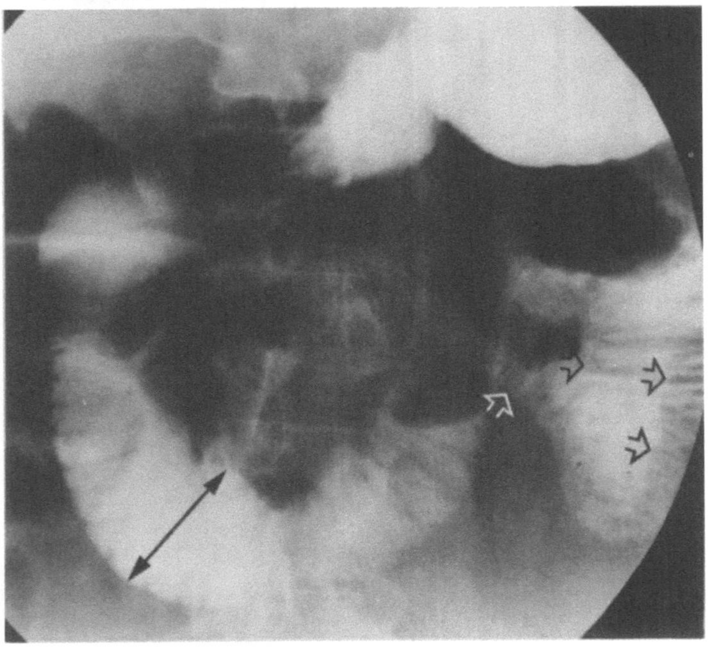

b

Fig. 177a–c. Localized mesenteric thrombosis of jejunal veins. Diagnosis by UGI series. Menopausal woman, 46 years old, experienced sudden vomiting and epigastric pain. Clinical examination showed a nonrigid, nontender abdomen with normal peristalsis; pulse 92/min. **a** *Supine film* shows mild, nonspecific distension of the small and large bowel with an irregular, sawtooth gas pattern in the left upper quadrant (jejunum?) (⇨). Left lateral film (not shown) excluded free air and showed duodenal and gastric distension with fluid levels (signifying mechanical obstruction?), otherwise no new findings. Further investigation by *UGI series* using water-soluble contrast (**b**) showed dilatation of the duodenum (↔) and proximal jejunum and swelling of Kerckring's folds (⇨).

Fig. 177 (continued)
c Markedly dilated, uncoiled jejunum with fold edema (⇒), otherwise normal transit. *Operation* disclosed localized mesenteric thrombosis of jejunal veins; 30 cm of jejunum was resected and continuity restored by end-to-end anastomosis. The patient survived

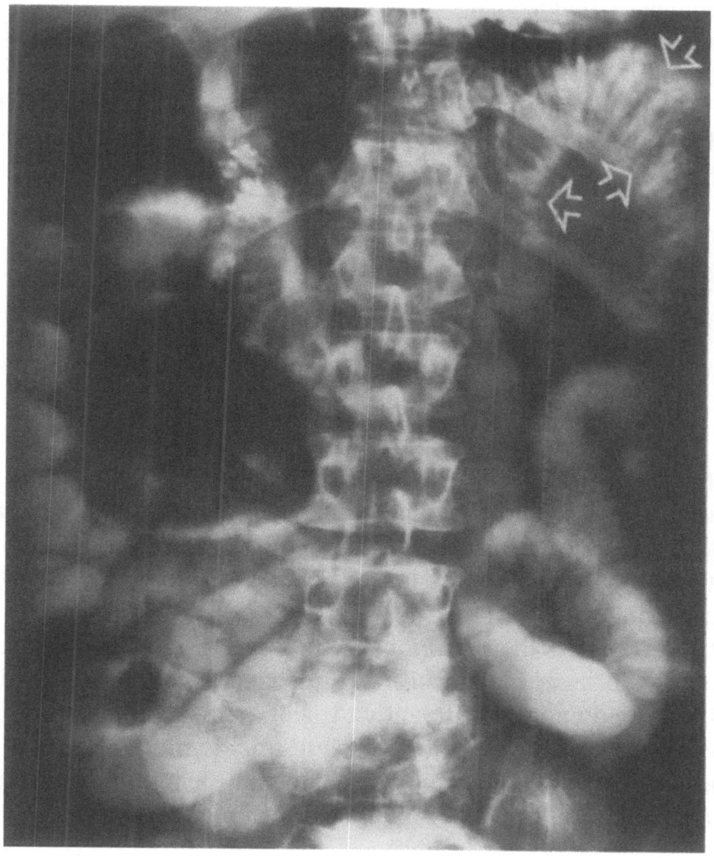

c

Computed Tomography

In some cases a bolus injection will demonstrate an embolus or thrombus lodged in the superior mesenteric artery or vein (Figs. 175, 176). CT can also demonstrate the thickened, edematous wall of the affected bowel (Fig. 36b) and intramural gas collections (Figs. 75f., 210f.) as well as gas in the portal veins (Fig. 210e).

> *Note:* CT is the most dependable means of detecting intramural or intravascular gas in the transition from the latent to the end stage. Therefore it is recommended as an adjunct in selected cases, especially when the course is protracted.

Angiography (Figs. 173c, 175c, 178c, 179b, c)

Angiography is indicated as soon as there is the *slightest suspicion* of occlusive vascular disease so that the patient can be referred for life-saving surgery as quickly as possible, even when symptoms appear to be regressing.

Angiography is the *only* modality that can differentiate central from peripheral segmental occlusions and exclude nonocclusive ischemia, which is managed entirely differently. Angiography is all the more justified when we consider that the majority of intestinal ischemias relate to arterial occlusions, 75% of which involve the main stem of the superior mesenteric artery and thus are accessible to surgical management.

Differential diagnosis of bowel wall thickening: see Sect. 3.2.
Differential diagnosis of distension limited to the small bowel: see Sect. 3.1.3.
Differential diagnosis of paralytic ileus: see Sect. 3.1.5.
Differential diagnosis of intramural and intravascular gas collections: see Sect. 3.5.4.

> *Note:* Bowel wall thickening and its accompanying signs are *absent* in traumatic and nonocclusive ischemia!
> The *primary imaging modalities* in the diagnosis of intestinal ischemia are plain radiography and sonography, as well as mesenteric angiography when there is clinical or radiologic suspicion of ischemia.
> The value of CT in suspected ischemia is limited to the differentiation and localization of questionable gas collections.
> The *main concern* in this type of disease is *to consider the possibility of a mesenteric infarction* in the first place!

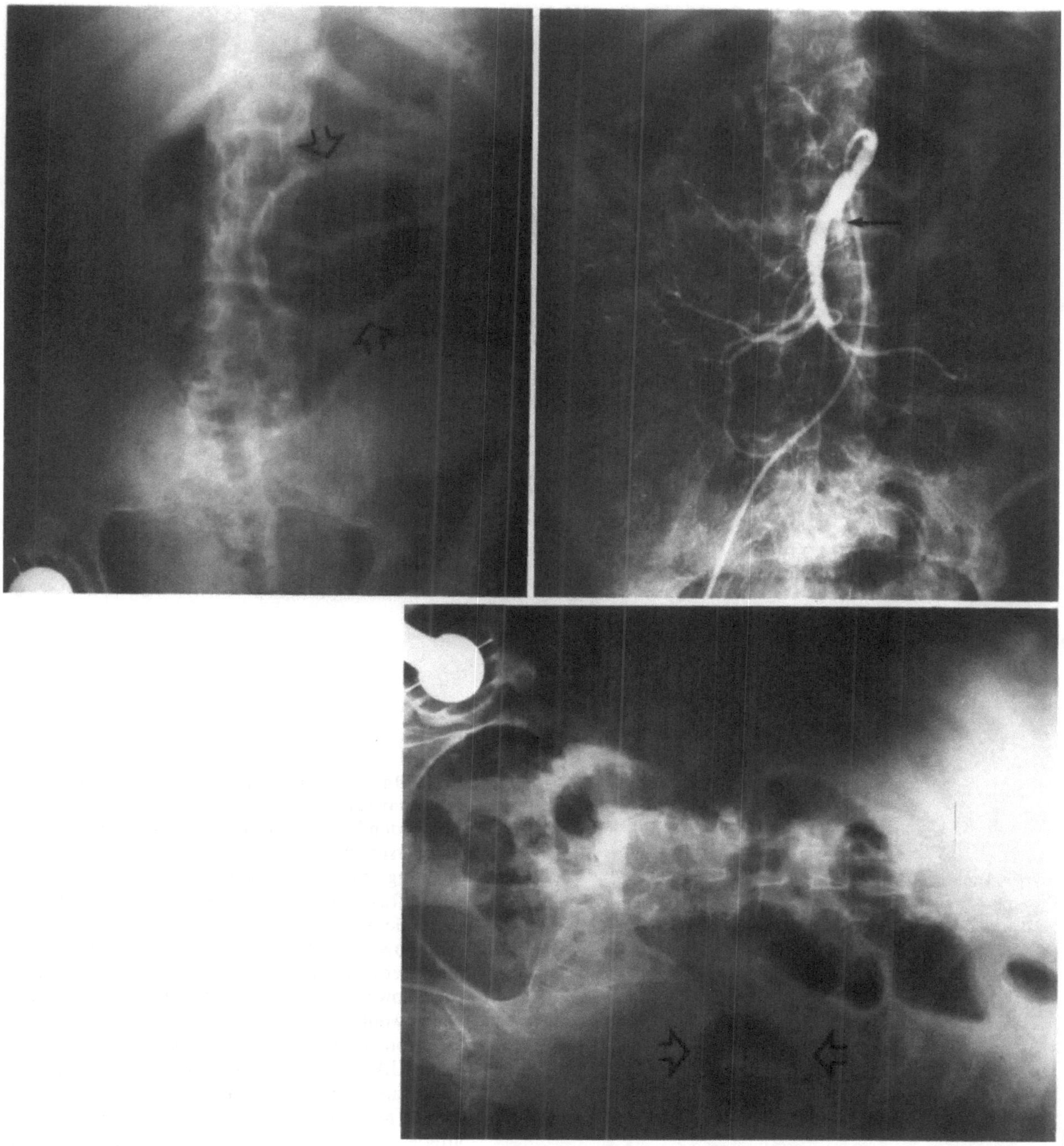

a c b

Fig. 178 a–c. Angiography of mesenteric arterial embolism in a 64-year-old man with severe abdominal pain of sudden onset. Known ventricular aneurysm was present as an underlying disease. *Clinical findings:* abdomen diffusely tender and nonrigid, decreased bowel sounds, pulse rate 130/min with pulse deficit, no leukocytosis. **a** *Supine film* taken about 8 h after initial symptoms shows isolated small-bowel distension with segmental wall thickening in the jejunum (⇨). **b** *Left lateral film* shows scattered fluid levels and marked wall thickening of the aforementioned jejunal loop (⇨). **c** *Selective mesenteric angiogram* shows central embolic occlusion of the jejunal branches (←). *Operation* disclosed incipient hemorrhagic necrosis of 1.2 m of jejunum with marked wall edema. Patient survived resective surgery

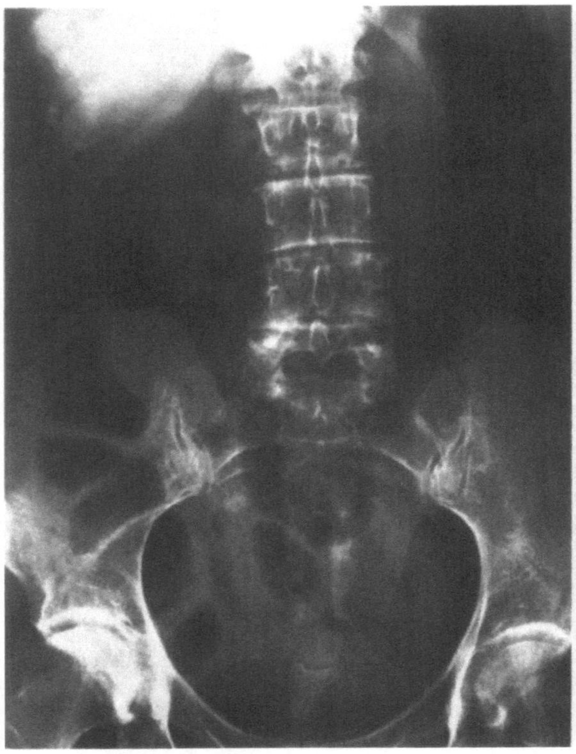

a

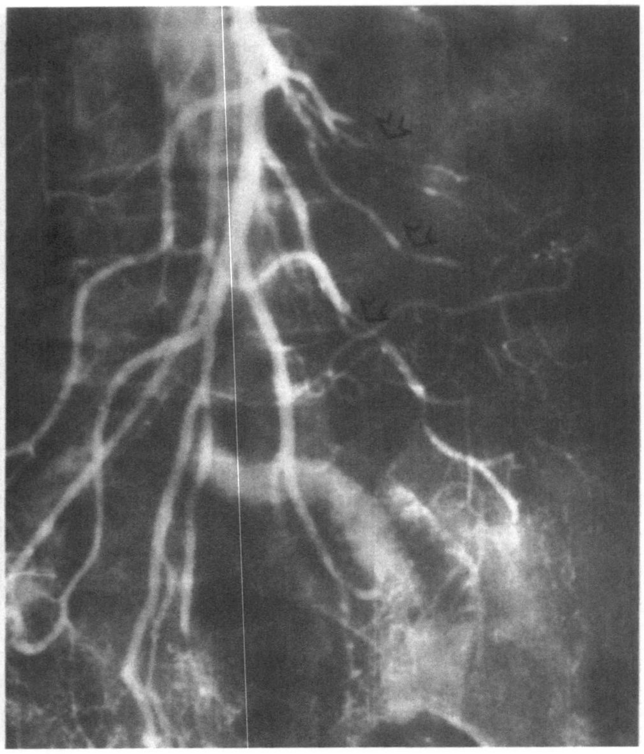

b

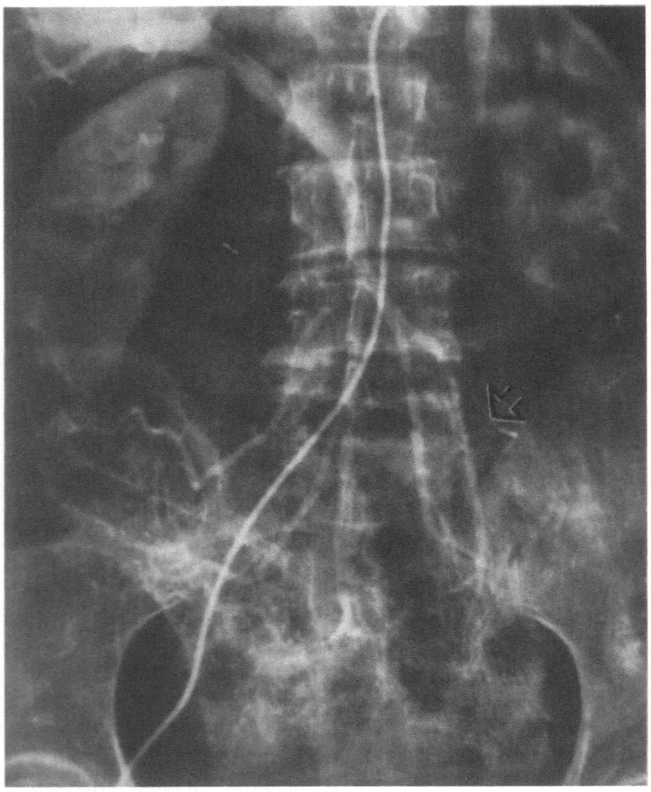

c

Fig. 179 a–c. Nonocclusive bowel ischemia from digitalis intoxication in a 78-year-old man who had recurring abdominal pain for months. At examination he had persistent and slowly increasing colics and severe vomiting of about 16 h duration. *Clinical symptoms:* soft, diffusely tender abdomen, faint bowel sounds, arrhythmic pulse of 120/min, no leukocytosis. **a** *Supine film* shows nonspecific bowel gas pattern with moderate distension of the ascending colon. Left lateral, film (not shown) depicted no fluid levels and no free air which would indicate a perforation. Clinical signs were consistent with vascular disease, and the digitoxin-RIA test was performed, confirming suspicion of digitalis overdose. **b** *Selective mesenteric angiogram, arterial phase:* segmental constrictions of the jejunal arteries with fluctuations of caliber (△). **c** *Selectivce mesenteric angiogram, venous phase:* stasis of contrast flow in a jejunal artery (⇒) with otherwise normal venous drainage. *Operation* disclosed segmental ischemia and edema of the small bowel; a 1.2 m length of small bowel was resected. *Histology* showed incipient hemorrhagic mucosal necrosis and segmental wall necrosis with no evidence of arterial or venous obstruction. Patient died of renal failure 3 days after surgery

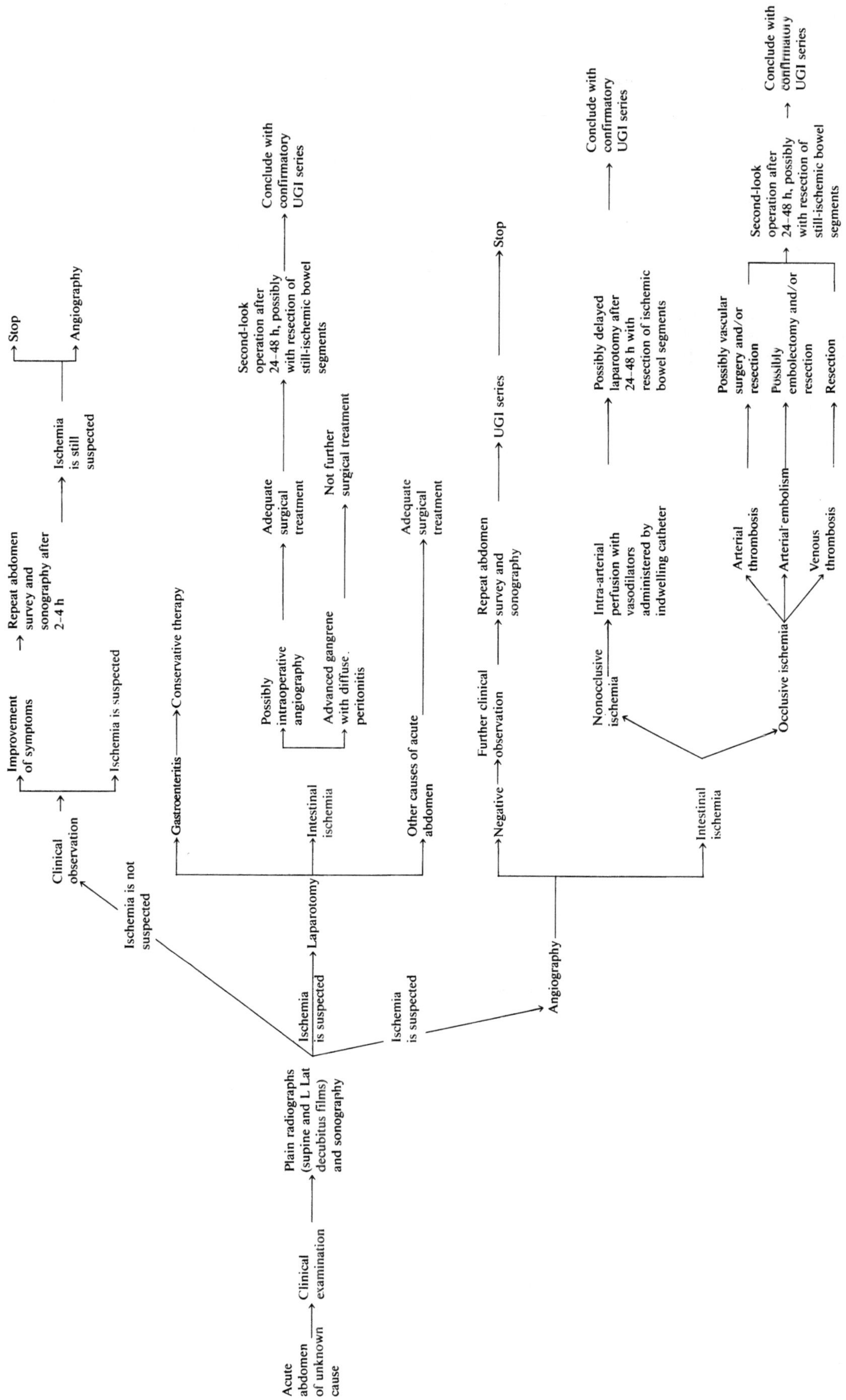
Acute abdomen of unknown cause
Clinical examination
Plain radiographs (supine and L Lat decubitus films) and sonography
Ischemia is not suspected
Clinical observation
Improvement of symptoms
Repeat abdomen survey and sonography after 2-4 h
Ischemia is still suspected
Stop
Angiography
Ischemia is suspected
Ischemia is suspected
Laparotomy
Gastroenteritis
Conservative therapy
Intestinal ischemia
Possibly intraoperative angiography
Adequate surgical treatment
Second-look operation after 24-48 h, possibly with resection of still-ischemic bowel segments
Conclude with confirmatory UGI series
Advanced gangrene with diffuse peritonitis
Not further surgical treatment
Other causes of acute abdomen
Adequate surgical treatment
Angiography
Negative
Further clinical observation
Repeat abdomen survey and sonography
UGI series
Stop
Intestinal ischemia
Nonocclusive ischemia
Intra-arterial perfusion with vasodilators administered by indwelling catheter
Possibly delayed laparotomy after 24-48 h with resection of ischemic bowel segments
Conclude with confirmatory UGI series
Occlusive ischemia
Arterial thrombosis
Possibly vascular surgery and/or resection
Arterial embolism
Possibly embolectomy and/or resection
Venous thrombosis
Resection
Second-look operation after 24-48 h, possibly with resection of still-ischemic bowel segments
Conclude with confirmatory UGI series

References

Beyer D, Horsch S (1980) Röntgendiagnostik bei akuter Darmischämie. Zentralbl Chir 105: 1005

Beyer D, Köster R (1984) Bildgebende Diagnostik akuter intestinaler Durchblutungsstörungen. Ein klinisch-radiologisches Konzept. Springer, Berlin Heidelberg New York Tokyo

Beyer D, Schultze P (1983) Sonographie des Magen-Darm-Traktes. In: Bücheler E, Friedmann G, Thelen M (eds) Real-time Sonographie des Körpers. Thieme, Stuttgart

Beyer D, Horsch S, Bohr M, Schmitz T (1980) Röntgensymptomatik der experimentellen Darmischämie beim Hund nach Ligatur der A. mesenterica superior. Fortschr Röntgenstr 132/4: 377

Boley JS, Schwartz SS, Williams LF (1971) Vascular disorders of the intestine. Appleton Century-Crofts, New York

Nelson SW, Eggleston W (1960) Findings on plain roentgenograms of the abdomen associated with mesenteric vascular occlusion with possible new sign of mesenteric venous thrombosis. AJR 83: 886

Swart B, Meyer G (1974) Die Diagnostik des akuten Abdomens beim Erwachsenen - ein neues klinisch-radiologisches Konzept. Radiologe 14: 1

Tomchik FS, Wittenberg J, Ottinger LW (1970) The roentgenographic spectrum of bowel infarction. Radiology 96: 249

4.2.5 Toxic Megacolon

D. Beyer

The term for this disease is misleading, and it would be more accurate to speak of an acute fulminating stage of colitis with deep, extensive damage to the bowel wall and total or segmental dilatation with systemic toxicity.

Etiology
The cause is not known. Predisposing factors are:
- Narcotics, opiates
- Anticholinergic drugs

Exacerbation of any severe form of colitis, usually without transmural cicatrizing processes in the early stages:
- Ulcerative colitis
- Granulomatous colitis
- Amebic colitis
- Ischemic colitis
- Pseudomembranous colitis
- Typhus
- Cholera
- Bacterial dysentery
- Antiobiotic-induced colitis
- Methotrexate - and vincristine-induced colitis

Note: The mortality rate of toxic megacolon is 25%-30% despite optimum utilization of intensive medical and operative treatment. With perforation of the colon, the mortality rate reaches 80%!

Clinical Symptoms
Signs of acute colitis with
- Cramping abdominal pain
- Diffuse abdominal tenderness without rigidity
- Copious bloody diarrhea with absent or decreased peristalsis
- Toxemia with fever, tachycardia, leukocytosis, and shock symptoms
- Also: hypotension, dehydration, electrolyte disorders, anemia, and hypoalbuminemia

Caution: If diffuse muscular rigidity is noted, the patient should be assumed to have parietal peritonitis due to a free perforation!

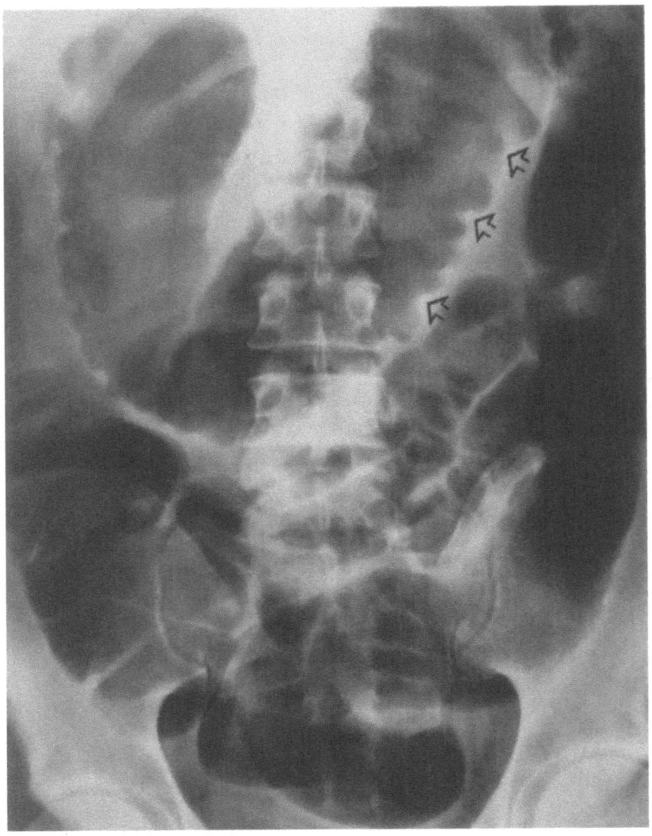

a

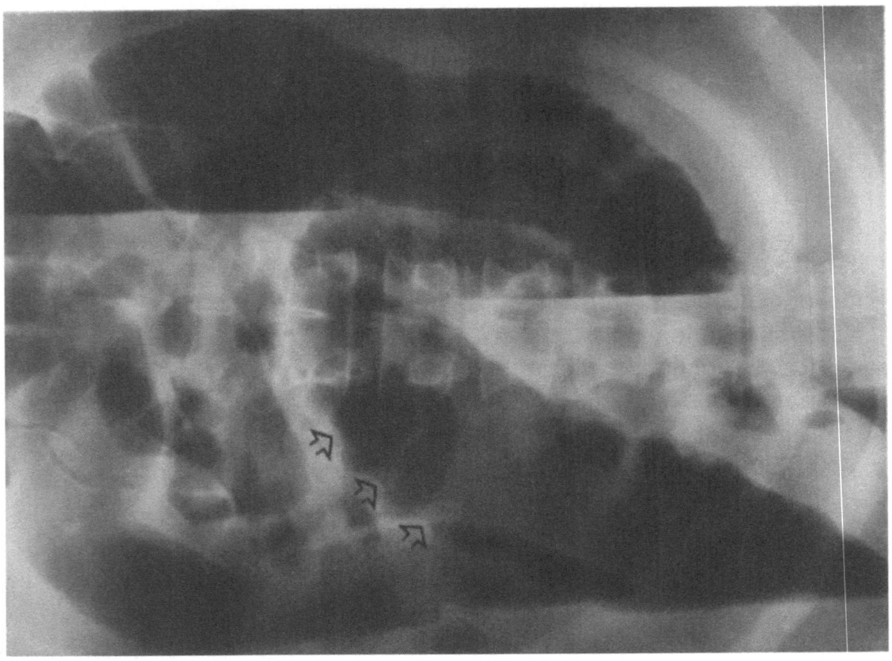

b

Fig. 180 a, b. Toxic megacolon in a 36-year-old woman with a 12-year history of **ulcerative colitis.** Patient had cramping abdominal pain, diffuse abdominal tenderness, severe bloody diarrhea, aperistalsis, and shock. **a** *Supine film* shows combined small- and large-bowel distension; it is most pronounced in the colon from the cecum to the rectum. The haustra (⇒) are markedly thickened in the transverse colon (thumbprints), but elsewhere haustrations are lost. **b** *Left lateral film* shows generalized dilatation of the colon accompanied by moderate small-bowel distension with long fluid levels in the ascending, transverse, and descending colon. The left lateral film likewise shows marked thickening of the colonic mucosa (thumbprints) (⇒)

Fig. 181 a, b. Toxic megacolon in granulomatous colitis. Woman, 27 years old, known to have had Crohn's disease for 8 years experienced cramping abdominal pain, diffuse abdominal tenderness, severe bloody diarrhea, aperistalsis, and shock symptoms. **a** *Supine film* shows isolated colonic distension with an irregular wall contour, especially in the aboral transverse hemicolon and descending colon. **b** *Left lateral film* shows no free air, generalized colonic distension with several fluid levels in the ascending and transverse colon, and loss of haustrations with multiple „thumbprints" (⇒) in the transverse colon and especially the descending colon

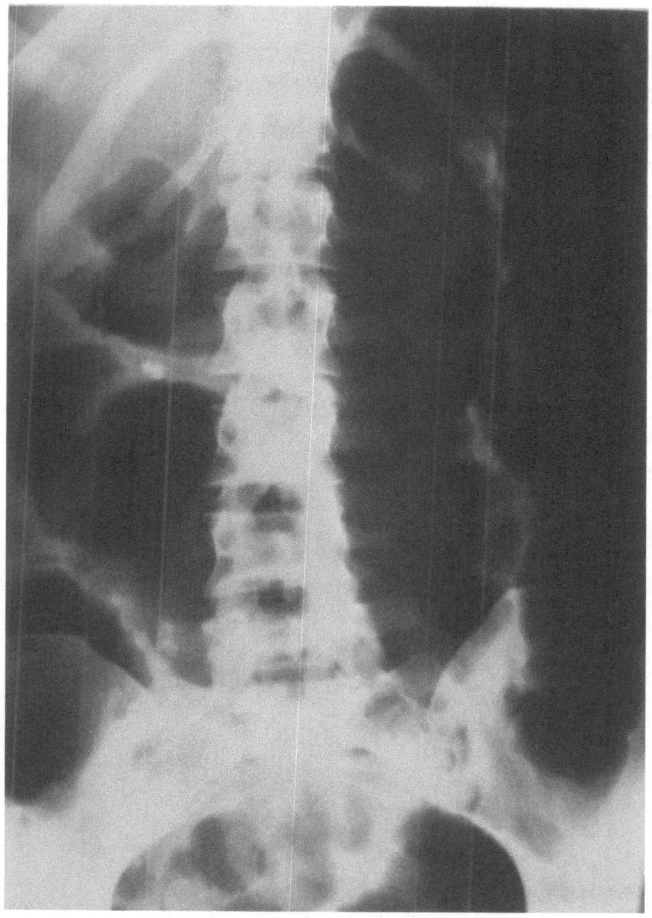

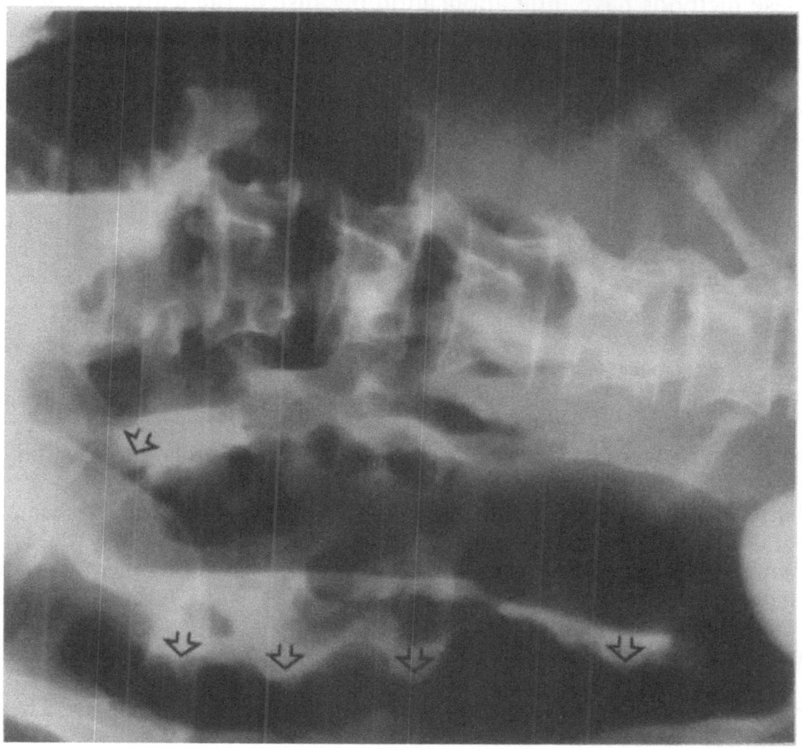

b

Radiologic Signs

Plain Radiographs (Figs. 180, 181)
Supine film
Marked colonic distension by paralysis of the smooth muscles resulting from transmural inflammation; loss of haustrations with smoothing and inversion of wall contours; altered contour of the colonic mucosa ("thumbprinting") caused by edema of residual islets of mucosa (pseudopolyps); there may be concomitant small-bowel distension due to reflux or accompanying paralysis.

L Lat decubitus film
Marked colonic distension with few fluid levels; free air may be present as evidence of a perforation; concomitant small-bowel distension with fluid levels.

Note: Frequent plain films of the abdomen should be obtained to evaluate the *efficacy* of nonoperative treatment. These will demonstrate an increase or decrease in dilatation, mucosal changes, and any life-threatening *perforation!* Single supine views of the abdomen obviously are not sufficient, since a perforation can be missed.

Caution: Contrast examinations and especially contrast enemas are contraindicated in the acute fulminant stage due to the risk of perforation.

Sonography and Computed Tomography
These methods have little application because of the extreme gaseous distension of the colon and because the plain film signs and clinical features are diagnostic.
Abscess formation is common after surgery, however, and both sonography and CT are of value in this setting.

References

Beyer D, Köster R (1984) Bildgebende Diagnostik akuter intestinaler Durchblutungsstörungen. Ein klinisch-radiologisches Konzept. Springer, Berlin Heidelberg New York Tokyo

Fazio VW (1980) Toxic megacolon in ulcerative colitis and Crohn's colitis. Clin Gastroenterol 9: 389-407

Marshak RH, Lester LH, Friedman AJ (1950) Case reports: Megacolon, a complication of ulcerative colitis. Gastroenterology 16: 768-772

Swart B (1977) Die Röntgendiagnostik der Colitis ulcerosa. In: Kremer K, Kivelitz H (eds) Colitis ulcerosa. International Symposium, Düsseldorf, June 1976. Thieme, Stuttgart

Swart B, Meyer G (1974) Die Diagnostik des akuten Abdomens beim Erwachsenen - ein neues klinisch-röntgenologisches Konzept. Radiologe 14: 1

Truelove SC, Marks CG (1981) Toxic megacolon. Pathogenesis, diagnosis and treatment. Clin Gastroenterol 10: 107-117

4.3 Acute Hemorrhage

4.3.1 Upper Gastrointestinal Hemorrhage

K. F. R. NEUFANG, D. BEYER, P. E. PETERS

Definition: Bleeding site proximal to the ligament of Treitz.
Prevalence: about 50 hospitalizations per 100000 population/year in the United States of America for acute upper GI hemorrhage

Major symptoms: Hematemesis, non rigid abdomen, regular perstalsis
Associated symptoms: shock (pallor, cold sweats, palpitation, tachykardia, dizziness, hypotension, dyspnea)
Prognosis: Mortality rate has remained at 10% for 30 years.

Causes (Fig. 182)
Gastroduodenal ulcer (60%), superficial gastric erosions (15%). Less frequently (10%): tumor, e.g., leiomyoma, malignoma; hernia; intussusception; duodenal diverticulum; Mallory-Weiss syndrome; Boerhaave's syndrome; angiodysplasia; anticoagulant medication; hemorrhagic diathesis (Fig. 187); hematobilia (Fig. 183); bleeding from the pancreas, ruptured aneurysm of splenic or gastroduodenal artery.

Primary measures: symptomatic therapy (intravenous line, volume replacement, acid-base balance); nasogastric intubation, aspiration, irrigation

Note: Rapid clearing of the irrigating fluid indicates that the bleeding has stopped → expectant approach → further diagnostic evaluation and causal therapy. If the irrigating fluid remains pink or bright red, hemorrhage is continuing → acute measures → emergency diagnosis and therapy.

Emergency Diagnosis
Usually the bleeding site cannot be localized clinically. The history can give important clues (peptic ulcer disease, cirrhosis of the liver).

Endoscopy
Fiberoptic endoscopy is the primary diagnostic procedure of choice and will localize the bleeding site in 80%–85% of cases. Usually the nature of the hemorrhage can be ascertained, and immediate transendoscopic therapy (coagulation, injection of sclerosing solution) can be performed at the time of diagnosis.

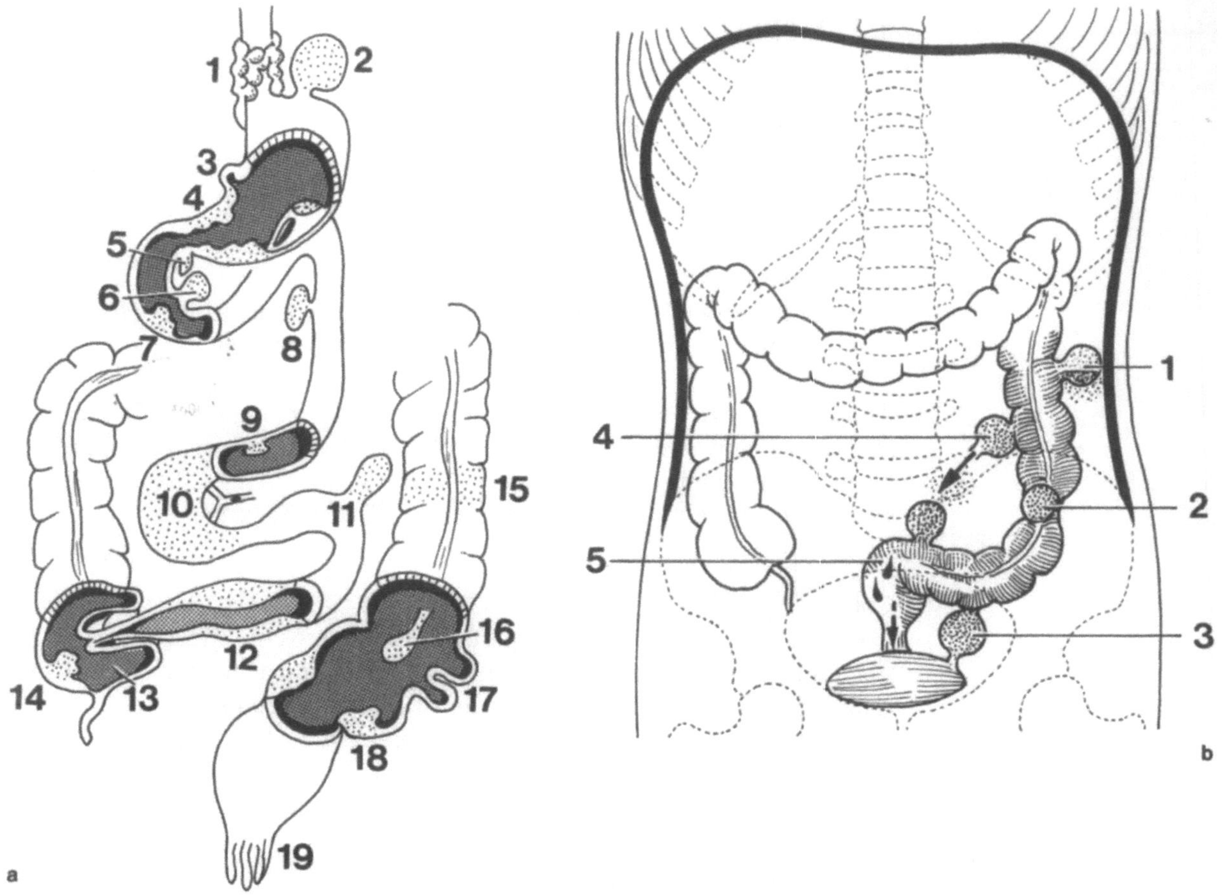

Fig. 182. a Frequent causes of acute upper and lower gastrointestinal bleeding: *1,* esophageal varices; *2,* paraesophageal hernia; *3,* gastric ulcer; *4,* gastric carcinoma; *5,* duodenal ulcer; *6,* duodenal diverticulum; *7,* duodenal tumor; *8,* duplication of the bowel (children); *9,* small-bowel tumor; *10* mesenteric vascular disease; *11,* Meckel's diverticulum; *12,* terminal ileitis; *13,* ileocecal intussusception; *14,* cecal tumor; *15,* ulcerative colitis; *16,* colonic polyp; *17,* diverticulum, diverticulitis; *18,* rectosigmoid carcinoma; *19,* anal fissure, hemorrhoids, anal tumor; **b Complications of colonic diverticulum that may be accompanied by an acute abdomen or lower gastrointestinal hemorrhage:** *1,* peridiverticulitic abscess; *2,* obstruction; *3,* vesicosigmoid fistula; *4,* perforation into the free abdominal cavity; *5,* rectal bleeding. (Modified from Botsford and Wilson 1981)

Angiography

Note: Improvements in endoscopic techniques have curtailed the indications for angiography. Today the study is limited to cases in which endoscopy is unavailable, not practicable, or unrewarding.

Indications for angiography in acute upper gastrointestinal hemorrhage (after Athanasoulis, Interventional Radiology, Saunders, 1982)

Main indications are continued active bleeding, signs of shock (tachycardia, hypotension), sustained need for a large transfusion volume, red or red-tinged gastrointestinal aspirate, and fall of hematocrit, under the following conditions:

1. Endoscopy is not available
2. Endoscopy is contraindicated or problematic
   - Perforation
   - Previous upper gastrointestinal surgery
   - Restricted pulmonary function
   - Too rapid bleeding
3. Endoscopy is technically precluded by:
   - Neck injury
   - Osteophytes
   - Kyphoscoliosis
   - Esophageal stricture
   - Endotracheal tube
   - Cricopharyngeal muscle spasm
4. Endoscopy is not diagnostic (15%–20%)

The bleeding point can be indentified only if bleeding persists. The limit of detectability is 0.5–1.0 ml/min following selective catheterization.
Usually angiography does not disclose the nature of the causative lesion. It does provide a route for interventional procedures, however (vasopressin infusion, embolization).

Note: Angiography is *contraindicated* by intermittent hemorrhage and by arrest of the hemorrhage. If angiography is indicated, the study should be performed without delay.

The angiography is performed in a systematic way, based on the prevalence of specific bleeding sites (see table on p. 312, Fig. 182).
If the proper equipment is available and the patient is cooperative (see Sect. 2.4), the technique of intra-arterial digital subtraction angiography (IA DSA) may be applied in selected cases. Intravenous DSA is *not* diagnostic!

Angiographic Evaluation of Acute Upper Gastrointestinal Bleeding
(after Athenasoulis, Interventional Radiology, 1982)

---

1. Selective celiac angiography (routinely done first): the catheter should not be advanced so far that it blocks the origin of the left gastric artery.
2. If step 1 demonstrates *extravasation* of contrast medium from the left gastric artery or gastroduodenal artery: selective catheterization and therapy (embolization, vasopressin).
3. If step 2 *does not* show contrast extravasation: selective visualization of the gastroduodenal artery and hepatic artery (20 ml contrast medium at 3-4 ml/s).
4. If step 3 *does not* show contrast extravasation: selective visualization of the left gastric artery (15-20 ml contrast medium at 2-4 ml/s). Series in LPO position so that the spine is not superimposed on the stomach.
   Caution: In some individuals the artery may arise directly from the aorta above the celiac trunk or the left hepatic artery.
5. If step 4 *does not* show contrast extravasation, and the clinical picture, history, and endoscopic findings are inconsistent with esophagogastric varices: selective opacification of the inferior and superior phrenic arteries.
   Caution: Do not mistake adrenal blush for a bleeding site!
6. If step 5 *does not* show contrast extravasation: selective superior mesenteric angiography to opacify the distal duodenal arteries via the pancreaticoduodenal arcades.
7. Abdominal aortogram, AP, and L Lat views (only with suspicion of aortoenteric fistula; then they are performed as initial series).

Note: When selective IA DSA is used, the amount of intravascular contrast medium can be reduced by about half without sacrificing the benefits of higher contrast resolution.

Other Imaging Procedures

Abdomen plain films on two planes do *not* contribute to the diagnosis. They can exclude free perforation, intestinal obstruction, and intramural intestinal bleeding.

Sonography rarely contributes to the diagnosis. It can exclude intraperitoneal, retroperitoneal, parenchymatous, and intramural bleeding.

UGI series does not contribute to the diagnosis in the acute stage (clots, poor wall coating, limited patient cooperativeness). Later, the study can demonstrate ulcers, esophageal varices, diverticulum, tumor.

Nuclear medicine, such as scintigraphy with ^{99m}Tc-labelled sulfur colloid is more sensitive than angiography for detection of acute bleeding and identification of small bleeding sites. Its sensitivity can be further increased when in vitro-labelled erythrocytes are used, and delayed scans are obtained up to 24 h after tracer injection. The method is hampered by a significant number of false positive results, i.e., low specificity. It is rarely indicated in acute upper gastrointestinal bleeding.

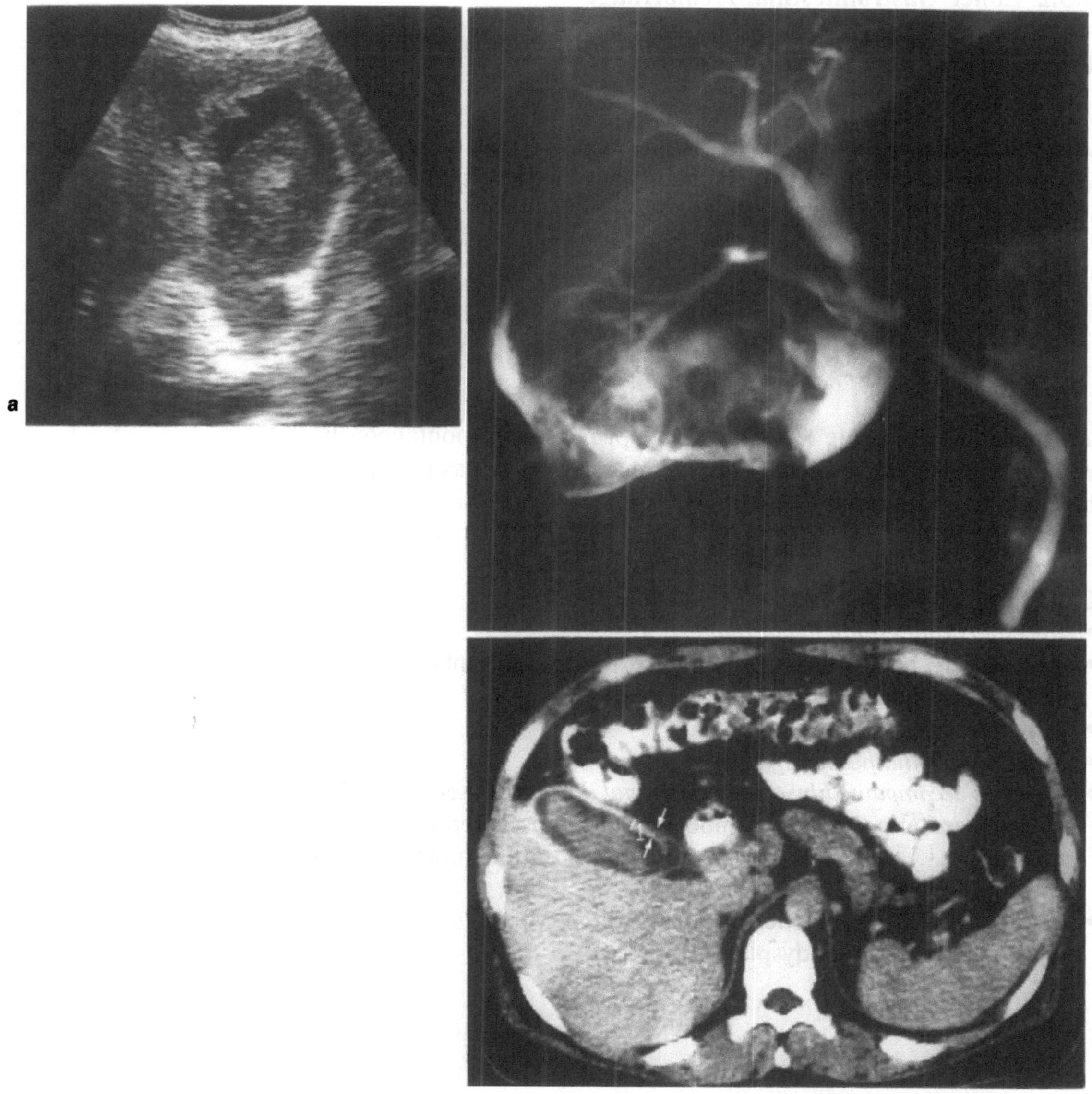

Fig. 183 a–c. Hematobilia with bleeding into the gallbladder in a patient with hemophilia A, presenting as an upper gastrointestinal hemorrhage. Man, 31 years old, with colicky pains in the right upper quadrant and a tarry stool. **a** *Sonogram* shows a slightly enlarged gallbladder with a thickened wall and hypoechoic border. The gallbladder contains echogenic material devoid of acoustic shadow. The bile duct caliber is normal. **b** *ERCP* shows no acute bleeding from the papilla. The pancreatic and common bile ducts are normal in size; the gallbladder is markedly enlarged and contains a nonhomogeneous material. **c** *CT scan* shows a hyperdense thickening of the gallbladder wall (→←) and high-density material in the lumen. Cholecystectomy disclosed massive bleeding into the gallbladder wall and lumen with multiple clots

4.3.2 Lower Gastrointestinal Hemorrhage

K. F. R. Neufang, D. Beyer, P. E. Peters

Definition: Bleeding site distal to the ligament of Treitz
Major symptom: gross rectal bleeding (occult bleeding is excluded)
Associated symptoms: nausea, shock

Note: The lighter the blood color, the lower the bleeding site or the more massive the hemorrhage! With bloody rectal discharge plus hematemesis, look for a bleeding site proximal to the ligament of Treitz.

Prognosis: 75% of acute rectal bleeding episodes stop spontaneously, 25% recur. Emergency operations for acute, massive lower gastrointestinal bleeding have a mortality rate of 20%-50%.

Causes (see Fig. 182)
- *Upper gastrointestinal hemorrhage* (q. v.)
- *Anal disease:* hemorrhoids, anal fissure, perianal thrombosis, erosive periproctitis, tumor, lymphoma
- *Infectious disease:* diarrhea, dysentery
- *Hemorrhagic diathesis* (Fig. 187)
- *Diseases accompanied by acute abdominal distress:* mesenteric infarction (q. v.), mesenteric venous thrombosis (q. v.), intussusception (q. v.), volvulus (q. v.), Meckel's diverticulum, (ulcer, inflammation), Henoch's purpura, periarthritis nodosa
- *Colorectal diseases:* diverticula (diverticulitis), Meckel's diverticulum (Figs. 182b, 185), angiodysplasia (Fig. 186)

Note: Although diverticula become more prevalent in the aboral direction, bleeding from diverticula tends to occur more proximally in the ascending or transverse colon.

- Rectal carcinoma, ulcerative colitis, regional granulomatous (ileo-) colitis (Crohn's disease), polyp (familial polyposis), endometriosis (cyclic bleeding!), perforated pancreatic tumor or abscess
- *Vascular lesions:* hemangioma, teleangiectasis (Osler, Turner), varices, perforated abdominal aortic aneurysm, perforated aneurysm of the splenic, hepatic, or gastroduodenal artery (highly acute!), perforated aortoilliac graft, sequel to colon surgery (see Figs. 184, 185).

Primary Therapeutic Measures
Symptomatic treatment (intravenous line, volume replacement, acid-base balance), nasogastric tube. When bleeding stops → further diagnostic procedures: rectoscopy, contrast edema, Sellink's double-contrast small-bowel study.

Emergency Diagnosis

1. *Exclusion of:* upper gastrointestinal hemorrhage (nasogastric tube), anal bleeding source (inspection, history, palpation, anoscopy), infectious disease (fever, diarrhea, laboratory values, history: travel abroad?)
2. (Trial of emergency) rectosigmoidoscopy (??endoscopy?? → danger of perforation, obscured vision, difficult interpretation of subsequent angiography)
3. *Angiography* is indicated when the causes listed under (1) have been definitely excluded.

Goals of emergency angiography:

- *Accurate preoperative localization of the bleeding site*

> *Note:* The surgeon can easily overlook smaller bleeding sites in the intestine during surgery!

- Attempt to control persistent bleeding preoperatively by vasopressin infusion or embolization (so that surgery can be done electively, with an improved hemodynamic status)

Advantages for the surgeon:

- Shorter operating time with more rapid localization of the bleeding site
- Resection limited to the area of the bleeding site
- Unobscured field (less bleeding)
- More stable circulatory status at operation (less blood loss) → lower overall operative risk

> *Caution:* Intermittent hemorrhage *contraindicates* angiography, and radionuclide imaging may be considered. Angiography should *not* be done after bleeding has stopped! Exception: Angiodysplasias which are often missed on endoscopy due to their submocosal localization may be demonstrated angiographically also in the asymptomatic interval. Typical findings: vascular tuft and early draining vein. Always perform subtraction angiograms or use selective intra-arterial (IA) DSA.

Preparation for angiography: Urinary bladder is catheterized to avoid superimposition of contrast medium in the bladder (visualization of the sigmoid and rectum).

> *Caution:* If the bowel has been irritated by a cleansing enema or prior colonoscopy, the resulting hyperemia can mimic an AV malformation. Hence with intermittent bleeding and stable condition of the patient angiography should be deferred for 48 h after a cleansing enema or colonoscopy (i.e., previous colonoscopy greatly lessens the change that angiography will localize the bleeding site and increases the risk of misinterpretation when findings are subtle).

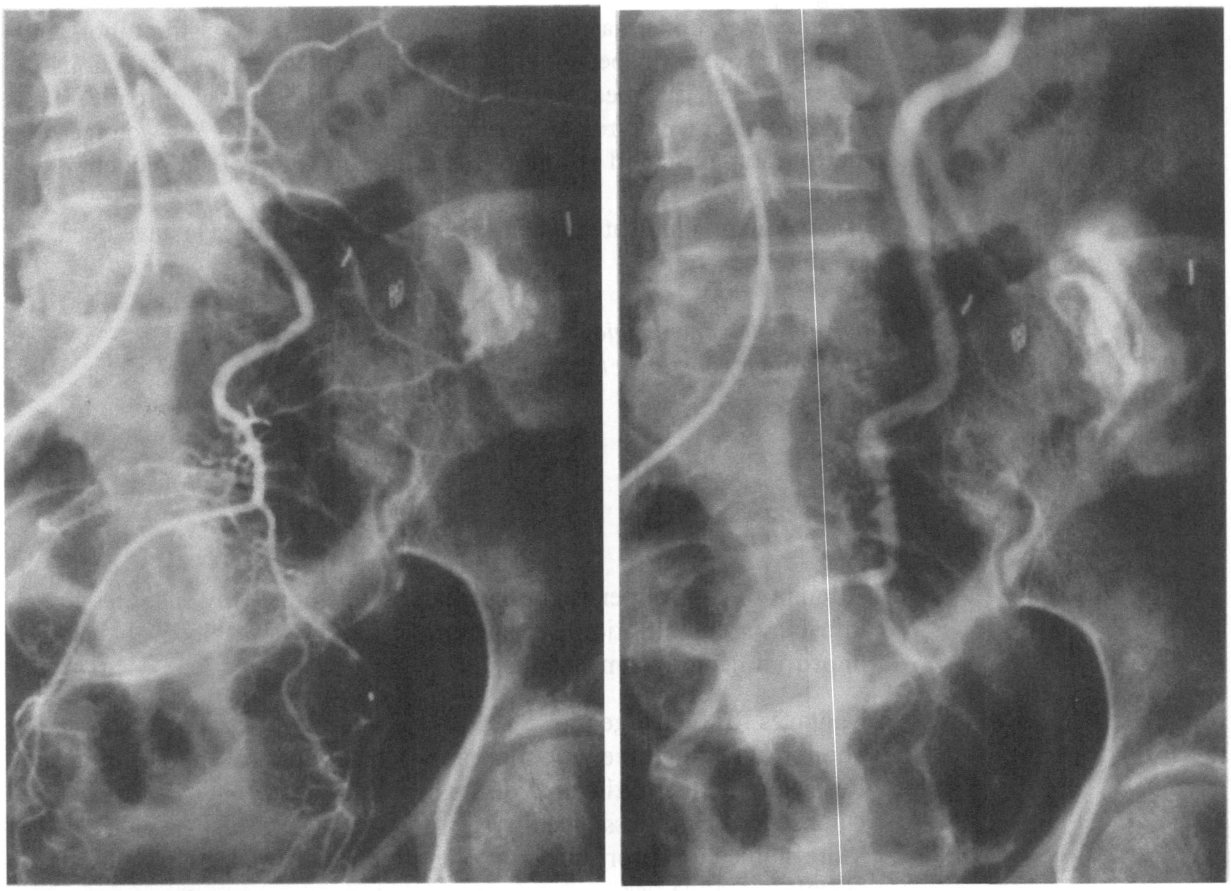

a b

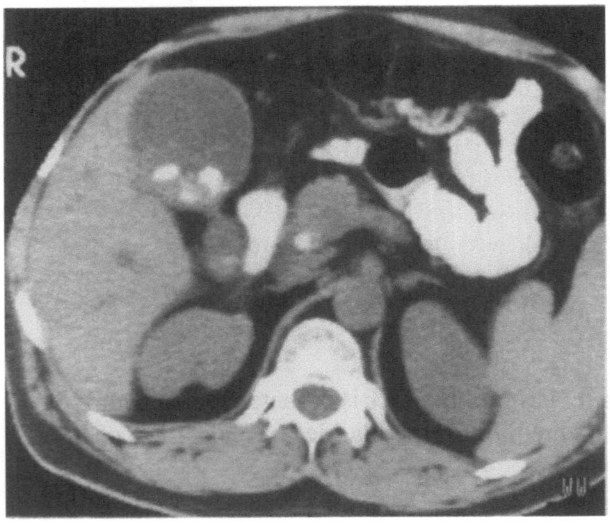

c

Fig. 184. Vascular erosion in an anastomosis with acute lower gastrointestinal bleeding.
a, b Woman, 54 years old who had undergone left-sided hemicolectomy for carcinoma of the left colic flexure 4 weeks earlier developed acute lower gastrointestinal hemorrhage with progressive shock symptoms. Superior mesenteric angiogram showed no sign of active bleeding. *Inferior mesenteric angiogram* (**a, b**) shows massive extravasation of blood into the bowel lumen in the area of the lower anastomosis. Operation disclosed vascular erosion in the lower anastomotic area. **c Hemobilia in a patient with hemophilia.** Man, 42 years old, with known hemophilia and violent pain in the right upper quadrant. *Sonogram* shows cholelithiasis and additional floating, complex echoes within the gallbladder. *CT scan* shows stones in the gallbladder and fresh bleeding into the gallbladder and bile ducts (hemobilia)

Angiographic problem cases

1. Contrast extravasation in the right upper quadrant on superior mesenteric arteriography.
   Differential diagnosis: bleeding site in the duodenum or right colic flexure. An extravasation in the duodenum can be fed by branches of the lower pancreatic arcade via the superior mesenteric artery and may be projected over the area of the right flexure. Doubts can be settled by carefully analyzing the courses of the blood vessels, e.g., by obtaining an oblique series or by repeating after insufflating air into the colon.
2. Hepatic artery arising from the superior mesenteric. Catheter placement for selective vasopressin infusion can present difficulties:
   - Too far proximal: a portion of the vasopressin enters the liver, and its vasoconstrictive action is diminished.
   - Too selective catheterization places an excessive concentration in the bowel, with a danger of necrosis and stricture.

Other Imaging Procedures

Plain abdominal radiographs in two planes do *not* contribute to the diagnosis in the acute stage; they can exclude free perforation and intestinal obstruction.
Films should precede contrast enema - performed in the free interval - for exclusion of free perforation.

Sonography does *not* contribute to the diagnosis. Rarely, it may show a target lesion (bowel wall thickening, edema, inflammation, bleeding, tumor). It can exclude intraperitoneal, retroperitoneal, and parenchymal hemorrhage or fluid collection, aneurysms of the abdominal aorta or major abdominal vessels.

Contrast enema does *not* contribute to diagnosis in the acute stage and carries the danger of perforation *(no barium!).*
Later, if perforation cannot be excluded (history; toxic colon in ulcerative colitis; diverticula, perforation; biplane abdominal films to exclude free air) → water-soluble contrast agents. Study can demonstrate inflammatory lesions, diverticula, tumors, stenoses.

Sellinck double-contrast small-bowel study does *not* contribute to diagnosis in the acute stage. Later it can demonstrate tumors, inflammatory lesions, Meckel's diverticula (may be done after radionuclide imaging).

Nuclear medicine
(see Upper GI Hemorrhage)
Whenever available, use of scintigraphy is advocated before angiography is contemplated in acute and chronic lower gastrointestinal hemorrhage of unknown origin. In acute bleeding, however, angiography is superior as it is quicker and offers selective intravascular therapy.

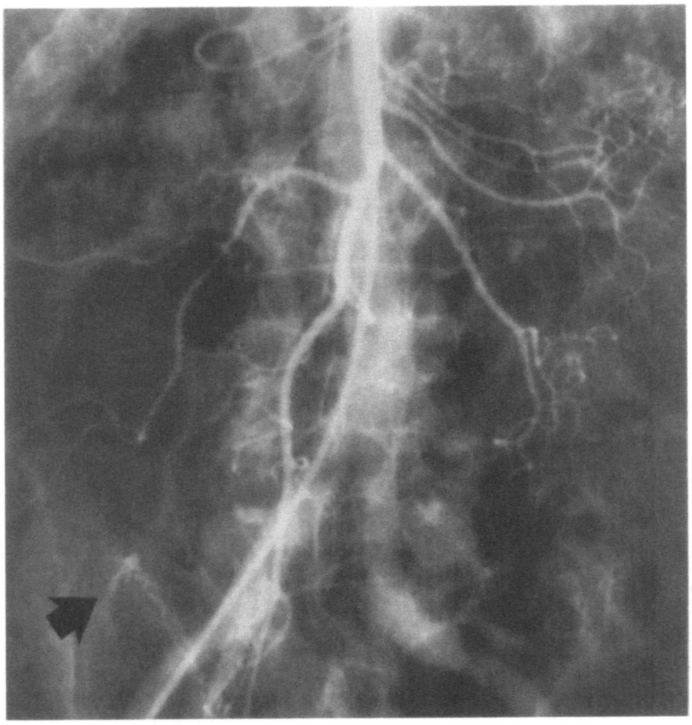

a

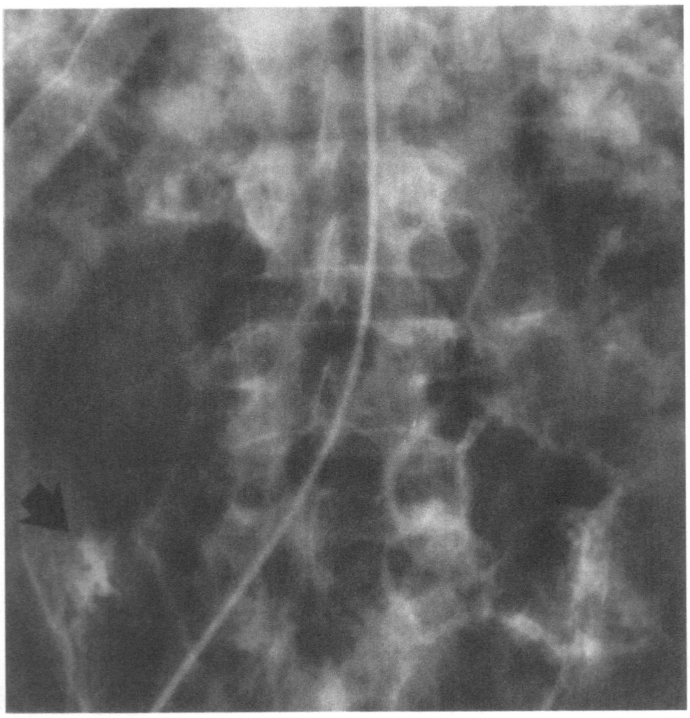

b

Fig. 185 a–d. Bleeding Meckel's diverticulum. Man, 54 years old, with acute lower gastrointestinal bleeding of more than 48 h duration with a corresponding fall of hemoglobin and shock symptoms. Gastroduodenoscopy and rectal examination did not demonstrate a bleeding site. *Superior mesenteric angiogram* shows contrast extravasation (➧) from a terminal branch of the ileocecal artery (**a**) that is visible in the late arterial phase (15 s after start of injection) (**b**). *Diagnosis:* bleeding Meckel's diverticulum 60 cm oral to the ileocecal valve. *Histology:* ulcerated heterotopic gastric mucosa with vascular erosion at the ulcer base.

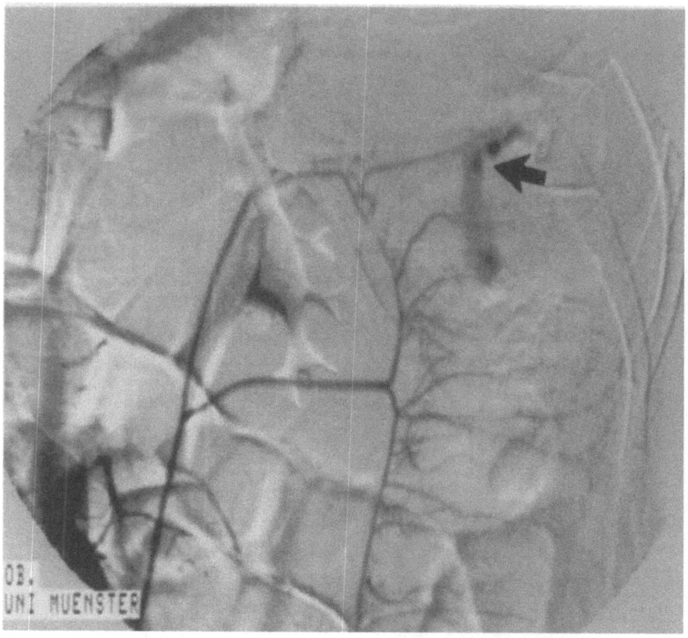

c

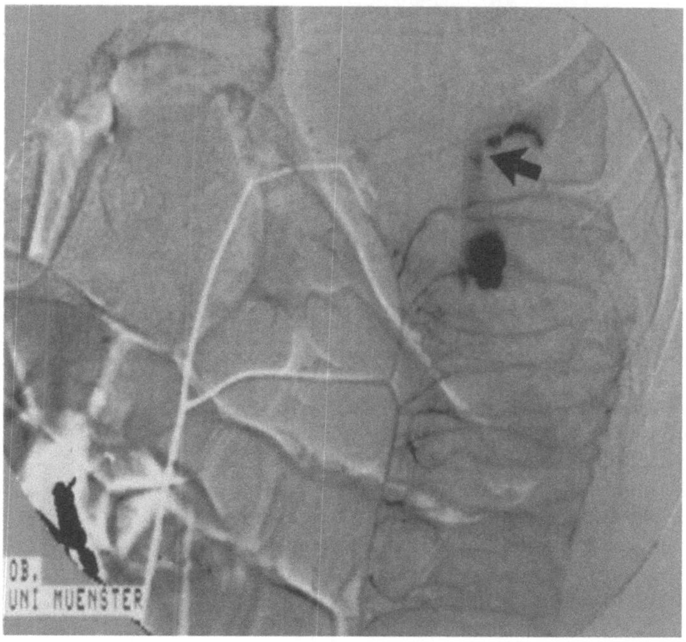

d

Fig. 185 (continued)
c Acute lower gastrointestinal bleeding. Operatively (total colectomy) and histologically confirmed bleeding in a 30-year-old man with necrotizing colitis. *Selective IA DSA of inferior mesenteric artery* (15 ml, 200 mg I/ml) shows contrast extravasation in the area of the left colic flexure (➧). Early phase. **d** Late phase. Increased amount of extravasated contrast medium (➧)

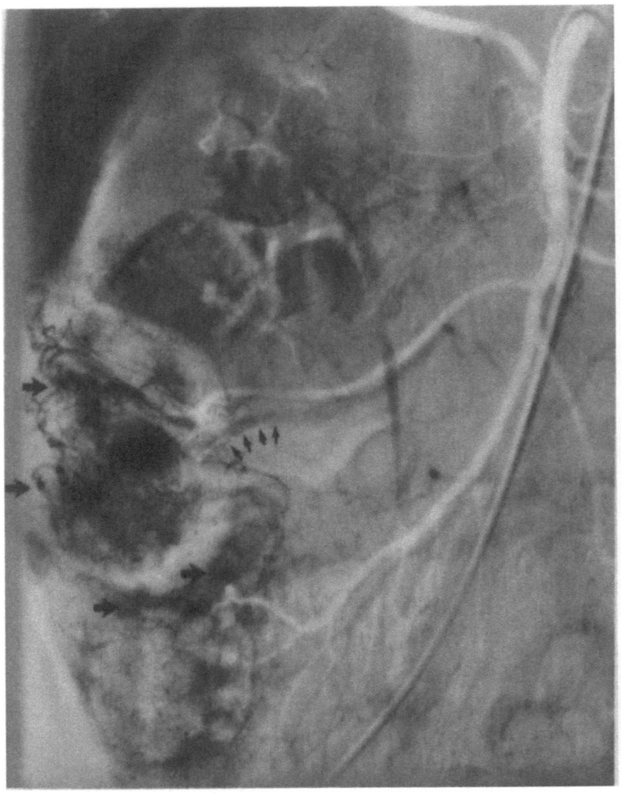

a

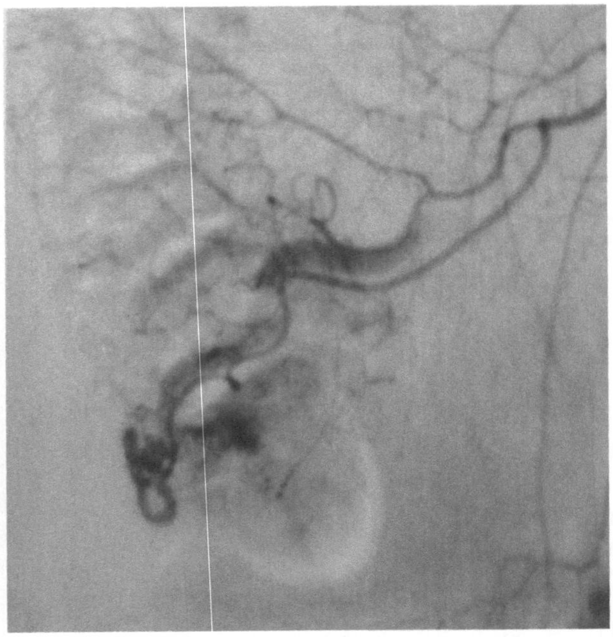

b

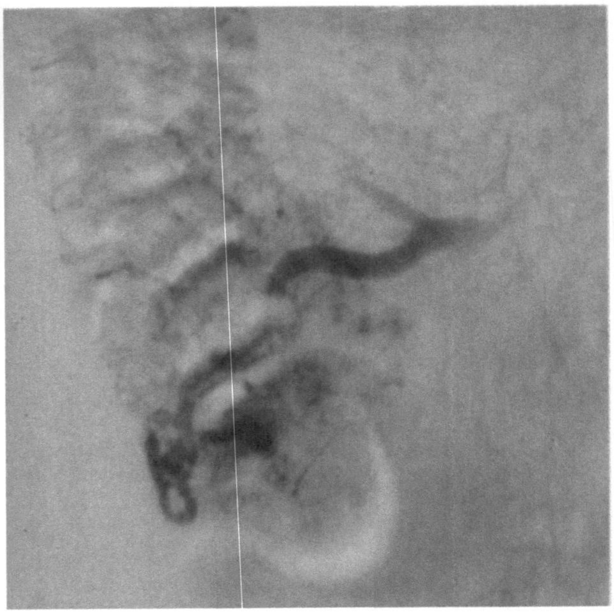

c

Fig. 186a–c. Angiodysplasia of the colon. Man, 73 years old, massive lower gastrointestinal bleeding. **a** *Selective superior mesenteriogram,* late arterial phase. Typical finding: vascular tuft and intensive, patchy staining in the ascending colon (➧) and early filling of a large draining vein (→). **b, c** *Superselective mesenteric angiogram* demonstrates coiled and enlarged feeding vessels and an early draining vein; filling of the vein persists into the venous phase. Extravasation of contrast material into the lumen of the colon

Fig. 187a–d. Hemophiliac disease with multiple bleeding sites. Woman 26 years old, massive intestinal hemorrhage for 8 days, requiring packed red cells five times per day. Scintigraphic study, repeat gastroduodenoscopy, and colonoscopy without evidence of bleeding source. **a** *Selective superior mesenteriogram,* venous phase. Acute bleeding and contrast material extravasation into the bowel lumen. Selective arterial infusion of vasopressin stops bleeding. **b** New bleeding site next morning in the lower jejunum. Repeat infusion of vasopressin. **c** Bleeding continues from another site in the upper jejunum 2 h later. **d** New bleeding sites emerge under continuous infusion of vasopressin. Laparatomy and resection of the jejunum. Shock, followed by death. Resected specimen and autopsy reveal multiple bleeding ulcers in the esophagus, stomach, and small and large bowel. *Diagnosis:* hemophiliac disease due to blocking antibodies ▷

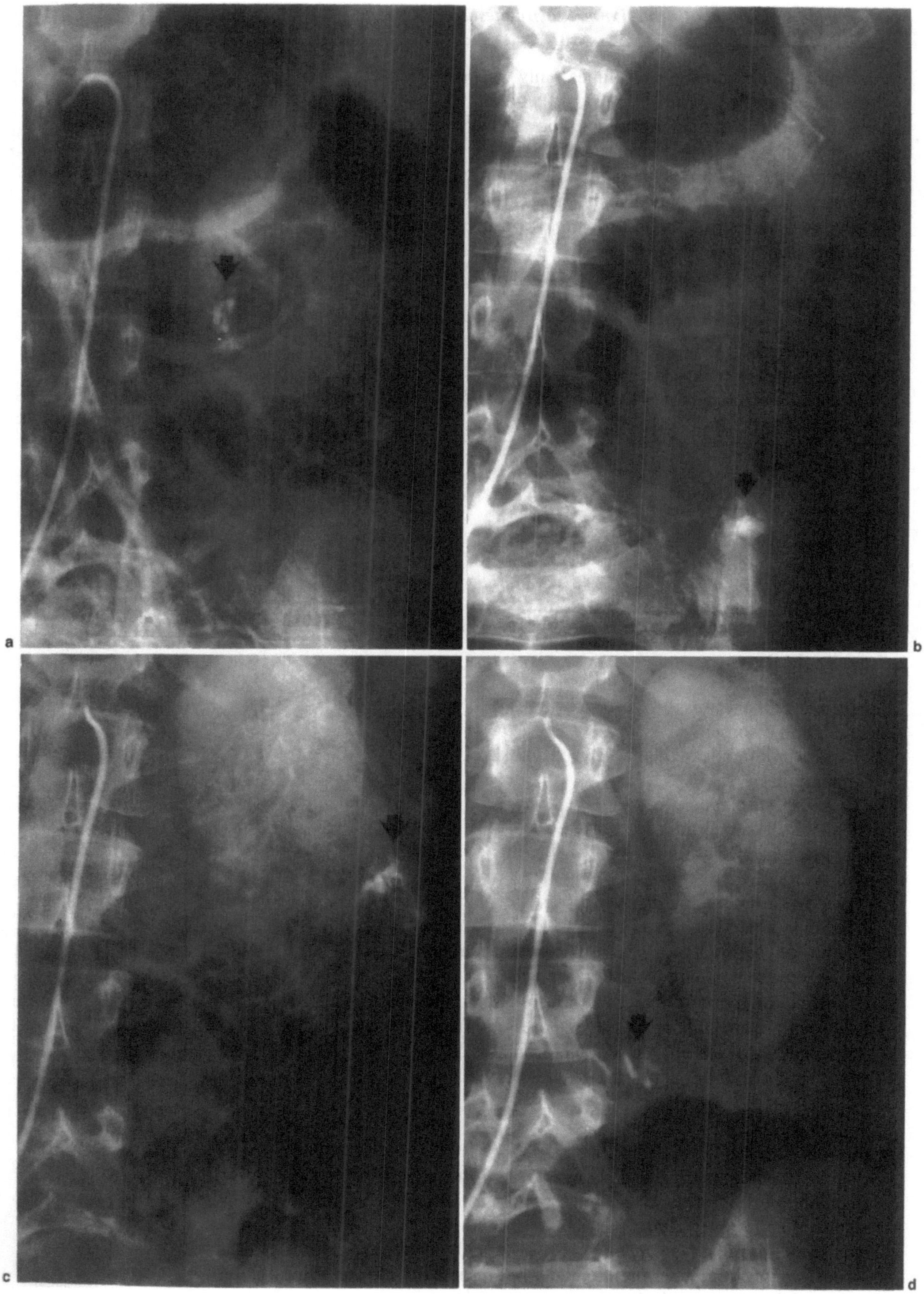
a
b
c
d

Angiographic Evaluation of Acute Lower Gastrointestinal Bleeding

1. Abdominal plain films in two planes: only with suspicion of aorto-iliacoenteric fistula
2. Selective superior mesenteric angiography: film centered on right half of abdomen; if positive: selective therapy
3. If step (2) *does not* show contrast extravasation: selective inferior mesenteric angiogram that covers the rectum; a second injection may be needed to demonstrate the left flexure. If positive, selective therapy (vasopressin)
4. If step (3) *does not* show contrast extravasation: selective celiac angiography
   - to exclude duodenal ulcer
   - because (rarely) the middle celiac artery may arise from the celiac trunk (supplies transverse colon)
   - to exclude a splenic arterial aneurysm or pancreatic tumor that has eroded into the transverse colon

4.3.3 Intramural Intestinal Hemorrhage

R. LORENZ, D. BEYER

Etiology and Pathogenesis

- Coagulation disorders
  - Therapy with anticoagulants (e.g., dicoumarol)
  - Hemophilia
  - Thrombocytopenic purpura
  - Schönlein-Henoch purpura
  - Paraneoplastic syndrome
  - Pancreatitis
  - Hypoprothrombinemia in liver disease
  - Childhood bleeding tendency of unknow cause (rare)
  - Hemorrhagic duodenitis after myocardial infarction (rare)
- Ischemia due to vascular occlusion (see Sect. 4.2)
  - Ischemic infarction of the bowel causes anoxic damage to the vessel walls with edema, allowing seepage of blood into the bowel wall (especially with mesenteric venous thrombosis).
- Trauma (blunt abdominal trauma)

Localization

- *Duodenum and mesentery* (usually a sequel to *trauma)* (Fig. 188): The descending portion of the duodenum is most commonly affected because of its retroperitoneal fixation.
- *Small bowel* (usually *coagulopathy*) (Figs. 189, 190): Trauma is rare; the ileocecal region is affected preferentially because of the retroperitoneal fixation of the cecum with the iliac crest as a fulcrum.

Fig. 188a–c. Posttraumatic intramural duodenal hematoma in a 31-year-old man with acute abdomen and decreased bowel sounds following a traffic accident. **a** *Erect abdominal film* shows a fluid level in the superior duodenal flexure (⇒) and a right paravertebral soft-tissue density with a curved right contour (→). The right renal shadow and right psoas muscle are not visualized. **b** *Left lateral film* shows isolated duodenal distension with a long fluid level (➧). **c** *UGI series* with water soluble contrast shows the contrast column terminating in the distal horizontal portion of the duodenum (⇨). Duodenal hematoma was found at *operation*

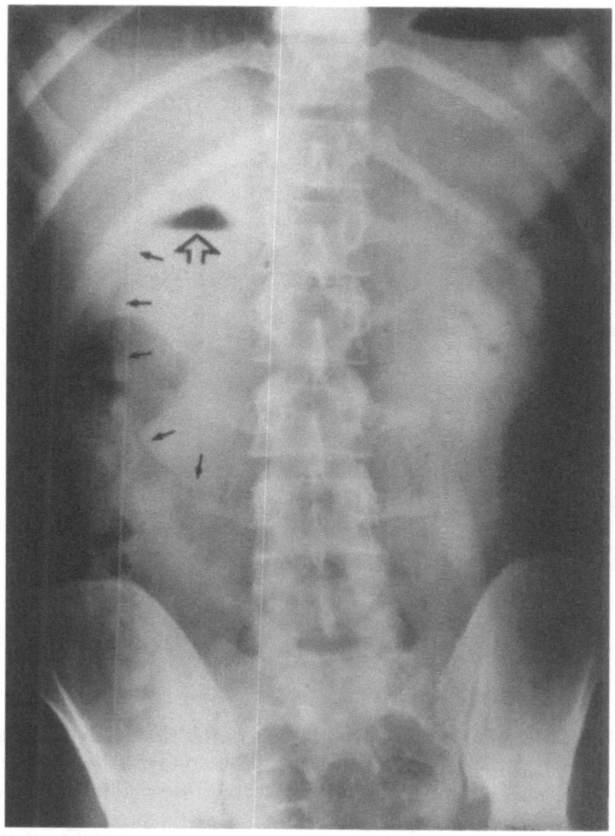

a

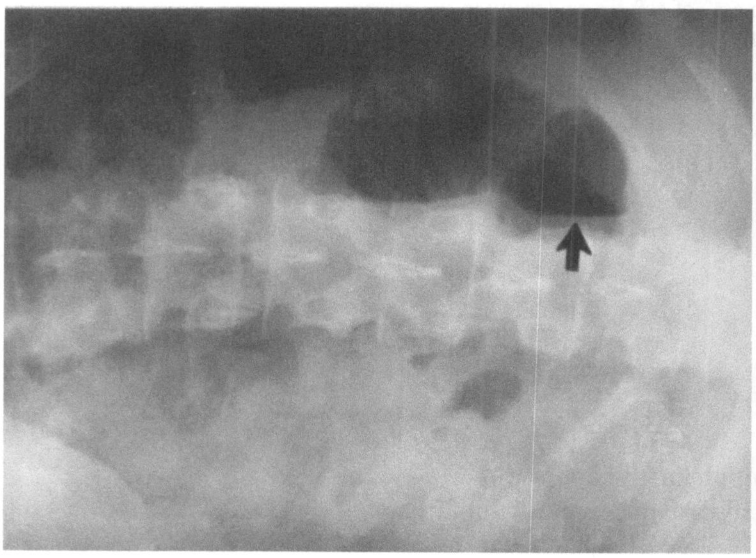

b

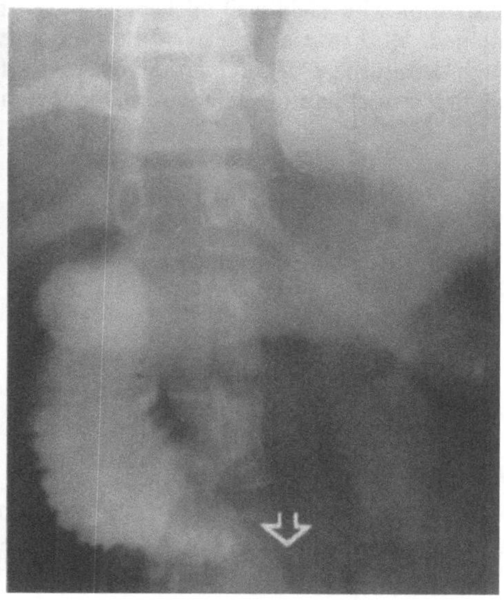

c

- *Large bowel* (usually *ischemia*) (Fig. 191): A common site is the left flexure between the superior and inferior mesenteric arteries, but any other localization is possible. Women in the second half of life and younger women taking contraceptive drugs are predisposed.

Note: Spontaneous hemorrhages relating to coagulation disorders *do not* show sites of predilection!

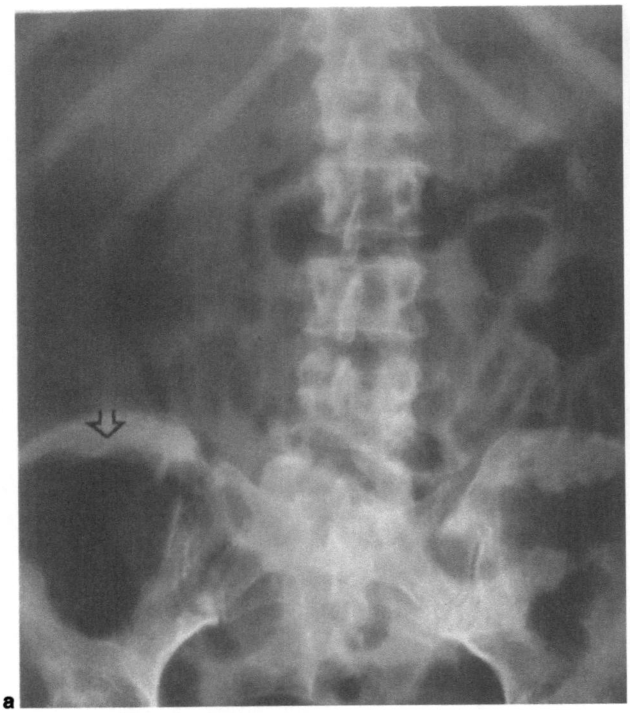

a

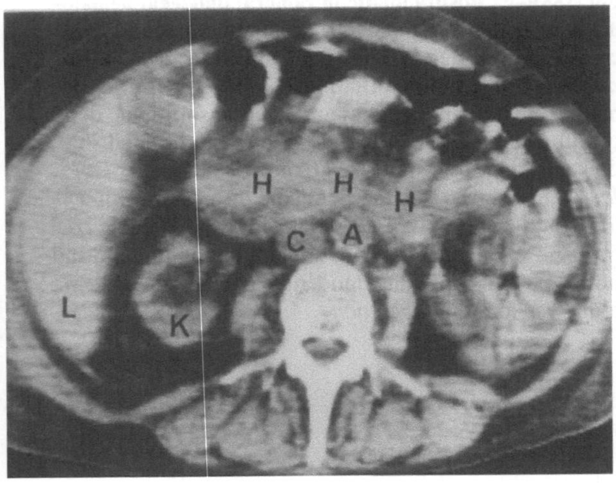

b

Fig. 189 a, b. Intramesenteric bleeding after thrombolytic therapy in a 47-year-old man with acute pelvic vein thrombosis. While on lytic therapy the patient experienced sudden, acute abdominal discomfort with diffuse rigidity and tenderness and an absence of bowel sounds. **a** *Supine film* shows an air-filled cecal pole (⇨), moderate small-bowel distension with slight wall thickening, and a "mass" of soft-tissue density in the midabdomen. **b** *CT scan* at the level of the inferior renal border shows a large, intramesenteric, high-density mass *(H); C,* inferior vena cava; *A,* aorta; *K,* right kidney; *L,* liver. *Diagnosis and course:* intramesenteric hematoma with spontaneous regression

Clinical Symptoms

- History: Trauma? Coagulopathy (hemophilia, therapy with anticoagulants)? Antecedent vascular disease or myocardial infarction? Contraceptive use?

Duration of complaints: may be acute (do not delay diagnosis!), subacute or intermittent (differentiate between inflammatory or ischemic process).

- Local or diffuse tenderness to palpation
- Nonrigid abdomen
- Peristalsis normal or diminished with coagulopathy
- Peristalsis diminished or absent with ischemia
- Palpable mass (need not be present)
- Shock symptoms associated with extensive bleeding, oozing with hypovolemia, or protracted ischemia
- Bloody diarrhea (in some cases)
- Coagulation abnormalities (platelets ↓, PT ↓, PTT ↑)

Radiologic Signs

- Diffuse wall thickening (Figs. 190 a, 191 a) (coagulopathy, ischemia)
- Localized intramural mass (trauma is almost always the cause)
- Combination of both symptoms (trauma with localized or diffuse intramural bleeding)

Plain Radiographs

- Localized separation of air-filled small-bowel loops by wall thickening (segmental involvement is evidence against ascites) (Fig. 190 a)
- Local alteration or inversion of the inner contour of the small bowel loops with thickening of Kerckring's folds (Fig. 190 a) or haustra (Fig. 191 a)
- Segmental small-bowel distension with fluid levels proximal to the segmental luminal narrowing (Fig. 190). With coagulopathy, the lumen will be only partially obstructed, never completely occluded
- Gastric distension with bleeding into the duodenum or proximal jejunum ("double bubble sign") (Fig. 188)
- Soft-tissue density displacing air-filled bowel loops (bleeding into the mesentery, frequent in coagulopathy) (Fig. 189). Intramural masses with ill-defined margins are uncommon; most result from traumatic hemorrhage
- Obliteration of the psoas shadow signifying bleeding into the duodenal wall (Fig. 188)

Note: Wall thickening from intramural hemorrhage is not appreciated on plain films in the absence of small- and large-bowel distension.

UGI Series with water-soluble contrast (Figs. 188 c, 190 c, 191 c)

Do *not* give barium if abdominal findings are questionable!

- Luminal narrowing, possibly with blockage of the contrast medium proximal to the segmental wall change
- Demonstration of a mass lesion arising from the wall
- Demonstration of an extraluminal, compressive mass (bleeding into the mesentery or mesocolon)

Sonography (Figs. 190 b, 191 f–i)

- Ill-defined *target-lesions* produced by wall thickening at the bleeding site
- Semisolid intestinal mass (intramural hemorrhage or mesenteric lesion). Difficult to interpret
- With local atony of bowel loops: fluid-filled lumen
- Sonography may be negative if there is marked gaseous distension of the bowel. Therefore, all scans should be done from the flank

Computed Tomography (Figs. 189 b, 191 b)

Segmental wall thickening or localized mass. CT is rarely necessary because the pattern of involvement is nonspecific; it is indicated only of sonography is restrained.

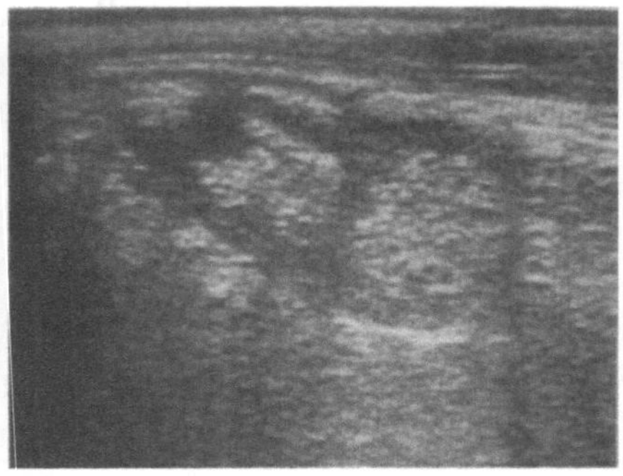

b

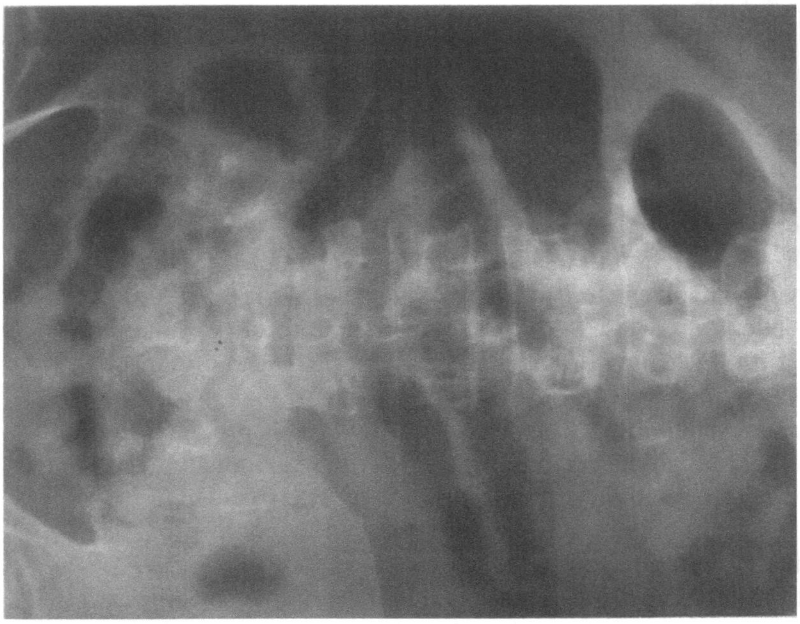

a

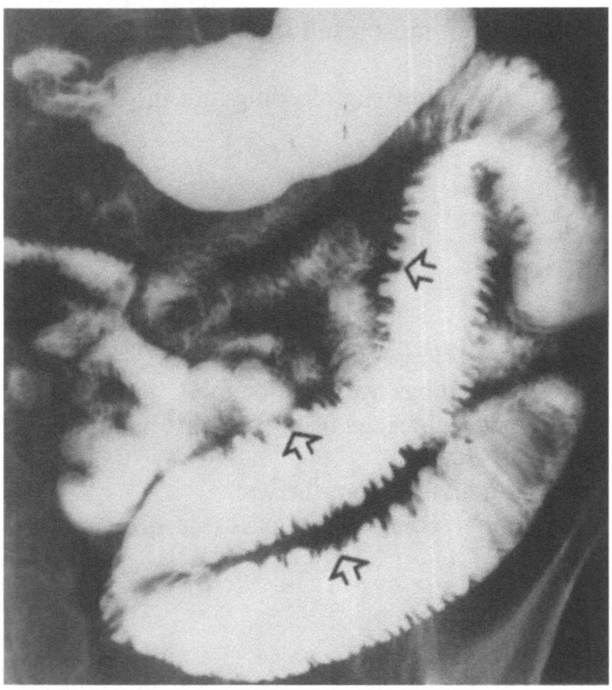

c

Fig. 190a–c. Intramural intestinal bleeding following anticoagulant overdose in a 60-year-old man on medication for myocardial infarction. The prothrombin test fell below 10% on the day before the examination. Patient experienced diffuse abdominal pain with a full sensation and vomiting; no diarrhea. *Clinical findings:* soft abdomen, epigastric tenderness, hypoperistalsis, pulse 120/min; no leukocytosis. **a** *Left lateral film* (supine film not available) shows isolated, small-bowel distension with pronounced wall thickening and a rigid loop sign. **b** *Sonogram* (longitudinal scan through left lower quadrant) shows multiple dilated and wall-thickened loops of small bowel. Presumptive diagnosis of intramural anticoagulant bleeding prompted conservative therapy. **c** *UGI series* (2 days after abdomen plain film) shows segmental dilatation of the proximal jejunum with marked thickening of the plicae conniventes by submucosal hematomas (⇒)

Angiography
Used when there is suspicion of ischemia from the occlusion of a mesenteric vessel (see Sect. 4.2).

Caution: Traumatic duodenal wall hemorrhage is often overlooked initially and treated too late!
In many cases intramural intestinal bleeding is only diagnosed retrospectively from the course (resolution of wall thickening or local mass with clinical improvement) or at operation, because the radiologic signs are nonspecific, and an ischemic cause cannot be definitely ruled out.

Differential Diagnosis of Segmental Wall Thickening
- Inflammatory edema: small- and large-bowel involvement by Crohn's disease, amebiasis
- Tumor: involvement of the bowel by malignant lymphoma
- Wall thickening secondary to storage disease (e.g., amyloidosis); here the changes involve a lengthy segment of bowel

---

Flowchart for evaluating patients with a history of *coagulopathy*

Abdomen plain films in two planes
⇩
If wall thickening or mass is noted
⇩
Real-time sonography
(exclusion of ascites, confirmation and localization of mass)
⇩
UGI series with water-soluble contrast medium: If circulatory status and leukocytes remain
stable (no evidence of ischemia) → no further evaluation
⇩
Conservative therapy

Flowchart for patients with a history of *trauma*

Abdomen plain films in two planes
⇩
Negative result: real-time sonography
If positive → CT may be done to exclude associated trauma
⇩
With gastric distension or double bubble sign (negative sonogram)
UGI series with water-soluble contrast medium
⇩
If all three investigations are negative: CT
⇩
Surgery

Flowchart for patients with *suspected ischemia* (see Sect. 4.2.4)

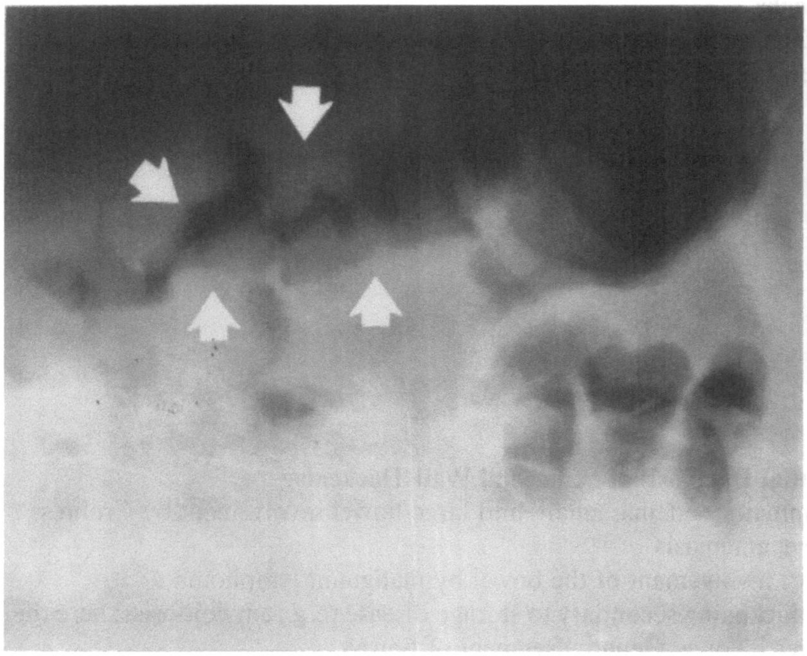
a

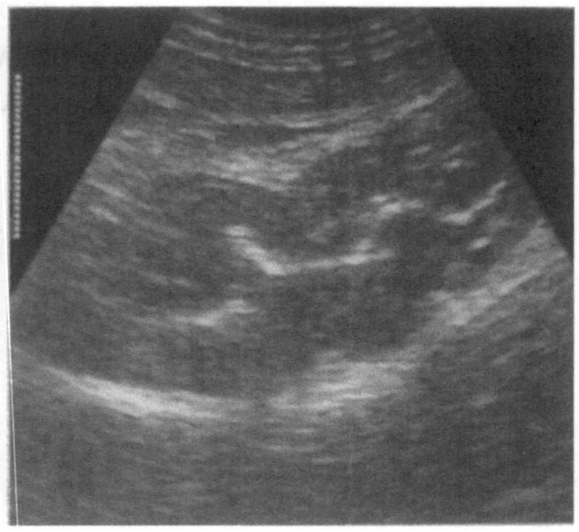
b

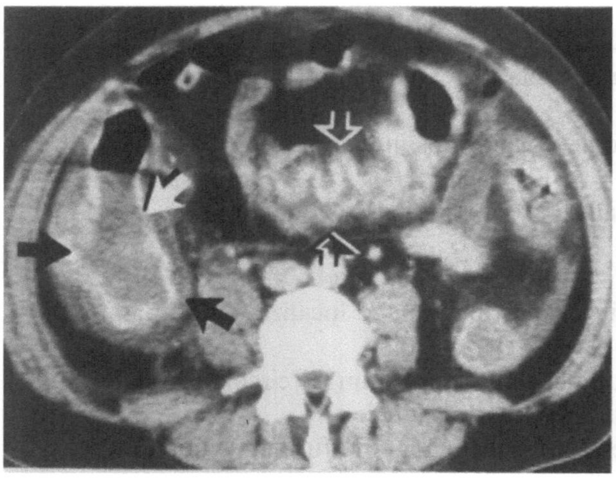
c

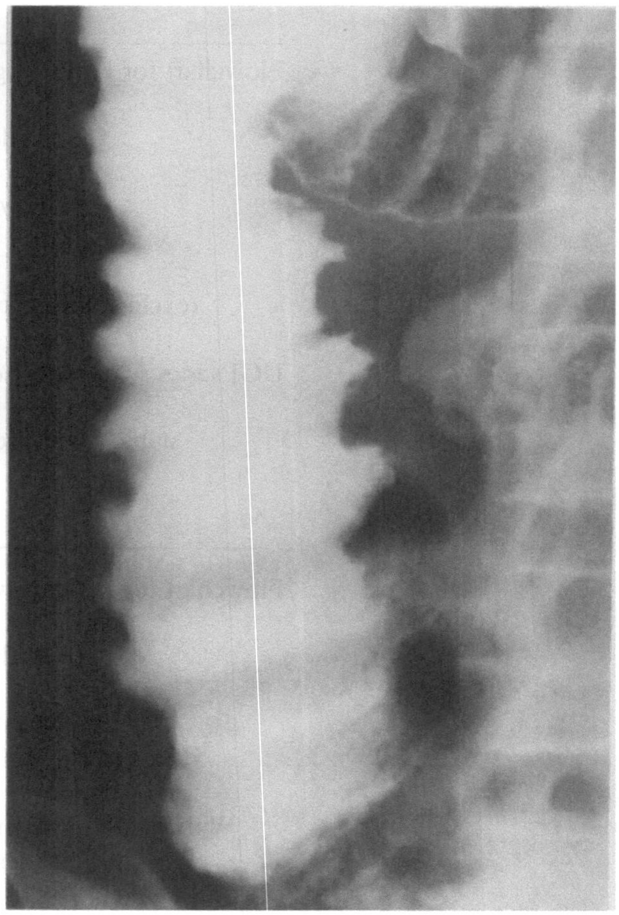
d

Fig. 191 a–i. Intramural colonic bleeding related to thrombocytopenia in a 21-year-old man with acute lymphocytic leukemia. Patient had pain of acute onset in the midabdomen and right lower quadrant with a platelet count of 26000. **a** *Left lateral film* (detail) shows irregular, air-outlined lumen of the ascending colon with massive polypoid wall thickening (➧). **b** *Sonogram* shows marked thickening of the wall and haustra of the ascending colon with extreme luminal narrowing. **c** *CT scan at the level of the lumbar spine* shows high-density, target-like wall thickening of the ascending colon solid arrows by fresh hemorrhage. Fluid- and air-filled colon; similar findings in transverse colon (⇨). **d** *Enema* with water-soluble contrast shows massive mucosal swelling and haustral thickening in the ascending colon and decreased distensibility.

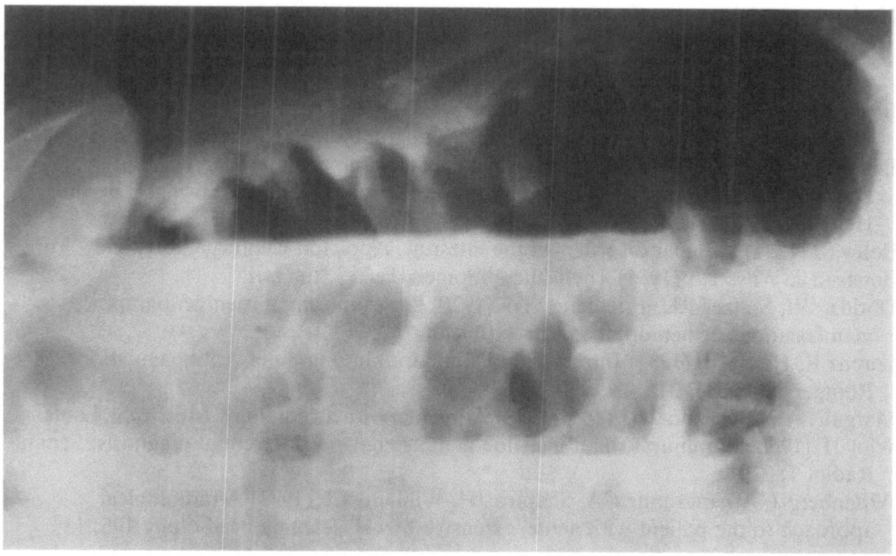

e

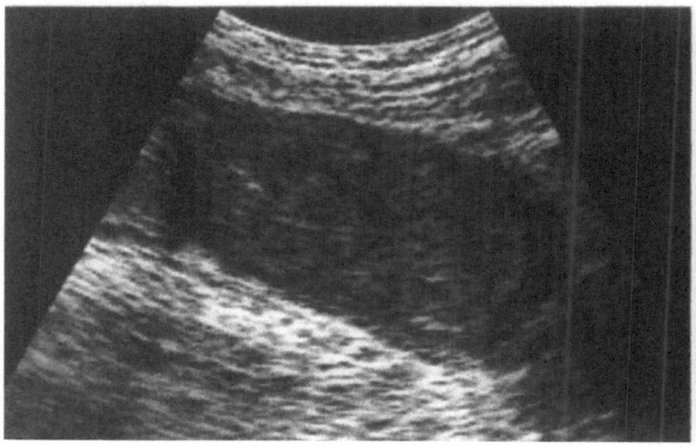

f

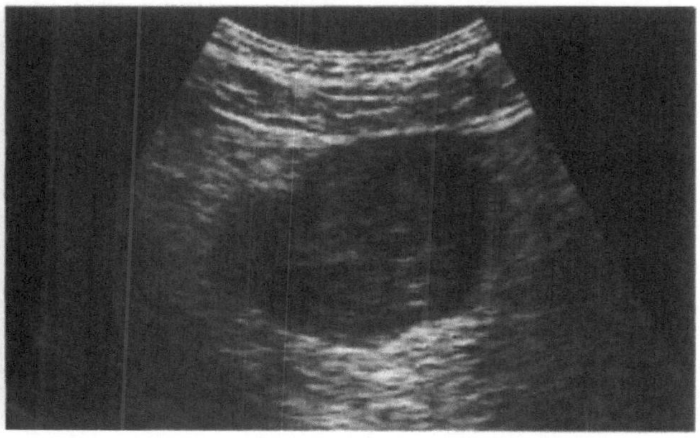

g

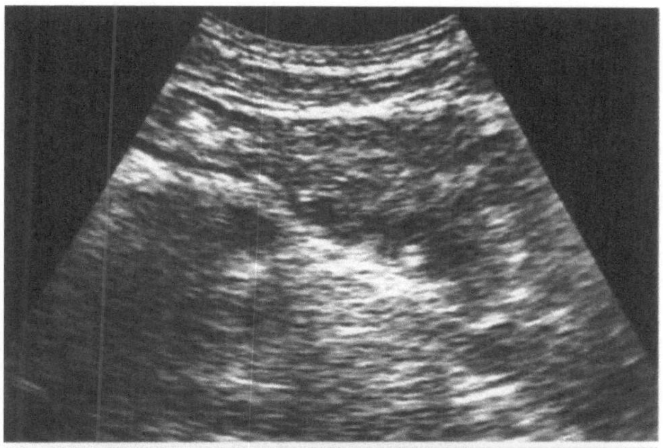

h

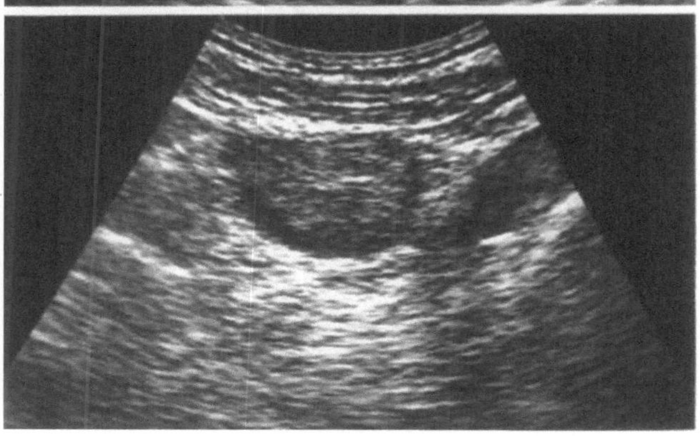

i

Fig. 191 (continued)
e *Repeat left lateral film* 2 days later shows regression of mucosal swelling with residual thumbprinting. **f** Bleeding into the sigmoid colon due to anticoagulant overdose in a 61-year-old man with bloody stools, acute pain in the left lower quadrant, and obstipation. *Sonogram* (longitudinal scan) shows a sausage-shaped mass in the left lower quadrant with no visible lumen. **g** *Sonogram* (transverse scan) shows target pattern with only a slight indication of a central lumen. **h** *Sonogram* (longitudinal scan) 6 days after the acute episode shows a marked regression of sigmoid-wall thickening with reexpansion of the lumen. **i** *Sonogram* (transverse scan) shows more clearly the residual wall thickening of the sigmoid colon

References

Beyer D, Friedmann G (1983) Sonographie des Magen-Darm-Traktes. In: Bücheler E, Friedmann G, Thelen M (eds) Real-time Sonographie des Körpers. Thieme, Stuttgart
Beyer D, Köster R (1984) Bildgebende Diagnostik akuter intestinaler Durchblutungsstörungen - Ein klinisch-radiologisches Konzept. Springer, Berlin Heidelberg New York
Boley SJ (1971) Vascular disorders of the intestine. Appleton-Century-Crofts, New York
Botsford J, Wilson A (1981) The acute abdomen. Enke, Stuttgart
Dodds, WJ, Spitzer RU, Friedland GW (1970) Gastrointestinal roentgenographic manifestations of hemophilia. AJR 110: 413
Lorenz R, Heuser L (1981) Intramurale Dünndarmblutung unter Antikoagulation. Röntgenblätter 34: 316
Margulis AR, Burhenne HJ (eds) (1983) Alimentary tract radiology. Mosby, St. Louis
Wiot JF (1966) Intramural small intestine hemorrhage - a differential diagnosis. Semin Radiol 1: 219
Wittenberg J, Athanasoulis CA, Shapiro JH, Williams LF (1973) A radiological approach to the patient with acute, extensive bowel ischemia. Radiology 106: 13

4.3.4 Acute Intraperitoneal Hemorrhage (of Nontraumatic Cause)

K. F. R. Neufang, D. Beyer, P. E. Peters

Major symptom: Signs of hemorrhagic shock and peritoneal irritation

Note: With a protracted course, abdominal symptoms are predominant; with an acute course, circulatory symptoms.

Clinical Symptoms
Pain may have an acute onset or may develop slowly. Initially, it may be localized or diffuse and radiate to the shoulder region. Abdominal rigidity may be local, diffuse, or absent. Bowel sounds are diminished.

Radiologic Signs
Demonstration of free intraperitoneal fluid is essential. With all imaging procedures, acute free intraperitoneal hemorrhages have the same features:
- *Plain film* shows signs of free intraperitoneal fluid (see Sect. 3.3)
- *Sonogram* shows signs of free fluid
- *CT* scan demonstrates free intraperitoneal blood (densitiometry)

In equivocal findings only: definitive confirmation through peritoneal lavage.

Note: The more acute the event and the more pronounced the hypovolemic shock, the less time is available for diagnostic imaging. Sonography provides the fastest result. When the presence of free fluid or blood has been shown, treatment must not be delayed by further imaging procedures.

Causes (Fig. 192)

Note: The major causes of acute intraperitoneal hemorrhage are:
- Penetration and rupture of an abdominal aortic aneurysm
- Ruptured ectopic pregnancy

The cause of the hemorrhage cannot be established preoperatively in all cases. Symptoms of massive intraperitoneal bleeding require that an immediate exploratory laparotomy be carried out as an emergency measure after the patient's circulatory status has been stabilized.

Ruptured Abdominal Aortic Aneurysm (Figs. 193 b, 201, 202) (see Sect. 4.4)

Ruptured Ectopic Pregnancy (see Sect. 4.7)
Many ectopic pregnancies terminate spontaneously and produce no symptoms. Intraperitoneal hemorrhage is most commonly associated with ectopic pregnancies at the following sites: ovarian surface, uterine tube, posterior uterine surface, sigmoid colon.
Suggestive clinical findings: onset of symptoms 2–4 weeks after the last missed period, abdominal pain of acute onset, hypovolemic shock, and possibly vaginal bleeding

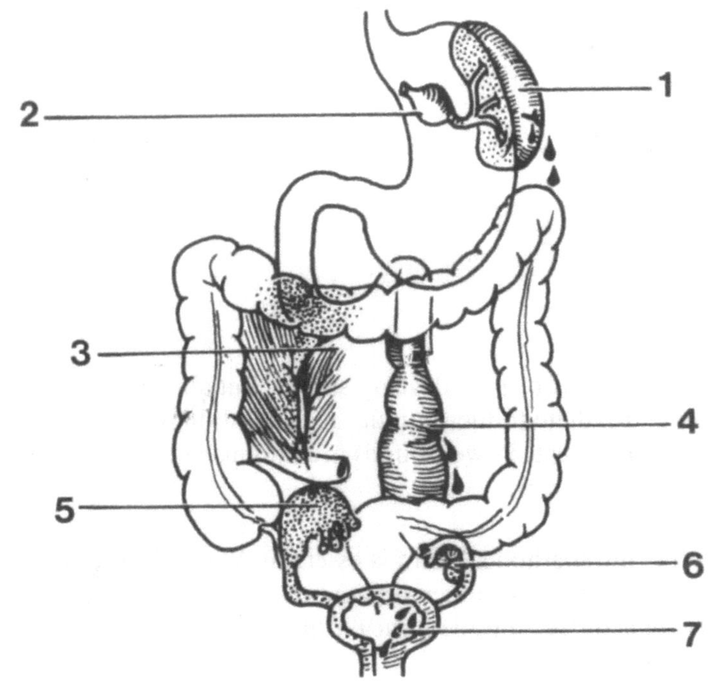

Fig. 192. Possible causes of acute extraluminal abdominal hemorrhage; *1*, splenic rupture; *2*, rupture of splenic artery aneurysm; *3*, traumatic bleeding; *4*, perforation of abdominal aortic aneurysm; *5*, ruptured ectopic pregnancy; *6*, ovulation, *7*, uterine rupture. (Modified from Botsford and Wilson 1981)

a

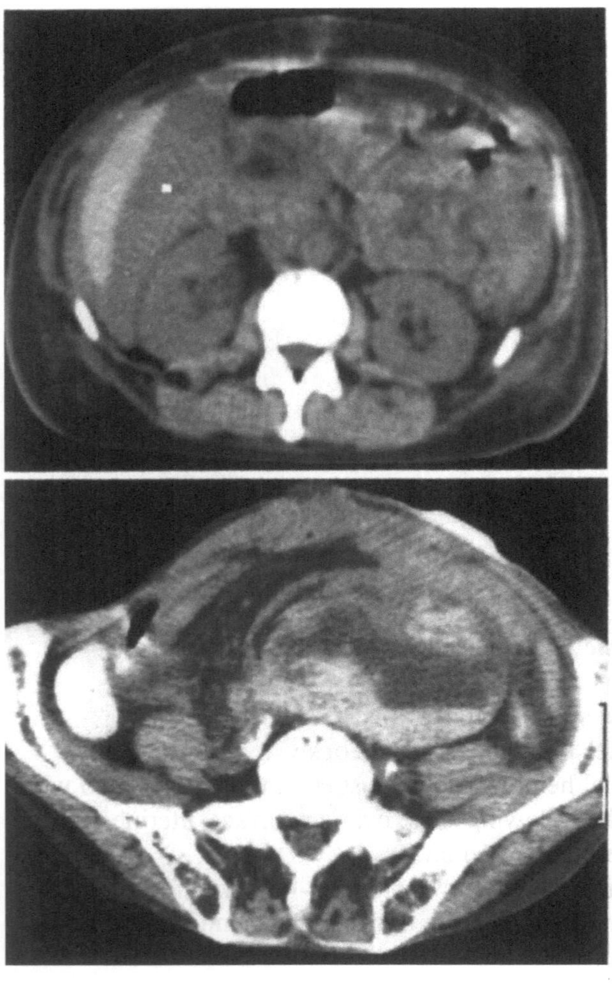

b

Fig. 193a–e. Hemoperitoneum secondary to thrombopenic bleeding in the setting of leukemia. a Shock symptoms and fall of Hb in a woman with acute lymphocytic leukemia. *Plain CT scan* shows free fluid in the perihepatic space and between the bowel loops. Attenuation values are consistent with hemorrhage. **b Predominantly retroperitoneal hematoma from a penetrating abdominal aortic aneurysm.** Man, 78 years old, had undergone a colostomy 4 years earlier for sigmoid carcinoma. For 10 days he had increasing back pain of varying intensity; 14 h ago he experienced an acute exacerbation with agonizing pain and incipient shock; hypertonicity. On *plain CT scan* the aorta is obscured by a large retroperitoneal mass projecting far into the pelvis. The mass consists of at least three layers of varying density. The mesenteric vessels are displaced

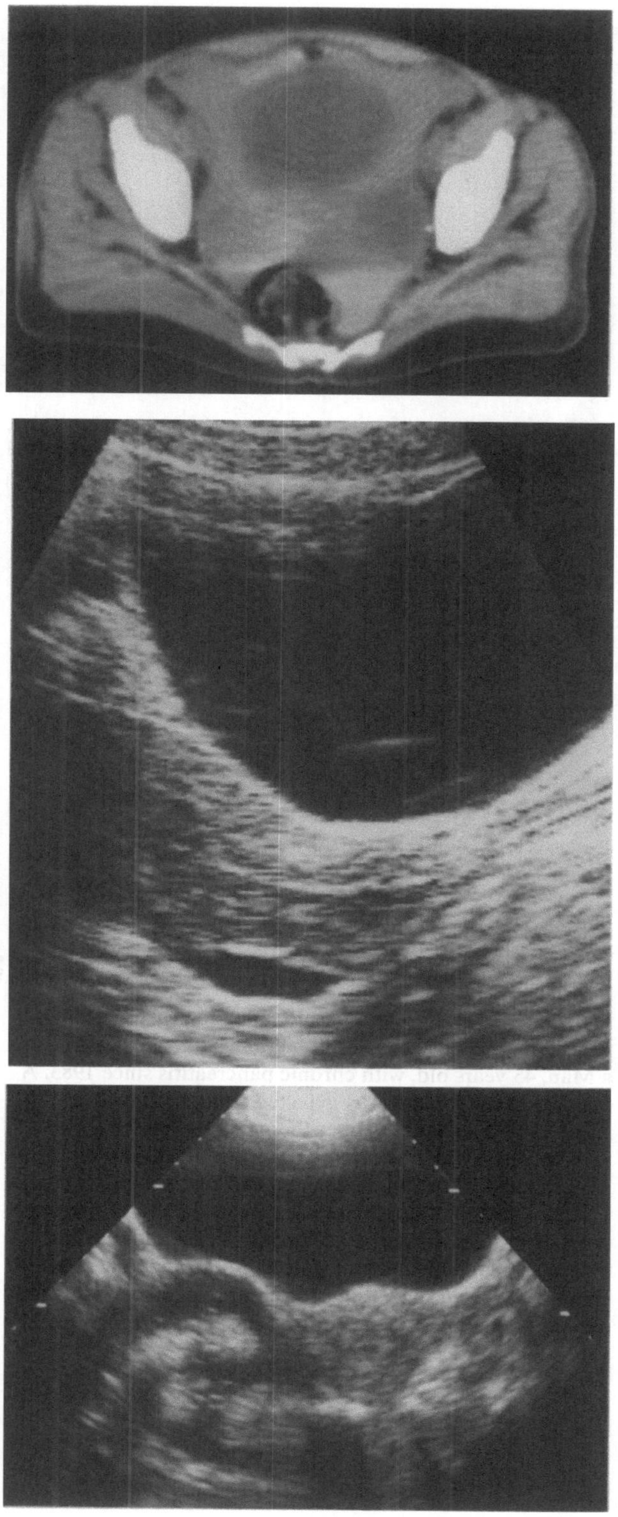

c

d

e

Fig. 193 (continued)
Intraperitoneal bleeding from spontaneous rupture of an ovarian cyst. c Acute abdomen in a 44-year-old woman that began with twinging and stabbing pains in the lower abdomen. *Plain CT scan* shows large amounts of free fluid in the peritoneal cavity filling the cul-de-sac and pelvic peritoneal recesses. The urinary bladder and cystic masses in the region of both ovaries appear in „negative contrast" (larger on the left than on the right). *Histology:* corpus luteum cyst. **d** "Acute" abdomen in a 15-year-old girl following ovulation **(midcycle pain)**. *Sonogram* (longitudinal scan) shows a small fluid collection in the cul-de-sac. **e Ruptured corpus luteum cyst** on the right side with bleeding into the cul-de-sac. Woman, 28 years old, with cystic transformation of the right ovary. The uterus and left ovary appear normal. Bloody track entering the cul-de-sac behind the rectum *(R)*. (Prof. Dr. H. Hackeloer, Department of Gynecology, Barmbeck General Hospital, Hamburg)

a b c d

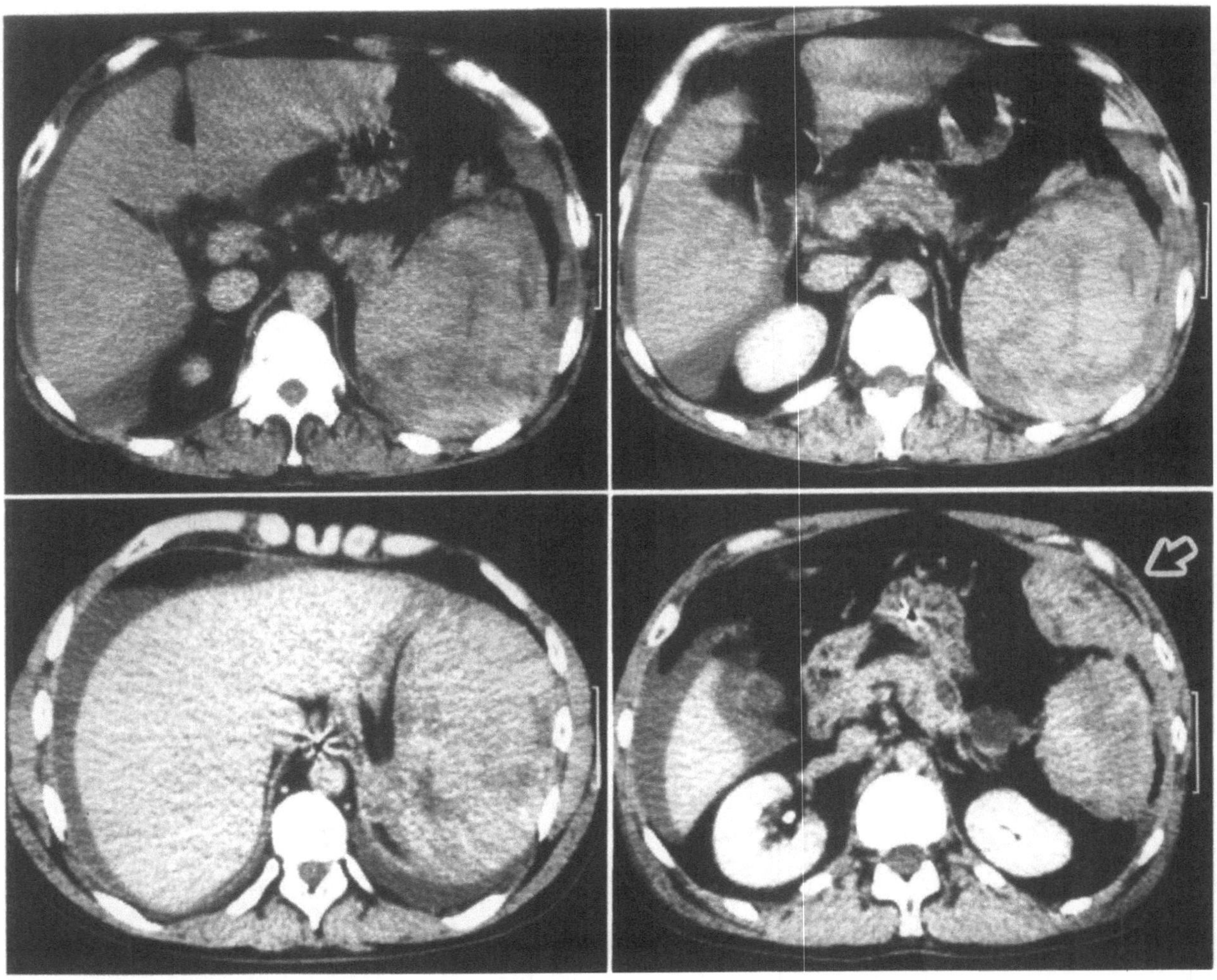

Fig. 194a–d. Rupture of the spleen due to penetration of pancreatic pseudocysts and intraperitoneal hemorrhage. **a** Man, 45 years old, with chronic pancreatitis since 1983. A pancreatic pseudocyst was detected sonographically in April 1984. Five months later the patient experienced severe epigastric pain, nausea, and vomiting with an Hb of 7.5 g%, leukocytosis of 28 000, and elevated serum amylase. *CT scan* shows intracystic bleeding into the tail of the pancreas. The splenic hilus is no longer clearly defined. Rupture and enlargement of the spleen. **b Intraperitoneal hemorrhage.** *CT scan* shows signs of chronic pancreatitis in the remaining pancreas, pancreatic ascites, and intraperitoneal hemorrhage. **c** Man, 32 years old, with chronic pancreatitis, in September 1985 experienced acute pain in the left upper quadrant radiating to the left shoulder. Laboratory results showed Hb of 6.3 g%, leukocytosis of 18 600, and markedly elevated serum lipase and amylase. *CT scan* shows a markedly enlarged spleen with hemorrhagic areas, pancreatic ascites, and left-sided pleural effusion. **d** *CT scan* shows a pancreatic pseudocyst extending to the hilus of the spleen. Intraperitoneal hemorrhage. (Prof. Dr. B. Kramann, Department of Diagnostic Radiology, University of Homburg/Saar)

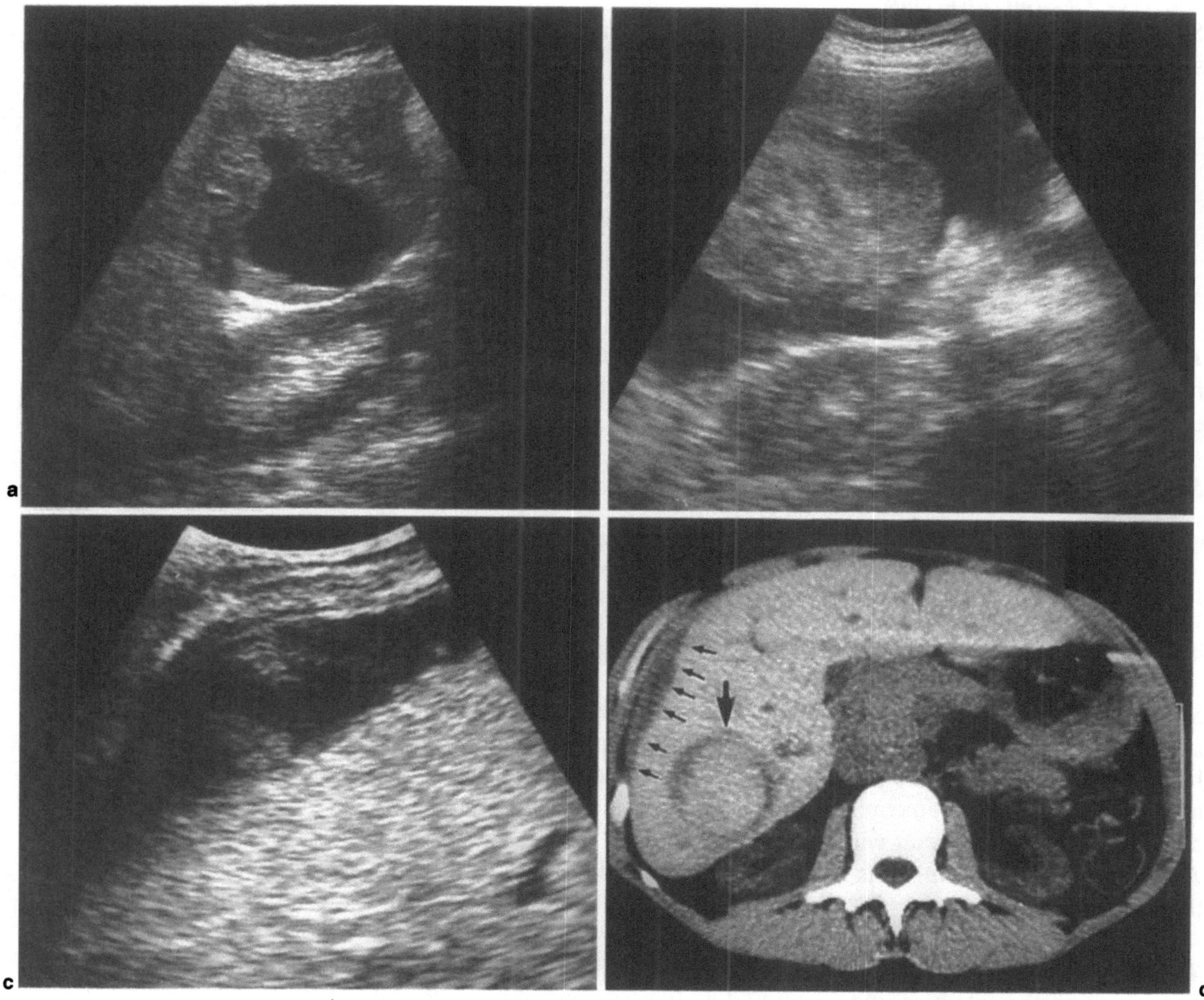

Fig. 195 a–d. Spontaneous intraperitoneal and subcapsular hemorrhages without trauma. a Spontaneous intraperitoneal hemorrhage due to rupture of a hepatic metastasis of malignant melanoma. *Sonogram* shows a centrally necrotic metastatic tumor in the left lobe of the liver with massive expansion of the inferior hepatic border. **b** Twenty-four hours later the patient presented with shock and an acute abdomen. *Sonogram* shows significant free fluid in the upper abdomen. The left hepatic lobe and the metastatic tumor were markedly reduced in size, and the fluid content of the lesion was no longer visible. **c Spontaneous subcapsular hematoma of the liver in a 27-year-old dialysis patient with multiple hepatic hemangiomas.** After completion of dialysis, she experienced severe pain in the right upper quadrant with a fall of blood pressure and hemoglobin level. *Sonogram* (transverse subcostal scan) shows a subcapsular, hypoechoic, liquid mass containing echogenic coagula. **d** *CT scan* (at a somewhat lower level than the sonogram) shows a subcapsular, band-shaped mass of low density (➧). Subcapsular hemorrhage from a hepatic hemangioma (→)

Ruptured Visceral Aneurysms
Sites of occurrence: celiac trunk, hepatic artery, splenic artery, renal artery, superior mesenteric artery and its branches.

Note: The splenic artery aneurysm is the most common of the visceral aneurysms, which on the whole are rare. Unlike the other types of visceral aneurysm, splenic artery aneurysm appears to affect women of childbearing age preferentially; ruptures have been described during pregnancy an the postpartum period.

Diagnostic features: The clinical course is usually dramatic. Fremitus is noted on palpation, and usually a bruit is audible throughout the epigastrium.

Splenic Rupture (Figs. 194–196)

Note: The spontaneous rupture of a normal-sized spleen is extremely rare. Splenomegaly, in the other hand, carries a significant potential for rupture

Splenic ruptures have been associated with the following causes of splenomegaly: infections (mononucleosis, typhus, syphilis, malaria, kala-azar), cysts, Gaucher's disease, amyloidosis, Hodgkin's disease, malignant lymphoma, leukemia, traumatic subcapsular hematoma, bleeding into a splenic cyst with secondary rupture.
Diagnostic features: Pain starts in the left upper quadrant and radiates to the left shoulder.

Tumors
Erosive or perforative bleeding associated with intra- and retroperitoneal tumors. Large, heavily vascularized, hepatic tumors are most susceptible: hemangioma, adenoma, focal nodular hyperplasia, hepatic metastases (Fig. 195).

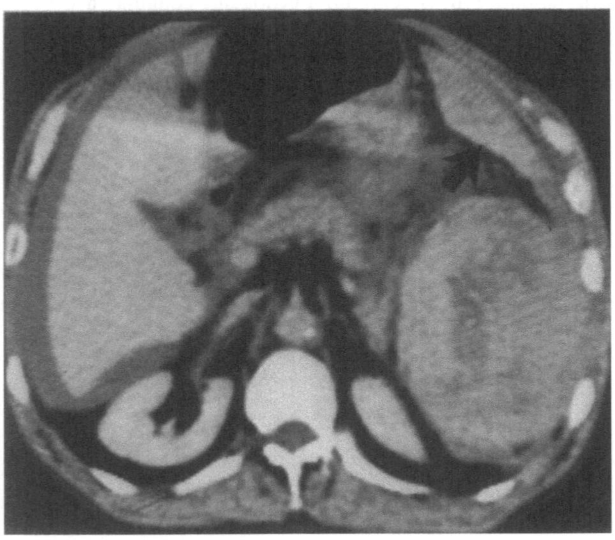

Fig. 196. Acute bleeding into the abdominal wall. Man, 42 years old, who had necrotizing pancreatitis involving the tail of the pancreas 7 weeks previously. Now the experienced a recurrence of severe left upper quadrant pain consistent with a recurrence of the pancreatitis. On *CT scan* the lobulated body of the pancreas is well delineated, still showing evidence of a slight, streaky-edematous, ambient tissue reaction and a relatively wide main duct. There is marked splenomegaly with central, irregular, low-density areas. Fresh hemorrhage (➧) into the lateral and anterior parts of the abdominal wall is apparent, and there is free ascites in the perihepatic space (13 HV). *Postoperative diagnosis:* acute bleeding into the abdominal wall associated with splenomegaly; no evidence of recurrent pancreatitis

Gynecologic Causes Dependent on the Menstrual Cycle (see Sect. 4.7)
Mittelschmerz: Local peritoneal irritation associated with the rupture of a Graafian follicle
Reflux of menstrual blood through the uterine tube: Fluid collection at the fibriated end of the tube
Bleeding into a follicular cyst with secondary rupture
Rupture of a chocolate cyst of the ovary (endometriosis)
Bleeding due to hemorrhagic diathesis: consumption coagulopathy, thrombopenia, leukemia, anticoagulant therapy

References for Sects. 4.3.1-4.3.2 and 4.3.4

Alavi A, Ring EJ (1981) Localization of gastrointestinal bleeding. Superiority of 99mTc sulfur colloid compared with angiography. Am J Roentgen 137: 741
Athanasoulis CA (1982a) Lower gastrointestinal bleeding. In: Athanasoulis CA, Pfister RC, Green RE, Roberson GH (eds) Interventional radiology. Saunders, Philadelphia
Athanasoulis CA (1982b) Upper gastrointestinal bleeding of arteriocapillary origin. In: Athanasoulis CA, Pfister RC, Green RE, Roberson GH (eds) Interventional radiology. Saunders, Philadelphia
Athanasoulis CA, Waltman AC, Novelline RA (1976) Angiography, its contribution to the emergency management of gastrointestinal hemorrhage. Radiol Clin North Am 14: 265
Bookstein JJ, Greenway GD (1981) Gastrointestinal hemorrhage: angiography and transcatheter therapy. In: Teplick JG, Haskin ME (eds) Surgical radiology. Saunders, Philadelphia
Briley CA Jr, Jackson DC, Johnsrude IS, et al. (1980) Acute gastrointestinal hemorrhage of small-bowel origin. Radiology 136: 317
Federle MP, Jeffrey RB Jr (1983) Hemoperitoneum studied by computed tomography. Radiology 148: 187
Lewin JR, Patterson EA (1980) CT recognition of spontaneous intraperitoneal hemorrhage complicating anticoagulant therapy. AJR 134: 1271
Myerovitz MF, Fellows KE (1984) Angiography of gastrointestinal bleeding in children. Am J Roentgen 143: 837
Orecchia PH, Hensley EK, McDonald PT, Lull R (1985) Localization of lower gastrointestinal hemorrhage: experience with red blood cells labeled in vitro with technetium Tc99m. Arch Surg 120: 621
Scherer K, Kramann B (1987) Rupture of the spleen by penetration of pancreatic pseudocysts. Eur J Radiol 7: 67-69
Sing AK, Agenant MA, Hausman R, et al. (1980) Vascular ectasis (angiodysplasias) of the cecum and ascending colon. Fortschr Röntgenstr 132: 534
Thoeni RF, Venbruc AC (1983) Value of colonoscopyand double contrast barium-enema examination of patients with subacute and chronic lower intestinal bleeding. Radiology 146: 603
Wenz W, Roth FJ, Bruckner U (1969) Die Angiographie bei der akuten Gastrointestinalblutung. Experimentelle Voraussetzungen und klinische Ergebnisse. Fortschr Röntgenstr 110: 616
Wetzel E, Strauss LG, Hoevels J, Georgi M (1986) Nachweis und Lokalisation von Blutungen im Intestinaltrakt. Vergleich zwischen 99m-T-Kolloid-Szintigraphie und selektiver Angiographie der viszeralen Gefäße. Dtsch Med Wsch 111: 203
Wilson SE, Stone RT, Christie JP, et al. (1979) Massive lower gastrointestinal bleeding from intestinal varices. Arch Surg 114: 1158
Winn M, Weissmann HS, Sprayregen S, Freeman LM (1983) The radionuclide detection of lower gastrointestinal bleeding sites. Clin Nucl Med 8: 389

4.4 Acute Retroperitoneal Disorders

R. Lorenz, D. Beyer, U. Mödder

Note: Flank pain is a symptom of retroperitoneal disease. It should not be mistaken for pain from other organic processes radiating to the flank.

Causes

Kidney, Ureter
- Urolithiasis (Fig. 197)
- Inflammation (Figs. 198, 199)
- Abscess (renal, perirenal) (see Sect. 4.1.5.2) (Figs. 198, 199)
- Hemorrhage [tumor, cyst, therapy with anticoagulants (Fig. 200), bleeding into the collecting system with clot formation]
- Renal infarction (embolic occlusion of segmental arteries or renal artery)
- Papillary necrosis (diabetes)
- Rupture of cyst (simple renal cyst, posttraumatic cyst, echinococciasis)
- Trauma (see Sect. 4.5)

Adrenals
- Hemorrhage (tumor, cyst)
- Infarction
- Abscess
- Rupture of cyst (traumatic cyst, echinococciasis)

Blood Vessels
- Abdominal aortic aneurysm, renal artery aneurysm: perforation, penetration (Figs. 201, 202)
- Graft aneurysm or infection
- Renal venous thrombosis (usually coagulation disorder)
- Renal infarction (see above)
- Angiitis (Takayasu's syndrome)
- Arteriovenous fistula
- Trauma (see Sect. 4.5)

Connective Tissue, Musculature (see Sect. 4.6)
- Abscess
- Inflammatory fibrosis (benign, malignant: Ormond's disease)
- Tumors (sarcoma)
- Hematoma (trauma, see Sect. 4.5)

Pancreas (see Sect. 4.1.2)

Clinical Symptoms

Acute flank and/or back pain, scoliosis, palpable mass, nonspecific abdominal symptoms, abdominal tenderness, colicky symptoms with urolithiasis, papillary necrosis, or clot formation. Acute "agonizing pain" with ruptured abdominal aortic aneurysm. Fall of blood pressure with massive bleeding. Septic temperatures with abscess formation and inflammation; acute pain episode with ruptured cyst.

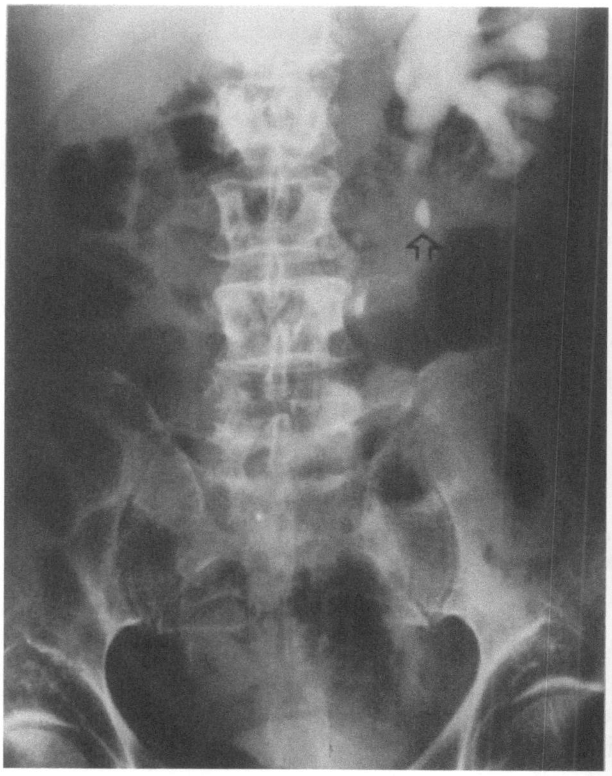

a

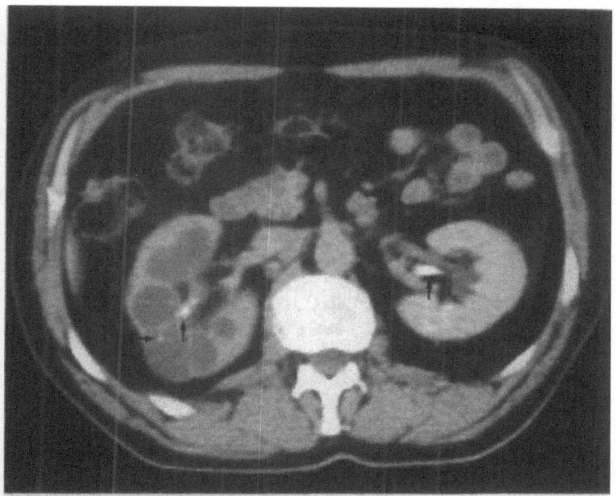

c

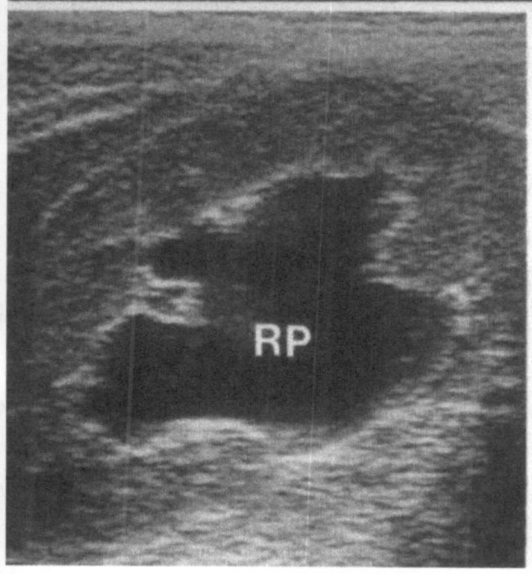

d

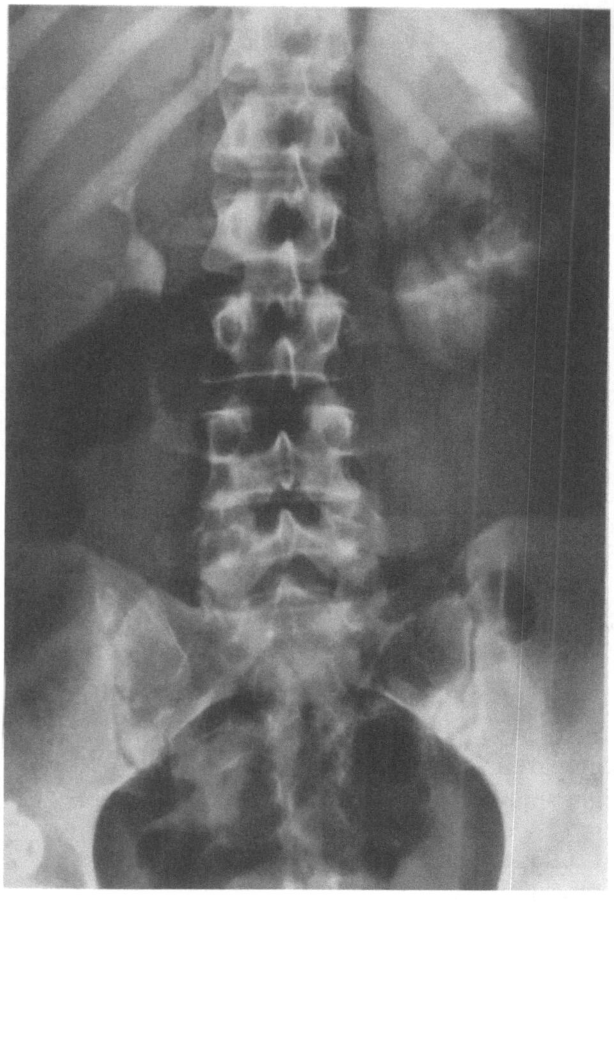

b

Fig. 197 a–d. Acute renal colic, pain in the right renal bed. **a** Radiopaque stone in the left ureter. *Urogram* (4 h after contrast medium) shows marked dilatation of the collecting system of the left kidney with a small, arched, filling defect in the area of the proximal ureter; impacted stone of calcific density (⇨); moderate accompanying colonic distension. **b** Radiolucent stone. *Urogram* (4 h after contrast medium): enlarged left kidney showing an increasing, prolonged, nephrographic effect with a nonopaque ureteral stone („large white kidney) and an absence of ureteral filling. There is marked accompanying distension of the colon. **c Hydronephrosis, nephrolithiasis.** *CT scan* shows enlarged hydronephritic right kidney with a markedly narrowed parenchymal border, small stones in the right collecting system, and a larger, bandlike calculus in the left renal pelvis (→). **d** Obstructed kidney with intact parenchyma. *Sonogram* (lateral longitudinal scan of the right kidney) shows a markedly dilated renal pelvis (RP) with distended calices as a sign of long-standing obstruction. The obstructing lesion is not visualized. Urogram (not shown) confirmed obstruction of the right kidney by a ureteral tumor

Radiologic Signs

Plain Radiographs

Major signs:

- Distension limited to the colon without long fluid levels on the L Lat film as evidence of retroperitoneal disease (Figs. 197a, b, 200b, c)
- Calculi, vascular calcification (aneurysm) (Fig. 197)
- Gas collections in atypical compartments: string-of-beads or linear gas collections in the area of the kidneys and ureters (emphysematous pyelonephritis or cystic ureteritis) (Figs. 198, 199)
- Soft-tissue mass (Fig. 200); obscured psoas shadow, positive flank sign; renal displacement, nonvisualization of normally present organ shadows (kidneys) (Figs. 199a, 201b)

Note: In some circumstances it will not be possible to localize gas and calculi to the peritoneum or retroperitoneum from standard plain films alone, and oblique views or film tomograms should be obtained.

Sonography (Figs. 197d, 198b, 200a, d, 201c)

- Obstructed renal collecting system, with or without demonstrable stones
- Mass that may or may not be assignable to a specific organ (solid, liquid, cystic)
- Gas in the mass or soft tissues, with acoustic shadowing and reverberations
- Aneurysm with a perivascular liquid mass signifying penetration or perforation

Note: A negative sonogram *does not* exclude urolithiasis or inflammation. Ureteral stones are rarely detected with ultrasound, and ureteral dilatation is apparent only pas a diameter of 2 cm.
Usually retroperitoneal masses are easily recognized, although extensive lesions can be difficult to assign to a particular organ, and it may be difficult to distinguish between liquid and solid structures.
With extensive retroperitoneal fat and massive overlying bowel gas, it can be difficult to detect aneurysmal penetration or perforation with ultrasound.

Contrast Examination

Urogram (Figs. 197a, b, 199a, 201a, b), *retrograde pyelography*

- Nonopaque stones
- Ureteral changes: stasis, tumor, displacement
- Renal pelvis: tumor, calculus, clot
- Inflammation: edematous enlargement of kidney compared with opposite side, delayed excretion, narrowing and slight splaying of the calices
- Papillary necrosis: medullary type with rice-grain-sized defect in the papilla; papillary type with sloughing of the entire papillary tip and appearance of a ring-shaped feature. Differential diagnosis: diabetes, sickle cell anemia, chronic pyelonephritis, obstructive uropathy.

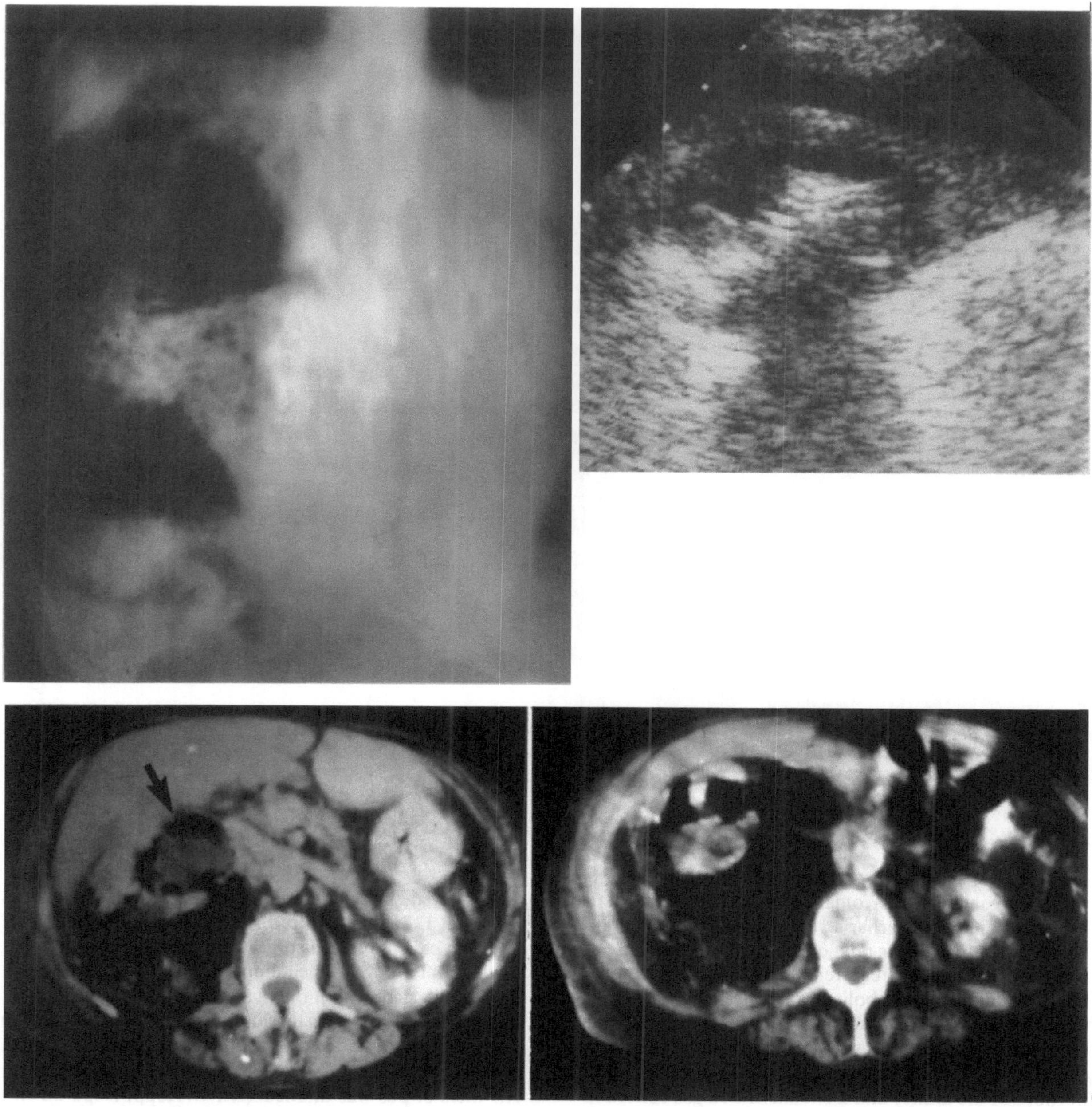

Fig. 198a-d. Acute emphysematous pyelonephritis. Woman, 67 years old, admitted with general malaise, fever, abdominal pain, and a tender, immobile mass in the right renal bed. Renal failure, leukocytosis, diabetes mellitus. **a** *Supine film* shows a large, retroperitoneal, vesicular gas collection projected in the right half of the abdomen. Normal structures appear obliterated in that region. **b** *Sonogram* (longitudinal scan of right renal bed) shows pronounced intrarenal and perirenal echo collections with acoustic shadowing and reverberations. **c, d** *CT scan* shows a huge gas collection occupying the right retroperitoneal space. Remnants of the renal parenchyma are displaced upward (→). A small, abscessed kidney was removed at *operation.* Considerable gas was found in the renal parenchyma and perirenal space. The upper third of the ureter was occluded by a phosphate stone. (Dr. P. Farr, Service de Radiologie, Clinique Cesar De Paepe, Brussels)

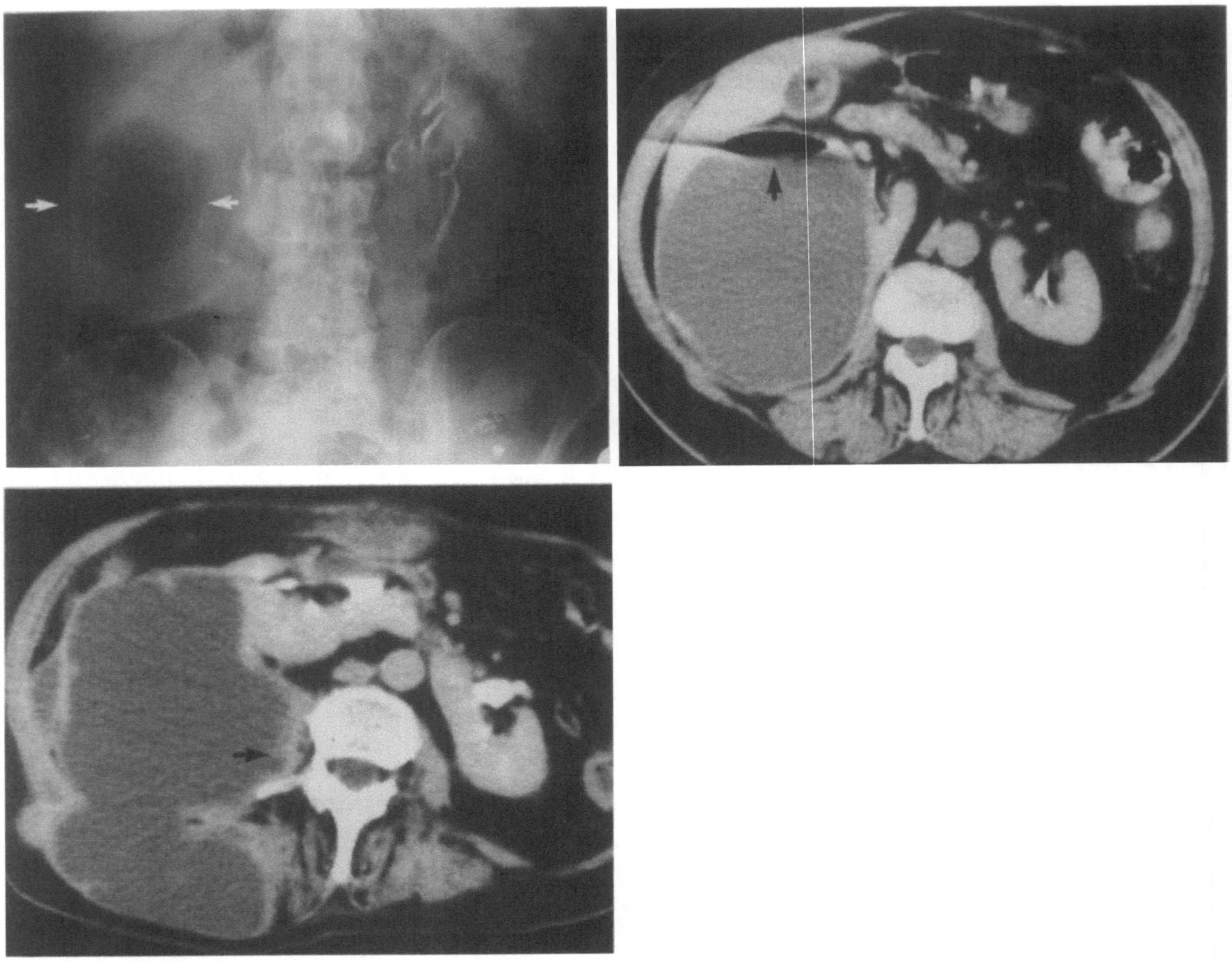

a b c

Fig. 199a–c. Spontaneous rupture of an infected renal cyst with pararenal abscess. Woman, 65 years old, with arterial hypertension. Years earlier a sonogram had revealed an 11 cm cyst at the upper pole of the right kidney. Patient was now experiencing recurrent bouts of fever with spikes up to 38°, diabetic metabolic disturbances, significant malaise, tenderness to pressure and percussion over the right renal area, and leukocytosis. **a** *Urogram* shows a horseshoe kidney with evidence of a mass lesion in the right portions of the kidney and a circumscribed gas collection in the right upper quadrant of the abdomen (→←) not associated with the bowel. **b** *CT scan* shows a 13.5 cm, thin-walled cystic mass in the right kidney with density values of about 33 Hn units, intracystic gas, and an air-fluid level (↓). The patient refused surgery and was discharged home with antibiotics. **c** Three months later she was readmitted in a septic state with a fluctuant, melon-sized swelling in the right flank. *CT scan* disclosed a pararenal abscess with extension to the paravertebral dorsal soft tissues and right psoas compartment (→). The abscess was incised, and 1.5 liters of pus was drained. (Dr. W. Kopp, Department of Radiology, Karl-Franzens University, Graz)

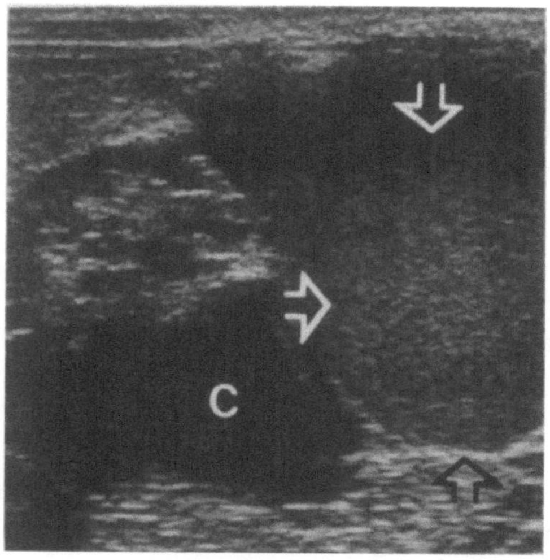

a

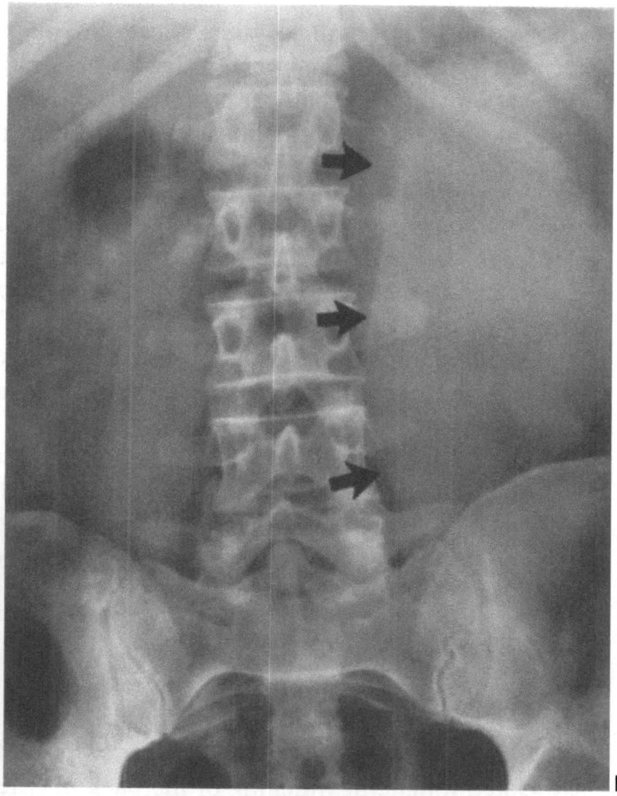

b

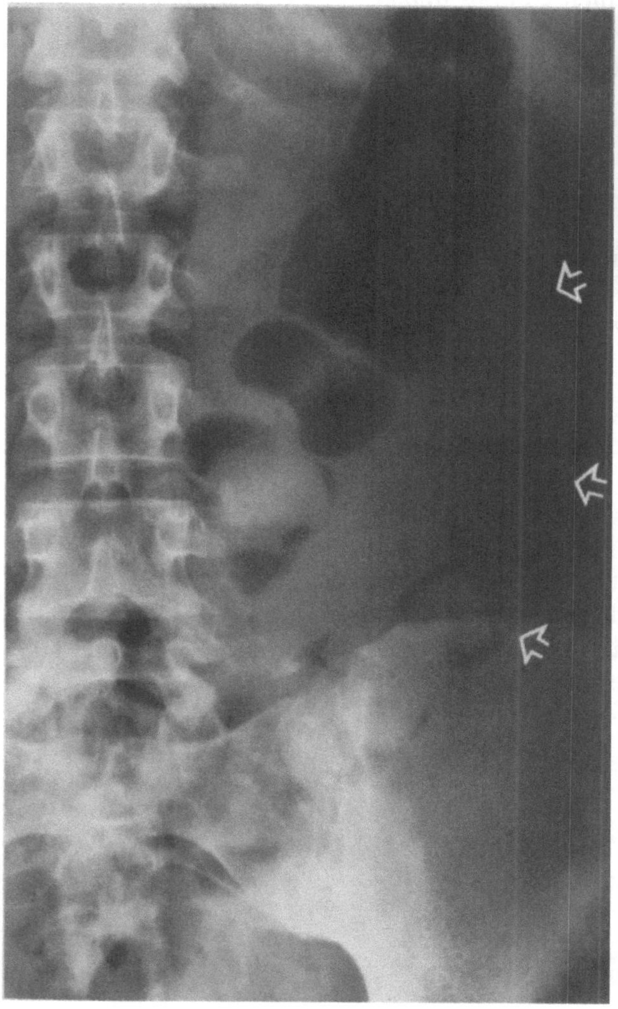

c

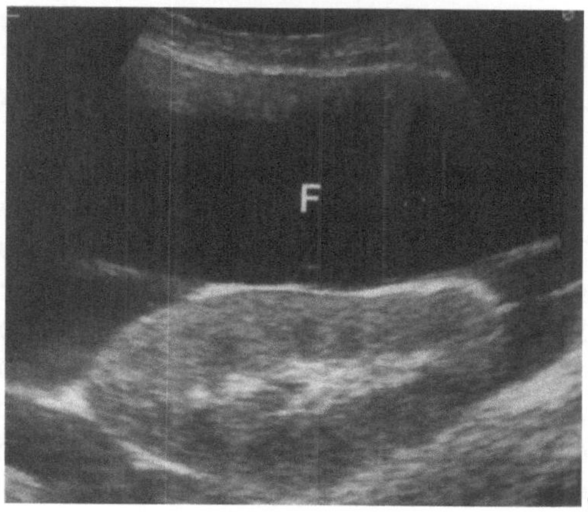

d

Fig. 200 a–d. Acute retroperitoneal hemorrhage.
a Bleeding into a cystic kidney following hemodialysis in a 32-year-old man with known cystic kidneys. Patient presented with marked abdominal distension, diffuse tenderness, and left flank pain. *Sonogram* from the left flank shows a large, somewhat rounded mass that contains echoes (⇨); cranial to the mass are echo-free cysts *(C)*.
b Acute renal hemorrhage following dialysis in a 35-year-old man with known cystic kidneys. Shortly after dialysis the patient developed massive abdominal distension with diffuse tenderness and marked left flank pain. *Supine film* without contrast medium shows a large soft-tissue density in the left paravertebral area (➡); the left psoas shadow is obscured. **c, d** Retroperitoneal hematoma in a 32-year-old man who developed an "acute abdomen" 7 h after renal transplantation with marked abdominal tenderness and a fall of hemoglobin level. *Supine film* shows a large retroperitoneal soft-tissue density on the left side (⇨) with obliteration of the flank stripe (**c**). **d** *Sonogram* from the left flank shows a large, hypoechoic, pararenal fluid collection *(F)* causing slight indentation of the lateral renal border

Angiography (DSA)
Aortic and renal artery aneurysms. Ulceration or contrast extravasation associated with aneurysmal penetration or perforation. Contrast extravasation with prosthetic graft infections. Delineation of vascular supply and vascular abnormalities associated with retroperitoneal tumors

Computed Tomography (Figs. 197 c, 198 c, 199 b, c, 202 a–c)
Permits a more accurate anatomic localization of pathologic processes:
- Confirmation of *abscess* with peripheral enhancement sign (abscess capsule)
- *Abdominal aortic aneurysm* or prosthetic graft aneurysm can be detected and its extent determined; perforation or penetration can be demonstrated
- *Prosthetic graft infection* with associated paravascular fluid and gas
- Retroperitoneal tumors can be demonstrated and their contrast uptake evaluated
- CT is the diagnostic procedure of choice for suspected adrenal disease.

Differential Diagnosis
Processes intrinsic to the vertebral column:
- Spondylodiscitis with paravertebral abscess
- Disc herniation with flank pain and reflex postural deviation and associated unilateral widening of the back muscles
- Rare neurogenic and osteogenic vertebral tumors with paravertebral and muscular spasm and flank pain
- Lesions of the back muscles (see Sect. 4.6)

Diagnostic Procedures
The first step is plain abdominal radiography in two planes, followed by sonography to localize the lesion and perhaps identify it as liquid or solid. Sonography is the procedure of choice for the detection and evaluation of abdominal aortic aneurysms. If circumstances restrict the use of ultrasound, alternatives are CT and angiography, with the benefits of contrast enhancement. Angiography is utilized in the acute diagnosis of trauma (see Sect. 4.5).

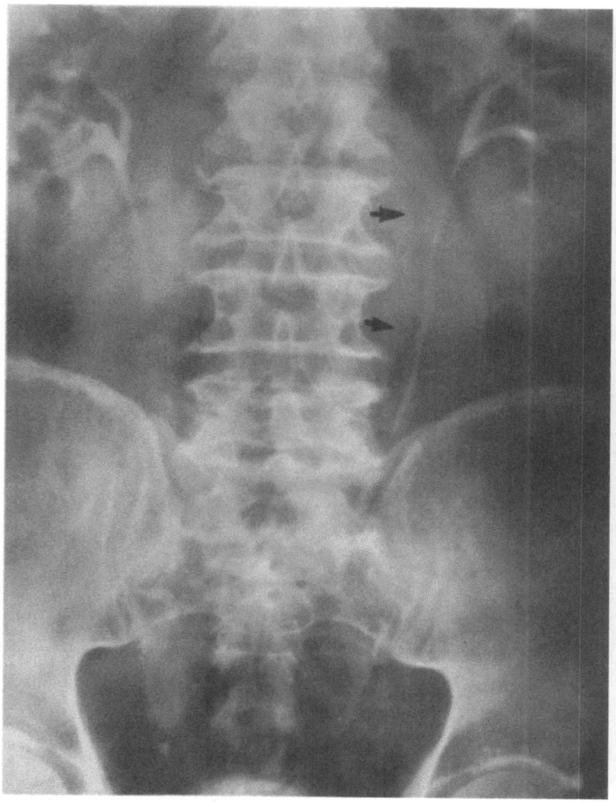

a

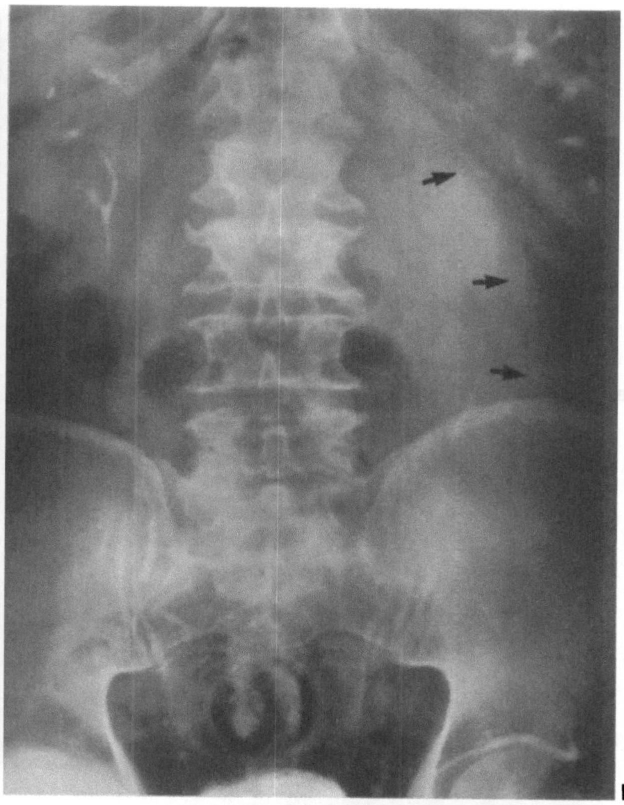

b

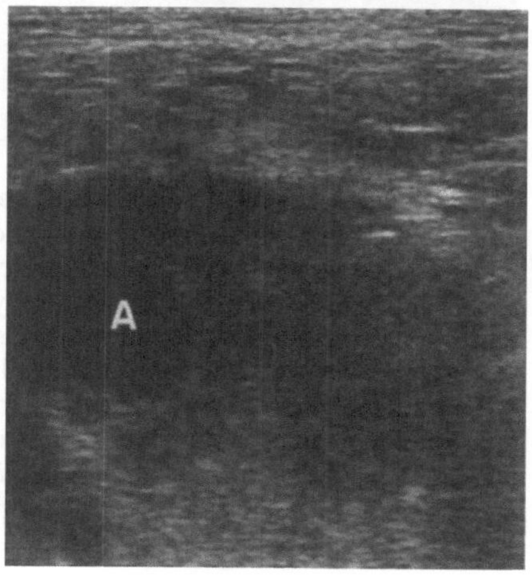

c

Fig. 201 a–c. Ruptured abdominal aortic aneurysm in a 71-year-old man with initially mild back pains; 4 h after hospital admission the patient experienced acute excruciating pain with diffuse abdominal tenderness. **a** *Urogram* on admission shows moderate left paravertebral soft-tissue expansion (→) by an abdominal aortic aneurysm; the left psoas muscle is well-defined. **b** *Radiograph 4 h later* shows large, arched, left, paravertebral, soft-tissue density (→) displacing the left ureter and obscuring the left psoas shadow. **c** *Sonogram* (transverse scan) shows a large, hypoechoic mass mainly in the left para-aortic area; A aorta. *Operation* disclosed perforation of an abdominal aortic aneurysm

References

Beyer D (1983) Retroperitoneal Raumforderungen. In: Bücheler E, Friedmann G, Thelen M (eds) Real-time Sonographie des Körpers. Thieme, Stuttgart

Brant-Zawadski M, Post MJD (1983) Trauma. In: Newton TH, Potts DG (eds) Computed tomography of the spine and spinal cord. Clavadel, San Anselmo

Farr P, van Hasselt C, Hurard T, Libert M, Litwin B (1985) Emphysematous pyelonephritis: CT diagnosis. JBR - BTR 68: 433-435

Federle MP, Goldberg HJ, Kaiser JA, et al. (1981) Evaluation of abdominal trauma by computed tomography. Radiology 138: 637

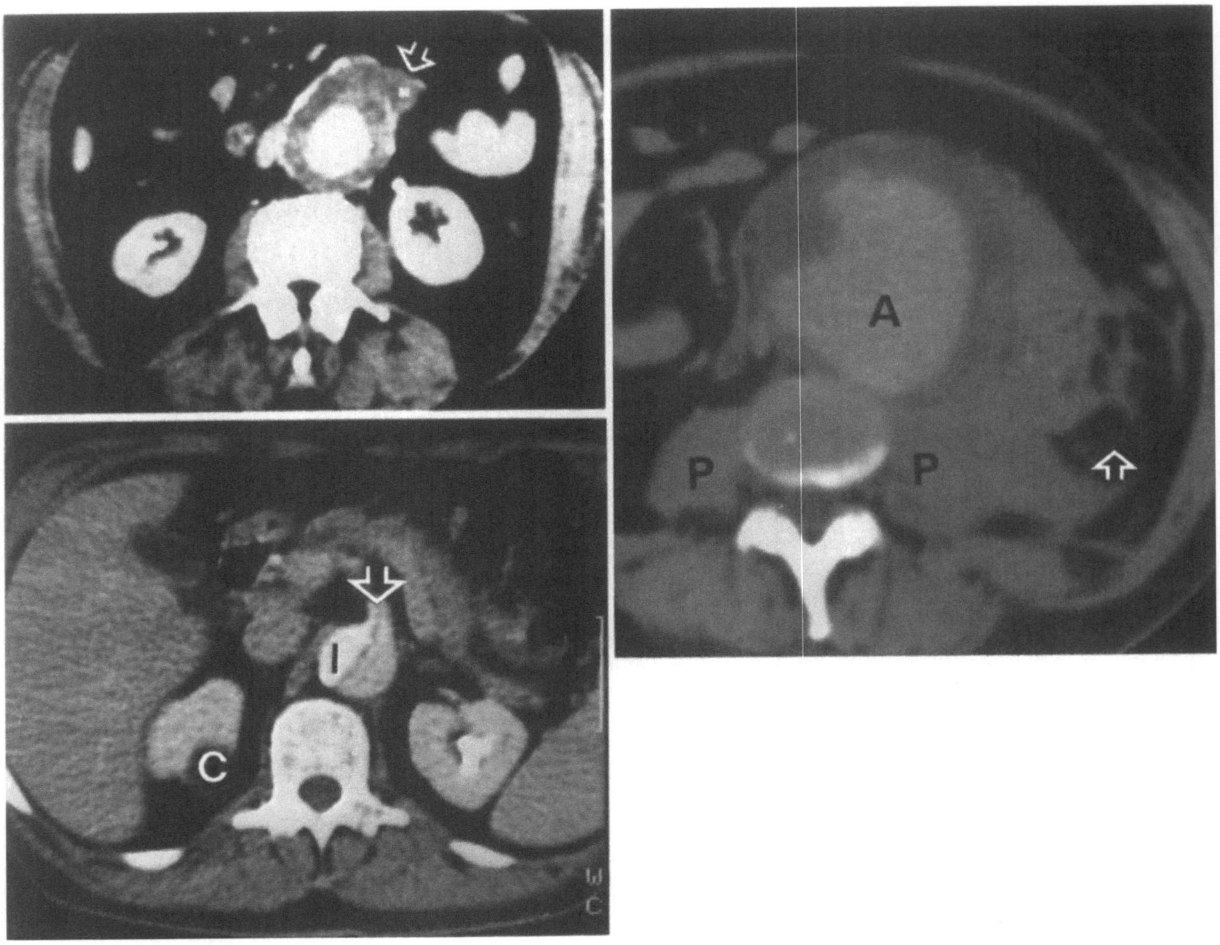

a b c

Fig. 202. a Penetration of an abdominal aortic aneurysm in a 64-year-old man with acute back pain and only moderate abdominal tenderness. *CT scan with i. v. contrast medium* shows an aortic aneurysm with a centrally perfused lumen and a peripheral thrombotic rim with a discontinuity in the left anterolateral wall caused by a protruding thrombus (⇨). **b Perforated abdominal aortic aneurysm** in a 71-year-old man with acute excruciating pain and marked abdominal tenderness. *CT scan with i. v. contrast medium* shows a large abdominal aortic aneurysm *(A)* with peripheral thrombosis perforating into the retroperitoneal soft tissues and left pararenal space. The left psoas muscle *(P)* is obscured by bleeding into the anterolateral tissues; note the blood-soaked perirenal fat (⇨). **c Dissecting abdominothoracic aortic aneurysm** in a 63-year-old man with excruciating chest pain radiating to the back and diffuse abdominal tenderness. *CT scan (with continuous i. v. contrast injection)* shows a dissecting abdominal aortic aneurysm with extension of the dissection into the superior mesenteric artery (⇨). *I*, true perfused lumen; *C* renal cyst

Friedmann G, Wenz W, Ebel-K-D, Bücheler E (1983) Dringliche Röntgendiagnostik. Traumatologie und akute Erkrankungen. Thieme, Stuttgart
Heuser L (1981) Nieren. In: Friedmann G, Bücheler E, Thurn P (eds) Ganzkörper-Computertomographie. Thieme, Stuttgart
Kopp W, Tölly E, Ebner F, Kullnig P (1986) Spontanruptur einer infizierten Nierenzyste. Röntgenblätter 39: 203-204
Lange S (1983) Niere und ableitende Harnwege. Thieme, Stuttgart

4.5 Acute Abdominal Trauma

R. LORENZ, D. BEYER

Causes

Blunt trauma: crush injury, rupture, hematoma, or perforation of abdominal viscera; skeletal fractures (usually from car accidents and occupation-related injuries)
Penetrating trauma: gunshot and stab wounds, splinters, anogenital impalement (usually an act of brutality in adults, a play- or sport-related injury in children)

Note: Blunt trauma in peacetime is about 10 times more prevalent than penetrating trauma.
The organs most frequently injured in abdominal trauma, in decreasing order of incidence, are: spleen, kidney, liver, gastrointestinal tract, bladder, diaphragm, and pancreas (two-cavity injuries in about 2%) (Fig. 203).

Caution: In patients with multiple injuries (skull, chest, pelvis, extremities), diagnostic evaluation may be hindered by the patient being unconscious. One must be alert to the possibility of exsanguination, peritonitis, and sepsis.

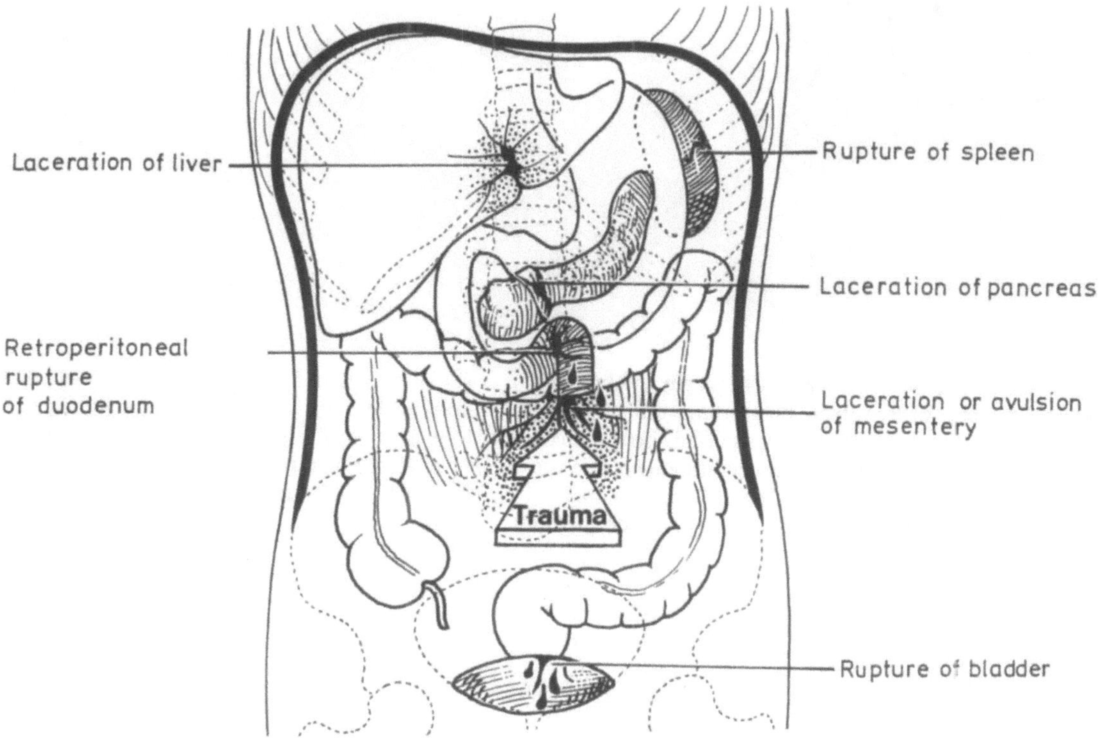

Fig. 203. Typical injuries associated with blunt abdominal trauma. (Modified from Botsford and Wilson 1981)

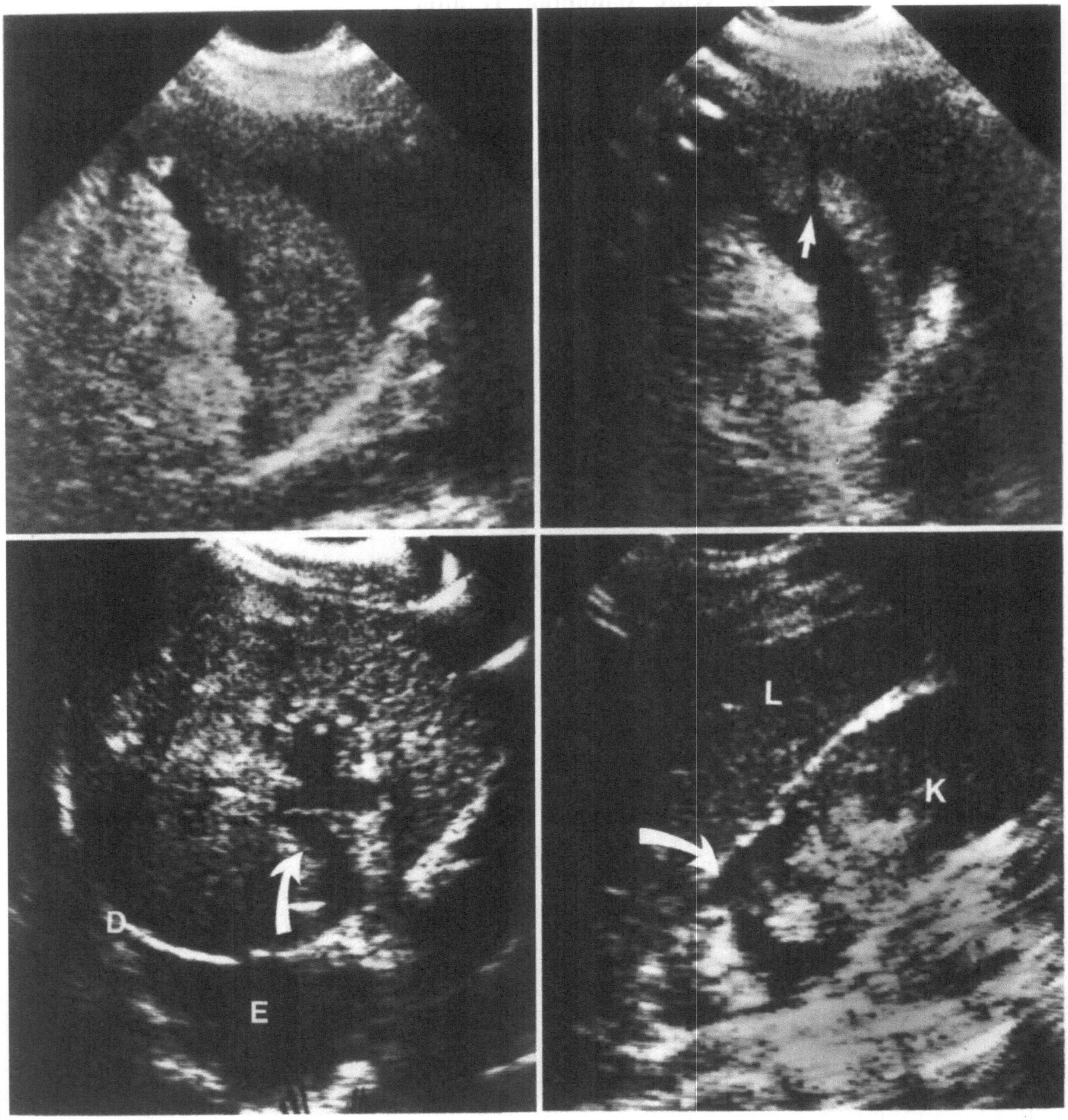

a b c d

Fig. 204 a–d. Diagnostic value of sonography in blunt abdominal trauma. **a** Perisplenic hemorrhage due to splenic rupture. The rupture itself is not visualized. Left intercostal scan. **b** Left intercostal scan demonstrating a splenic rupture (→). **c** Rupture of the right lobe of the liver (→). Transverse subcostal scan through the right upper quadrant (*D*, diaphragm; *E*, pleural effusion). **d** Renal rupture involving the right upper third of the kidney (→). *L*, right lobe of liver; *K*, right kidney. Longitudinal subcostal scan through the right upper quadrant (Priv. Doz. Dr. F. P. Kuhn, Department of Radiology, University of Düsseldorf)

Splenic Trauma (Figs. 204 a, b, 205)

- The spleen is the most commonly injured organ in blunt abdominal trauma. Associated injuries are generally present (isolated splenic rupture in only 25% of cases)
- Acute splenic rupture with a capsular tear and immediate intraperitoneal bleeding
- Delayed splenic rupture (20% of cases) with an enlarging hematoma below the initially intact capsule that eventually ruptures after a period of hours or days, causing intraperitoneal bleeding
- Traumatic cyst (old colliquated hematoma)

Clinical Symptoms (Fig. 205 a)
Pain in the left upper quadrant and left shoulder (Kehr's sign), respiratory difficulties, restricted diaphragmatic motion, peritonitis, hemorrhagic shock with delayed rupture, pain-free interval

Radiologic Signs

Plain Radiographs
Elevated left diaphragm, displacement of gastric shadow, enlarged splenic shadow (Fig. 205 a). Posterobasal rib fractures may be apparent.

Sonography (Figs. 204, 205)
Demonstrates an initially echogenic, nonliquid, subcapsular mass. Usually the rupture itself is not visualized, with scans depicting instead the parasplenic fluid. With splenic rupture, extensive bleeding can mimic a large parasplenic tumor.
Free intra-abdominal fluid (especially in the left paracolic space and cul-de-sac)
Older hematoma: liquid, hypoechoic, cystic mass with smooth margins

Computed Tomography (Fig. 205 c)
Can localize the bleeding and establish its nature by densitometry. However, where there is extensive hemorrhage with splenic rupture or a ruptured cyst, CT may be unable to localize the lesion to the spleen.

Angiography
Signs include vascular cutoff, contrast extravasation, absence of parenchymal opacification, and the direct demonstration of a laceration or fragmentation of the spleen.
(Angiography is indicated only if sonographic and/or CT findings are inconclusive.)

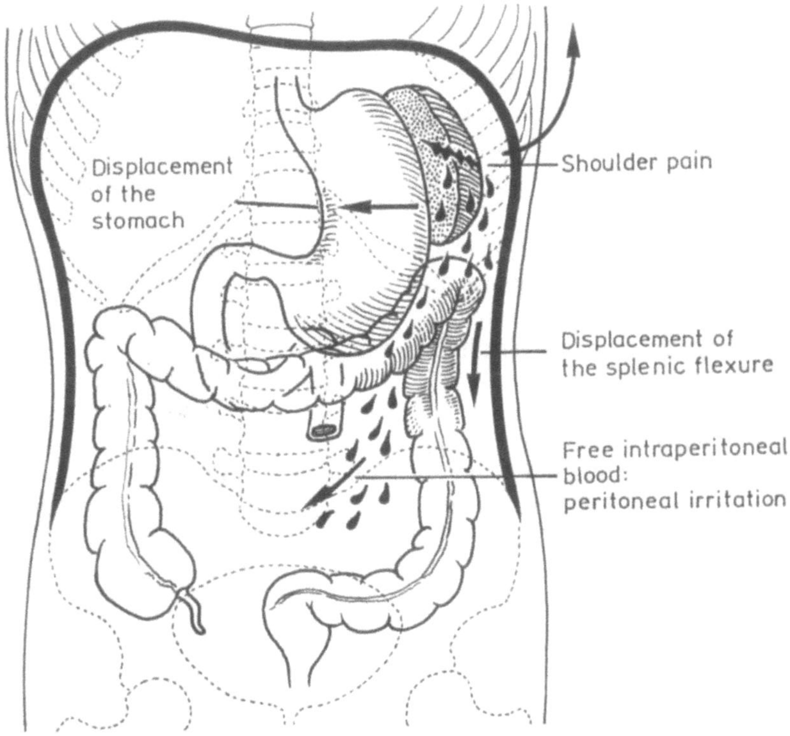

a

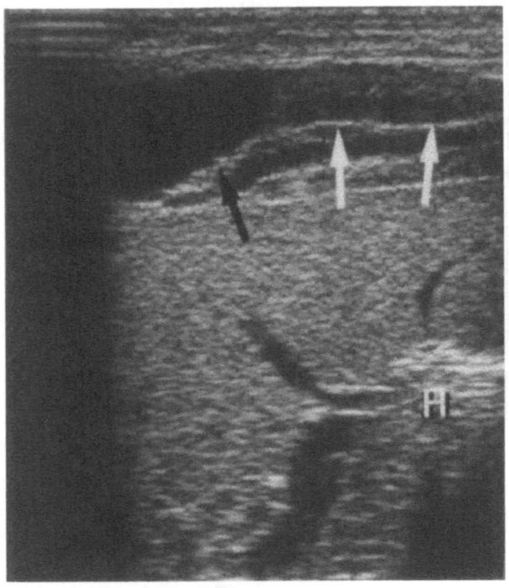

b

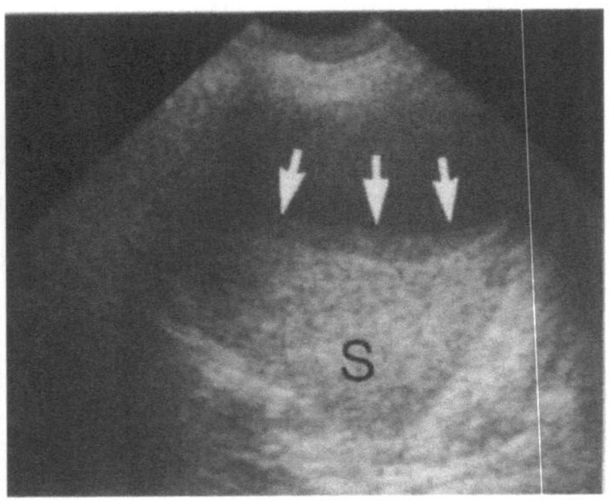

c

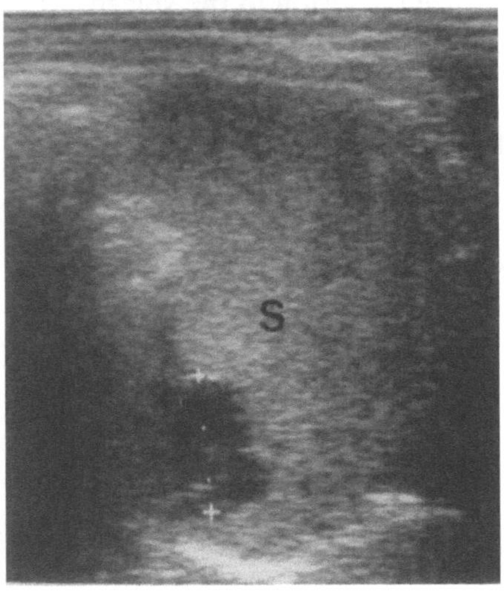

d

Fig. 205 a–e. Blunt splenic trauma.
a Clinical and radiologic signs of splenic rupture with intraperitoneal bleeding. (Modified from Botsford and Wilson 1981). **b** Subcapsular splenic hematoma about 10 h after blunt abdominal trauma in a 35-year-old man involved in a traffic accident. Patient had abdominal pain and distension with incipient muscular rigidity. *Sonogram* from the left flank shows a hypoechoic, bandlike liquid mass under the splenic capsule (➧) (*H*, hilus of spleen). Additional fluid in the cul-de-sac (not shown) indicates free bleeding into the abdominal cavity. **c** Iatrogenic subcapsular splenic hematoma in a 52-year-old man who underwent percutaneous aspiration of a malignant pleural effusion. Patient had marked left upper quadrant tenderness with no muscular rigidity. *Sonogram* from the left flank shows an extensive subcapsular, almost echo-free mass (➧) displacing the splenic parenchyma *(S)*, with sedimentation of cellular elements. **d** Small intraparenchymal hematoma 24 h after blunt abdominal trauma in a 32-year-old man involved in a traffic accident. Patient had marked left upper quadrant tenderness. *Sonogram* from the left flank shows a small, irregular mass in the posterosuperior portion of the spleen *(S)*.

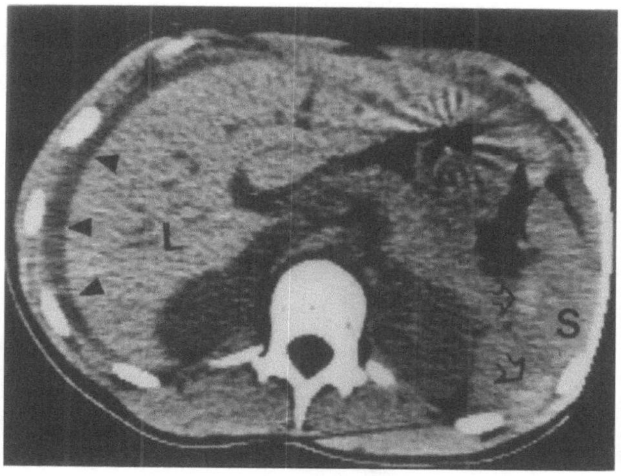

e

Fig. 205 (continued)
e Fresh splenic hematoma in a 23-year-old man injured in a traffic accident. Patient had marked left upper quadrant tenderness with increasing muscular rigidity. *CT scan* shows small, high-density hemorrhages (⇨) into the splenic parenchyma *(S)*, hemorrhagic ascites (45 Hn units) (▶); *L*, liver

Renal Trauma

- Predominantly blunt trauma
- Types (Fig. 206)
  - Contusion (80%)
  - Parenchymal rupture with intra- or perirenal hematoma and hematoma in the pyelon.
  - Tear or avulsion of hilar vessels
  - Pelvic rupture with urinoma formation
  - Complications after trauma (Fig. 206 c)

Clinical Symptoms

Flank pain, gross or microscopic hematuria, shock symptoms

Radiologic Signs

Plain Radiographs

Usually nonspecific. With a larger hematoma there is obliteration of the psoas shadow and a large soft-tissue density obscuring the renal outline (Fig. 207 e) and displacing the colon and fat stripe.

Contrast Examination Urography and angiography can directly demonstrate the laceration (Fig. 207 e, f), contrast extravasation from a rupture, and absence or renal opacification with a vascular avulsion (silent kidney). The urogram demonstrates the rupture of the ureter best (Fig. 208).

Note: Hematuria should always raise suspicion of a renal, ureteral, or bladder injury. A contusion may produce no signs on urography.

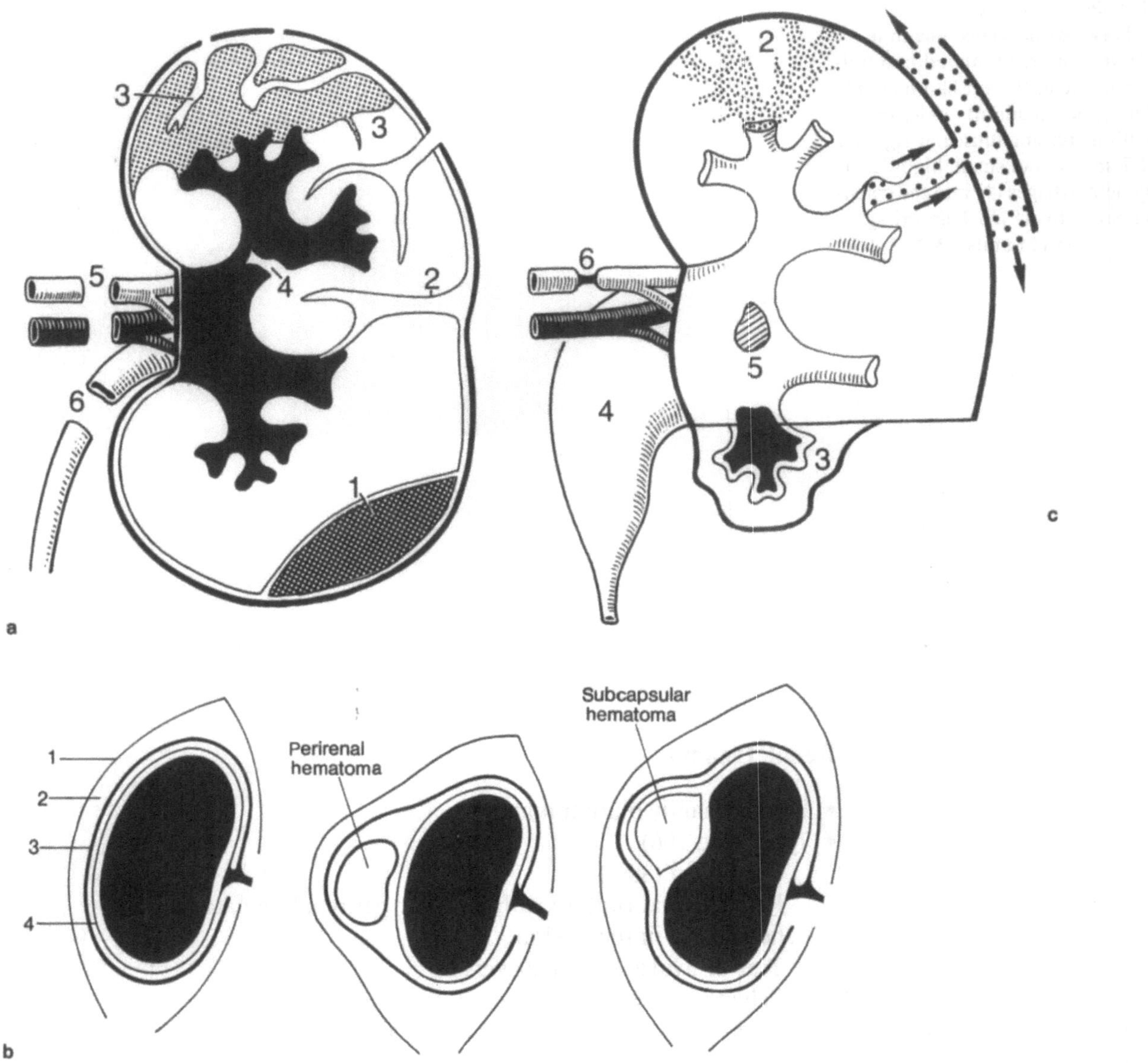

Fig. 206. a Sites of occurrence of renal trauma: *1,* subcapsular hematoma; *2,* subcapsular parenchymal rupture; *3,* contusion with capsular laceration; *4,* central rupture with involvement of the renal pelvis; *5,* avulsion of vascular pedicle; *6,* ureteral avulsion (rare) (modified from Burri 1976). **b Normal anatomy of the renal fasciae and the topography of hematomas:** *1,* renal fascia (of Gerota); *2,* adipose capsule (perirenal fat); *3,* capsular artery; *4,* fibrous capsule (true renal capsule); *perirenal hematoma,* hematoma within the fascia of Gerota; *subcapsular hematoma,* hematoma under the true renal capsule (characterized by displacement of the renal parenchyma - does not occur with perirenal hematoma) (modified from Meyers 1982). **c Posttraumatic complications of renal trauma:** *1,* urinary phlegmon; *2,* infection with abscess formation; *3,* atrophy of parenchyma; *4,* urinary stasis; *5,* stone formation; *6,* constrictive hypertension; *7,* rare-aneurysms, fistulas, perirenal calcifications. (Modified from Burri 1976)

Sonography (Figs. 204e, 207a, b, g, 208a)
Echogenic, nonliquid, subcapsular mass (fresh hematoma, Fig. 207b; older hematoma, hypoechoic liquid mass, Fig. 207a). A rupture appears as a bandlike disruption of the parenchyma (demonstration of pararenal fluid/hematoma, urinoma) and can be difficult to demonstrate. Vascular avulsions are not visualized. Sonography is the procedure of choice for monitoring progress.

Computed Tomography
Intraparenchymal hemorrhage; peri- or pararenal blood collection (densitometry enables differentiation between hematoma and urinoma) (Fig. 207c, d).
Renal displacement by the hematoma
Renal nonvisualization due to vascular avulsion
Nonvisualization of parenchyma that is unperfused or damaged by contusion.
Direct visualization of renal laceration or fragmentation.

Note: Whenever there is suspicion of renal contusion or other injury, it is important that the patient's progress be followed closely, for small parenchymal tears may escape both urographic and sonographic detection. With enlargement of the tear of further bleeding secondary to rupture or avulsion of the kidney, a retroperitoneal hematoma may form and grow rapidly, leading to shock. A severe renal contusion with parenchymal bleeding or edema may produce no sonographic signs initially, whereas urography may already demonstrate a silent kidney. When changes are advanced, edema may sometimes be apparent from enlargement of the organ and loss of contrast between the central echo complex and the surrounding parenchyma.

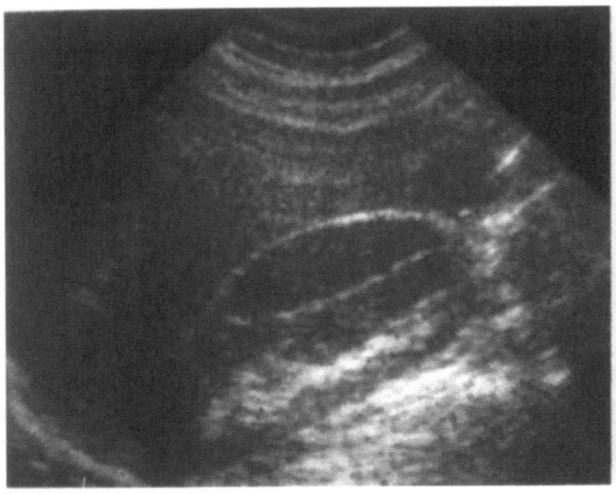

a

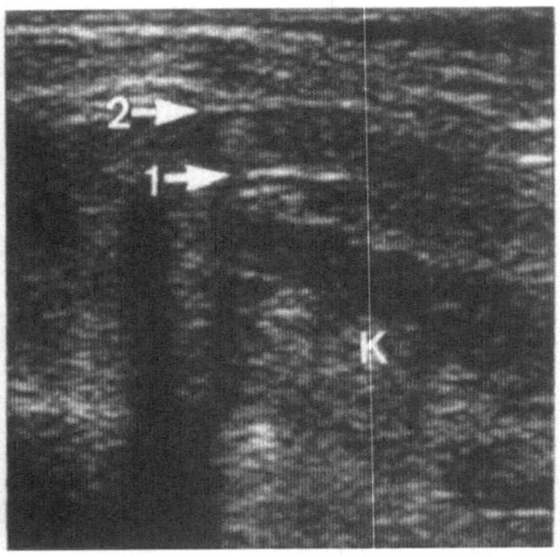

b

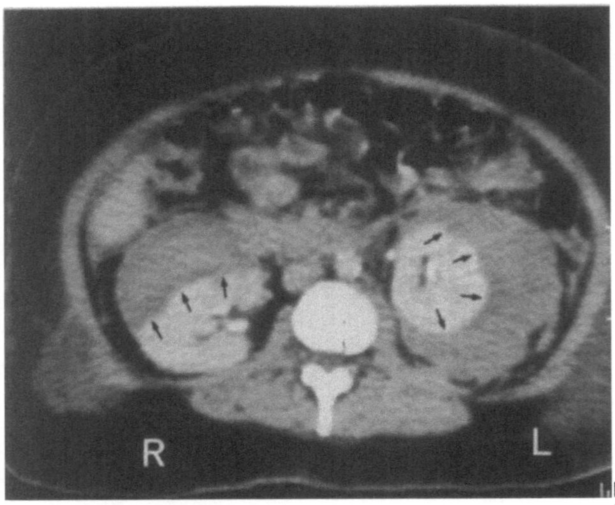

c

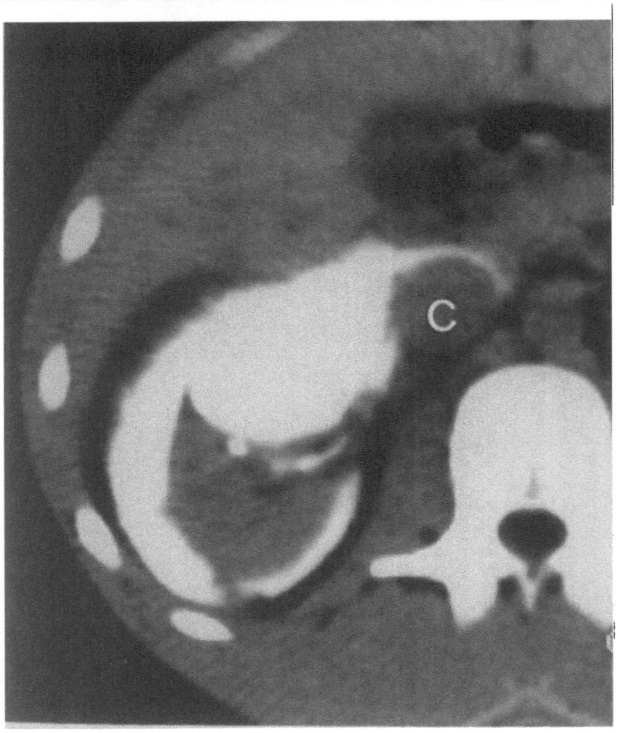

d

Fig. 207 a–g. Blunt renal trauma.
a Subcapsular renal hematoma in a 30-year-old man involved in a motorcycle accident. Patient had marked abdominal distension and tenderness with pronounced right flank pain. *Sonogram* from the right flank shows an echo-free, subcapsular fluid collection with displacement of the renal parenchyma. **b Renal rupture with subcapsular and perirenal hematoma** in a 27-year-old man involved in a traffic accident. Patient had an "acute abdomen" with pronounced left flank pain and gross hematuria. *Sonogram* from the posterolateral side: The kidney *(K)* is not clearly delineated. Large, hypoechoic, perirenal mass between the fibrous renal capsule *(1)* and renal fascia *(2)*.
c Subcapsular and perirenal hematoma in a 47-year-old woman who fell from a horse. Patient had massive back pain and slight abdominal tenderness. *CT scan: (right side)* subcapsular hematoma (→), no longer fresh, producing slight displacement of the renal parenchyma; *(left side)* low-density perirenal hematoma (→), no longer entirely fresh. **d Rupture of renal pelvis** with contrast extravasation in a 31-year-old man injured in a traffic accident. Patient had an "acute abdomen" with marked right flank tenderness and gross hematuria. *CT scan* at the level of the right renal pelvis after i.v. contrast medium (detail) shows contrast medium escaping into the perirenal space, outlining the renal parenchyma, and also anteriorly outlining the inferior vena cava *(C)*.

Fig. 207 (continued)
e, f Renal rupture sustained by a 19-year-old man, in a motorcycle accident. Patient had an "acute abdomen" with exquisite right flank tenderness and gross hematuria. *Urogram* shows faint and incomplete opacification of the right renal collecting system with outflow of contrast medium through the displaced right ureter. There is a large soft-tissue density at the lower pole of the right kidney; the left kidney appears normal (**e**). *Corresponding renal arteriogram* (arterial phase) shows a transverse rupture through the midportion of the kidney and an injury of the upper renal pole with filling of fine, displaced capsular vessels (**f**). **g** *Sonogram* shows perirenal hematoma. The "step" at the center of the kidney is caused by a transverse tear (**g** courtesy of Dr. G. A. Stampfel, Leoben, Austria)

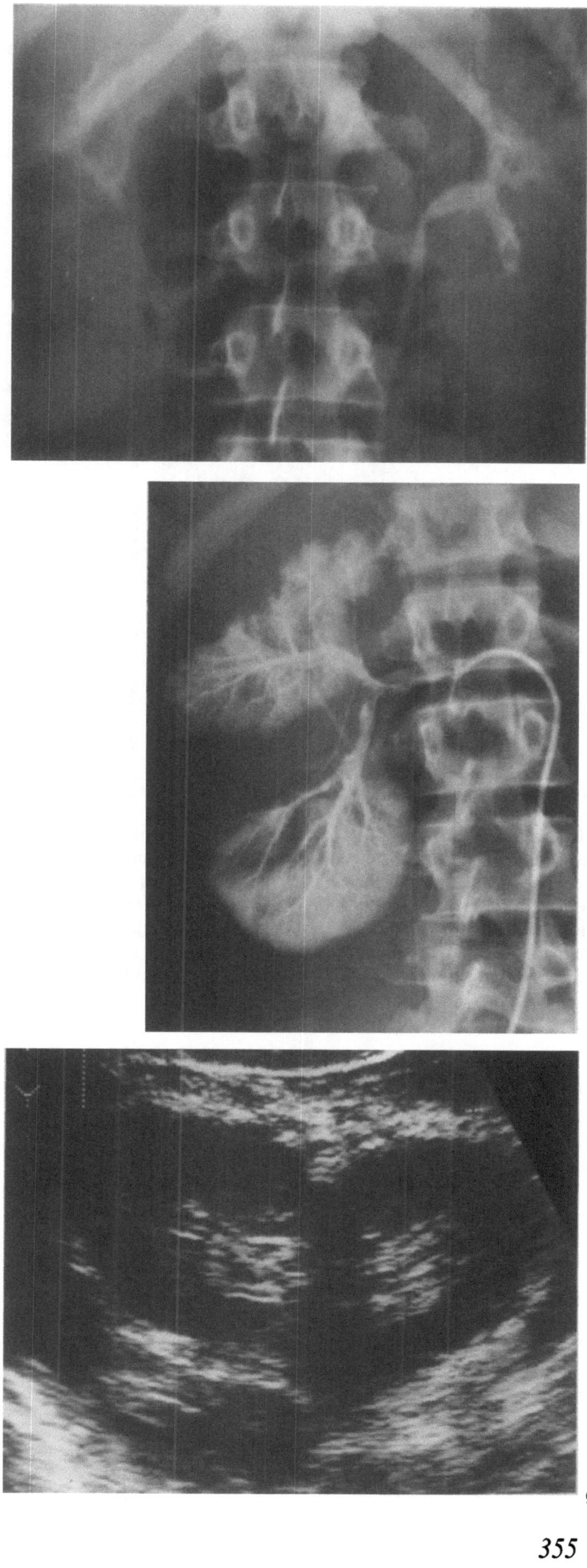
e

f

g

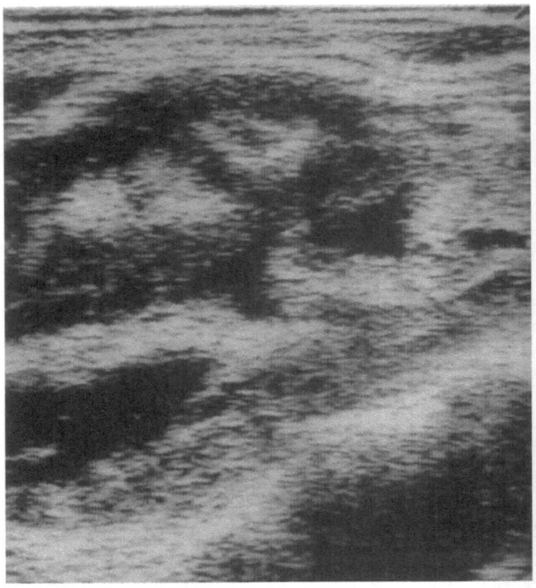

a

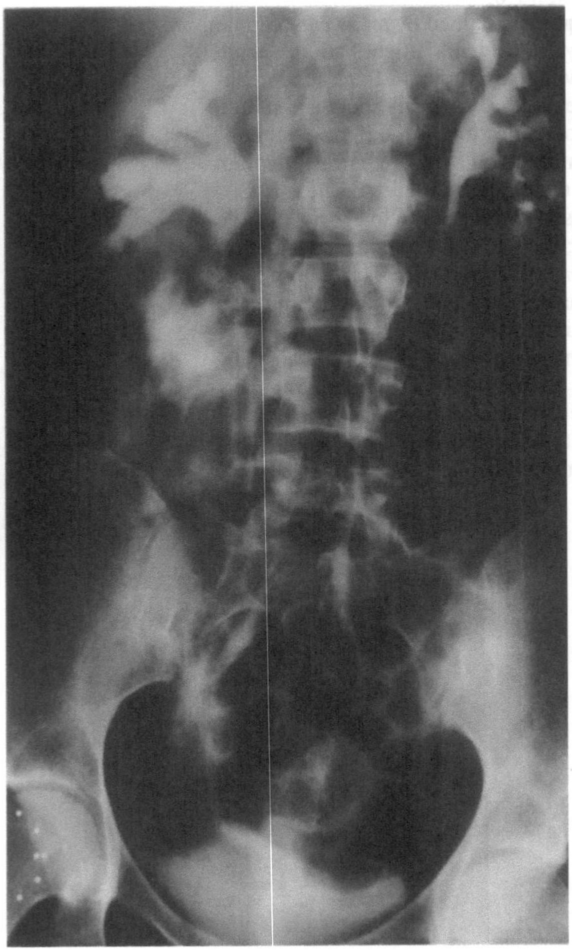

b

Fig. 208 a, b. Posttraumatic partial avulsion of the right ureter. Woman, 25 years old, fractured the right ribs in an automobile accident. No hematuria. **a** *Sonogram* shows a perirenal fluid collection on the right side separating the kidney from the psoas muscle *(P)*. **b** One day post injury the patient had gross hematuria and pain in the right renal bed. *Urogram* shows an irregular perirenal collection of contrast medium along the psoas muscle and ureter with mild ectasia of the right pyelocaliceal system. The left kidney appears normal. *Operation* disclosed a hematoma and urinoma within Gerota's fascia and a laceration of the right ureter at the ureteropelvic junction. Repaired by end-to-end anastomosis with splinting. (Dr. G. A. Stampfel, Loeben, Austria)

Hepatic Trauma (Figs. 204c, 209)

- Most patients have associated injuries: rib fractures, contused soft tissues, splenic rupture, head injury, limb injuries
- Types of hepatic injury:
  - Superficial, smooth parenchymal tears (Fig. 209d)
  - Partial avulsions
  - Central rupture (Fig. 209b, c)
  - Lacerations of hepatic veins and vena cava
  - Vasobiliary fistula (Fig. 209h)
  - Bilioma or bile ascites with bile duct laceration (Fig. 209e)
  - Laceration with intraperitoneal bleeding

Caution: Central hepatic ruptures, hepatic venous avulsions, and vena cava tears have a 50% mortality rate!

Clinical Symptoms
Shoulder pain, bradycardia, local tenderness, jaundice, hiccough, hemobilia, shock

Radiologic Signs

Plain Radiographs
Elevated hemidiaphragm, thoracic injury (right-sided), soft-tissue density in the right upper quadrant (Fig. 209a)

Sonography (Figs. 204c, 209b, c, d)
Small tears may escape diagnosis
Hematoma: an echogenic, nonliquid mass located below the capsule or centrally in the hepatic parenchyma (Fig. 209b–d)
Biloma: hypoechoic cystic mass
Parahepatic fluid collection: hematoma or biloma – these cannot always be differentiated with ultrasound
Nonvisualization of the hepatic veins with vascular avulsion.

Computed Tomography (Fig. 209g, e, f)
Permits clear visualization of bleeding sites or bilomas, classification of parahepatic fluid collections by their density, evaluation of vena cava and hepatic veins after i.v. administration of contrast medium, detection of coexisting injuries.

Cholescintigraphy
Used when there is suspicion of pathologic bile leakage – biloma (localized) or bile ascites – to demonstrate the leak when sonography and/or CT are unrewarding.

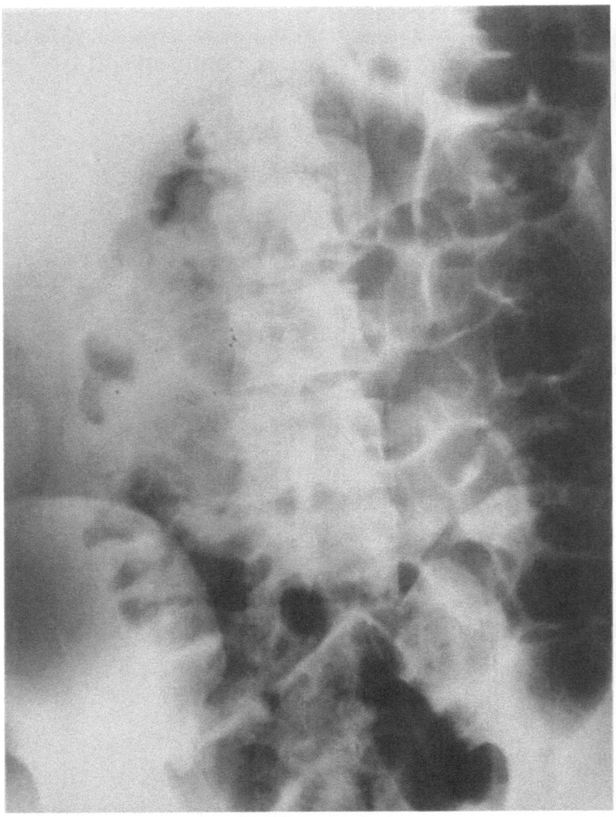

a

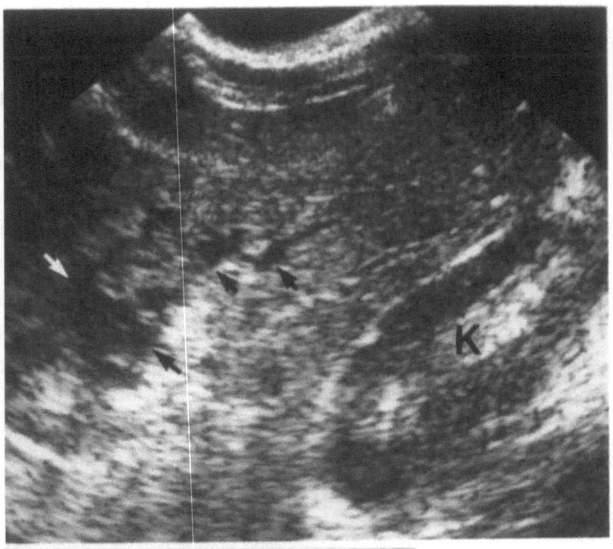

c

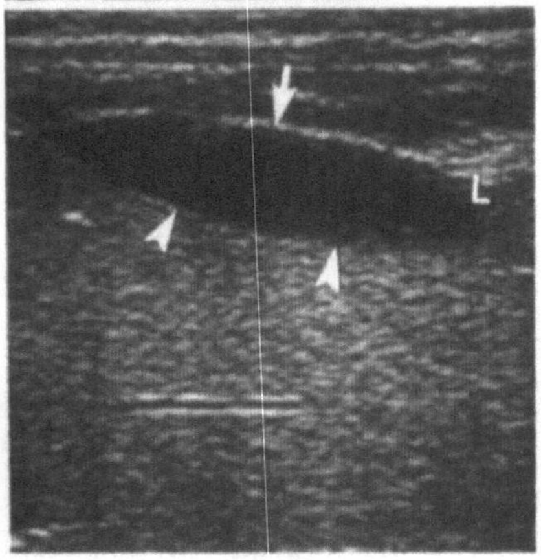

d

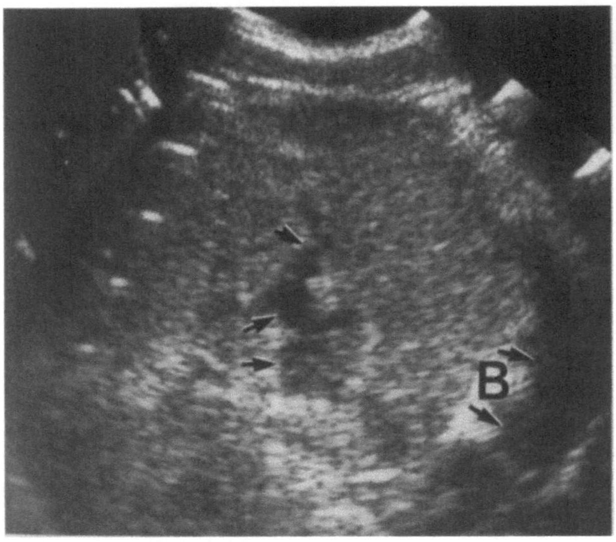

b

Fig. 209 a–h. Hepatic rupture in a 22-year-old man injured in a traffic accident. Patient had an "acute abdomen" with an elevated right hemidiaphragm, exquisite right upper quadrant tenderness; and a marked fall of hemoglobin. **a** *Supine film* shows a relatively gasless right upper quadrant with a soft-tissue density. The right lower margin of the liver is obscured. There is combined distension of the small and large bowel. **b** *Sonogram* (transverse scan) shows an obvious intrahepatic tear with hematoma (→) and a parahepatic collection of blood *(B)*. **c** Corresponding longitudinal scan shows a linear but tortuous mass (→) in the liver with associated acoustic shadowing; *K*, right kidney. **d Subcapsular hepatic hematoma** after blunt abdominal trauma in a 31-year-old man with marked abdominal distension and right upper quadrant tenderness. *Sonogram* (right subcostal scan) shows a spindle-shaped liquid mass (▶) (hematoma) under the echogenic hepatic capsule *(L)* (→). **e Postoperative intrahepatic hematoma and bilioma** in a 20-year-old woman who developed an acute abdomen with diffuse rigidity after undergoing surgery for hepatic rupture. *CT scan* shows a high-density hematoma *(H)* adjacent to a low-density bilioma *(B)*. **f Hepatic hematoma with abscess formation** after blunt abdominal trauma in a 33-year-old man. Patient had an "acute abdomen" with right upper quadrant tenderness. Sonogram shortly after the injury outlined two intrahepatic hematomas in the right lobe of the liver. Findings improved initially with conservative therapy, but 3 days postinjury the patient again developed an "acute abdomen" with septic temperatures. *CT scan* at this time shows a larger hematoma *(H)* with fresher, high-density components and an anterior fluid level with a gas collection (➧) and smaller gas bubbles below (→). Adjacent to this

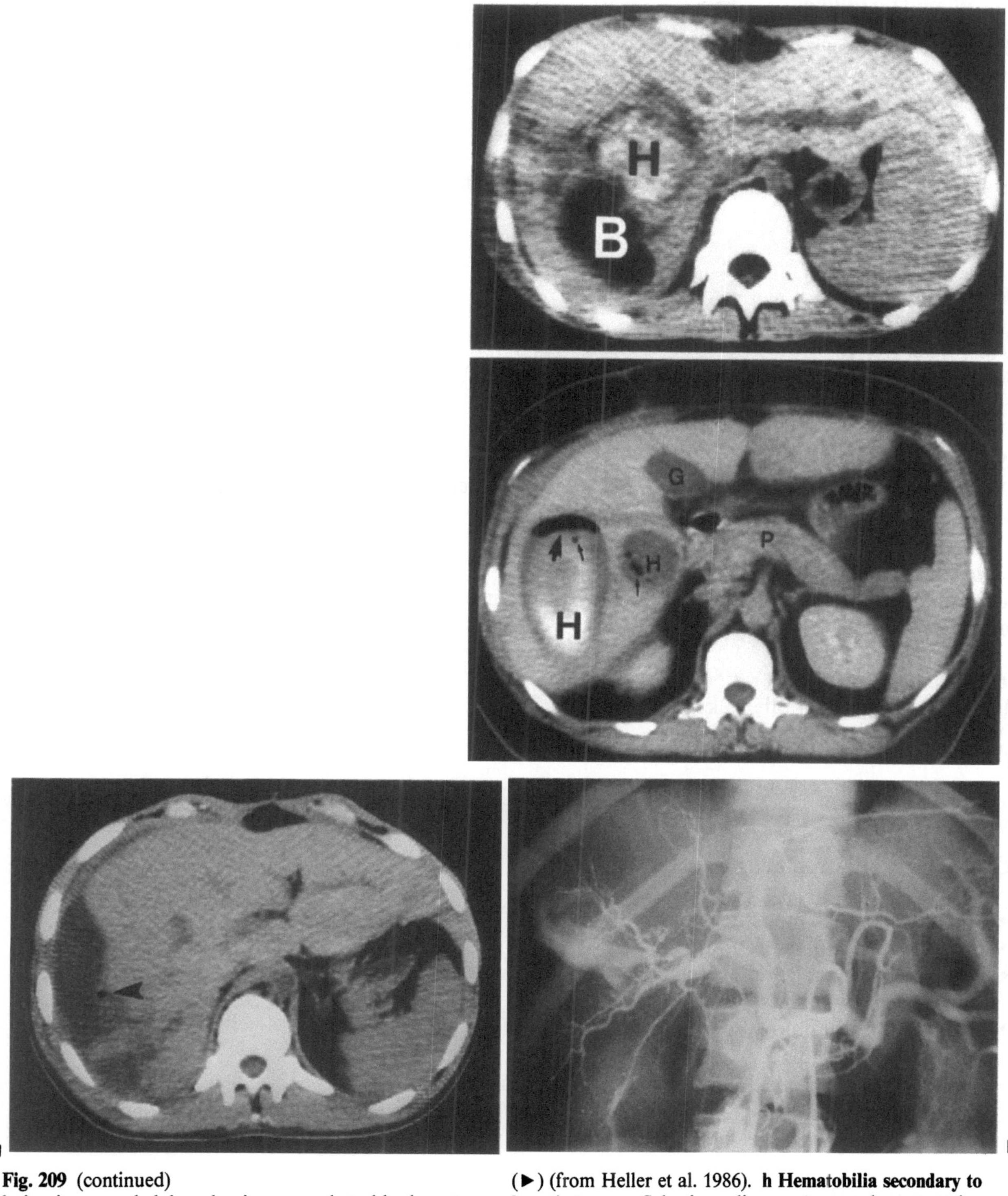

Fig. 209 (continued)
lesion is a rounded, low-density, somewhat older hematoma *(H)* with multiple small air bubbles (➧); *G,* gallblader; *P,* pancreas. **g** Infected subcapsular hepatic hematoma with gas inclusion after blunt abdominal trauma. *CT scan* shows the perihepatic fluid collection as a low-density border. Gas is present in the infected subcapsular hematoma (►) (from Heller et al. 1986). **h Hematobilia secondary to hepatic trauma.** Selective celiac *angiogram* shows massive extravasation of contrast medium from a side branch of the right hepatic artery (**h,** courtesy of Prof. Dr. W. Wenz, Department of Diagnostic Radiology, Albert-Ludwig University, Freiburg)

Gallbladder Trauma

Rupture of the organ with free bile leakage (bile ascites) or localized collection of bile (biloma). This is an extremely rare injury whose diagnosis is frequently delayed.

Clinical Symptoms

Signs of bile peritonitis, intestinal paralysis, oliguria, right upper quadrant pain.

Radiologic Signs

Plain Radiographs

May show gas in the bile ducts, right subphrenic air, soft-tissue density in the right upper quadrant, duodenal atony.

Sonography

Nonvisualization of the gallbladder, demonstration of free intraperitoneal fluid

Computed Tomography

Demonstrates parahepatic fluid of water density: biloma. Usually CT does not show the injury directly.

Cholescintigraphy

Direct visualization of bile leakage

Gastrointestinal Trauma (Figs. 210, 212)

- Subserosal or mesenteric hematoma
- Incomplete rupture or perforation
- Degloving trauma: circumferential avulsion of all wall layers but the mucosa, leaving an intact mucosal sleeve
- Intraperitoneal rupture or perforation: opens lumen to peritoneal cavity (danger of peritonitis)
- Confined retroperitoneal rupture (duodenum, cecum, ascending and descending colon): retroperitoneal phlegmons (80% mortality rate)
- Avulsion of the mesentery of the small bowel

Clinical Symptoms

Stomach: epigastric pain, hematemesis, peritonitis
Small bowel: bradycardia, bowel paralysis, diffuse abdominal rigidity (peritonitis), hemorrhagic shock with vascular avulsion
Large bowel: signs of peritonitis, fecal phlegmons

Fig. 210 a–g. Intestinal injuries after trauma.
a, b Intramural hematoma of the ascending colon in a 52-year-old man who sustained a seat-belt injury in car accident. The patient had an "acute abdomen" with marked tenderness in the right lower quadrant. **a** *Supine film* (4 h postinjury) shows an irregular air collection with wall thickening in the area of the hepatic flexure (►), no air in the ascending colon, a right paravertebral soft-tissue density, and obliteration of the right psoas shadow. **b** *Left lateral film* shows an absence of air filling of the ascending colon and a constriction of the air column just below the right flexure (►). **c Mesenteric hematoma** in a 35-year-old man who was thrown against the steering wheel in a car accident. Patient had marked midabdominal tenderness. *Sonogram* (transverse scan) shows a hypoechoic lesion in the area of the mesentery with an acoustic shadow denoting a liquid mass. **d Intraperitoneal encapsulated hematoma** in a 43-year-old woman taking anticoagulants who experienced a minor trauma. She displayed marked abdominal distension and left lower quadrant tenderness. *Sonogram* (longitudinal scan through the left lower quadrant) shows a smoothly marginated liquid mass with posterior echogenic components (fluid level) (➡).

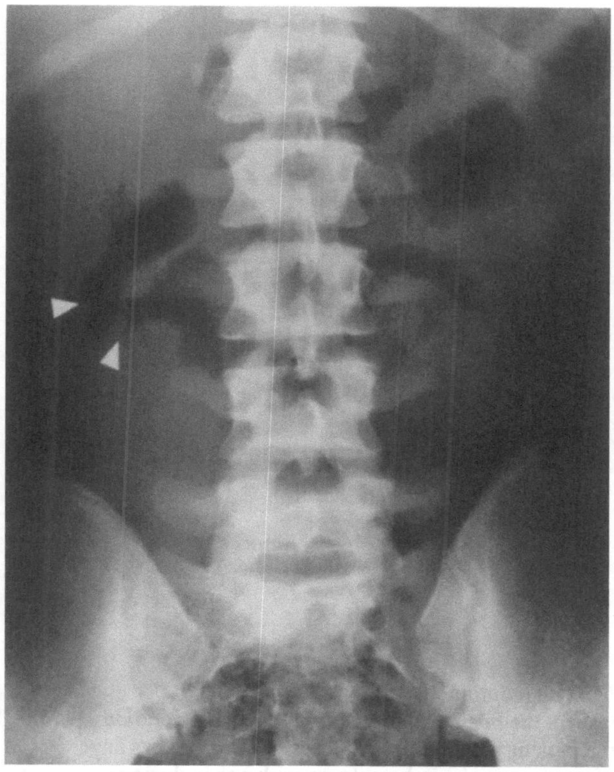

a

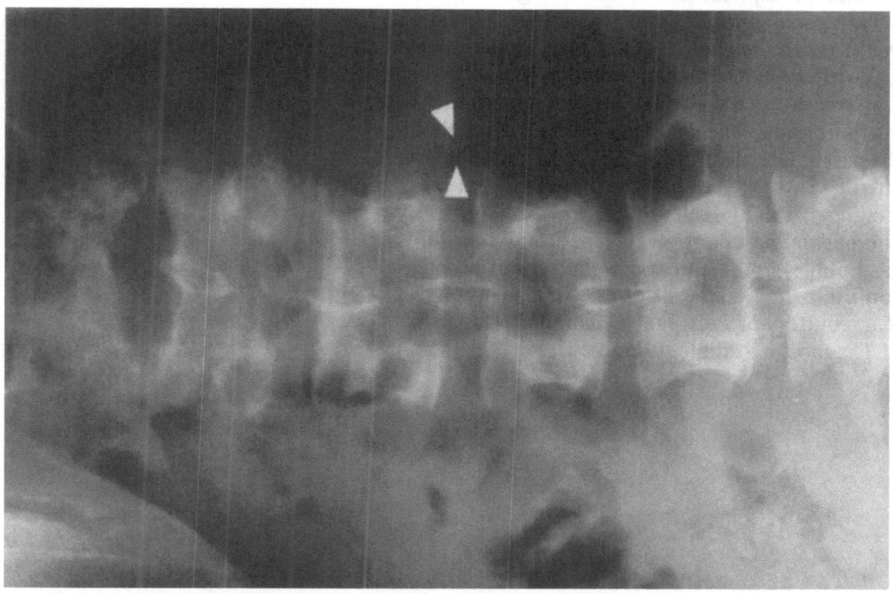

b

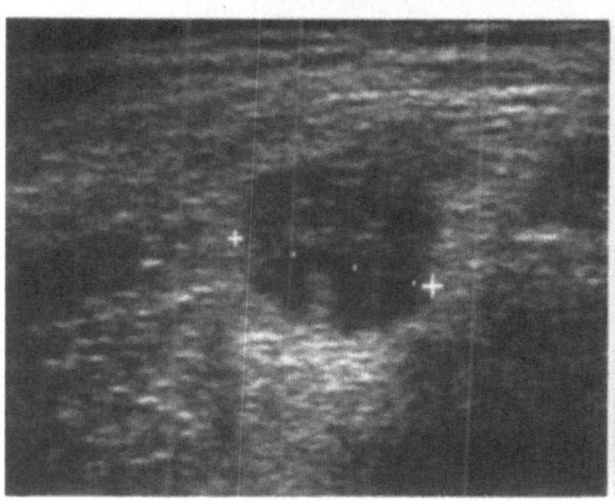

c

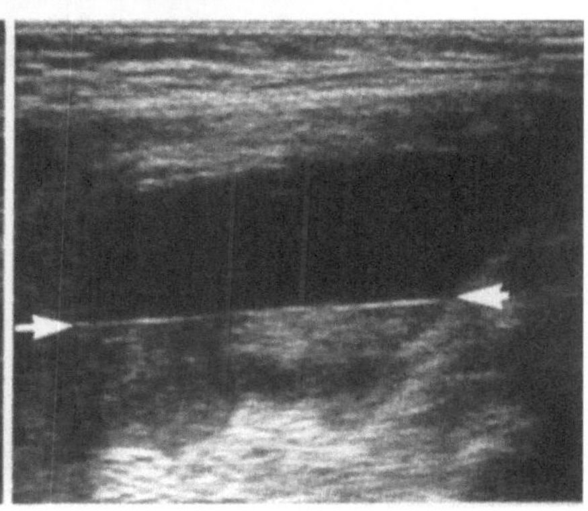

d

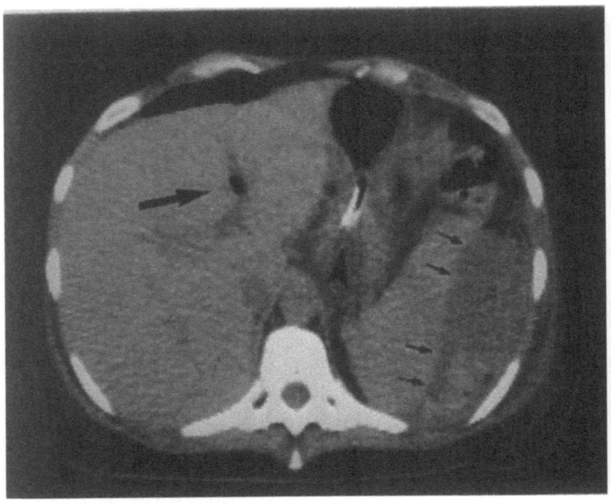

e

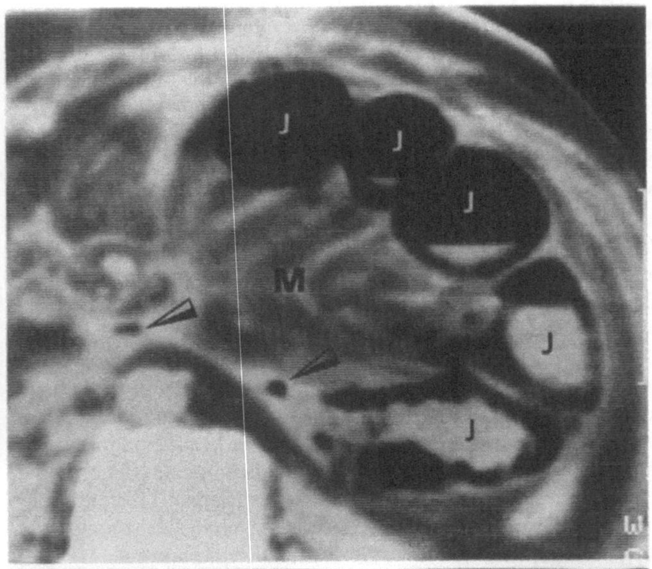

f

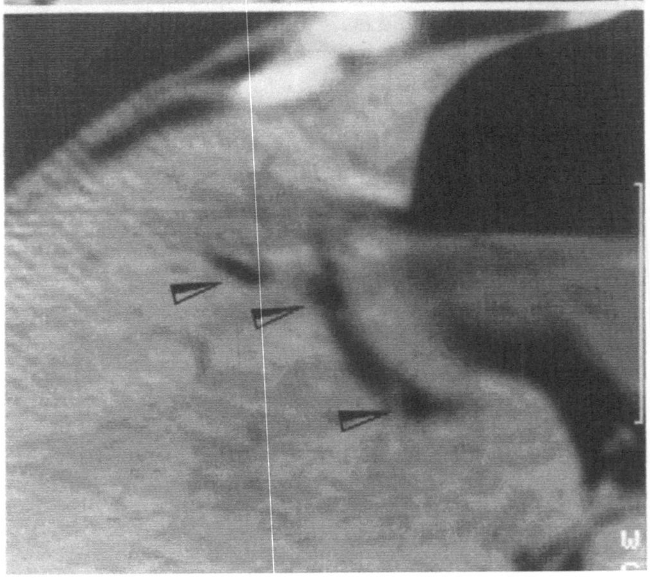

g

Fig. 210 (continued)
e Air in the bile ducts secondary to jejunal laceration in a patient with multiple injuries. *CT scan* shows an infected parasplenic hematoma with gas inclusions (→). A small amount of air is visible in a bile duct (➡) (from Heller et al. 1986). **f Small-intestinal gangrene after blunt abdominal trauma.** Midabdominal *CT scan* shows a distended loop of jejunum *(J)* with air-fluid levels. The small gas bubbles throughout the circumference of the bowel walls and in the mesenteric veins (►) are pathognomonic for intestinal gangrene. The mesentery *(M)* shows inflammatory and edematous changes. **g** Hepatic *CT scan* shows gas bubbles in the anterior portal venous branches, confirming the diagnosis of intestinal gangrene (**f, g,** courtesy of Prof. Dr. G. Schindler, Department of Diagnostic Radiology, University of Wurzburg)

Radiologic Signs

Plain Radiographs (Fig. 210 a, b)
Free air signifying the perforation of a hollow viscus, retroperitoneal air signifying a penetration or perforation of the aforementioned organ systems into the retroperitoneal space. Soft-tissue density or wall thickening (edema, hemorrhage) with mesenteric avulsion. Isolated duodenal distension signifying pancreatic injury. Obliteration of psoas muscle by retroperitoneal hematoma or retroperitoneal abscess.

Sonography (Figs. 210 c, d, 212 c)
Diagnosis is greatly hampered by overlying bowel gas. Scans may show a retroperitoneal or peritoneal mass (hemorrhage), a thickened bowel wall (edema), or a mesenteric mass (bleeding from avulsed mesentery). It may not be possible to assign a large mass to a particular organ system with ultrasound.

Angiography
Localization of bleeding sites or isolated vascular injuries.

Computed Tomography (Figs. 210 e, g, 212 d)
Thickened bowel wall, hemorrhagic mass in the region of the mesentery; gas collection in the retroperitoneum; tumorous mass in the area of the duodenum or colon (ascending, descending, cecum)

Caution:
- Intestinal bleeding can mimic a tumor!
- Mesenteric avulsions have a very high mortality and therefore may preclude angiographic evaluation.

Note: The oral administration of a water-soluble contrast medium gives information on the degree of obstruction caused by intramural bleeding if sonographic and/or CT findings are equivocal. Contrast studies are also useful in such cases for monitoring the regression of an intramural hematoma.

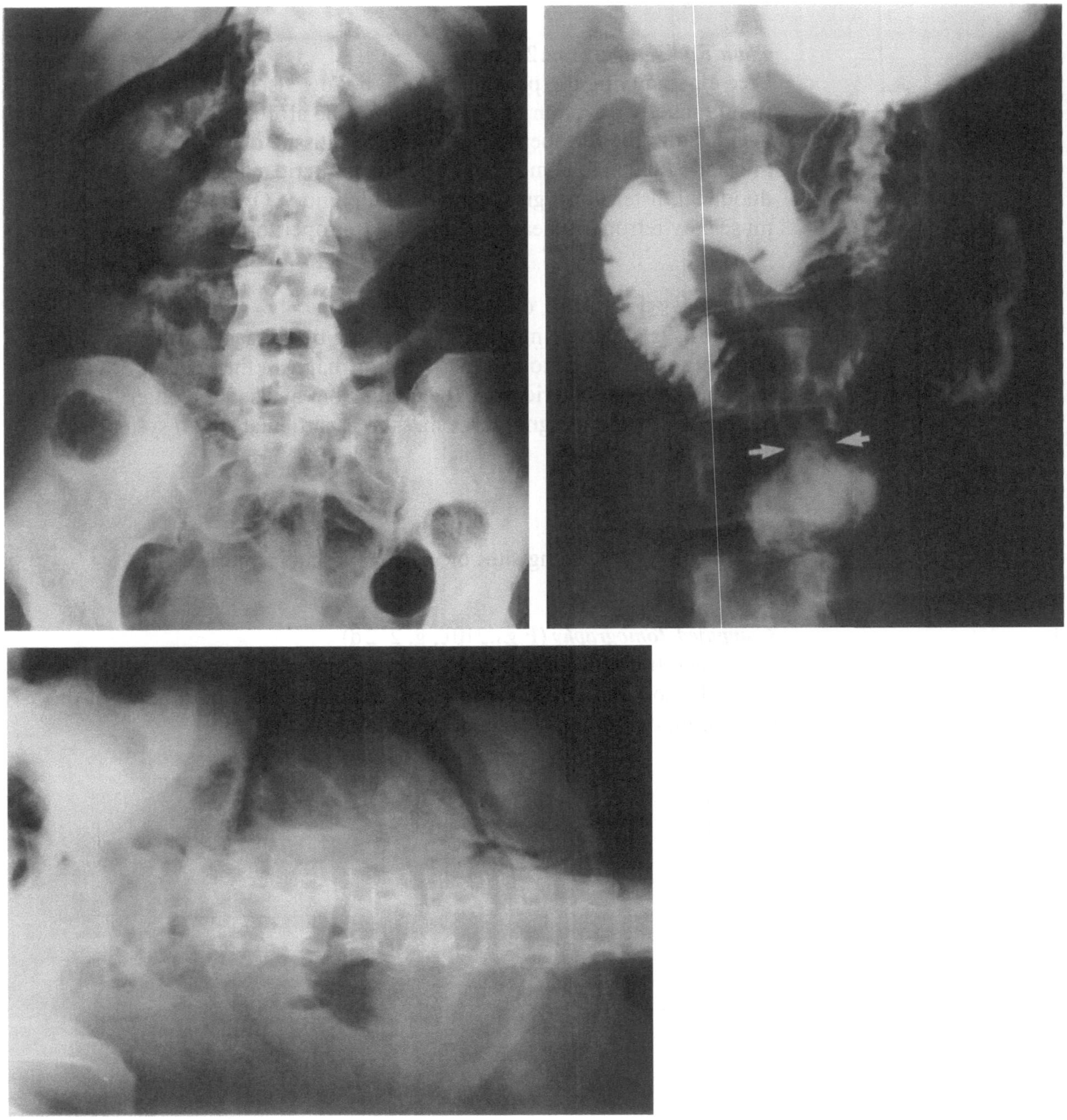

a c b

Fig. 211 a–c. Retroperitoneal duodenal rupture after blunt abdominal trauma. Sonogram in a 31-year-old female alcoholic who had been beaten disclosed a ruptured liver and signs of pancreatic contusion with a hematoma in the pancreatic region. The findings were confirmed at operation. No evidence of bowel perforation was apparent. A diffuse peritonitis developed overnight. **a** *Supine abdominal film* shows pneumoretroperitoneum with perirenal gas in the left renal bed. **b** *Left lateral film* shows postoperative pneumoperitoneum with no displacement of the retroperitoneal air in the perirenal space and no air-fluid levels. The radiologic diagnosis of retroperitoneal duodenal rupture was confirmed by a repeat laparotomy, which disclosed a gaping 4 cm tear in the posterior wall of the descending part of the duodenum. A bile-soaked aggregate tumor was found in the omental bursa, and the mesentery and abdominal wall were saturated with bile. The patient died 4 days postinjury from complications of the duodenal rupture (Dr. K. Tremmel, Department of Radiology, Municipal Hospital Esslingen/Neckar). **c Retroperitoneal duodenal rupture.** *Gastrografin UGI series* shows perforation of the ascending part of the duodenum with a rounded collection of extravasated contrast medium (→). There is edematous distortion of the bowel contour (from Hertel 1975)

Fig. 212 a–d. Confined rupture of the duodenum and ascending colon after blunt abdominal trauma. Woman, 23 years old, with protracted pain in the right upper quadrant and right flank and persistent septic temperatures at 7 days postinjury. **a** *Urogram* 10 min postinfusion) shows a pathologic gas collection projected onto the right kidney (→), which is displaced medially downward. **b** *Left lateral film* shows a fixed cluster of small gas bubbles projected onto the right kidney (→). **c** *Sonogram* (right kidney scanned from the right side) shows a broad, pararenal fluid collection (→); *K*, kidney; *P*, psoas muscle; *L*, liver. **d** *CT scan* shows a fixed pararenal gas collection (→); *A*, ascites; *K*, kidney

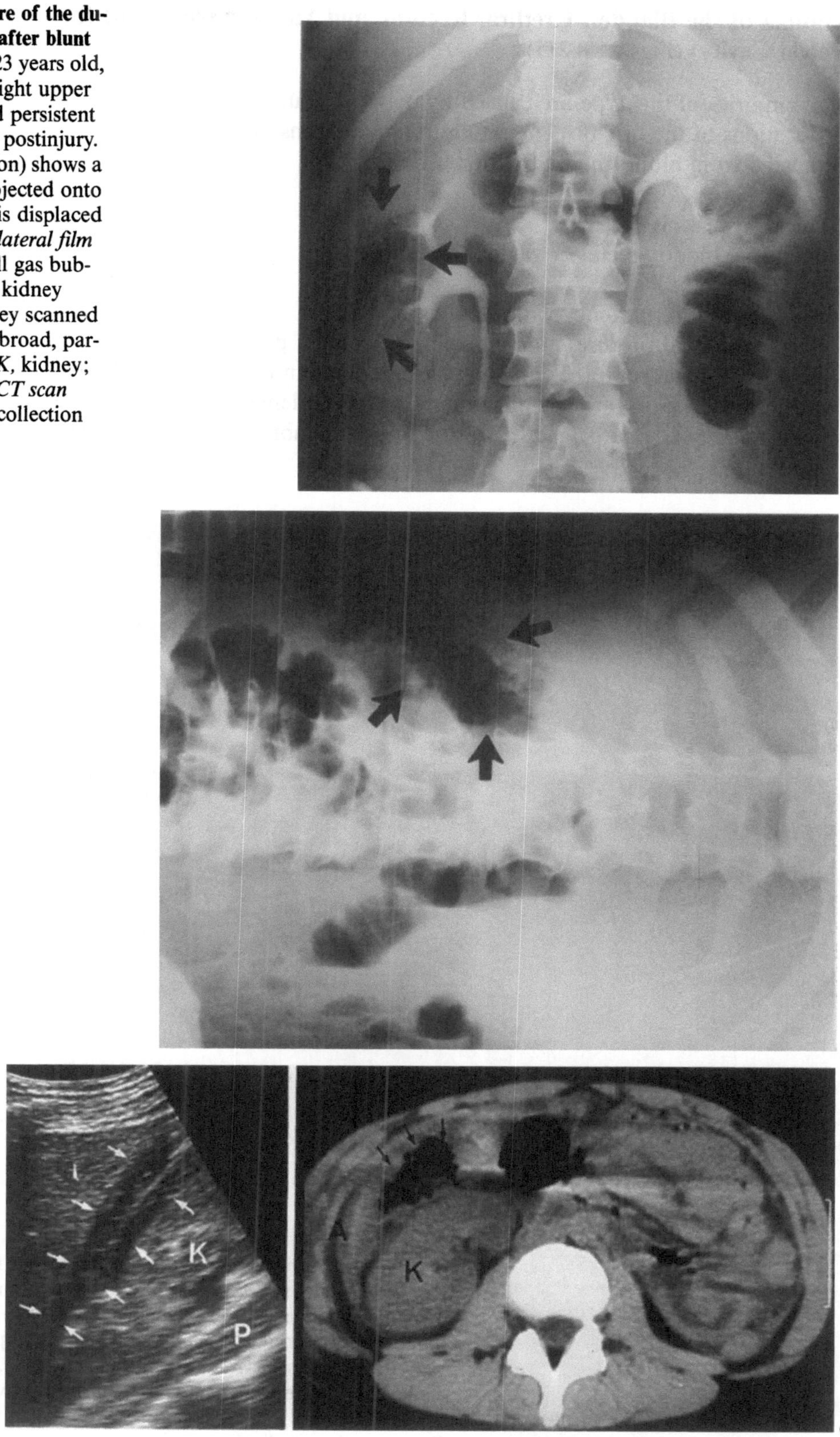

Trauma of the Bladder, Urethra, Rectum, and Vagina (Trauma of the Pelvic Cavity) (Figs. 213–215)

Most injuries of this type are caused by pelvic fractures, central dislocations of the hip, or penetrating trauma (organs are normally protected from blunt trauma by the pelvic ring).

Clinical Symptoms

Hematuria, bloddy rectal or vaginal discharge
Bladder trauma:

- Closed rupture: urgency with inability to void
- Intraperitoneal rupture: atonic bowel, meteorism, peritonitis
- Extraperitoneal rupture: doughy, painful edema in the suprasymphyseal or perineal region (urinary phlegmons), scrotal edema, elevated prostate with doughy edema; suggests rupture of the membranous portion of the urethra

Caution:
- Intraperitoneal bladder ruptures lead to urinary ascites with peritonitis
- Urinary phlegmons from extraperitoneal bladder or urethral rupture

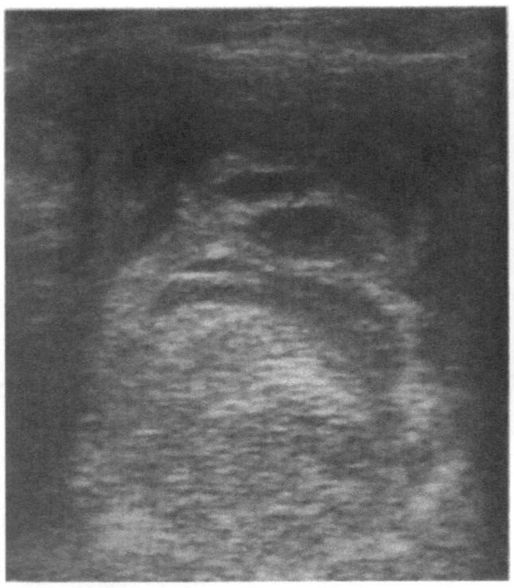
a

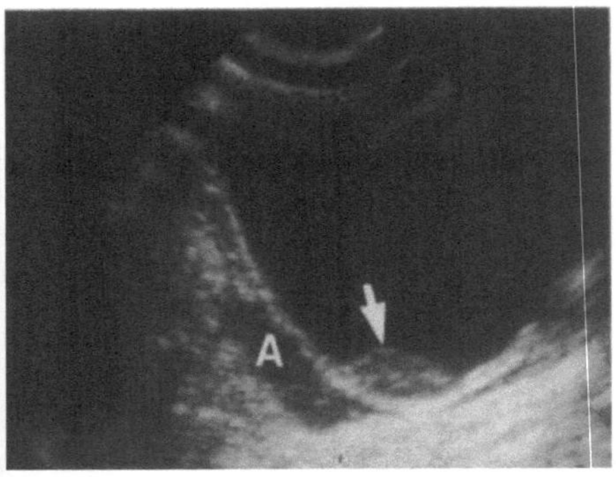

b

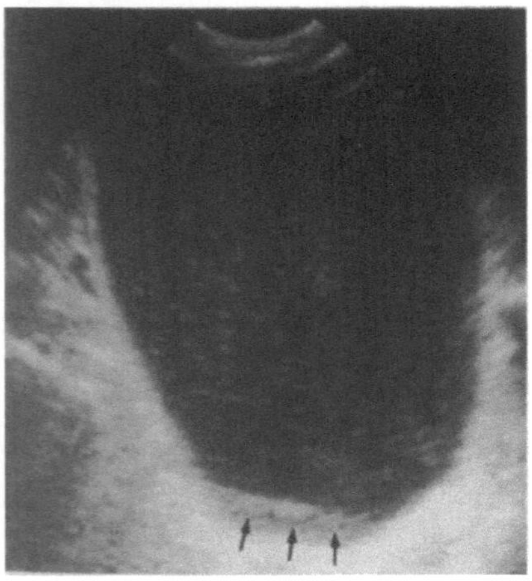
c

Fig. 213 a–f. Pelvic trauma. a Bladder tamponade following a pelvic ring fracture. After a motorcycle accident the 32-year-old man developed an acute abdomen with massive lower abdominal tenderness and anuria. Plain survey film of the abdomen (not shown) disclosed multiple pelvic fractures. *Sonogram* (transverse scan) reveals a large, hypoechoic, layered mass in the urinary bladder. **b Intravesical clot** in a 47-year-old man who jumped from a bridge (suicide attempt). Patient had an acute abdomen with massive left flank pain. *Sonogram* (longitudinal scan of right lower quadrant) shows an echogenic lesion on the posterior bladder wall (➧): clot following renal contusion, paravesical fluid collection *(A)* (hemorrhagic ascites?). **c Intravesical bleeding** in a 21-year-old man who sustaining a blunt renal contusion in a traffic accident. Right flank tenderness. *Sonogram* (longitudinal scan) shows multiple floating echo complexes with sedimentation of cellular elements on the bladder floor (→).

Fig. 213 (continued)
d–f Bladder rupture in a 24-year-old man who sustained a pelvic fracture in a motorcycle accident. Patient had an acute abdomen with marked lower abdominal tenderness and gross hematuria. *Supine urogram* shows cranial displacement of the distended small and large bowel (➧) by a large, rounded, soft-tissue mass in the pelvic region (**d**). *Pelvic survey (urogram)* shows marked elevation of the bladder floor (►), a left paravesical soft-tissue density, and a displaced fracture of the left pubic bone (➧) (**e**). *Spot film after cystogram* (detail) with Valsalva's maneuver shows contrast extravasation in the area of the left bladder wall, a short distance above the fracture (⇨) (**f**; Dr. Geppert, Norden)

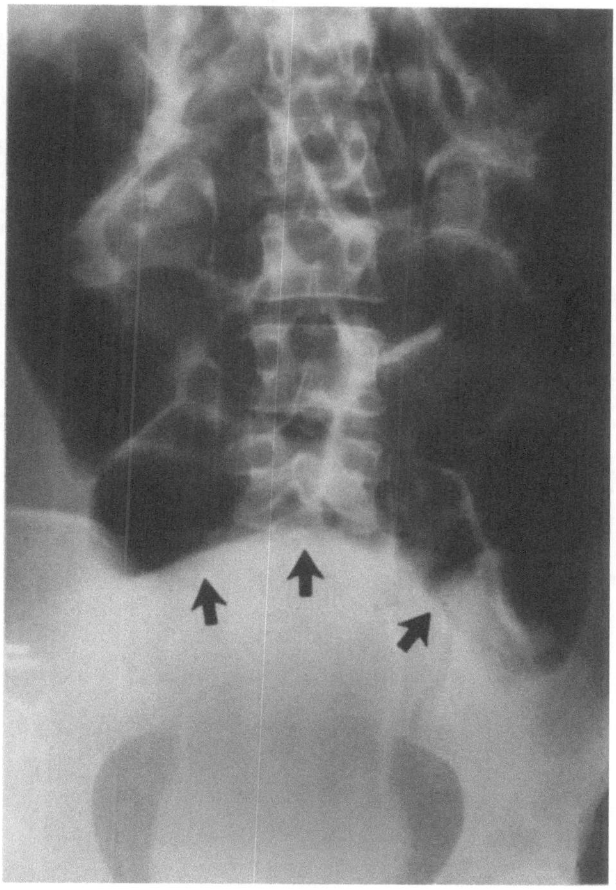
d

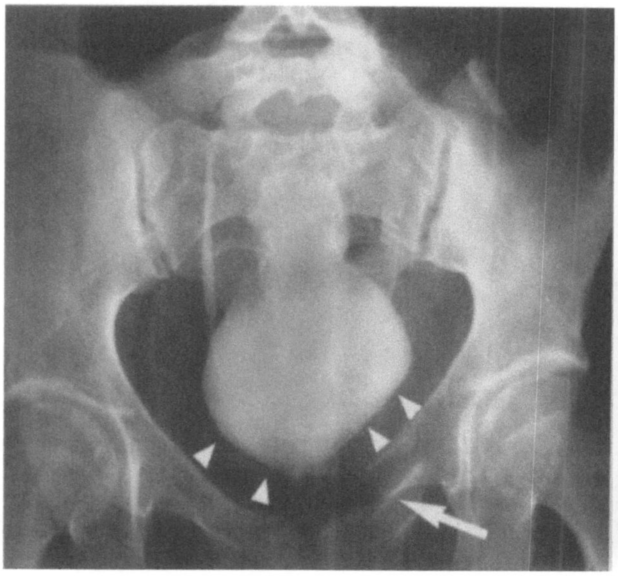
e

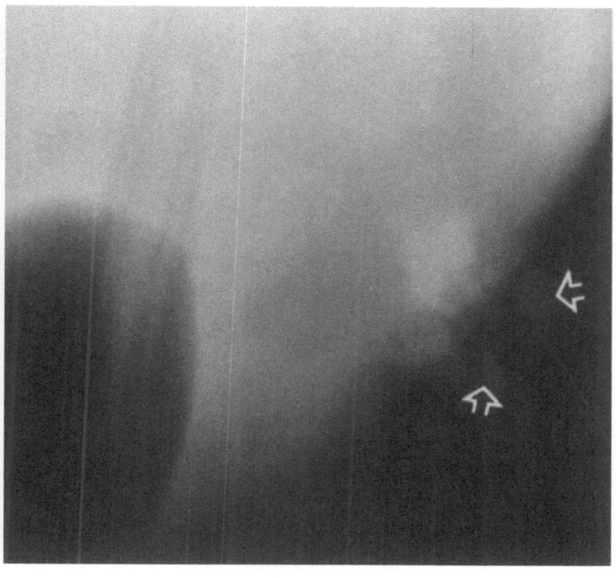
f

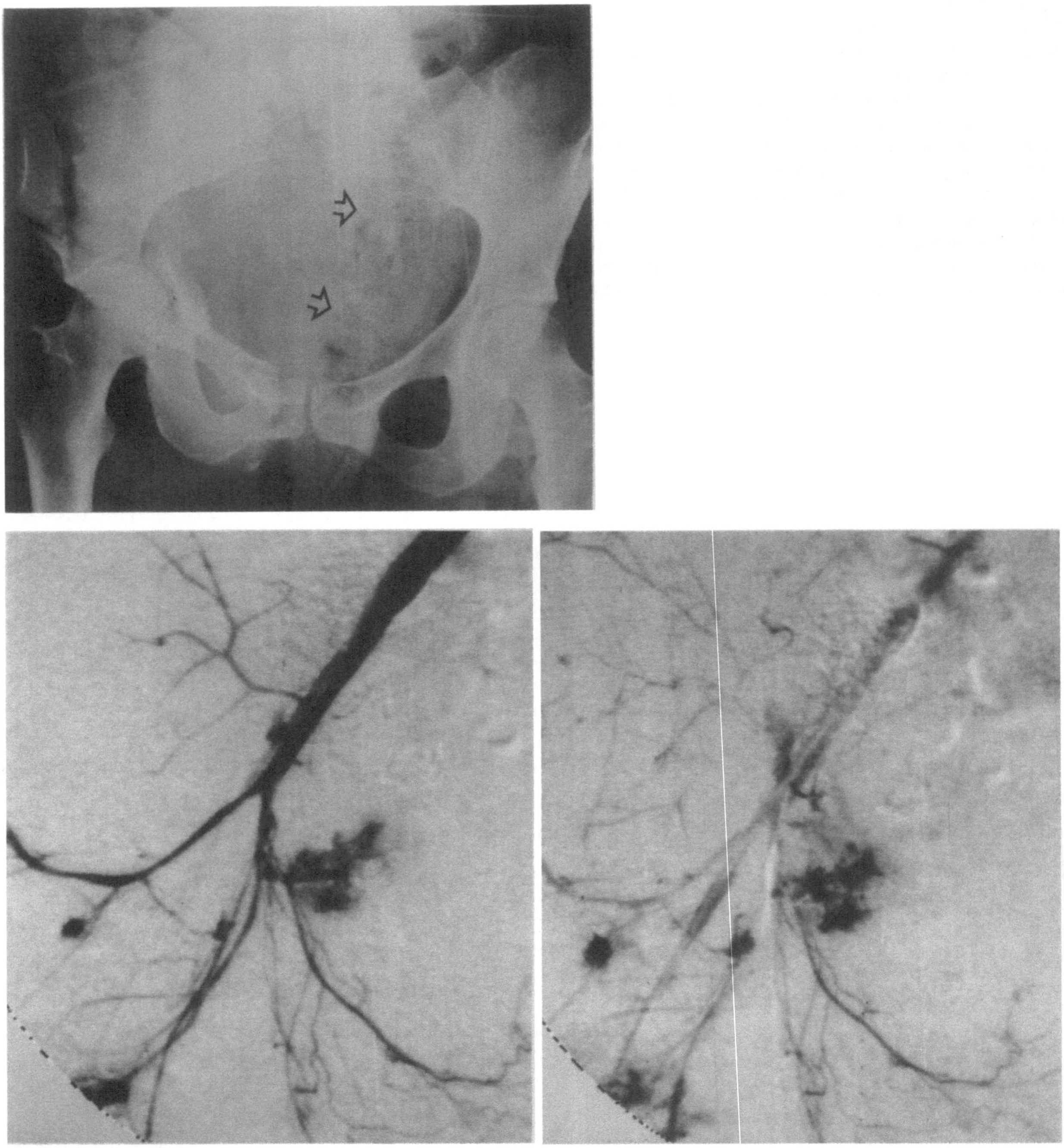

a b c

Fig. 214a–c. Pelvic hemorrhage in a patient with multiple injuries. **a** *Supine pelvic film* demonstrates anterior and posterior pelvic ring fractures on the right side with a hip fracture and avulsion of the iliac wing. The partially gas-filled rectum is displaced to the left by a mass of soft-tissue density (→) (hemorrhage). Intraarterial digital subration angiography: **b** *IA-DSA* selective catheterization of the right internal iliac artery shows multiple sites of contrast extravasation as evidence of the arterial hemorrhage. **c** Late arterial phase (Prof. Dr. K. J. Pfeifer, Department of Radiology, Surgical Hospital and Outpatient Clinic, University of Munich)

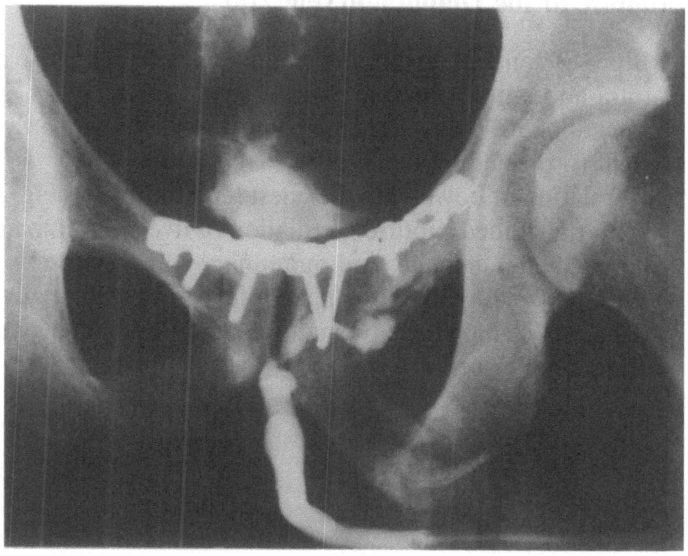

Fig. 215. Urethral rupture accompanying pelvic fracture in a multiply injured patient. Man, 21 years old, was involved in a traffic accident, sustaining anterior and posterior pelvic ring fractures that were managed by internal fixation. Urethrogram shows an imcomplete urethral rupture. Part of the contrast medium enters the bladder, and part is extravasated into the superficial perineal space (Prof. Dr. K.J. Pfeiffer, Department of Radiology, Surgical Hospital and Outpatient Clinic, University of Munich)

Radiologic Signs

Plain Radiographs (Figs. 213 d, 214 a, 215)
Skeletal injuries, dislocation with acetabular injury, soft-tissue density, shifting of phleboliths on repeat examinations as a result of increasing hematoma, intravesical air-collection, free air with intraperitoneal perforation of the vagina or rectosigmoid.

Contrast Examination (Cystography) (Figs. 213 e, f, 215)
(Instillation of 100–200 ml Amidotrizoate 65%): contrast extravasation
Enema with water-soluble contrast for suspected perforation of the rectum or vagina

Note: Barium-containing contrast medium is contraindicated when a perforation is suspected!
Contrast extravasation outside the peritoneal cavity often can be detected only by elevated intra-abdominal pressure during voiding.

Sonography (Fig. 213)
Soft-tissue density in the lesser pelvis (hematoma may be indistinguishable from blood-tinged urinoma)
Free intraperitoneal fluid with an intraperitoneal rupture
With hematuria: coagulated blood in the bladder

Computed Tomography
Soft-tissue mass, fluid in the lesser pelvis. Usually CT can differentiate fresh hematoma from urinoma. It can assign the mass to the pelvic organs and establish the extent of bony injuries (central hip dislocation, sacroiliac plate fracture). CT may disclose fractures that are not appreciated on conventional radiographic views.

Rupture of the Diaphragm (Fig. 216)

- Blunt abdominal or thoracic trauma with an acute rise of intra-abdominal pressure
- Location: 90% of ruptures are on the left side, and only 10% are on the right (protected by the liver!)
- Herniation of bowel into the chest (enterothorax) (Fig. 216 a)
- With right-sided rupture: herniation of liver with impaired perfusion, parenchymal damage, and pulmonary compression
- With perforating diaphragmatic injury from stab or gunshot wounds: danger of hemorrhage (hematopneumothorax, concomitant injury of abdominal viscera)

Caution: Herniation of the small bowel may be delayed for hours or days and may occur gradually as a result of negative intrathoracic pressure. Thus, *rupture of the diaphragm* with herniation of the bowel should be suspected in a trauma patient who develops respiratory difficulties or takes a downhill turn several days after the injury (auscultation will disclose bowel sounds in the left axilla).

Clinical Symptoms

Acute abdomen with cardiorespiratory disorders, free interval with bilateral rupture

Radiologic Signs

Plain Radiographs (Fig. 216 b, c)
Elevation of the diaphragm (in some cases), immobility of the diaphragm, multiple fluid levels in the chest, direct demonstration of air-filled bowel loops, wide soft-tissue density in the right basal area (basal atelectasis, lung injury)

Contrast Examination
Demonstration of contrast-filled bowel loops within the chest after oral administration of contrast medium

Sonography
Usually is unrewarding

Computed Tomography
Will not demonstrate the rupture directly but will disclose intrathoracic bowel segments or injuries of the liver and spleen

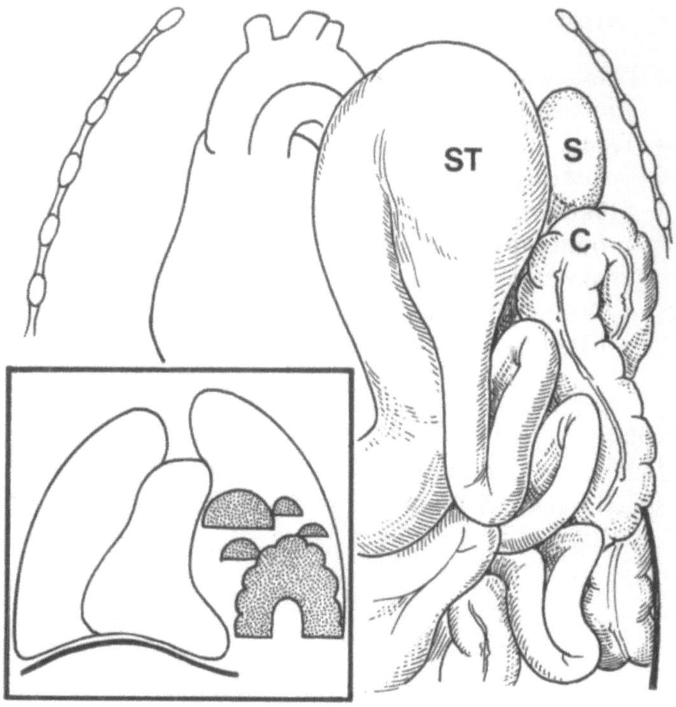

a

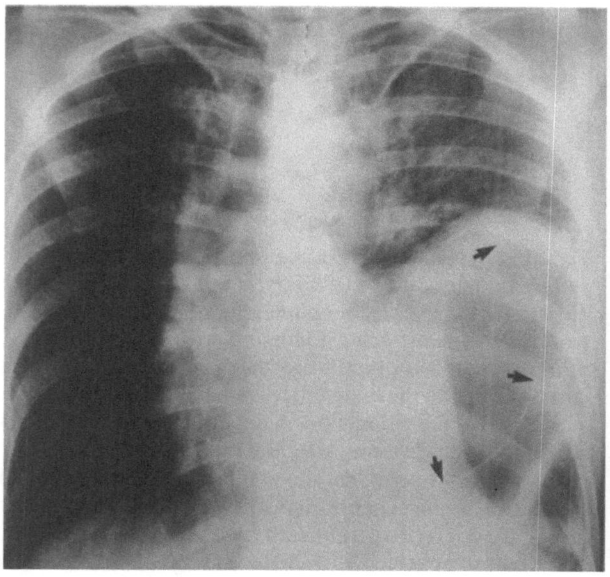

b

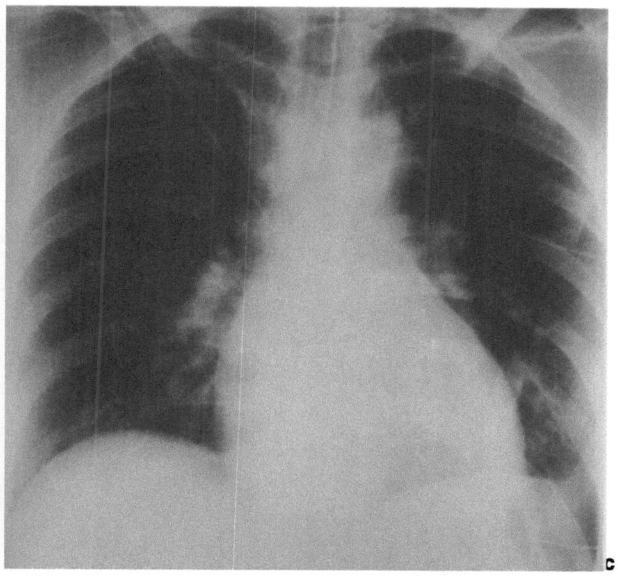

c

Fig. 216. a Left-sided diaphragmatic rupture with enterothorax (*St*, stomach; *S*, spleen; *C*, splenic flexure). The boxed diagram shows the typical radiographic signs: multiple fluid levels in the left half of the chest, nonvisualization of the left hemidiaphragm (modified from Reifferscheid 1977). **b, c Left-sided diaphragmatic rupture** in a 35-year-old woman after blunt abdominal trauma. **b** *Supine chest film* displays stomach and air-filled bowel loops in the chest cavity, dystelectasis of the left lung, and a mediastinal shift toward the right side; indwelling gastric tube (→). **c** *Supine chest film* following surgical repair of the diaphragm and placement of a chest tube (Prof. Dr. K. J. Pfeifer, Department of Radiology, Surgical Hospital and Outpatient Clinic, University of Munich)

Pancreatic Trauma (Fig. 217)

- Blunt crushing injury (steering-wheel injury in car accidents, handlebar injury of bicycle); multiple injuries are common
- Types
  - Contusion with hemorrhage and preservation of organ contour
  - Parenchymal tears, possible with injury to the pancreatic duct
  - Injury of the head of the pancreas with damage to the duodenum or common bile duct
  - Traumatic pancreatic pseudocyst
  - Bleeding into the omental bursa

Clinical Symptoms
Symptoms tend to be masked by other visceral injuries; there are no specific signs. Serum amylase has limited diagnostic value.

a
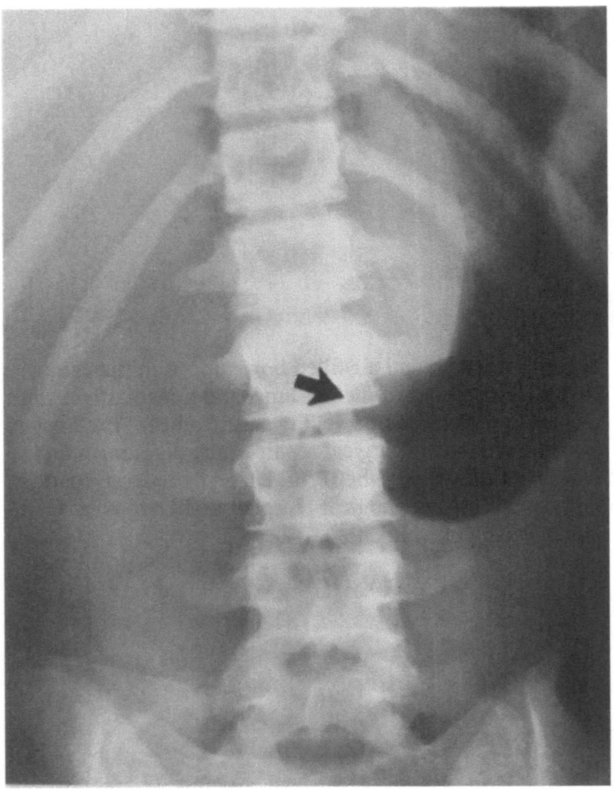

Fig. 217 a–f. Pancreatic trauma in a 13-year-old boy who suffered a perforating eye injury in a fall from a mini-bike. He was first treated in an ophthalmic clinic, where the patient developed an "acute abdomen" with massiv vomiting. **a** *Supine film* shows that the stomach is distended with gas and displaced to the left, with termination of the air column at the level of the pylorus (➧). A large soft-tissue density obscures the right psoas muscle; the rest of the abdomen is gasless. **b** *Left lateral film* shows a crescentic air collection in the area of the superior duodenal flexure (⇨) and a long gastric fluid level, superimposed by an external catheter and a button projected over the lower edge of the right 12th rib. **c** Pseudocyst in the region of the pancreatic head. *Sonogram* (longitudinal scan) shows a large, hypoechoic lesion under the right margin of the liver that is compressing the inferior vena cava *(C)*. Clotted blood and sediment are visible inside the cyst. **d–f** *Sonogram* taken after about 250 ml of blood-tinged fluid was aspirated from the cyst. Transverse scan at the level of the pancreatic head shows a marked diminution in the size of the cyst with floating echo complexes. The fluid-filled, atonic duodenum *(D)* is compressed into a crescent shape; *K*, right kidney (**d**). Corresponding longitudinal scan of the now smaller precaval cyst (⇨), which is causing less compression of the inferior vena cava *(C)* (**e**). Corresponding *CT scan* (**f**) shows a posttraumatic pseudocyst of the head of the pancreas *(Z)* flanked by two small areas of hemorrhage (→), *G*, gallbladder

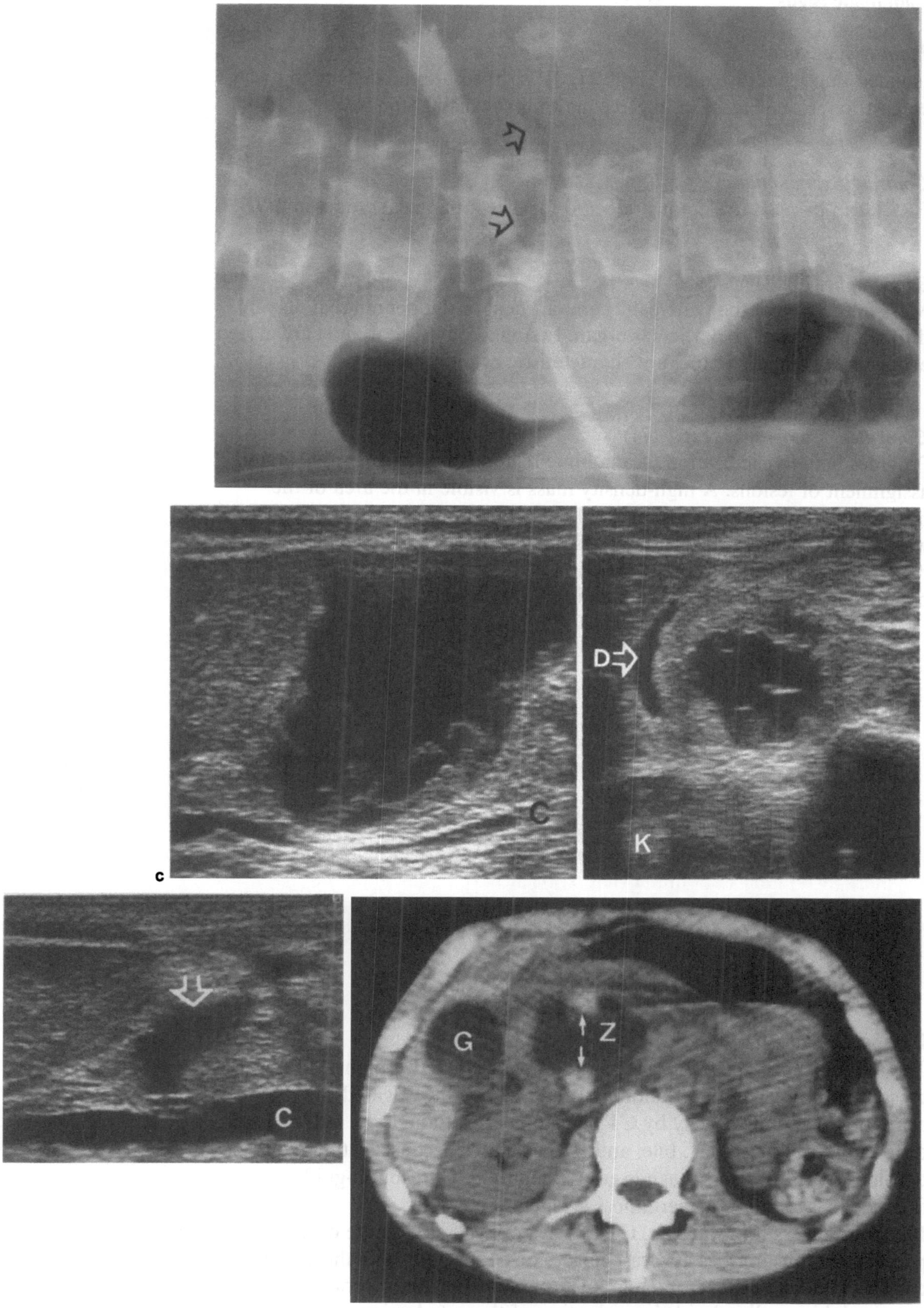

Fig. 217 b–f (Legend see page 372)

Radiologic Signs

Plain Radiographs

Isolated duodenal distension (Figs. 11, 217 a, b) soft-tissue density in the epigastric region (Fig. 217 a, b), free air with coexisting injuries.

Contrast Examination

ERCP can be used to demonstrate and localize a pancreatic duct injury.

Sonography (Fig. 217 c–e)

Mass in the area of the pancreatic compartment or duodenum that may be difficult to assign to a particular organ. Lesions from fresh trauma are more echogenic, while cystic foci are characteristic of older trauma.

Computed Tomography (Fig. 217 f)

Provides better visualization of anatomic relationships and permits organs assignment of lesions. A high-density mass is visible in the area of the pancreas with a fresh contusion and hemorrhage, and a low-density mass with an older contusion. A pseudocyst may form from leakage of pancreatic enzymes. A simple contusion is indistinguishable from a parenchymal tear or pancreatic duct injury in the early stages.

Caution: A traumatic "acute" pseudocyst from a pancreatic duct injury is strongly suggested by a continuous increase in the size of the cyst!

Note: Because coexisting injuries (see above) frequently dominate the picture, care should always be taken to consider pancreatic injuries in the differential diagnosis, especially when there is superficial evidence of blunt upper abdominal trauma.
Also, one should always consider the possibility of *bilateral* injuries (spleen, liver, diaphragm) even when complaints appear to be unilateral. Whenever an intra-abdominal fluid collection (blood, urine, bile) is detected sonographically in the trauma patient, injury to an internal organ should be suspected until proof to the contrary has been obtained.

Diagnostic Procedures

The first diagnostic procedure is plain radiography in two planes, followed by sonography. Free intra-abdominal fluid can be investigated by aspiration or noninvasively by CT densitometry, although the latter cannot differentiate among urine, bile, and serous ascites because of their equal densities. A fresh hemorrhage is easily identified. Ultrasound-guided, fine-needle aspiration or peritoneal lavage are possible.
If sonography is unrewarding, CT can be very valuable in the diagnosis of parenchymatous injuries and vascular lesions, especially with the use of i.v. contrast material. The peroral administration of contrast material (usually a water-soluble medium) aids in evaluation of the gut. Angiography is used when CT is unavailable or if the foregoing procedures are inconclusive; it is also used when there is a primary suspicion of vascular injury, or therapeutic embolization is being considered.

References

Ben-Menachem V (1981) Blunt Trauma. Radiol Clin North Am 19: 1

Botsford J, Wilson A (1981) The acute abdomen. Enke, Stuttgart

Burri C (1976) Trauma surgery. Springer, Berlin Heidelberg New York

Bowermann J (1977) Radiology and injury in sport. Appleton-Century-Crofts, New York

Braedel HV, Rzedak L, Schindler E et al. (1980) Computertomographische Untersuchungen bei Nierenverletzungen. RÖFO 132: 49

Brecht G, Lackner K, Janson R, Thurn P (1980) Die Computertomographie der Notfalldiagnostik. RÖFO 132: 272

Federle MP, Goldberg HI, Kaiser JA et al. (1981) Evaluation of abdominal trauma by computed tomography. Radiology 138: 637

Fischedick AR, Müller RP (1982) Bedeutung der Computertomographie bei Nierenverletzungen. Röntgenblätter 35: 218-221

Fischedick AR, Müller RP, Kramps H, Cramer B (1982) Computertomographie retroperitonealer Traumen. Fortschr Röntgenstr 136: 56

Friedmann G, Mödder U (1982) Computertomographie bei Bauchtraumen. Radiologe 22: 112

Friedmann G, Wenz W, Ebel K-D, Bücheler E (1983) Dringliche Röntgendiagnostik-Traumatologie und akute Erkrankungen. Thieme, Stuttgart

Greenbaum EI (1982) Radiology of the emergency patient. Wiley, New York

Heim U, Baltensweiler J (1981) Checkliste Traumatologie. Thieme, Stuttgart

Heller M, Jend HH, Genant HK (1986) Computed tomography of trauma. Thieme, Stuttgart

Hertel M (1975) Röntgendiagnostik viszeraler Verletzungen. Thieme, Stuttgart

Kuhn FP, Schreyer T, Schild H et al. (1983) Sonographie beim stumpfen Bauchtrauma. Fortschr Röntgenstr : 310

Lorenz R, Beyer D, Peters PE (1984) Detection of intraperitoneal bile accumulations: Significance of ultrasonography, CT and cholescintigraphy. Gastrointest Radiol 9: 213

Lorenz R, Beyer D, Buschsieweke U (im Druck) Rationelle Milzdiagnostik durch Einsatz von Sonographie und Computertomographie. Röntgenpraxis

Meyers MA (1982) Dynamic Radiology of the Abdomen. Springer, Berlin Heidelberg New York

Reifferscheid J (1977) Surgery. Thieme, Stuttgart

Sandler CM, Hall JT, Rodriguez MB, Corriere JN (1986) Bladder injury in blunt pelvic trauma. Radiology 158: 633-638

Stampfel G, Joost J (1984) Die Ureterruptur nach stumpfem Bauchtrauma. RÖFO 141 (5): 570-573

Stampfel G, Scheiber K, Rauschmeier H (1986) Sonographische Verlaufskontrolle bei zweizeitiger Nierenruptur. Röntgenblätter 39: 114-116

4.6 Soft-Tissue Lesions of the Abdominal Wall and Back That Produce Acute Symptoms

R. LORENZ, D. BEYER

Note: The diagnosis of a "soft-tissue lesion" should not divert attention away from a coexisting organic disease, and vice-versa. Thus *inspection* and *palpation* at the start of the examination are important in making a diagnosis. Local pain does not necessarily originate in the palpated area.
Because of the association between organic disease and the referral of pain to specific dermatomic areas, visceral disease should be sought whenever pain is accompanied by apparently normal local findings on inspection and palpation.

Hematoma (Fig. 218)

Causes
Trauma, therapy with anticoagulants, coagulopathy, penetration of a subcutaneous vascular prosthetis graft, fractures

Radiologic Signs

Plain Radiographs
Soft-tissue density, widening of flank stripe, obliteration of psoas shadow

Sonography
Localized echogenic (fresh hematoma) or hypoechoic (old hematoma) liquid mass (Fig. 218e, f, g).
Configuration: round or spindle-shaped, elongated with rectus sheath hematoma
Paravascular fluid collection (bleeding) associated with a suture aneurysm after the subcutaneous insertion of a prosthetic graft or with a perforation or penetration of an aneurysm.

Fig. 218a–g. Acute hemorrhage into the soft tissues of the abdominal wall and back with "acute abdomen." a Spontaneous rupture of intercostal artery with acute abdomen in a 65-year-old man. Patient developed massive swelling of the right chest wall 30 min after a severe coughing fit. *CT scan* shows marked expansion of the intercostal muscle by a tissue-isodense hemorrhage; *L*, liver. **b Spontaneous hemorrhage related to anticoagulants** in a 55-year-old man who underwent cardiac valve replacement. Patient had increasing weakness of the right leg, which began also to affect the left side. *CT scan* shows a high-density hematoma expanding the right iliacus muscle *(I)* and displacing the right psoas muscle *(P)*, which, like the left psoas, shows hemorrhagic expansion. **c, d Spontaneous hemorrhage related to anticoagulants** in a 70-year-old man following multiple episodes of pelvic vein thrombosis. Patient had an acute abdomen with a firm, progressive swelling in the right lower quadrant. *CT scan* shows an older, low-density hematoma in the area of the right rectus muscle and a fresher, high-density hematoma in the area of the left rectus abdominis (⇨); the hemorrhage on the left side extends through the musculature to the iliac crest. There is reactive bowel distension with multiple fluid levels (**c**). *CT scan* about 10 cm below the previous scan shows a large, tumorlike hemorrhage into the left anterior abdominal wall with a low-density, irregular center (→) (**d**). **e Bleeding into the abdominal wall following an axillofemoral bypass.** The 57-year-old man developed swelling and acute pains in the left lateral abdominal wall 2 months after implantation of an axillofemoral graft. *Sonogram* (longitudinal scan) shows the graft (►) ensheathed by an echo-free hematoma *(B)*. **f Acute rectus sheath hematoma secondary to anticoagulant overdose.** Man, 39 years old, with acute swelling of the lower left quadrant and severe pain following a pulmonary embolism. *Longitudinal sonogram* of the lower left quadrant shows a liquid, oval-shaped, predominantly echogenic mass (fresh hematoma) with sedimentation. **g** *Transverse sonogram* of the same area also demonstrates the sedimentation ▷

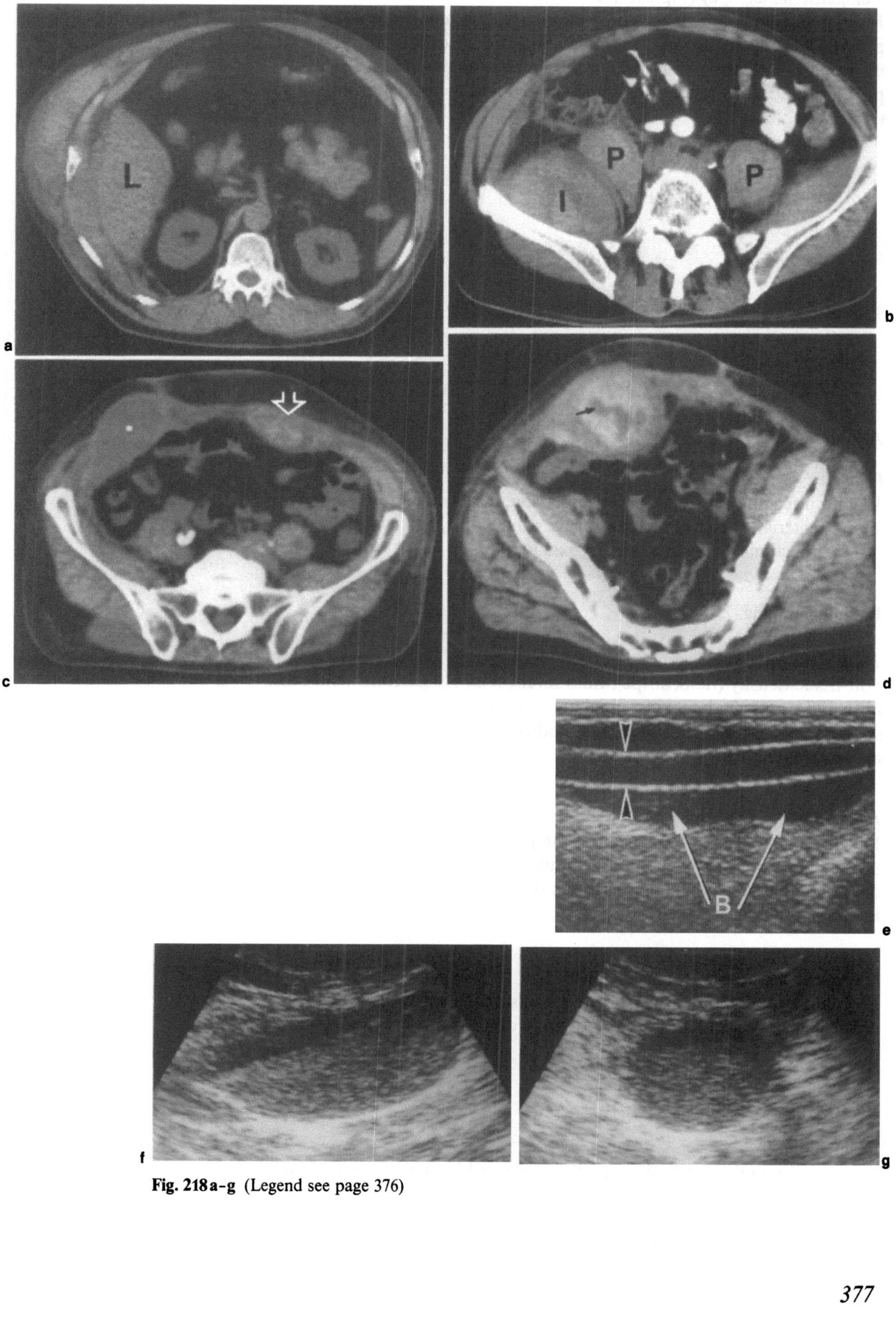

Fig. 218 a–g (Legend see page 376)

Computed Tomography (Fig. 218 a–d)
Fresh hematoma appears as a high-density feature and becomes progressively less dense with sedimentation and absorption of cellular elements. Contrast extravasation may be seen in the area of a vascular prosthesis. Osseous lesions are demonstrated and their relationship to soft tissues established.

Note: Soft-tissue lesions are visible on plain films only if they are struck tangentially by the X-ray beam (flank stripe). Hence, sonography and CT have a special role in detecting the lesions and evaluating their extent.

Abscess (Fig. 219)

Causes
Wound infection, previous surgery, injection, insect sting, foreign body, suture material; diabetes mellitus, acute pancreatitis, leukosis, cytostasis, AIDS, infection of subcutaneous bypass graft

Radiologic Signs

Plain Radiographs
Soft-tissue density (flank stripe), fluid levels, possibly gaseous inclusions, obscured psoas shadow with spinal and paravertebral abscess, signs of spondylodiscitis, radiopaque foreign bodies, calcium inclusions (older abscess, tuberculosis)

Sonography (Fig. 219 a, b)
Localized liquid mass. Expansion of the psoas muscle with paraspinal abscess, possibly gaseous inclusions (multiple floating echo complexes). As the lesion matures, it becomes easier to delineate on account of its thick, irregular wall.

Computed Tomography (Fig. 219 c, d)
Low-density mass and/or soft-tissue expansion, capsular contrast enhancement in an older lesion; gas, bony destruction, foreign body

Incarcerated Hernia (see Fig. 163)

Localization
Inguinal, femoral, umbilical, epigastric incisional hernia; rarely lumbar hernia (triangle between obliquus externus and latissimus dorsi muscles above the iliac crest); ischiatic, obturator, perineal hernia (see Sect. 4.2.1)

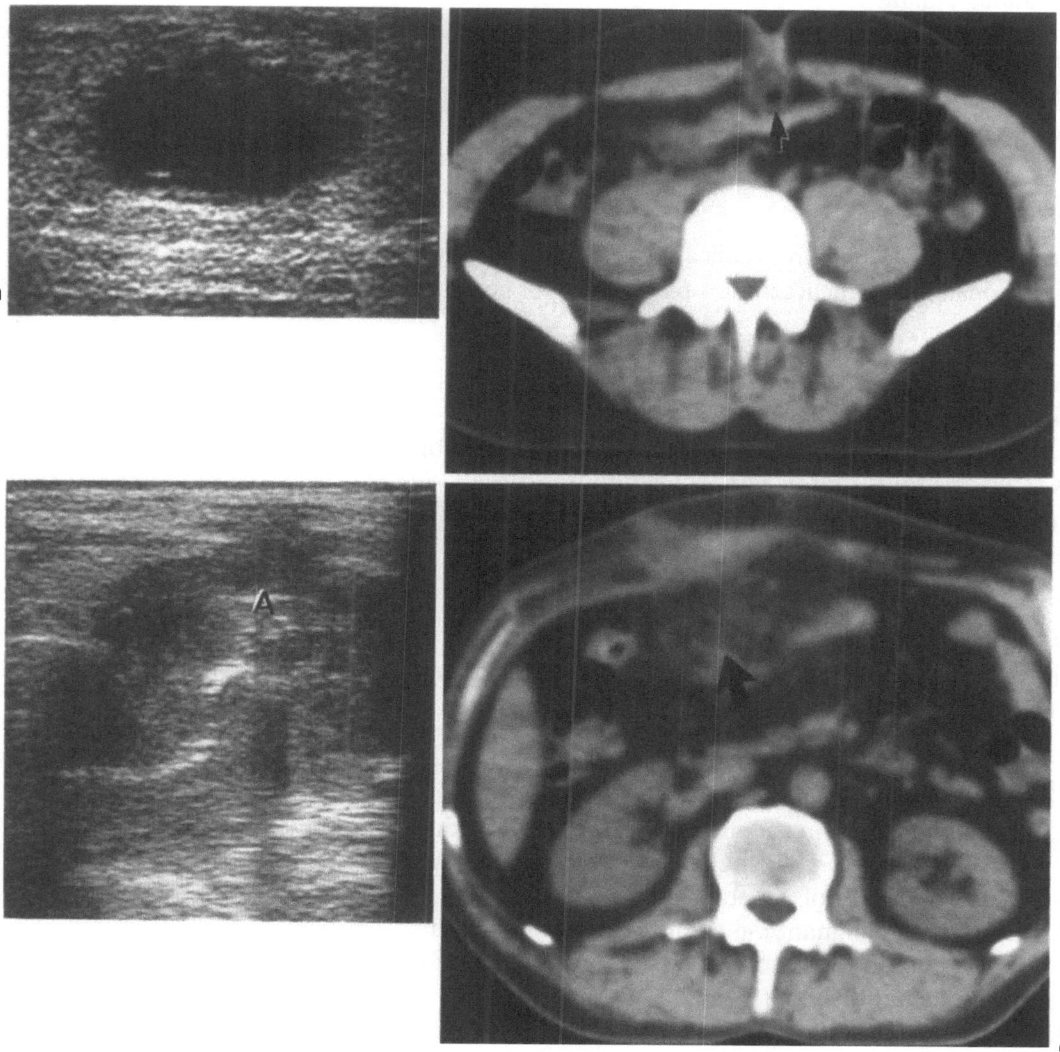

a c b d

Fig. 219 a–d. Abdominal wall abscesses with acute symptoms.
a Abdominal wall abscess after cholecystectomy in a 34-year-old man who had midabdominal pains of acute onset and marked local tenderness. *Sonogram* shows a hypoechoic, irregular, liquid mass in the abdominal wall. **b** Abdominal wall abscess in a 17-year-old man with known Crohn's disease. Patient developed symptoms of partial bowel obstruction with marked abdominal tenderness and distension. *Sonogram* shows an irregular mass with hypoechoic and hyperechoic elements and a central echo complex; *A*, air. **c** Periumbilical abscess in a 40-year-old man with a persistent omphaloenteric duct. Patient had acute tenderness in the umbilical region. *CT scan* at the level of the umbilicus shows a lesion of soft-tissue density with a small gaseous inclusion (➧). **d** Abdominal wall abscess after gastric surgery in a 45-year-old man who experienced acute midabdominal pain with marked tenderness and rigidity 3 weeks postoperatively. *CT scan* shows a reticulated area (➧) below the abdominal wall, which is thickened by scarring. *Operation* disclosed an abscess of the abdominal wall

Radiologic Signs

Plain Radiographs (see Fig. 163 a, b)
Soft-tissue density, atypical gas collection (inguinal, lumbar, abdominal wall, etc.)

Contrast Examination
Irrelevant and even contraindicated with acute symptoms (too time-consuming). Incarceration *blocks* entry of contrast medium into the hernial sac.

Sonography (see Fig. 163 c, d)
Liquid and partly gas-containing mass that may exhibit peristalsis and Kerckring's folds (in the early stage only)
In late stages: thickening of the bowel wall (edema) (Fig. 163 b)

Computed Tomography
Very rarely indicated (rare atypical hernia: obturator hernia, etc.). CT shows a low-density, fluid-containing structure and enhancement in the bowel wall (early stages).

Conditions That Are Relevant to Acute Diagnosis
1. Extranodal lymphomas: about 30% of non-Hodgkin's lymphomas are of extranodal origin; almost all extranodal lymphomas in Hodgkin's disease are a sign of generalization or recurrence
2. Metastases: malignant melanoma, breast carcinoma
3. Primary tumors: sarcoma, Kaposi's sarcoma (AIDS), carcinoma, hemangioendothelioma
4. Osseous lesions: accompanying soft-tissue reaction to trauma, inflammation, neoplasia (primary, secondary, metastatic)
5. Vascular lesion: superficial thrombophlebitis (Mondor's syndrome), prosthetic graft aneurysm
6. Skin disorders: herpes zoster, allergies, burns
7. Spinal processes: spondylodiscitis (Fig. 220), paravertebral abscess

Note: Soft-tissue lesions frequently present a nonspecific sonographic and CT pattern, and it is often impossible to differentiate among hematoma, abscess, lymphoma, leukemic infiltration, and tumor from image features alone!

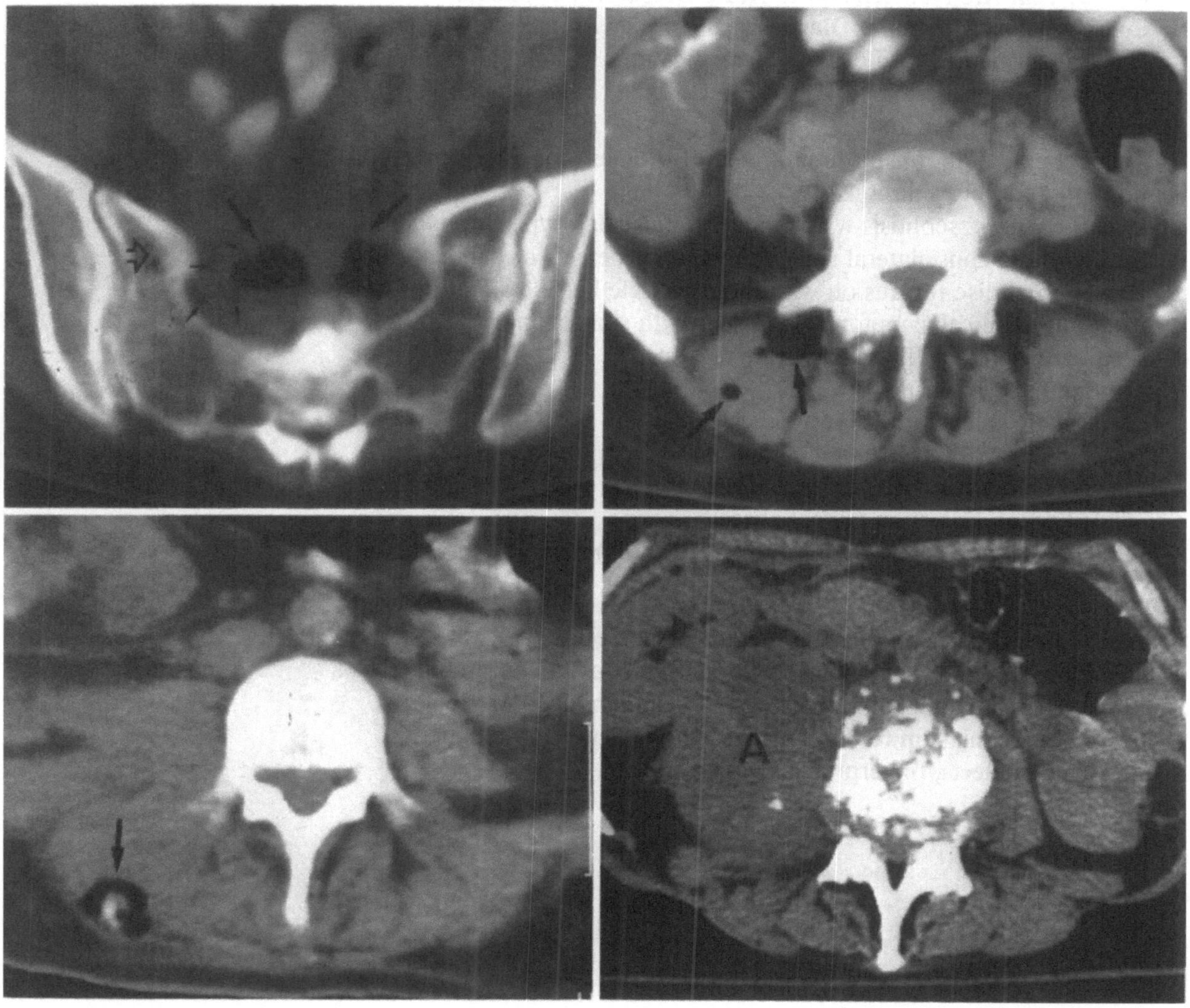

a b c d

Fig. 220a–d. Abscesses of the dorsal and pelvic soft tissues with acute abdominal symptoms. Abscess-forming recurrence of rectal carcinoma, with an abscess ascending through the paraspinal muscles. Woman, 42 years old, with a tender and distended abdomen and left paraspinal tenderness in the back. **a** *CT scan* shows a presacral soft-tissue density with two large air inclusions (➧), smaller right-sided air inclusions (→), and two intraosseous air bubbles in the right lateral portion of the sacrum (⇨). **b** *CT scan* above the iliac crest shows multiple gaseous inclusions in the right erector spinae muscle (→). **c** Paraspinal injection abscess in a 41-year old man with recurring lumbago. Patient developed "abdominal pain" 2 weeks after a right paraspinal injection. *CT scan* through the lower lumbar spine shows expansion of the right erector trunci with a gas collection (➧) and a small central hemorrhagic area. **d** Tuberculous spondylitis with a gravitation abscess in a 55-year-old woman with progressively limited motion in the right leg and acute abdominal pain. *CT scan* through the midlumbar spine shows destruction of the vertebral body by tuberculous spondylitis. The paraspinal musculature is markedly expanded by a large abscess of partly low density *(A)* on the right side of the spine

Conditions That Are Not Relevant to Acute Diagnosis but Should Be Considered in Differential Diagnosis

1. Scar, scar formation with extensive calcifications (usually after midline laparatomy)
2. Lipoma, fibroma, angioma
3. Benign skin alterations: birthmark, neurofibromas (consider spinal cord and peripheral nerve lesions)
4. Skeletal changes: scoliosis with unilateral muscular hypertrophy and atrophy of the contralateral side with postural defects or deformities
5. Intervertebral disc protrusion with reflex muscle hardness and postural deviation; identical symptoms can occur with spinal tumors
6. Calcifications (plain films, sonogram, CT scan):
   - Idiopathic calcinosis
   - Metastatic calcifications in hypercalcemia
   - Ossifying myositis, calcified hematoma
   - Parasites: cysticercosis, guinea worm
   - Calcified postinjection gluteal abscess
   - Phleboliths in AV malformations (see Sect. 3.7)

Sources of Error in Plain Film Interpretation (see Sect. 3.7)

Calcifications, foreign bodies, and soft-tissue changes can be simulated by:

1. Exteral foreign matter: ointments, dyes (containing lead or zinc)
2. Dressing material, skin folds, clothing, objects beneath the patient
3. Film-screen defects, fingerprints, scratches

Note: A soft-tissue lesion that cannot be definitively classified by noninvasive imaging should be investigated by ultrasound- or CT-guided aspiration or biopsy.

References

Miller EI, Rogers A (1982) Sonography of the anterior abdominal wall. Semin Ultras 3: 278

Osborn AG, Koehler R (1982) Computed tomography of the paraspinal musculature: normal and pathologic anatomy. AJR 138: 93

Peters PE, Beyer D (1983) Weichteile. In: Bücheler E, Friedmann G, Thelen M (eds) Real-time Sonographie des Körpers. Thieme, Stuttgart

Yiu-ChiuKV, Chiu L (1982) Multiple imaging modalities in the evaluation of musculoskeletal masses. CT 6: 201

4.7 Acute Diseases of the Lesser Pelvis

D. BEYER, W. STEINBRICH

Causes

Males

Acute prostatitis
Acute prostatic abscess (Fig. 225 c)
Postoperative changes (Fig. 226)

Females

Acute endometritis
Acute adnexitis
Acute salpingitis with pyosalpinx (Fig. 223 a–c)
Abscess in the cul-de-sac (Fig. 225 b)
Tubal rupture in ectopic pregnancy (Fig. 221 a)
Torsion of tumors of pelvic organs (ovarian cyst, subserous myoma) (Fig. 222 c–e)
Mittelschmerz (Fig. 221 c)
Hematocolpos (Fig. 222 a)
Polycystic ovary after hormonal overstimulation (Fig. 222 b)
Postoperative changes

Males and females

Postoperative abscess in the cul-de-sac or extraperitoneally in the lesser pelvis (Figs. 225 a, b, 226)
Acute cystitis
Bladder tamponade (see Sect. 4.5)
Trauma (see Sect. 4.5)

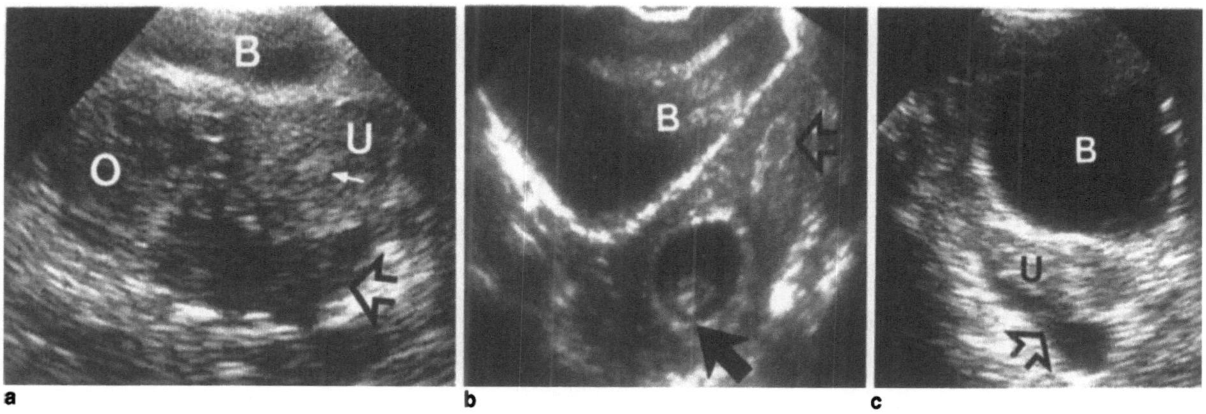

Fig. 221 a–c. Acute pain in the lesser pelvis in young women. a Tubal rupture after 7 weeks of amenorrhea. *Sonogram* (transverse scan) shows a slightly enlarged uterus *(U)* with a pseudogestational sac (→) situated behind the bladder *(B)*; right-sided adnexal tumor *(O)*; free fluid in the cul-de-sac (blood) (⇨). **b** An **intact tubal pregnancy** is shown for comparison. Vaginal bleeding. *Sonogram* (oblique scan) shows a displaced and slightly enlarged uterus with a pseudogestational sac (⇨) behind the bladder *(B)*; intact tubal pregnancy with embryo (➧) in the adnexal region. **c Mittelschmerz, ovulation.** *Sonogram* (longitudinal scan) shows a normal-sized uterus *(U)* behind the bladder *(B)* and small amounts of free fluid in the cul-de-sac (⇨) (Figs. 221 a–c, 222 a, b, c and 223 a, courtesy of Prof. Dr. B. J. Hackelöer, Dept. of Gynaecology and Obstetrics, Barmbeck General Hospital, Hamburg)

Common Clinical Symptoms

Pain in the lower abdomen, often of sudden onset (tumor torsion, tubal abortion), followed by nausea, vomiting, and shock; fever or subfebrile temperatures (in all inflammatory processes); often local muscular guarding in the lower abdomen; attenuated bowel sounds; absence of peristalsis is frequent with tubular abortion and pyosalpinx; menorrhagia with endometritis; dysuria with cystitis and prostatitis

Radiologic Signs

Female Pelvis

Plain Radiographs

Plain radiographs in two planes contribute little to the diagnosis of many lesser pelvic disorders. They may document the reaction of the intestine to the extraperitoneal process, showing typical fluid levels in the L Lat position and in rare cases atypical gas bubbles projected over the lesser pelvis as evidence of an abscess.

Sonography

Sonography has become the primary diagnostic tool. Scans of the lesser pelvis must be performed through the "acoustic window" of the full urinary bladder.

Note: Ectopic pregnancy (EP) can simulate *any* cystic or solid process that may occur in the lesser pelvis! It is imperative that the possibility of EP be considered, therefore.
Sonography is not absolutely reliable. It can exclude EP in 75% of cases, and it can diagnose EP in 80%. This emphasizes the central importance of *clinical presentation* (dramatic course, signs of peritoneal irritation) in the diagnosis of EP.

1. Ectopic pregnancy

- Pseudogestational sac in the uterine cavity mimicking a true gestational sac (Fig. 221 a, b)

Caution: An intact EP may be projected onto the midline and displace the small, nondistended uterus to one side, giving the impression of an intact pregnancy! One should always establish the relationship between the gestational sac and the uterine cervix to verify that the pregnancy is intrauterine!

- Demonstration of an intact EP in the cul-de-sac or adnexal region (rare: 1%–5% of all EPs). Signs of viability from a live, intact fetus (Fig. 221 b)
- Tubal abortion, tubal rupture: blood (free fluid) in the cul-de-sac with some solid components. A solid-looking mass is often seen with a confined rupture (Fig. 221 a). Distended, blood-filled uterine tube (hematosalpinx)

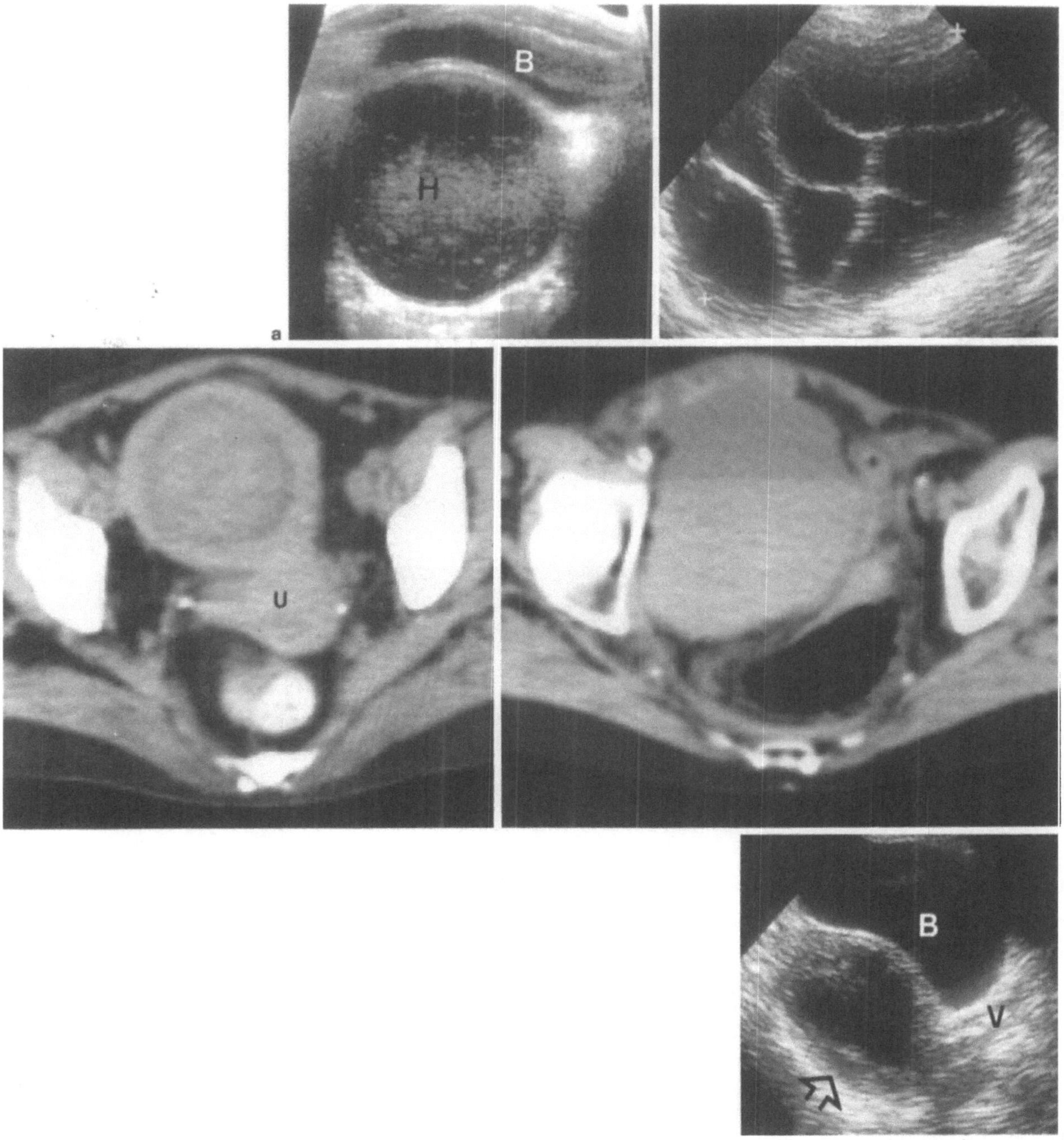

Fig. 222 a–e. Pain in the lesser pelvis with a space-occupying lesion and no fever. a Girl, 14 years old, had increasing pain in the lower abdomen. *Sonogram* shows a hypoechoic, rounded mass behind the bladder (*B*, displaced anteriorly) with floating echo complexes and posterior acoustic enhancement: hematocolpos *(H)* in hymenal atresia (source as in Fig. 221). **b** Right lower quadrant tenderness and full sensation in a 32-year-old woman following overstimulation with HMG-HCG. *Sonogram* shows a polycystic ovary with giant follicles. No cystoma: Patient was treated nonoperatively (source as in Fig. 221). **c** Woman, 50 years old, experienced acute hypogastric pain 3 days earlier that slowly subsided, leaving a dull pain in the lower abdomen; hypoperistalsis. *CT scan* shows a round mass with a central, low-density area communicating directly with the uterus *(U)*. *Operation* disclosed a large, subserous uterine myoma with a twisted pedicle and central necrosis. **d** Woman, 43 years old, experienced sudden right lower quadrant pain, aperistalsis, and nausea. *CT scan* shows a large, soft-tissue density in the right anterior hemipelvis with a fluid level caused by bleeding and sedimentation (56 Hn units). *Operation* disclosed an ovarian cyst with a twisted pedicle. **e** Postmenopausal woman, 62 years old, had lower abdominal tenderness and no fever. *Sonogram* shows a large, fluid-filled mass with a thick wall in the uterine position (⇨) above the vagina *(V)* and posterior to the bladder *(B)*. *Operation* disclosed hematometra secondary to endometrial carcinoma (source as in Fig. 221)

Note: Ovulation can likewise produce lower abdominal pain and sonographic signs of free fluid in the cul-de-sac (Fig. 22c)!

2. Tubo-ovarian abscess

This lesion is easily demonstrated by virtue of its cystic features, while echogenic elements and thick walls give clues to the presence of purulent debris. Gas bubbles will be apparent in a gas-forming abscess, and frequently the cul-de-sac will contain small amounts of inflammatory exudate (Fig. 223).

Often it is necessary to differentiate between adnexitis and appendicitis. With negative adnexal findings, the psoas region should be examined to exclude the possibility of perityphlitic abscess (see Sect. 4.1.4).

a b c

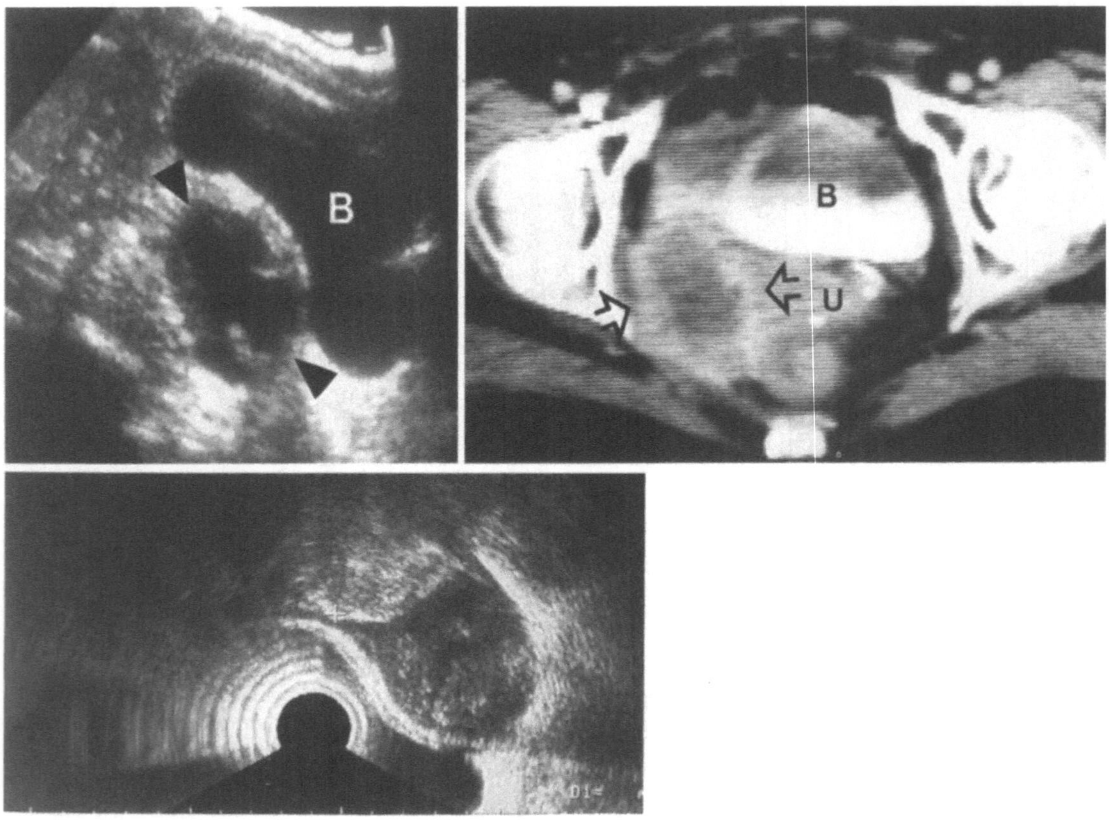

Fig. 223 a–c. Tubo-ovarian abscesses.
a Woman, 27 years old, with suspected adnexitis, fever, and tenderness in the right lower quadrant. *Sonogram* (right paramedian longitudinal scan) shows a large liquid mass with thick walls (►◄) in the ovarian position posterior to the filled bladder *(B)*. Tubo-ovarian abscess; nonoperative treatment (source as in Fig. 221). **b** Woman, 31 years old, with same clinical symptoms. *CT scan (bolus injection)* shows a low-density mass with marked peripheral enhancement (⇨⇦) behind the bladder (*B*, partly filled with opacified urine) and adjacent to the normal-sized uterus *(U)*. Moderate small-bowel distension with fluid levels. **c** Tubo-ovarian abscess of the right ovary in a 35-year-old woman with unexplained lower abdominal pain. The patient was afebrile, and her ESR was high. Transvaginal sonogram shows a cystic-solid mass in the cul-de-sac with highly positive inflammatory parameters. Needle aspiration identified the mass as an abscess (Prof. Dr. J. Hackeloer, Department of Gynecology, Barmbeck General Hospital, Hamburg)

3. Pedicular torsion in genital tumors
This condition is difficult to confirm with ultrasound as a cause of acute abdomen. CT is advised (Fig. 222 c, d).

Computed Tomography
CT has few indications in the acute abdomen with pain in the lesser pelvis. Tubo-ovarian abscesses are demonstrated as clearly with CT as with ultrasound (Fig. 223 b).
Pedicular torsion in genital tumors is evidenced by bleeding and central necrosis (Fig. 222 c, d).
CT is excellent for demonstrating small gas bubbles in the lesser pelvis associated with an abscess (Figs. 224, 226 c)

Male Pelvis
The only disorder worth mentioning in this context is *prostatic abscess,* which is readily demonstrated with ultrasound (Fig. 225 b). Simple prostatitis may not produce sonographic signs other than enlargement of the gland.

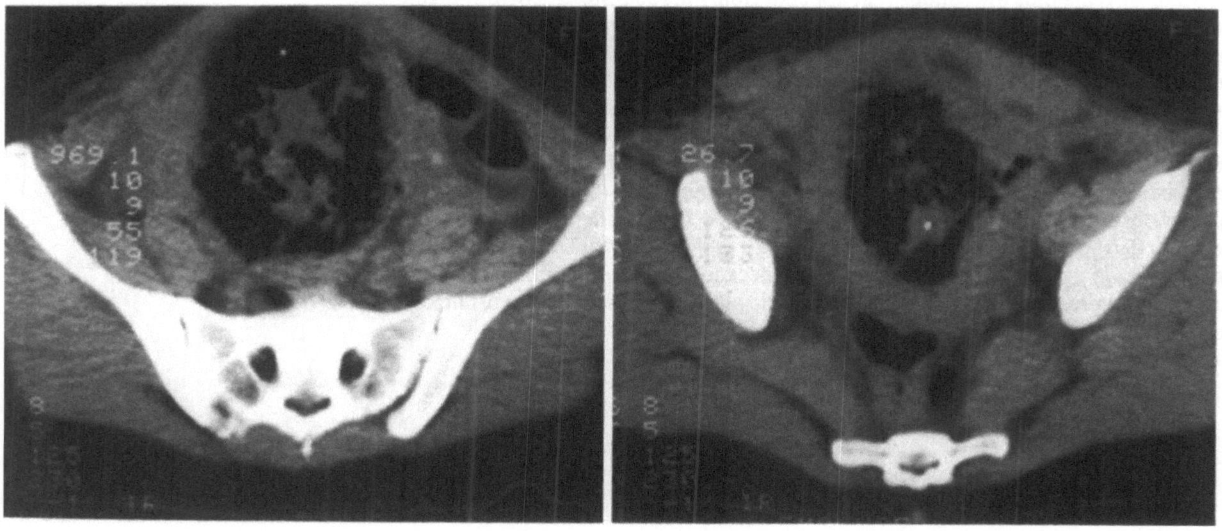

a b

Fig. 224 a, b. Puerperal endometritis caused by gas-forming bacteria. Meteorism and a fall of hemoglobin were noted 1 day after cesarean section in a 28-year-old primipara. Other findings were elevations of bilirubin and alkaline phosphatase, bilious vomiting, and increasing jaundice of the skin; no fever. **a** *CT scan* shows a large, atonic uterus that extends past the umbilicus and contains a massive central gas collection. Uterine wall has a thickened, mottled appearance. No ascites. Moderate small-bowel distension with fluid levels. **b** *CT scan* at a more caudal level shows gas and debris in the uterine cavity. *Operation* disclosed a necrotic, flaccid, gray-colored uterus with diffuse endomyometritis. *Bacteriology* demonstrated aerobic spore-forming organisms, presumably clostridial. (Courtesy of Prof. Dr. H. Kiefer, Department of Radiology, German Clinic für Diagnostics, Wiesbaden)

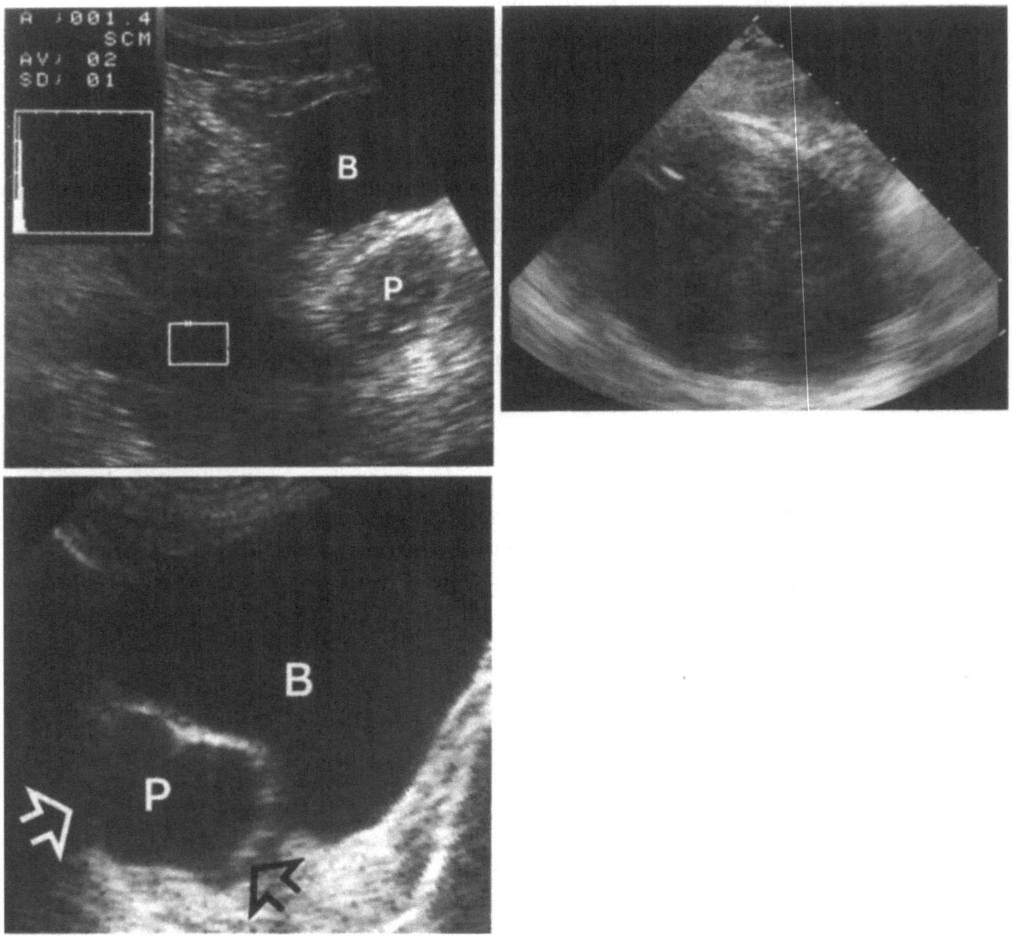

a b c

Fig. 225 a–c. Acute pelvic pain with fever.
a Man, 24 years old, who underwent appendectomy abroad presented with high fever, right lower quadrant tenderness, and intestinal atony. *Sonogram* (longitudinal scan) shows an echo-free mass with maplike borders situated above the bladder *(B)* and prostate *(P)* between loops of bowel. Gray scale measurement confirms a cystic mass. *Operation* disclosed a large intraperitoneal abscess in the right lower quadrant between bowel loops. **b** Cul-de-sac abscess in a patient with unexplained lower abdominal pain and fever. *Sonogram* shows anterior displacement of the uterus *(U)*. The cul-de-sac is occupied by a large, predominantly liquid mass. A drainage tube *(D)* is introduced from the posterior fornix under ultrasonic guidance (Prof. Dr. J. Hackelöer, Department of Gynecology, Barmbeck General Hospital, Hamburg). **c** Man, 28 years old, with fever and perineal pain aggravated by urination and defecation. *Sonogram* (oblique scan) shows an enlarged prostate *(P)* pushing upward on the bladder floor *(B)*. The prostate contains echo-free fluid (⇨). *Diagnosis:* large prostatic abscess

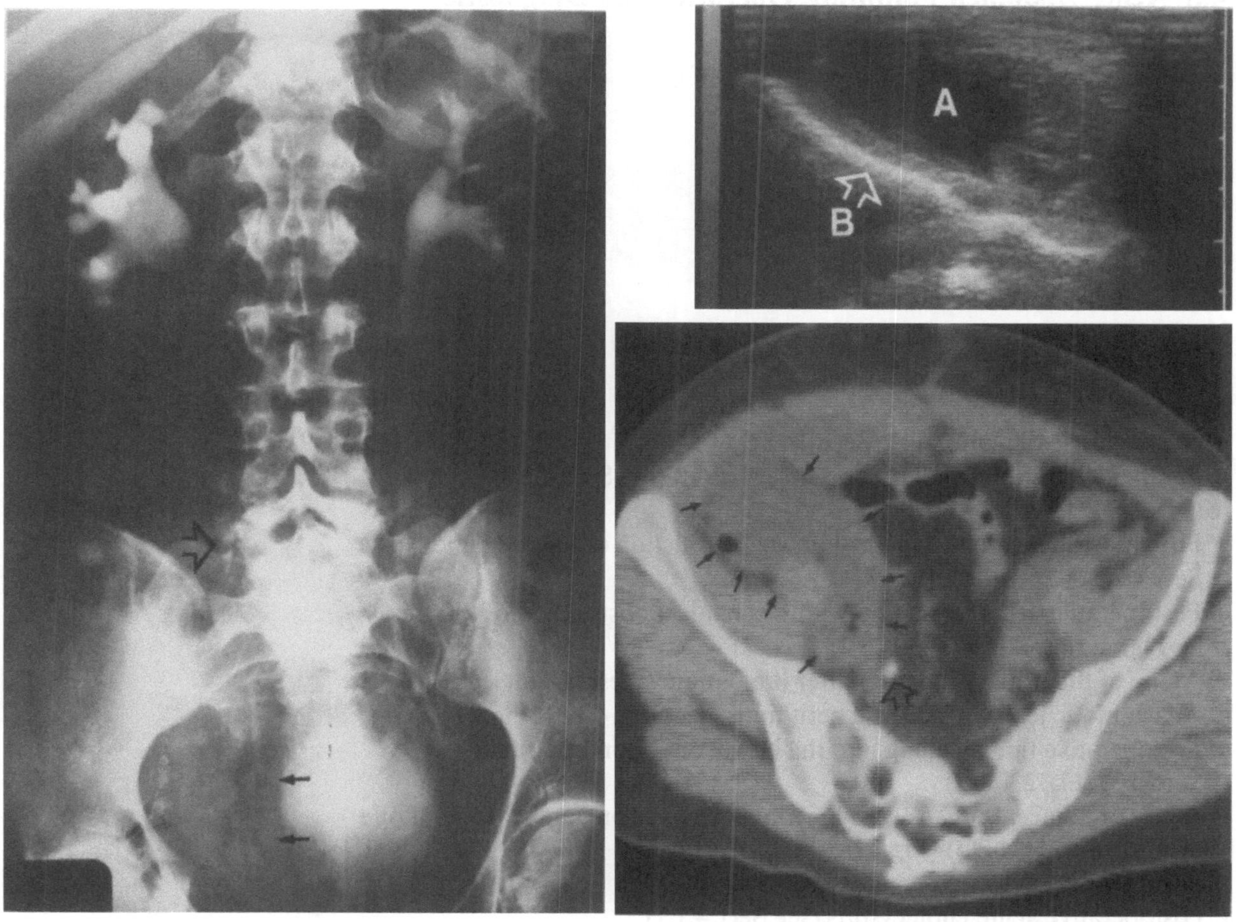

a b c

Fig. 226a–c. Abscess on the pelvic wall. Man, 24 years old, who had undergone right-sided inguinal lymphadenectomy for a teratoma of the right testicle developed right flank pain radiating to the groin, burning on urination, and fever in the 3rd postoperative week. **a** *Urogram* shows congestion of the right renal collection system and right ureter to the level of S1 (⇨). There is a mass in the right side of the lesser pelvis displacing the bladder to the left (→). **b** *Sonogram* (transverse scan) shows a thick-walled hypoechoic mass *(A)* anterior to the right iliac wing *(B)* (⇨) and iliopsoas muscle. Right-sided renal congestion is also present (not shown). **c** *CT scan* shows an abscess anterior to the right iliac wing gaseous inclusions (→). Dilatation of the right ureter (⇨). ***Operation*** disclosed an abscess on the pelvic wall anterior to the right iliopsoas muscle causing ureteral compression with right-sided outflow obstruction and bladder displacement

References

Hansmann M, Hackelöer BJ, Staudach A (1984) Ultraschalldiagnostik in Geburtshilfe und Gynäkologie. Springer, Berlin Heidelberg New York

Kiefer H, Berle P, Harding P (1982) Computertomographische Diagnose einer Endometritis puerperalis durch gasbildende Bakterien. Fortschr Röntgenstr 137/4: 476–478

Screevinas VJ (1980) Acute disorders of the abdomen. Diagnosis and treatment. Springer, Berlin Heidelberg New York

Skaane P, Katre SP (1981) Spontaneous rupture of a massive physopyometra presenting as a acute abdominal emergency. Fortschr Röntgenstr 134: 697–698

Steinbrich W (1982) Computertomographie des weiblichen Genitale. Normale Anatomie und Ergebnisse bei gynäkologischen Tumoren. Inauguraldissertation, Univ. Köln

4.8 Acute Abdomen Following Operative and Diagnostic Procedures

P. E. Peters, D. Beyer

Note: The major causes of acute abdomen in the postoperative setting are paralytic ileus, mechanical bowel obstruction, peritonitis, abscess, and hemorrhage, usually accompanied by cardiopulmonary complications.

Causes
- Acute gastric dilatation (see Sect. 3.1.1)
- Paralytic ileus (intestinal pseudo-obstruction) (see Sect. 4.2.3) (Fig. 227 a, b)
- Early postoperative mechanical bowel obstruction (adhesive bands) (see Sect. 4.2.1)
- Postoperative fecal impaction with mechanical obstruction of the small and large bowel (see Sect. 4.2.2)
- Atony of the urinary bladder (after lumbar anesthesia) (see Sect. 3.6)
- Anastomotic leak with diffuse peritonitis (see Sect. 4.1.3) (Fig. 227 c, d)
- Postoperative free bleeding into the bowel or abdominal cavity (see Sect. 4.3) (Fig. 227 f, g)
- Injury of adjacent organs with bleeding, perforation, and leakage of bile or urine (see Sect. 3.3) (Fig. 228)
- Postoperative acute pancreatitis (see Sect. 4.1.2)
- Postoperative acute cholecystitis (see Sect. 4.1.1)
- Postoperative abscess (see Sect. 4.1.5) (Fig. 231)
- Postoperative obstructive jaundice
- Cardiopulmonary complications, some associated with abdominal pain (postoperative pneumonia, pleurisy, pulmonary embolism, myocardial infarction)

Note: With unexplained postoperative abdominal complaints or fever, the abdominal survey should always be supplemented by a chest radiograph!

Diagnostic Problems
Diagnostic imaging is hampered by
- the seriously ill and bedridden condition of most patients, and lack of patient cooperation
- dressings, suture material, drains, catheters
- postoperative free residual air and atonic gastrointestinal distension
- difficult clinical examining conditions

The postoperative acute abdomen is a serious entity with a high mortality rate. Diagnostic evaluation must be rapid, atraumatic, and efficient!

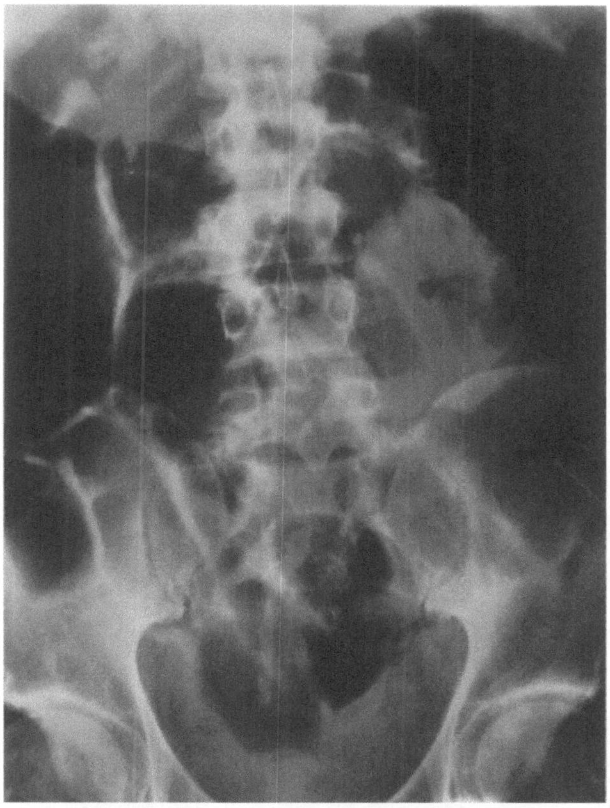

a

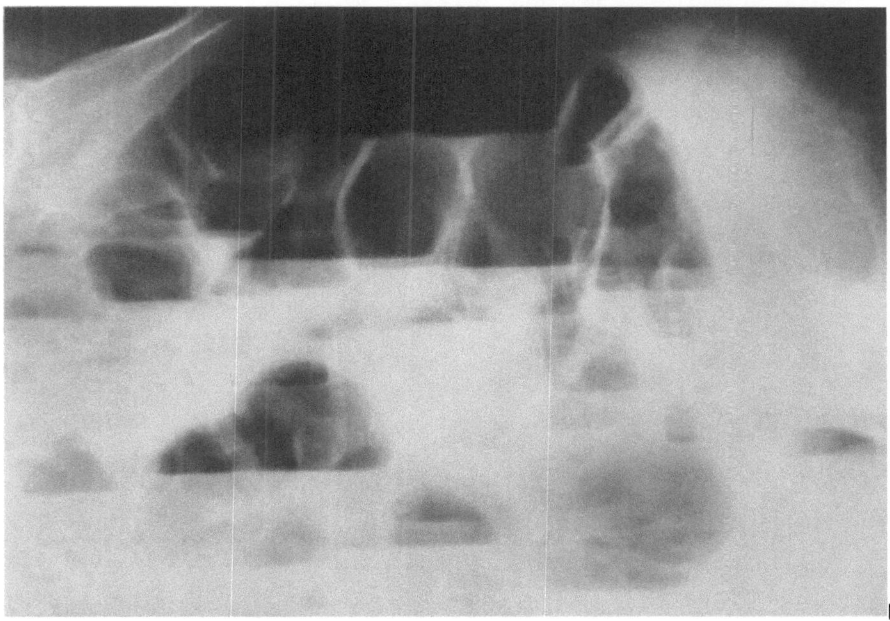

b

Fig. 227 a–g. Postoperative lesions following surgery of the gastrointestinal tract.
a Man, 56 years old, developed abdominal distension and aperistalsis following gastric surgery. *Supine film* shows marked concurrent distension of the small and large bowel. **b** *Left lateral film* shows multiple fluid levels in the small bowel and colon. Postoperative free air is no longer evident. Diagnosis: postoperative paralytic ileus.

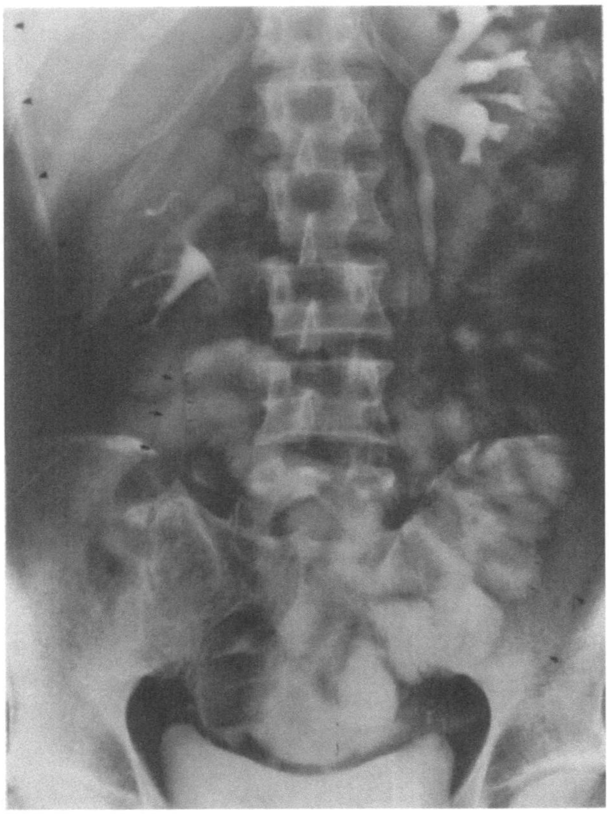

c

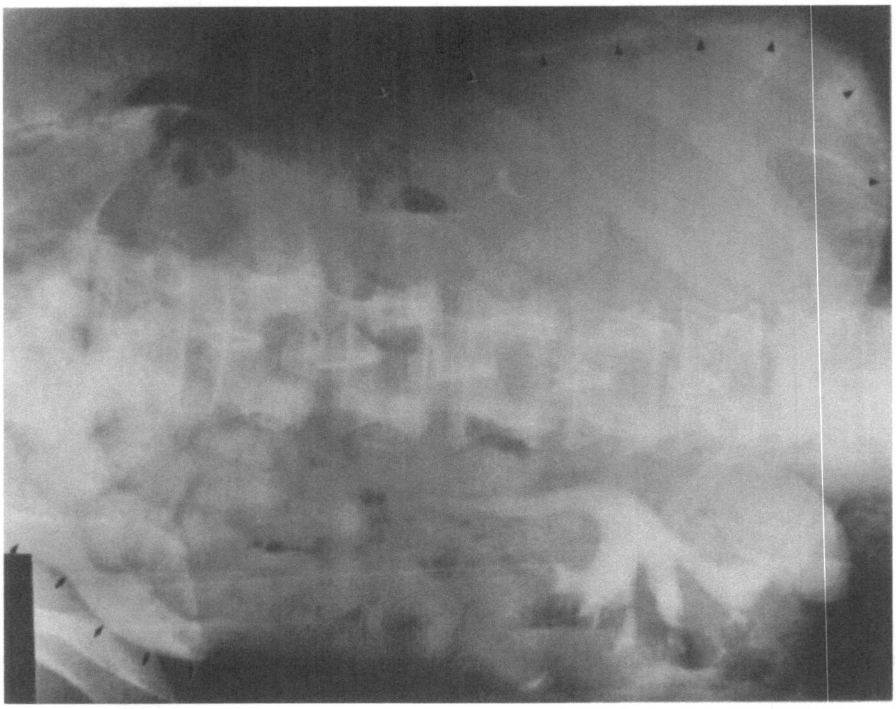

d

Fig. 227 (continued)
c Man, 48 years old, who underwent gastrectomy for carcinoma and subsequent bougienage of a constriction in the upper part of the anastomosis; perforation. Water-soluble contrast was given *orally* to check for anastomotic leak: *Supine film* shows contrast medium in the right and left paracolic gutters (◀←) and around the opacified small bowel loops (→). Renal excretion of the medium into the bladder is apparent. **d** *Left lateral film* shows obvious contrast accumulation in the right parahepatic space (▶) and left paracolic gutter (→).

Fig. 227 (continued)
e Man, 23 years old, with 3-year history of Crohn's disease developed symptoms of partial bowel obstruction. *Supine film after* giving water-soluble contrast p.o. shows *heterotopic* contrast excretion via the kidneys (faintly opacified) into the bladder (heavily opacified). There is no evidence of perforation. **f** Woman, 68 years old, who had undergone gastrostomy for bleeding presented with massive upper gastrointestinal hemorrhage. *Selective angiography of the superior mesenteric artery* (emergency) shows a five-mark-sized, ringlike area of contrast accumulation in the early arterial phase (→). **g** The contrast extravasation (→) is markedly accentuated in the capillary phase. *Diagnosis after reoperation:* bleeding leiomyoma of the duodenum

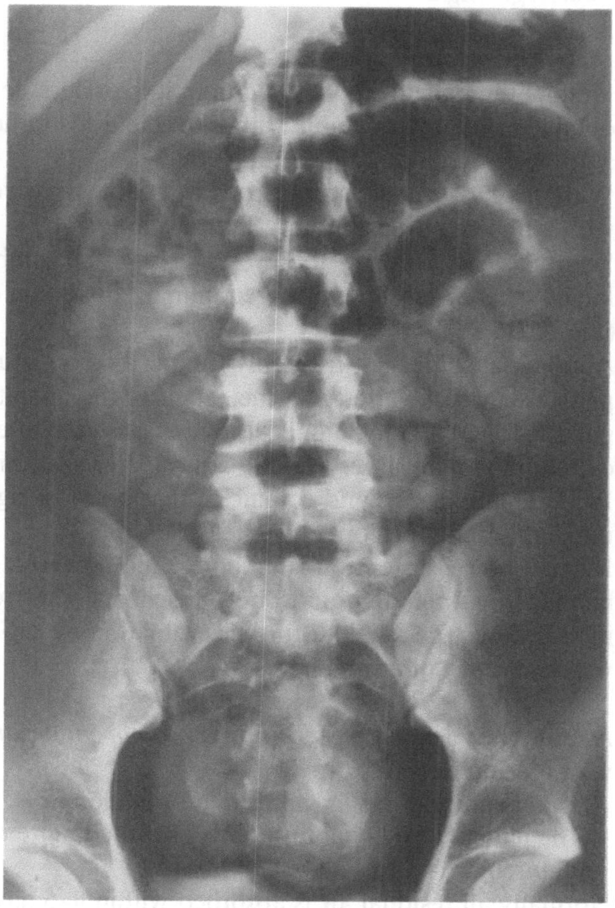

e

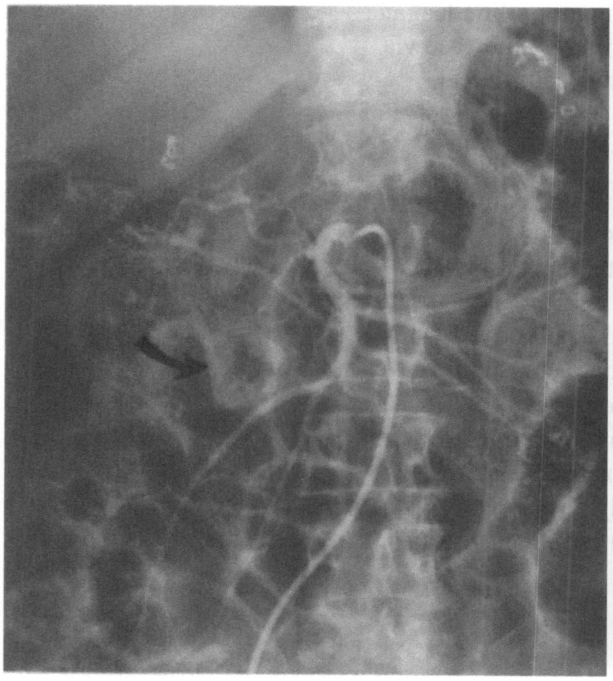

f

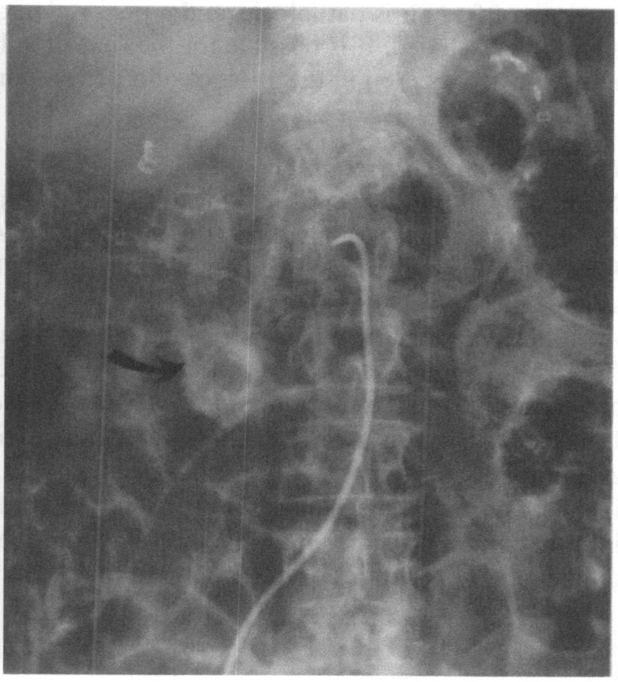

g

Radiologic Signs

Plain Radiographs

Despite the patient's poor condition, it is preferable that plain films be obtained on an X-ray table with movable grids rather than at bedside with a grid cassette and mobile X-ray unit.

With *acute gastric dilatation,* films will show massive gastric enlargement with long fluid levels in the L Lat position.

With *paralytic ileus* (silent bowel) there will be combined small- and large-bowel distension with predominant dilatation of the colon (Fig. 227 a, b).

Abdominal surgery is invariably followed by a disturbance of intestinal peristalsis which varies with the extent of the operation. Gastric atony persists for 24–72 h. Colonic atony persists 16 h after trauma and extra-abdominal surgery, and 4–5 days after gastrointestinal surgery. Predominant gastric and colonic distension most signifies an uncomplicated "postoperative ileus."

If small-bowel distension is predominant, however, differentiation must be made between peritonitis, bowel ischemia, electrolyte disorder, and incipient obstruction, and further evaluation by *UGI series* with water-soluble contrast is necessary!

Another problem ist *postoperative pneumoperitoneum.* The duration is variable and depends on:

- The quantity of air introduced at operation
- The patient's body habitus (air is obsorbed more rapidly in asthenics and children).

Normally all residual air is absorbed within 4-5 days after surgery. An increase of free air is pathologic, and a perforation or suture line leakage should be excluded. It is possible for the free air volume to increase via indwelling tubes even in the absence of a perforation or suture leak.

UGI Series with water-soluble contrast

Normal small-bowel transit time for this kind of contrast medium is 30-90 min; normal postoperative transit time is 1.5–4 h.

Recall that the hyperosmotic contrast agents stimulate peristalsis in the atonic bowel.

A prolonged transit time of 3–5 h, a dilated proximal small bowel with fluid levels, and an absence of contrast medium in the distal small bowel are suggestive of a *postoperative mechanical obstruction.*

Delayed transit with dilated small-bowel loops proximal to an obstruction and normal-sized, contrast-filled loops distally are suggestive of an incipient or partial mechanical obstruction. The study also given information on proximal anastomotic leaks from the esophagus, stomach, duodenum, or oral third of the small intestine.

Excretion of the contrast medium (Fig. 227 c–e)
Renal excretion of the orally administered contrast medium as established by pyelography or bladder filling signifies:
- Perforation or suture line leak (the water-soluble contrast medium is absorbed by the serosa and excreted via the kidneys: *"Gastrografin" test*)
- Heterotopic excretion or a normal variant (the water-soluble contrast medium is absorbed from the intestine and excreted via the kidneys; a perforation is *not* present)

Note: The *"Gastrografin test"* for perforation or anastomotic leak is *unreliable*. Heterotopic contrast excretion in the absence of a perforation is noted in about 5% of postoperative oral contrast studies.

Caution: Small postoperative anastomotic leaks are easily overlooked in the UGI studies with water-soluble contrast (e.g., 25%–50% of esophageal perforations). With an appropriate index of clinical suspicion and a *negative* study performed with water-soluble contrast, examination with *barium sulfate* is indicated. Here it is assumed that the small amount of extravasated barium sulfate can be removed during the subsequent operation. The benefit of pinpointing the leak in this situation outweighs the risk of barium peritonitis.

Sonography
Sonography is well-tolerated and can be performed at the bedside, but its value is often compromised by bowel distension, dressings, drains, wounds, and lack of patient cooperation.
It is useful in the diagnosis of:
- Bladder atony
- Postoperative free fluid collections (fresh blood, pus, bile, ascites, and urine cannot be differentiated) (Figs. 228, 230)
- Fluid-filled and dilated small-bowel loops, with or without wall edema, in examinations performed from the flank
- Subphrenic and subhepatic abscesses
- Postoperative cholecystitis
- Postoperative pancreatitis (not possible with marked distension of the stomach and transverse colon)
- Postoperative jaundice
- Pleural effusions, pericardial effusion

Computed Tomography
CT is the diagnostic method of choice in patients with unexplained clinical symptoms and suspicion of:
- Postoperative free fluid collections (pus, blood, bile) (Figs. 228 b, f, 229 d, g, 230 b)
- Postoperative pancreatitis – its detection and grading
- Postoperative abscesses (Fig. 231 a)
- Iatrogenic changes in the upper abdomen with displacement of bowel loops and equivocal plain film findings (Fig. 232)
- Foreign body

CT is far superior to sonography in the evaluation of postoperative states.

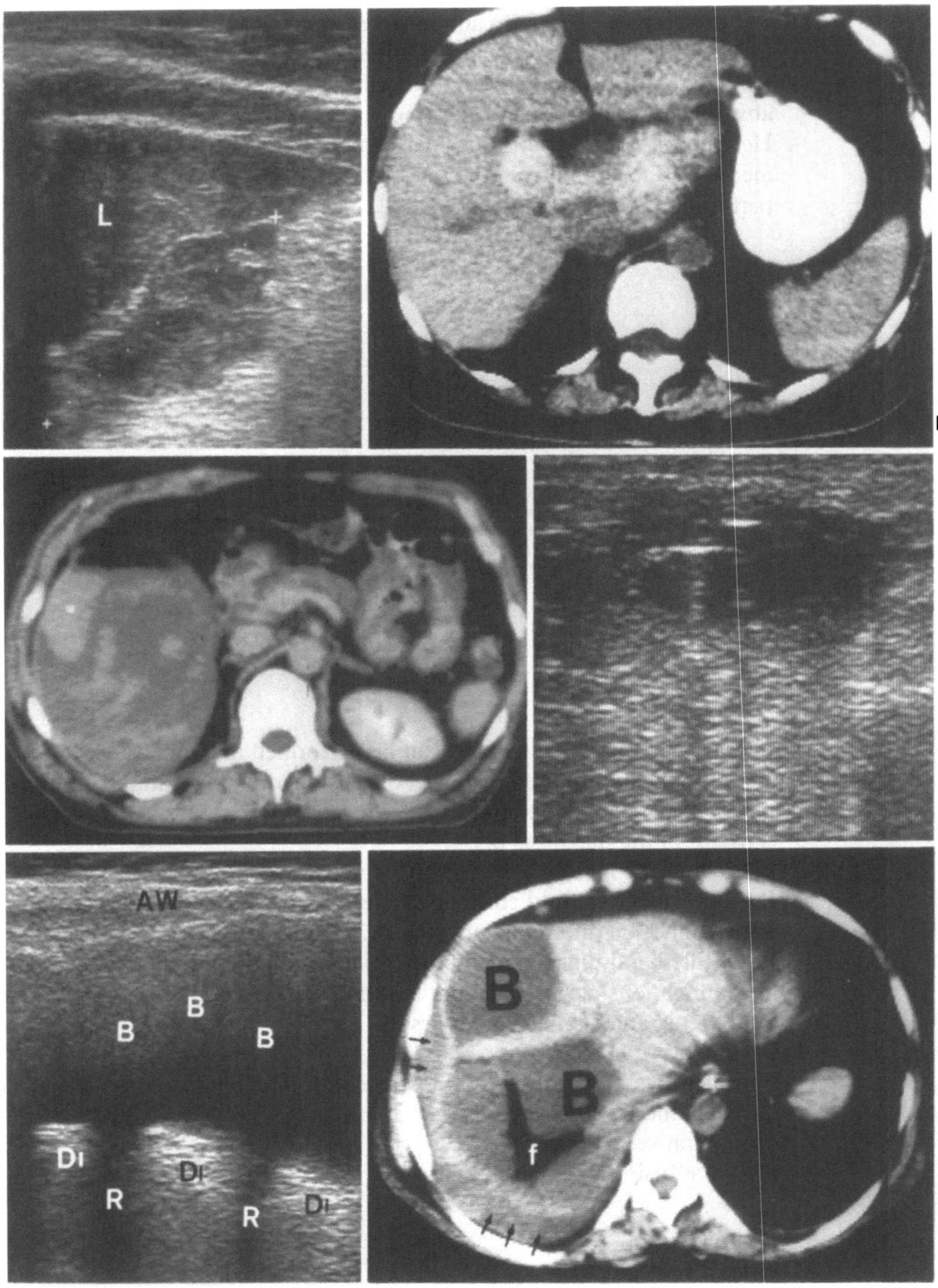

Fig. 228a–i. Postoperative lesions after hepatobiliary surgery.
a A fall of hemoglobin and right upper quadrant pain occurred in a 54-year-old woman who had undergone cholecystectomy 2 days earlier. *Sonogram* (longitudinal scan through the left hepatic lobe) shows a partly liquid and partly solid mass with lobular borders (+.....+) below the left lobe of the liver. **b** *CT scan* shows a high-density mass consistent with fresh postoperative hematoma in the area of the removed gallbladder, in the porta hepatis, and behind the left hepatic lobe. **c** A marked fall of hemoglobin occurred after cholecystectomy in a 46-year-old man, who had no fever. *CT scan* shows a large subhepatic mass with high- and low-density elements consistent with a large hematoma that is not entirely fresh. **d** A 42-year-old woman treated surgically for gallbladder empyema developed fever and tenderness below the right costal arch. *Sonogram* (longitudinal scan through the right hepatic lobe) shows a prehepatic liquid mass with anterior, mobile gas bubbles and an acoustic shadow displacing the tip of the right hepatic lobe. Gas-forming abscess.

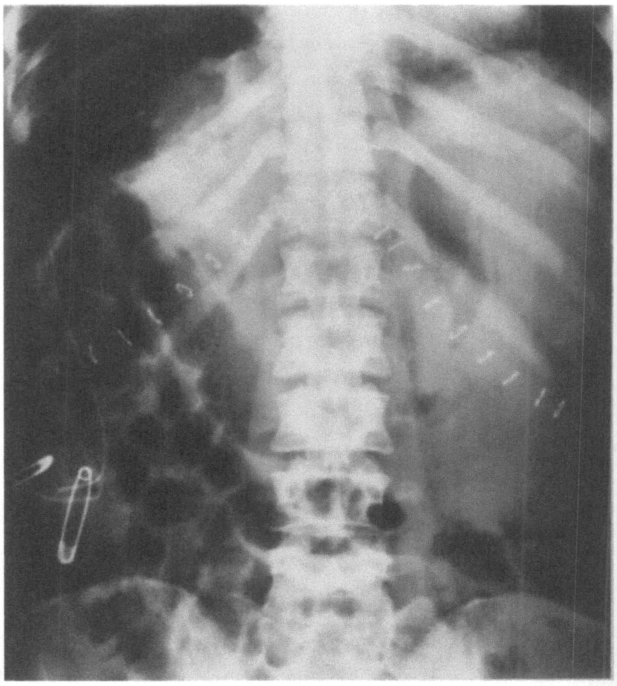
g

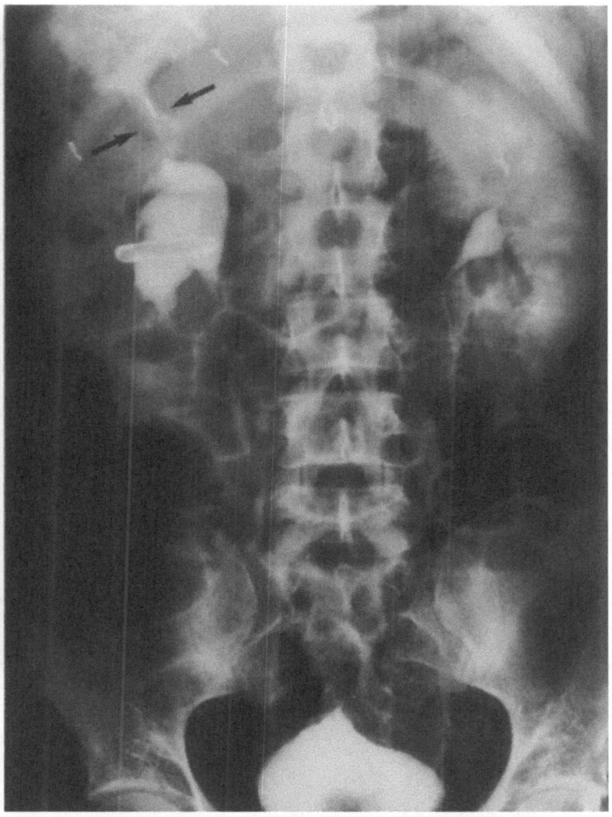
i

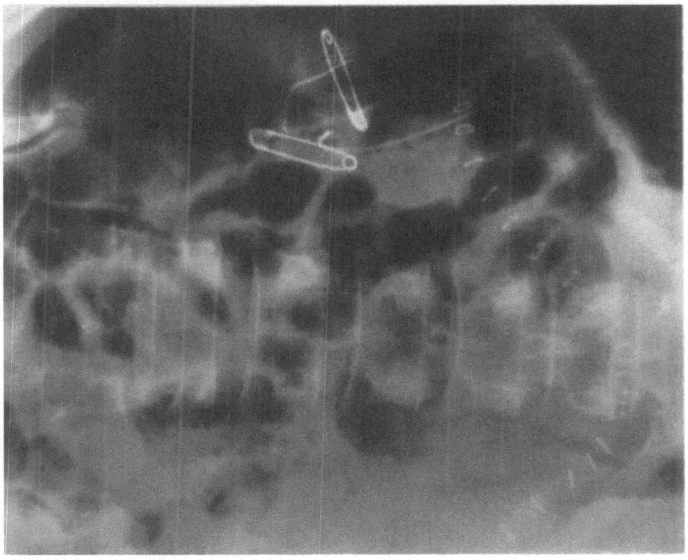
h

Fig. 228 (continued)
e Turkish man, 34 years old, who had undergone removal of a large echinococcal cyst. *Sonogram* (transcostal) shows a large subdiaphragmatic fluid collection *(B)*. Ultrasound-guided aspiration yielded bile (*AW*, abdominal wall; *Di*, diaphragm; *R*, rib shadows). **f** *CT scan* shows two, low-density, loculated, subphrenic fluid collections (*B*, bilioma). The low-density area *(f)* represents greater omentum that has become entrapped in the cyst. **g** Postoperative temperature elevation was noted after surgical resection of the right hepatic lobe for tumor. *Supine film* shows entry of a bowel loop into the space vacated by the right hepatic lobectomy and an indwelling drain. There is no significant pleural effusion. **h** *Left lateral film* shows no fluid levels, no extraintestinal gas bubbles, and no evidence of abscess. Sonography *cannot* be performed. **i** Postoperative urinary fistula following removal of a hydatid liver cyst involving the upper pole of the kidney. Man, 36 years old, of Mediterranean origin who had undergone removal of a large hydatid cyst from the right lobe of the liver. The cyst was in direct contact with the right kidney and had to be sharply separated from it at operation. There was copious fluid discharge postoperatively from the drainage tube. *Urogram* demonstrated leakage from the right upper caliceal group (→) into the cavity formed by the pericystectomy

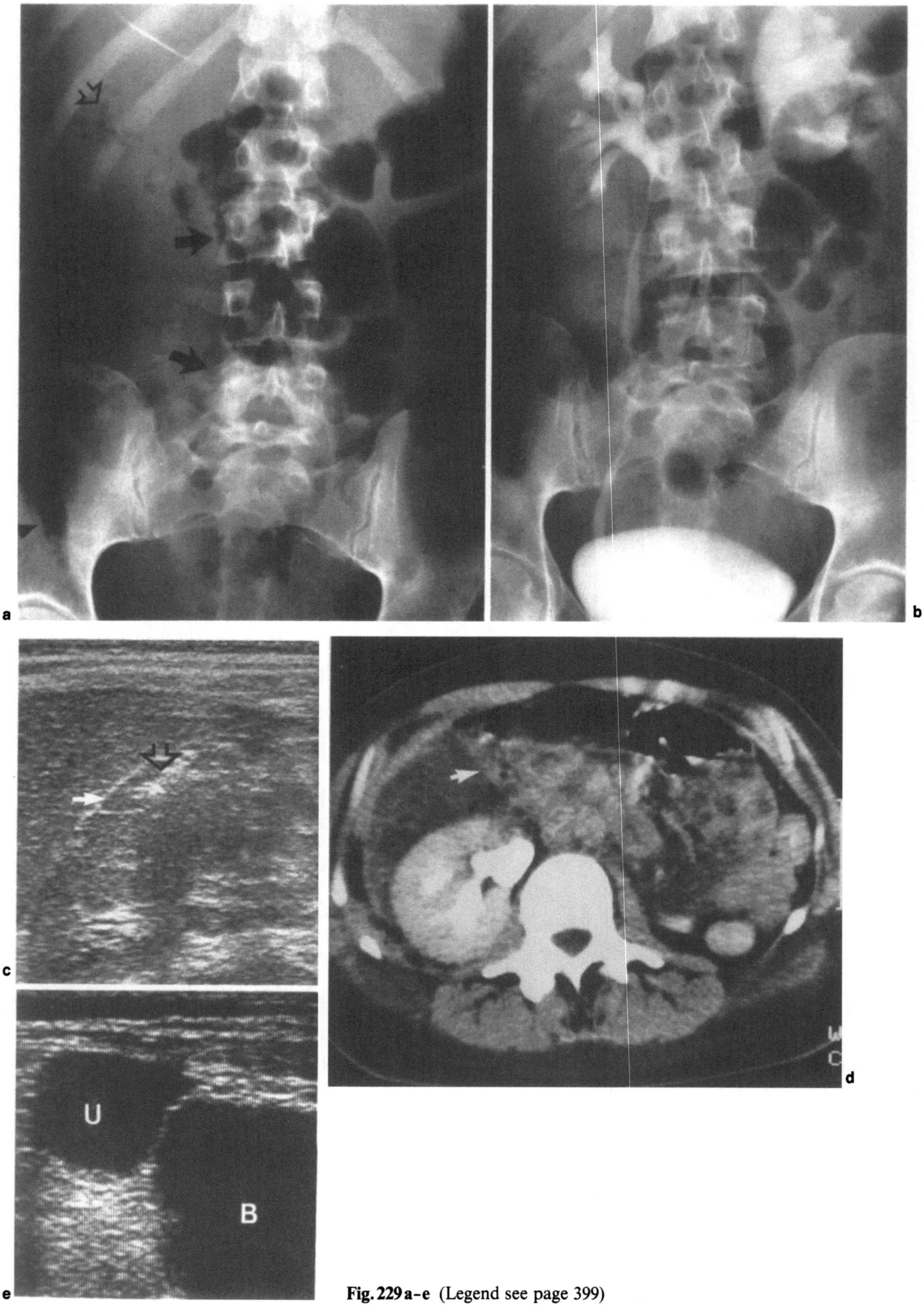

Fig. 229 a–e (Legend see page 399)

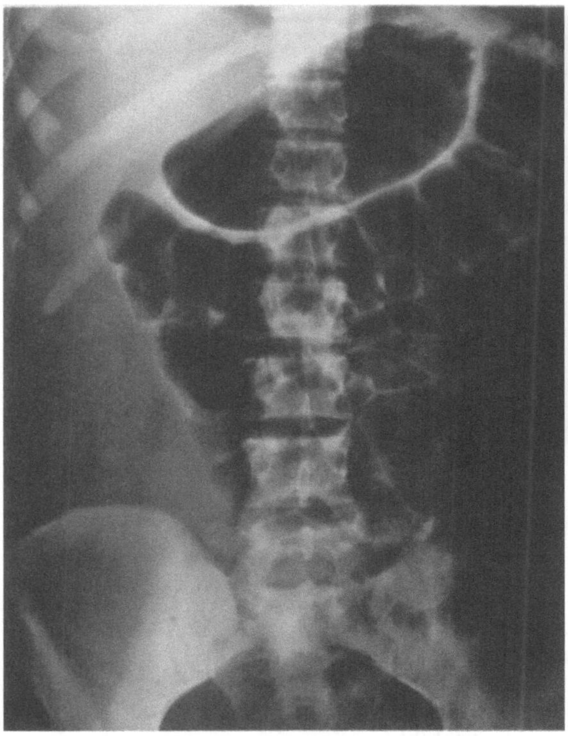

f

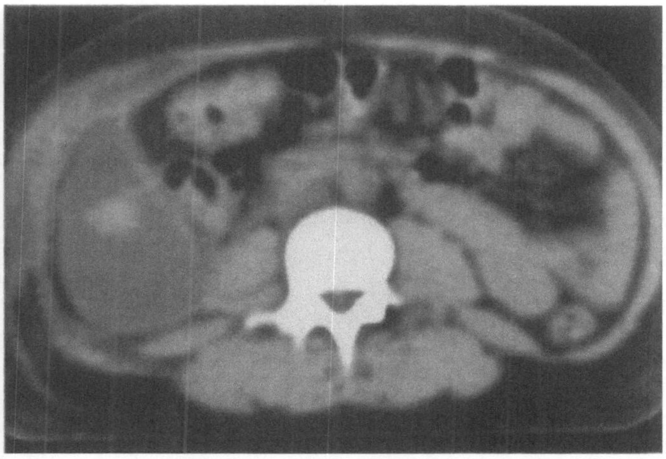

g

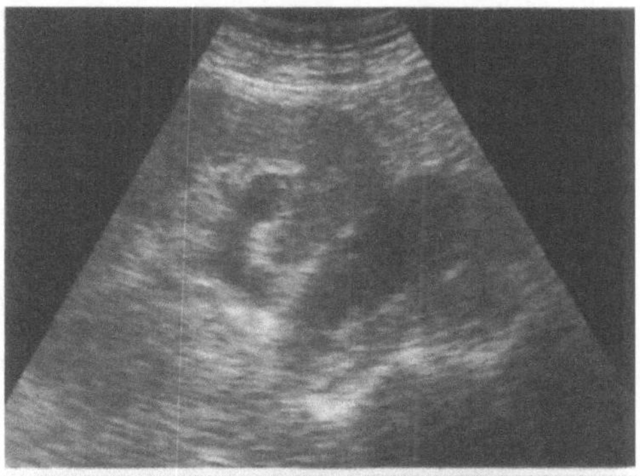

h

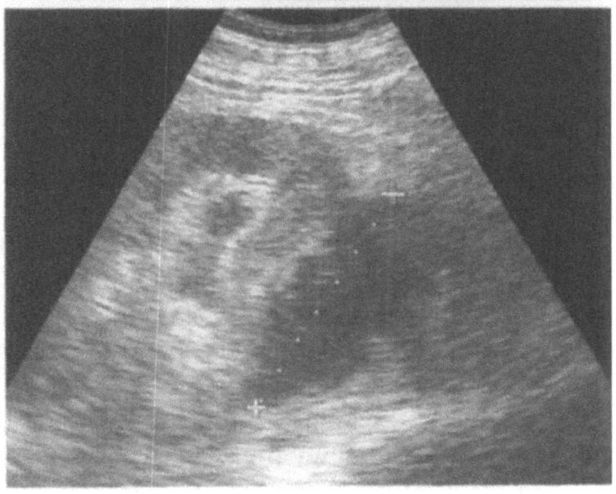

i

Fig. 229 a–i. Postoperative changes in the uropoetic system.
a Postoperative fall of hemoglobin and subfebrile temperatures occurred after operative treatment of ureteropelvic junction stenosis in a 28-year-old woman. Tenderness in the right renal bed. *Supine film* shows multiple small gas bubbles projected over the right renal bed (⇨) and gas in the right flank stripe (▶). Marked displacement of the distended small-bowel loops (➧). **b** *Postoperative urogram* shows a patent right ureteropelvic junction and a stenosed left ureteropelvic junction with an obstructed kidney. Slight medial displacement of the right kidney. The localization of the gas bubbles is unclear. **c** *Sonogram* (longitudinal scan through the right kidney from the flank) shows a hypoechoic mass (→) anterior to the right kidney with multiple gas bubbles and an acoustic shadow (⇨). **d** *CT scan* shows a low-density perirenal fluid collection that behaves like a mass lesion, displacing the small bowel to the left (→). Residual, postoperative, perirenal and pararenal gas bubbles. No abscess, but postoperative residual gas with perirenal hematoma. **e** Routine postoperative sonogram in an 18-year-old man following a ureterovesicoplasty for reflux. *Sonogram* [longitudinal scan through the bladder *(B)*] shows a relatively large fluid collection *(U)* above the bladder, presumably a urinoma. The lesion resolved completely in 4 days.
f Man, 28 years old, had undergone bilateral nephrectomy 2 years previously for renal atrophy; hemodialysis. Ten days earlier he had had a renal transplantation; the transplanted kidney ruptured and was removed. He presented now with acute, very violent, right-sided abdominal and back pain and manifestations of shock. *Supine film* shows combined distension of the stomach, small, and large bowel with a gasless area in the right flank. The ascending colon is displaced medially. The right flank stripe is obscured. *Diagnosis:* extensive retroperitoneal hemorrhage. **g** *CT scan* shows a large, predominantly low-density mass with high-density components in the right paracolic space. Bleeding into the abdominal wall has produced marked wall thickening with high-density zones. **h, i** Iatrogenic urinoma following retrograde pyelography. Man, 56 years old, with marked tenderness in the left renal bed, subfebrile temperatures, and a fall of blood pressure. **h** *Sonogram* (longitudinal scan from the left flank) shows a liquid, partially echogenic mass at the lower pole of the left kidney, which is displacing and elevating the kidney with a moderately dilated pelvicaliceal system. **i** *Sonogram* (repeat scan at 24 h) shows marked enlargement of the mass with further elevation of the kidney. Confident differentiation between hematoma and urinoma could not be made with ultrasound

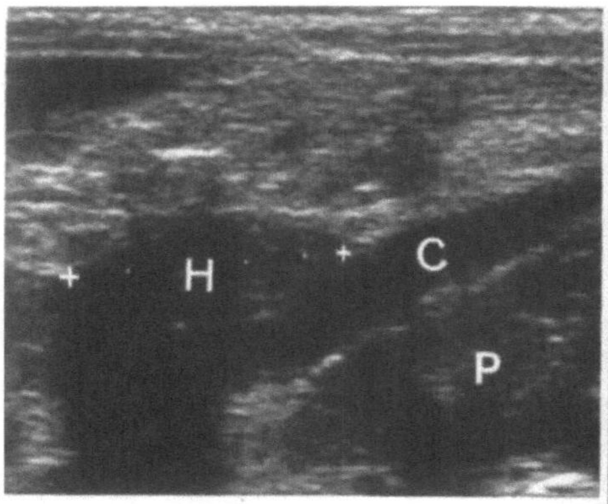

a

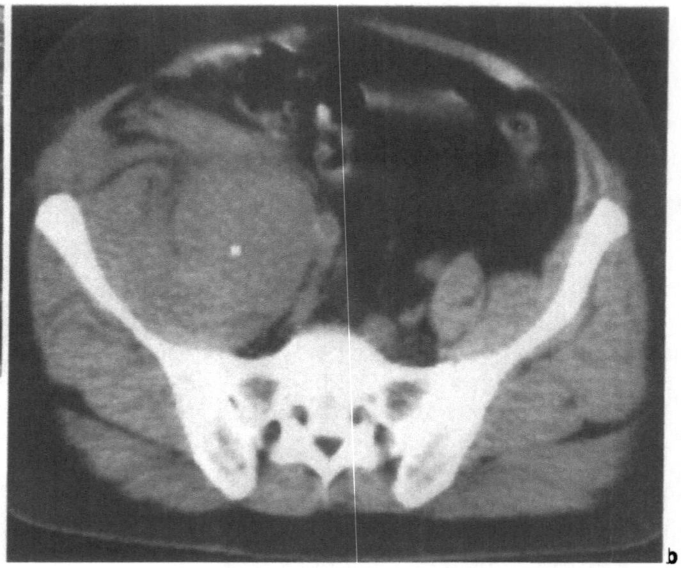

b

Fig. 230 a, b. Postoperative complications after vascular surgery.
a Fall of hemoglobin occurred in a 17-year-old man following vena cava reconstruction. *Sonogram* (right paramedian longitudinal scan) shows a hematoma *(H)* anterior to the vena cava prosthesis *(C); P,* psoas muscle. **b** A right lower quadrant mass developed after the insertion of an aortoiliac prosthesis in a 61-year-old man, and blood flow disturbances recurred. *CT scan* discloses a large suture aneurysm in front of the right iliac wing with bleeding into the psoas and iliacus muscles, which are obscured

References

Beyer D (1983) Sonographie des Peritonealraumes. In: Bücheler E, Friedmann G, Thelen M (eds) Real-time-Sonographie des Körpers. Thieme, Stuttgart

Burhenne HJ, Cooperberg P (1984) Complications of biliary tract surgery. In: Meyers MA, Ghahremani GG (eds) Iatrogenic gastrointestinal complications. Springer, Berlin Heidelberg New York

Burrell M, Jay BS (1984) Complications of gastric and duodenal surgery. In: Meyers MA, Ghahremani GG (eds) Iatrogenic gastrointestinal complications. Springer, Berlin Heidelberg New York

Clements JL Jr, Rogers JV Jr, Torres WE (1984) Complications of intestinal surgery. In: Meyer MA, Ghahremani GG (eds) Iatrogenic gastrointestinal complications. Springer, Berlin Heidelberg New York

Foley MJ, Gharhremani GG, Rogers LF (1982) Reappraisal of contrast media used to detect upper gastrointestinal perforations. Comparison of ionic water soluble media with barium sulfate. Radiology 144: 231

Janson R, Christ F, Schneider B, Engel C (1982) Wertigkeit der oralen Gastrografin-Passage in der Ileus-Diagnostik. Fortschr Röntgenstr 136: 641-648

Largiadėr F, Säuberli H, Wicki O (1983) Checkliste Viscerale Chirurgie. Thieme, Stuttgart

Oestmann J, Langenbruck K, Meyer HJ, Gerlings H (1985) Nachweis von Insuffizienzen enteroenteraler Anastomosen nach Gastrektomien durch Untersuchungen mit wasserlöslichen Kontrastmitteln. Zeitpunkt und Untersuchungsqualität. Röntgenblätter 38: 356-358

Riedl T, Dinstl K, Keminger K, Lechner G, Schiessl R (1976) Klinisch-radiologische Untersuchungen über die Treffsicherheit des Diatrizoat (Gastrografin)-Testes zum Nachweis von Anastomosen-Dehiszenzen und Perforationen des Gastrointestinaltraktes. Fortschr Röntgenstr 124: 48

Swart B, Meyer G (1974) Die Diagnostik des akuten Adomens beim Erwachsenen - ein neues klinisch-röntgenologisches Konzept. Radiologe 14: 1-57

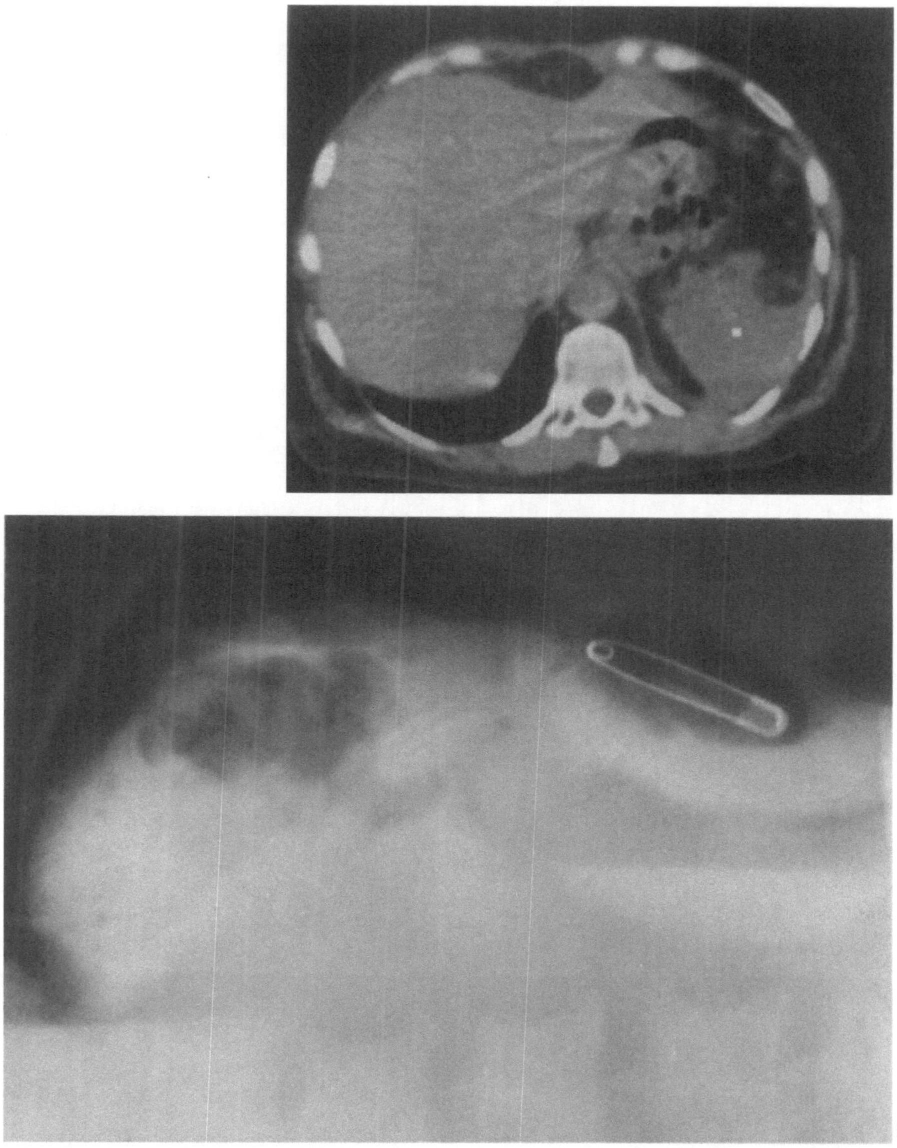
a

b

Fig. 231 a, b. Postoperative complications after splenic surgery. a A 60-year-old woman developed fever following a splenectomy. *CT scan* shows a left subphrenic mass with polycyclic contours in the former splenic bed, consistent with a hematoma that is no longer fresh. **b** A 44-year-old man became febrile after splenectomy. *Right lateral film* shows a localized gas collection in the left subphrenic space. The gas did not alter its position when the patient was moved to the left lateral position. *Operation* disclosed a left subphrenic abscess

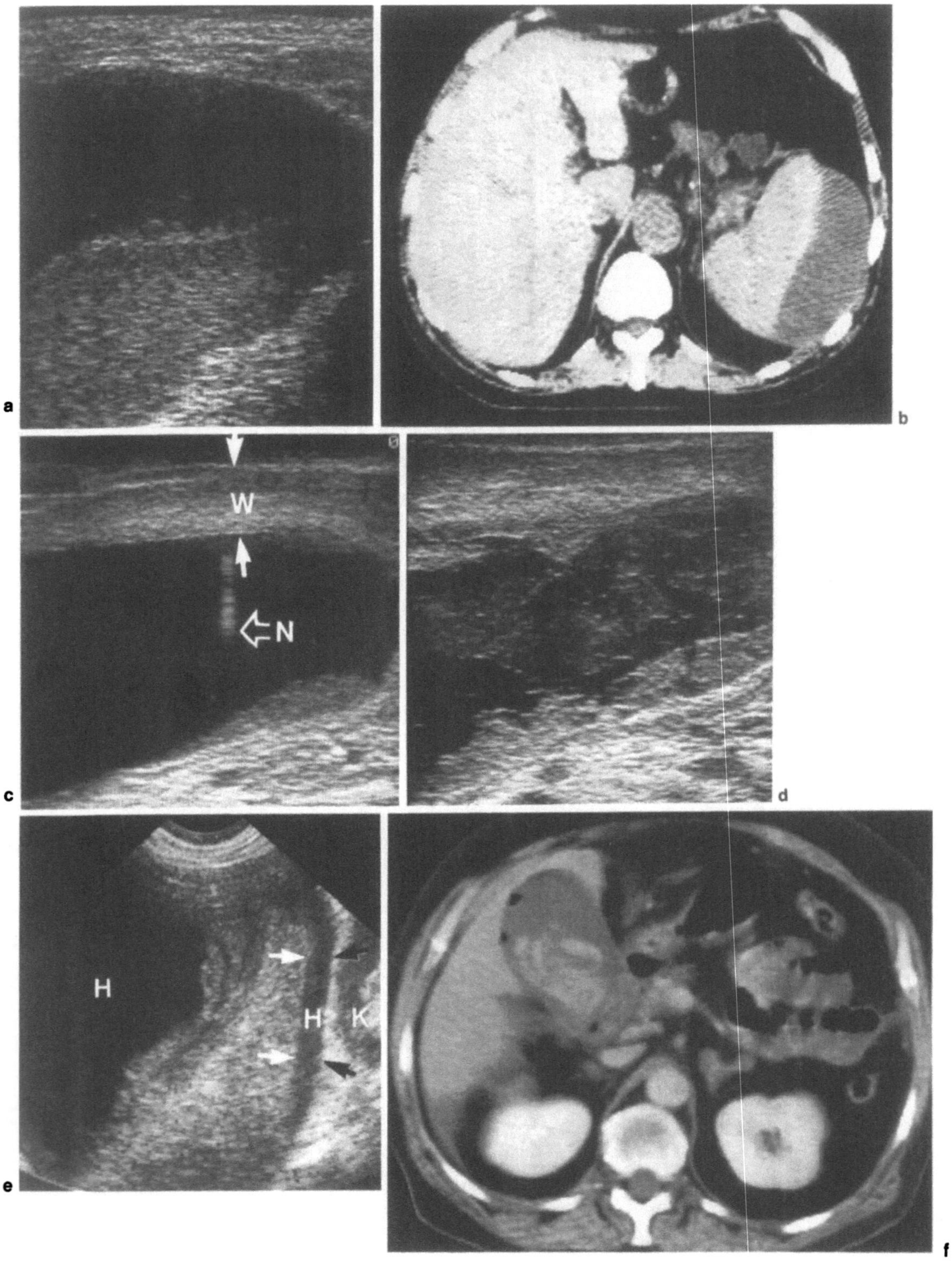

Fig. 232 a–f. Complications following abdominal punctures. **a** Thoracocentesis in this patient was followed by marked abdominal pain. *Sonogram* (longitudinal scan from the left side) shows a subcapsular fluid collection close to the chest wall with evidence of sedimentation. **b** *CT scan* (bolus) shows a low-density subcapsular fluid collection, consistent with an older subcapsular hematoma. **c** *Sonogram* shows a huge pancreatic pseudocyst with a thick wall (*W*, →←) and posterior sedimentary debris. The needle for ultrasound-guided aspiration (*N*, ⇨) is visible in the cyst lumen. The cyst was completely evacuated. **d** Follow-up scan was done 24 h after the puncture. Fall of hemoglobin. *Sonogram* shows that the cyst has refilled. Multiple floating echoes with posterior sedimentation signify a fresh hemorrhage. *Operation* disclosed bleeding into a large pancreatic pseudocyst; the bleeding source could not be identified. **e** *Sonogram* after blind needle biopsy of the liver (longitudinal scan with right kidney, *K*) shows a huge subcapsular

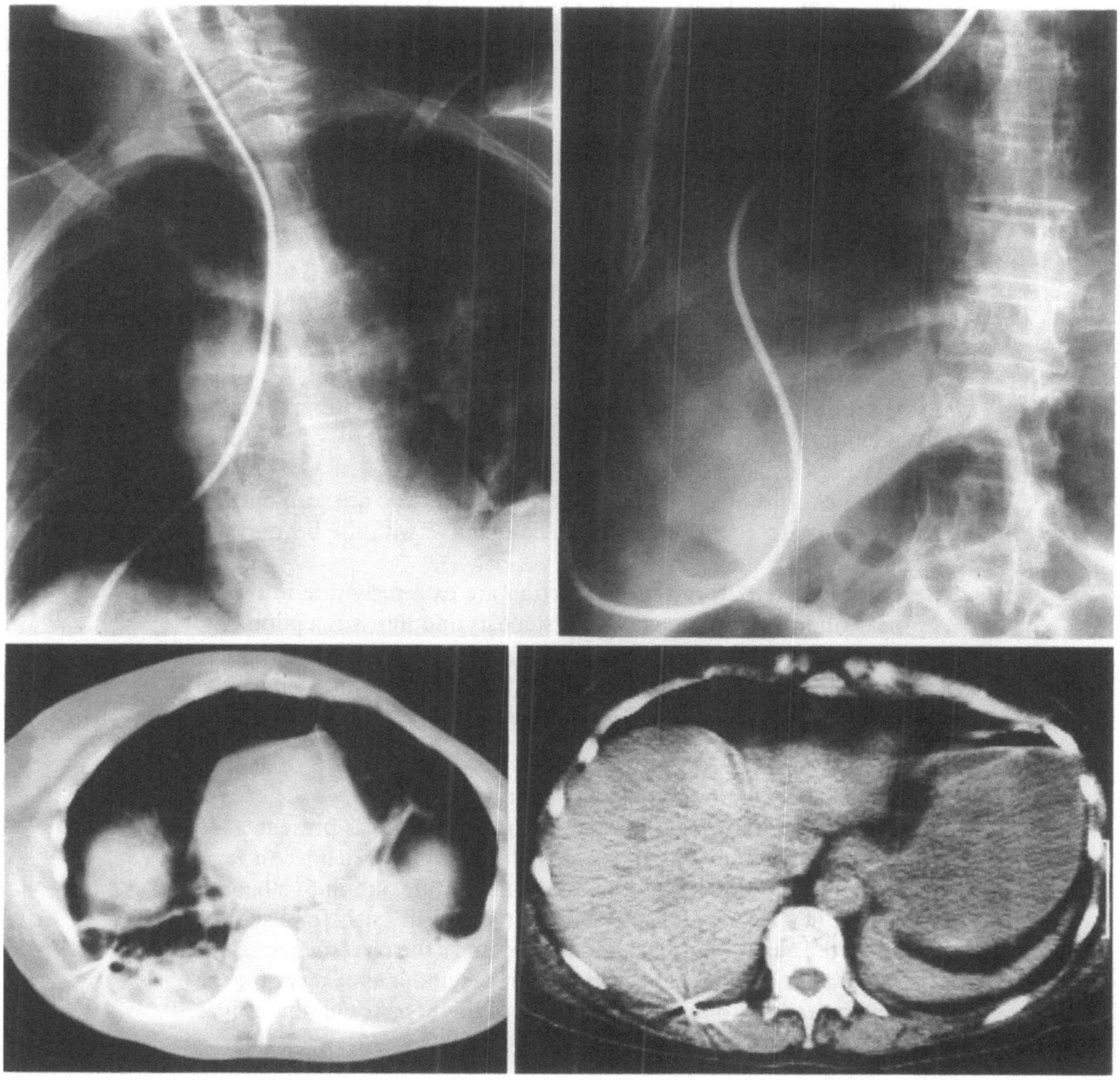

a b c d

Fig. 233 a-d. Esophageal perforation in the middle third with diaphragmatic perforation by a gastric tube. Difficult nasogastric intubation of a 72-year-old woman in ICU. Aspiration did not yield gastric contents. **a** *Chest film* after careful instillation of contrast medium confirms aberrant placement of the tube, which is projected onto the right mediastinum, lung, and liver. **b** On *supine abdominal film,* the tube can be traced into the retroperitoneal space on the right side. Contrast extravasation is noted in the right parahepatic area. **c** *CT scan* of the chest shows dystelectasis of the left lung and right-sided pleural effusion. The opacified gastric tube is visible posteriorly in the pleural space. **d** *CT scan* of the abdomen shows the gastric tube lying posterior to the liver in the peritoneal cavity

Fig. 232 (continued)
fluid collection *(H)* (→) representing a large hematoma. *Ultrasound-guided aspiration* yielded older blood.
f Increasing right upper quadrant pain, rigidity, and shock symptoms developed 4 days after a blind liver biopsy, performed at another hospital. *Emergency CT scan* after transfer to our institution shows free fluid around the liver and in Morison's pouch. Small low-density air bubbles and high-density material in the gallbladder. *Diagnosis:* perforation of the gallbladder, hematobilia, bile peritonitis

5 Special Features of Acute Abdominal Disorders in Children

G. BENZ-BOHM, A. E. HORWITZ

5.1 Acute Abdomen in Newborns

Definition of the Neonatal Period

For the classification of acute abdominal disorders in children, it is convenient to limit the neonatal period to the first 15 days of life for the following reasons:

1. The atretic forms of congenital intestinal obstruction are seen only in the first days of life, because they are incompatible with life beyond that period.
2. Several "acquired" forms of obstruction are extremely rare in the first 2 weeks after birth, such as pyloric stenosis and intussusception.

In addition, there is another group of diseases that can occur during as well as after the first 15 days of life and always present the same clinical and radiologic features (duodenal stenosis, necrotizing enterocolitis).

Normal Bowel Gas Pattern in the Newborn

Three hours after the newborn takes its first breath, air is present throughout the jejunum and in portions of the proximal ileum. Air reaches the cecum and ascending colon in 3-6 h, the left flexure in 6-8 h, and the rectum in 12 h at the latest. A physiologic meteorism exists for a short time, but by 48 h the aeration of the abdomen assumes the pattern characteristic of infancy; air is demonstrable throughout the abdomen except for the right upper quadrant due to the presence of the hepatic shadow (Fig. 234).

Absence of Air in the Gastrointestinal Tract (Fig. 235)

1. Cerebral cause
2. Heavy maternal anesthesia during delivery
3. Dehydration with electrolyte shift
4. Esophageal atresia without tracheoesophageal fistula (Fig. 236 a)

Note: The major cause of acute abdomen in the first days of life is congenital intestinal obstruction.
Bilious vomiting in newborns is suggestive of high intestinal obstruction.
Passage of meconium 24 h postpartum is suggestive of low intestinal obstruction.

Fig. 234. Normal distribution of intestinal gas in the newborn (drawing modified from Buffard and Deffrenne 1961): Air enters the stomach 10 min after birth, the duodenum at 30 min, the ileum at 3 h, and the rectum at 8 h

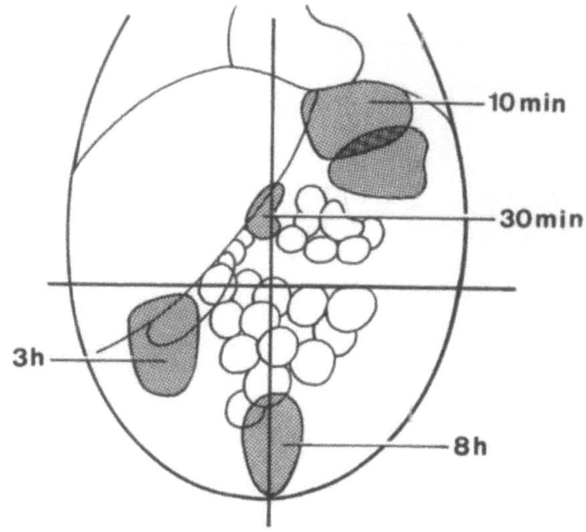

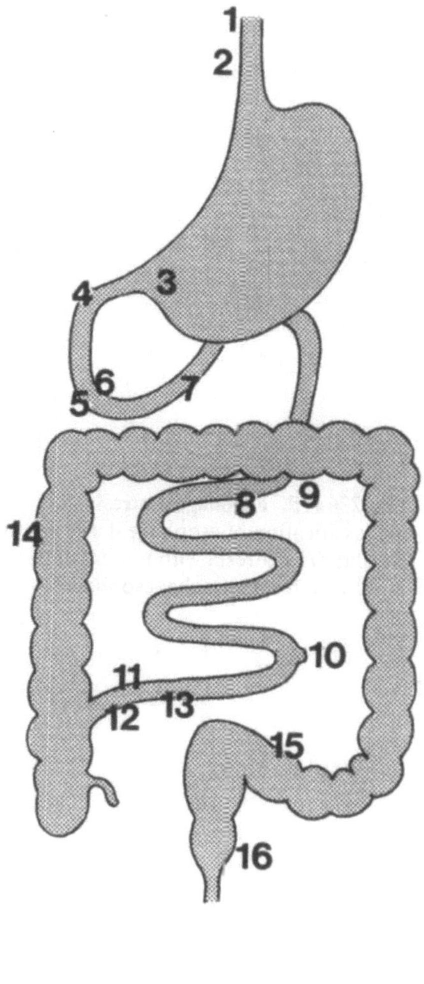

Fig. 235. Localization and relative frequency of gastrointestinal obstructive syndromes in newborns (drawing modified from Wolf 1971): *1*, esophageal atresia (with and without fistula); *2*, isolated tracheoesophageal fistula; *3*, pyloric membrane; *4*, suprapapillary (-ampullary) duodenal atresia; *5*, infrapapillary (-ampullary) duodenal atresia; 6, annular pancreas; *7*, external duodenal stenosis (anomalies of rotation); *8*, jejunal atresia; *9*, small-bowel volvulus; *10*, Meckel's diverticulum; *11*, ileal atresia; *12*, meconium ileus; *13*, meconium plug syndrome; *14*, colon atresia; *15*, congenital megacolon; *16*, anal atresia (stenosis)

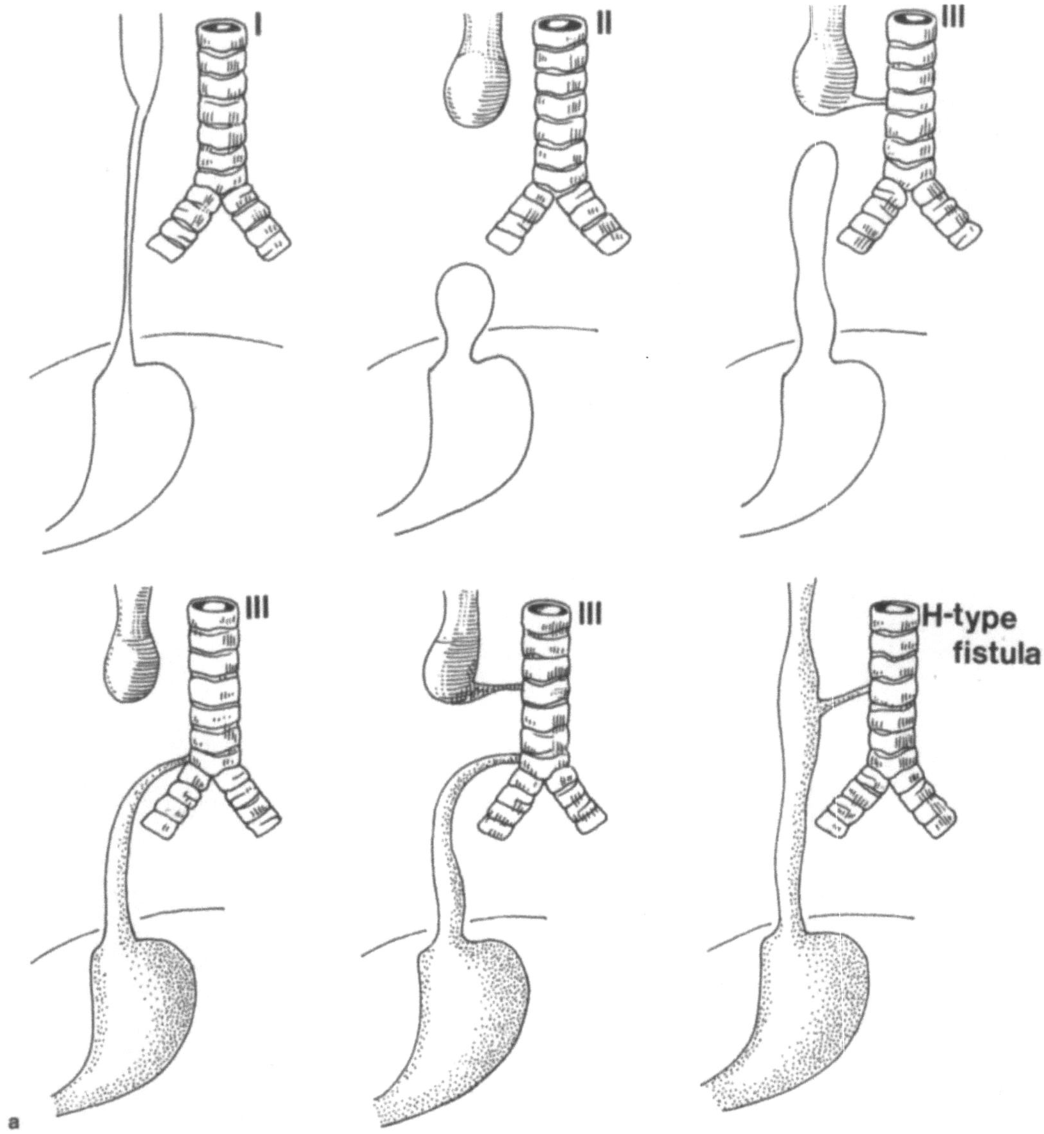

Fig. 236a–d. Esophageal atresia.
a Classification of esophageal atresias by the Vogt scheme: *I,* complete aplasia; *II,* atresia without fistula; *IIIa,* atresia with upper fistula; *IIIb,* atresia with lower fistula; *IIIc* upper and lower fistula. *H-type fistula,* tracheoesophageal fistula without atresia.

Fig. 236 (continued)
b Detail of *lateral radiograph* of upper blind pouch in Vogt III b esophageal atresia. Male newborn, 1st day of life. **c** *Upright thoracoabdominal film* of a 1-day-old newborn with Vogt type III c esophageal atresia. A gastric tube has been passed through the upper fistula into the upper lobe bronchus. **d** *Upright film* of the chest and abdomen shows isolated tracheoesophageal fistula (H-type fistula) in a newborn girl, 7th day of life, prior aspiration, meteorism

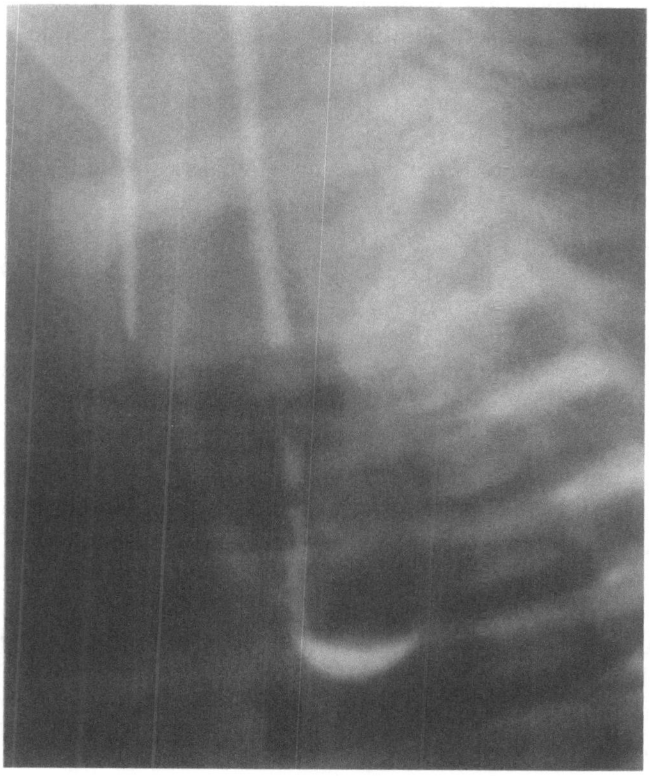
b

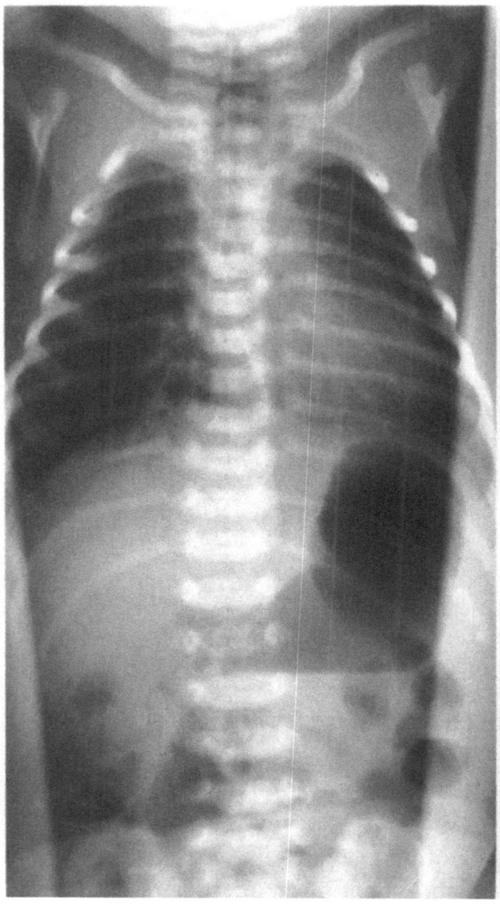
c

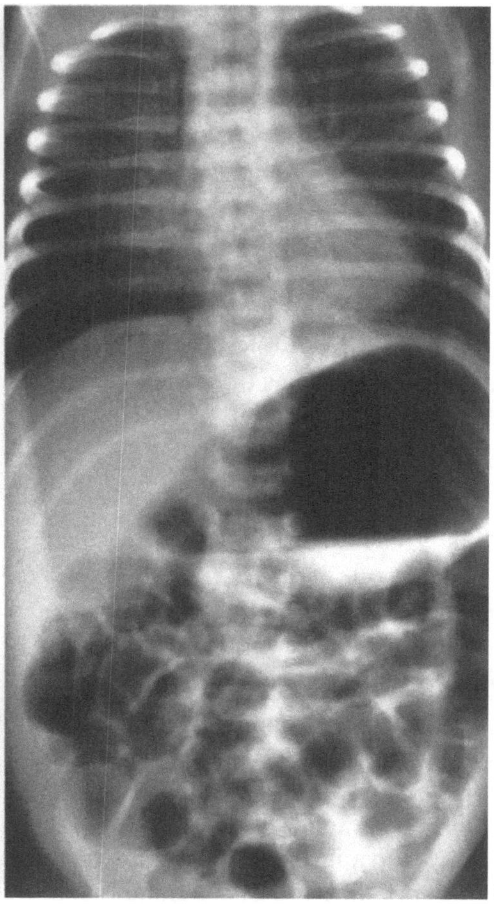
d

Examination of a Newborn with Intestinal Obstruction

1. Inspection of the abdomen: flat (esophageal atresia without tracheoesophageal fistula), distended (small-bowel obstruction)
2. Search for incarcerated external hernia (extremely rare in the first days after birth)
3. Evaluation of general findings (facial expression, skin folds, weight, skin color, temperature)
4. Gestational age
5. Assessment of amniotic fluid volume: polyhydramnios signifying a proximal obstruction
6. Associated anomalies (e.g., cardiac defects)
7. Exploratory catheterization (with a soft, well-moistened catheter): esophagus, rectum

Special Radiographic Studies

1. Upright AP sagittal film of the chest and abdomen (in a Babix sling)
2. Occasionally this view is supplemented with a lateral abdominal film, e.g., to check for air in the rectum and sigmoid when there is marked gaseous bowel distension

Alternatives if the infant's condition is so poor that upright films cannot be obtained:

1. Supine sagittal film of the chest and abdomen
2. Left lateral abdominal film with a cross-table beam

Note: The plain survey film of the chest and abdomen should precede contrast examination! This is because contrast medium is often unnecessary, and plain radiography enables the contrast examination to be performed selectively.

Radiographic Checklist

1. Air in the gastrointestinal tract intraluminal/intramural/extramural ("gas")
2. Fluid, space-occupying lesions ("mass")
3. Calcifications ("stones")
4. Skeletal anomalies (intestinal anomalies in conjunction with skeletal anomalies) ("bones")

5.1.1 High Intestinal Obstruction

Esophageal Atresia

Prevalence

Accounts for approximately one-fourth of all congenital obstructions of the digestive tract

Clinical Symptoms

Foamy saliva in the mouth and nose during the first hours of life, respiratory difficulties, coughing fits, indrawn abdomen in the absence of tracheoesophageal fistula, hydramnios; negative exploratory catheterization

Caution: Be alert for bending of a too-soft catheter, secretion from a blind sac, passage of gastric juice and bile through a lower fistulous tract, catheterization of the stomach via the trachea and fistula. Due to possible misinterpretation, radiographic evaluation is always indicated.

Radiologic Signs

1. *Upright survey film of the chest and abdomen* (sagittal projection): A narrow-gauge feeding tube with contrast medium (aqueous propyliodone or water-soluble isotonic medium) is introduced nasally until it meets resistance, then 0.5 ml of the contrast medium is injected shortly before exposing the X-ray film.
2. *Lateral chest film* (Fig. 236 b). Contrast medium is removed by aspiration after the second film is exposed.

Important:

Aspiration pneumonia, cardiac defect (associated malformation), position of aortic arch (operative approach)

If the gastrointestinal tract contains no air, three possibilities exist (Fig. 236 a):

Type I (very rare)
Type II (about 7% of cases)
Type III a (about 1% of cases)

If the gastrointestinal tract is filled with air, three other possibilities exist (Fig. 236 a):

Type III b (about 85%-90%)
Type III c (about 2%-3%)
Isolated tracheoesophageal fistula (H-type fistula; about 3%)

This lesion is often diagnosed later from recurrent episodes of aspiration and excessive air filling of the gastrointestinal tract (Fig. 236 c).

A lateral chest film will occasionally show air in the distal blind pouch. Otherwise the length of the distal blind pouch can be determined only through the gastrostomy following palliative surgery.

Membranous Atresia of the Pylorus

Prevalence

Very rare

Clinical Symptom

Nonbilious vomiting

Radiologic Signs

Upright survey film of the chest and abdomen in the sagittal projection shows an abnormal air pattern: enlarged stomach containing air and fluid, absence of air distal to the stomach (Fig. 237).

The diagnosis is confirmed by administering nonionic contrast medium (Metrizamide, Iopamidol, Iohexoe) through an indwelling stomach tube.

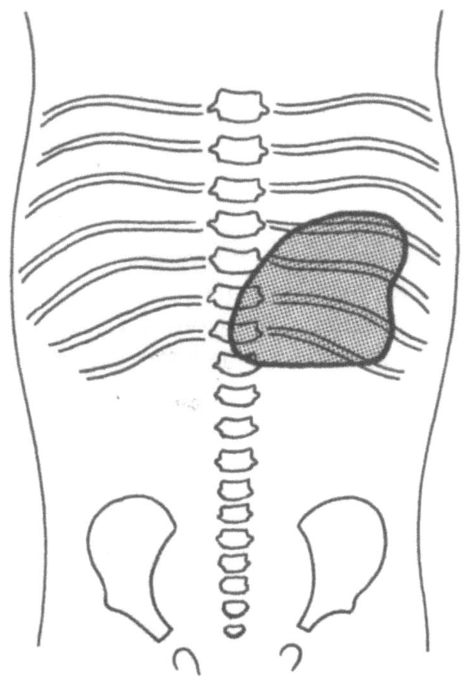

Fig. 237. Membranous atresia of the pylorus (drawing modified from Wolf 1971): Enlarged stomach containing air and fluid; no air distal to the stomach

Duodenal Obstruction

Duodenal Atresia

By membrane (common) or by total interruption of continuity (rare). Three types of congenital gastrointestinal atresia may occur:

1. Membranous atresia
2. Atresia in which intestinal continuity is preserved through a cordlike connection, with or without a mesenteric defect
3. Atresia with complete interruption of continuity and an associated mesenteric defect

Note: More than one atresia exists in over 8% of cases.

Prevalence
Reports vary widely from 1:9000 to 1:40000.

Clinical Symptoms
Vomiting, vomitus is bile-stained with an obstruction distal to the papilla; upper abdomen distended, mid- and lower abdomen scaphoid; hydramnios

Radiologic Signs
Upright film of the chest and abdomen in the sagittal projection shows an abnormal air pattern: marked air filled of the stomach and proximal duodenum with no air distal to the duodenum: "double bubble sign" (Fig. 238a).

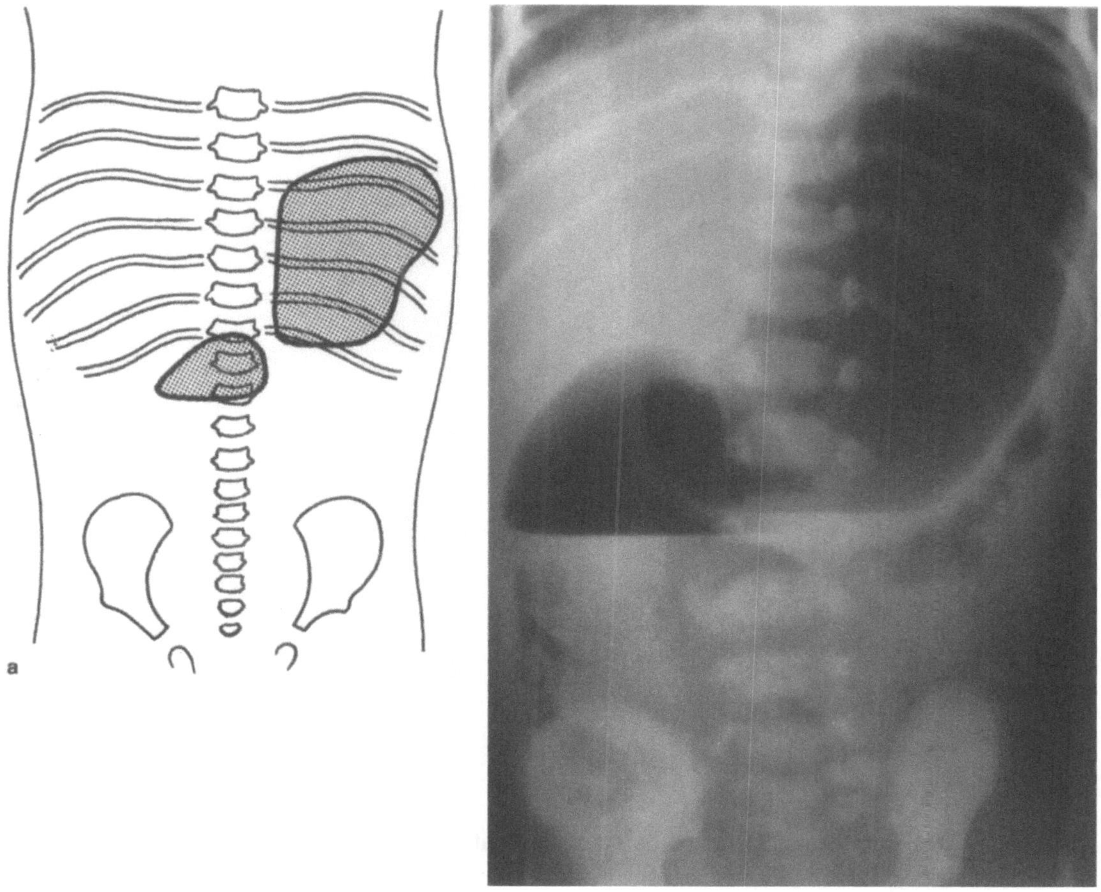

a b

Fig. 238a, b. Duodenal atresia.
a Drawing modified from Wolf (1971): "double bubble sign," no air distal to the duodenum. **b** *Upright film* of the chest and abdomen after aspiration of fluid and insufflation of about 25 ml of air by indwelling gastric tube in the left lateral position: "double bubble sign," air in the colon after repeated intestinal lavage. Male newborn, 3rd day of life

Caution: Fluid-filled stomach and fluid-filled proximal duodenum:
If the survey film shows only *one* fluid level, aspirate fluid from the stomach with a nasogastric tube and insufflate 20–30 ml of air in the L Lat position. Then repeat the upright film.

Note: Duodenal atresia can coexist with analogous malformations of the esophagus or rectoanal area.

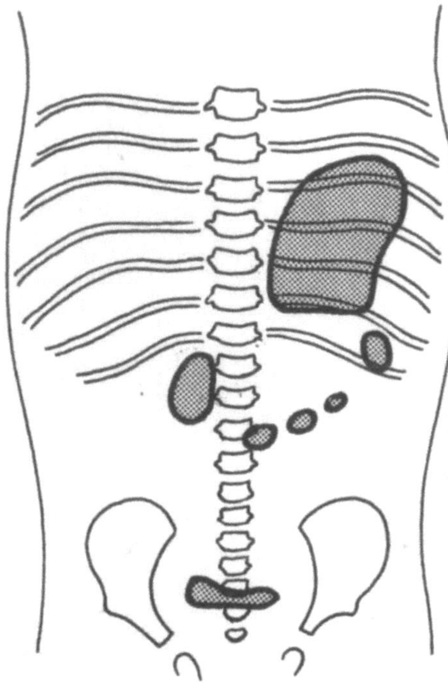

Fig. 239. Duodenal stenosis (drawing modified from Wolf 1971): marked air filling of the stomach and proximal duodenum, little air distal to the duodenum

Duodenal Stenoses

1. Internal forms: membrane stenosis, narrow segment
2. External forms: positional anomalies with adhesive bands or volvulus, thick Treitz ligament, aberrant vessels, aortomesenteric duodenal compression, duplications, annular pancreas, combined forms

Clinical Symptoms

Vomiting and dystrophic symptoms vary markedly in degree according to the underlying anatomy and often are present only periodically. Thus the time at which the diagnosis is made may vary.

Radilogic Signs

Upright survey film of the chest and abdomen in the sagittal projection shows abnormal air pattern similar to that in duodenal atresia but with a small amount of air distal to the duodenum (Fig. 239).

Note: Atresia and stenosis cannot be distinguished radiologically after irrigation of the bowel (Fig. 238 b).
Midgut volvulus is radiologically *indistinguishable* from duodenal atresia or stenosis.

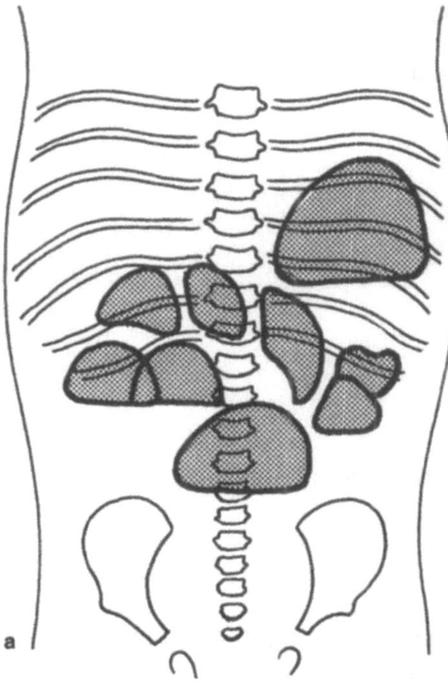

a

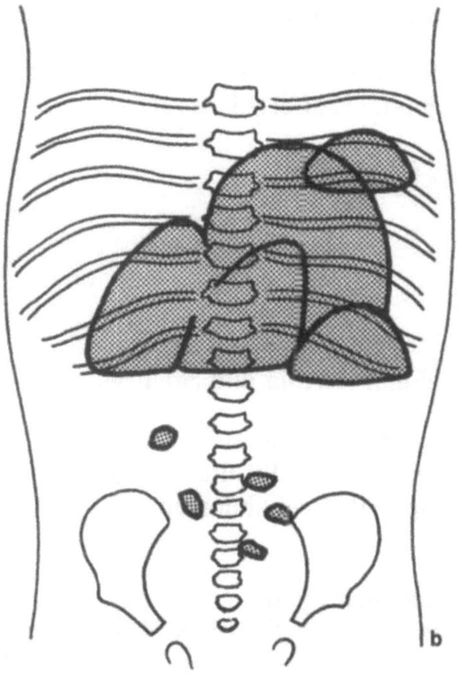

b

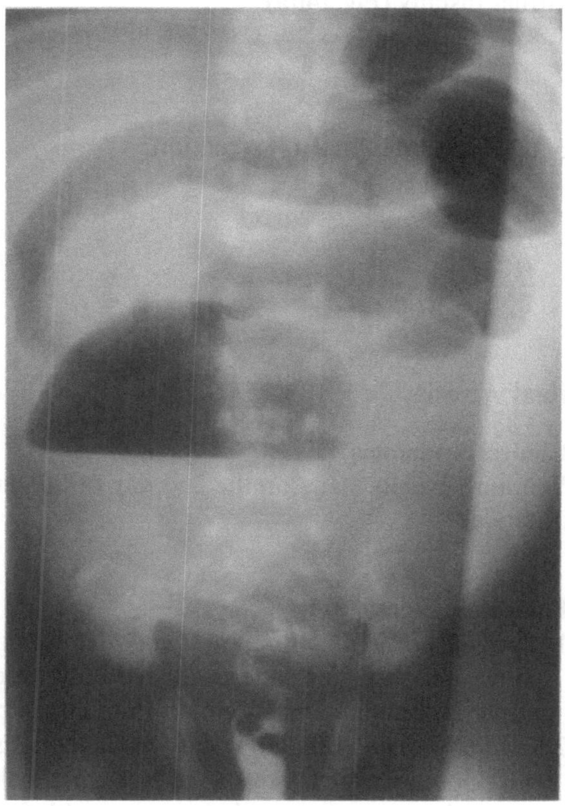

c

Fig. 240 a-c. Obstructions of the small bowel (drawings modified from Wolf 1971). **a Small-bowel atresia:** Dilated bowel loops in the upper and midabdomen with fluid levels, no air distally. **b Small-bowel stenosis:** Dilated bowel loops in the upper and midabdomen with fluid levels, air in the lower abdomen. **c** *Upright abdominal film* in sagittal projection of a 1-day-old newborn shows dilated bowel loops in the mid- and upper abdomen with an airless large bowel. Opacification of the colon is possible only to the rectosigmoid junction (microcolon). *Diagnosis:* ileal atresia

Other Obstructive Lesions of the Small Bowel

Most atresias of the small bowel occur in the lower ileum; occasionally the jejunum is affected.

> *Note:* The more distal the obstruction, the greater the number of air-fluid levels. Generally, one cannot distinguish between small-bowel and colonic fluid levels when intestinal obstruction is pronounced.

Jejunal Atresia and Stenosis

Clinical Symptoms
Vomiting, usually after the first feeding; distended upper abdomen; scaphoid lower abdomen

Radiologic Signs
Upright survey film of the chest and abdomen in the sagittal projection shows an abnormal air pattern: minimally dilated, air-filled bowel loops, especially in the left quadrants, with multiple fluid levels. No air is seen farther distally (Fig. 240 a).

5.1.2 Low Intestinal Obstruction

> *Note:* Unlike high obstructions, contrast enema is *always* required for the diagnosis of low intestinal obstructions.

Ileal Atresia

Clinical Symptoms
Vomiting usually starts on the 2nd day of life, and the abdomen is hugely distended.

Radiologic Signs
1. *Upright survey film of the chest and abdomen* in the sagittal projection shows abnormal air pattern: dilated bowel loops with fluid levels in the upper and midabdomen. No air in the large bowel (Fig. 240 c).
2. *Contrast enema* (diluted, water-soluble contrast medium). Early development of ileal atresia leads to microcolon from disuse atrophy (meconium passage: reaches cecum in 4th fetal month, rectum in 5th fetal month).

Radiologic Features of Microcolon
Threadlike or finger-thick bowel lumen that can be filled only under high hydrostatic pressure. Colon is shorter than normal and appears flattened at the flexures.

Note: Differential diagnosis of low small-bowel obstruction and microcolon:
1. Meconium ileus or meconium peritonitis
2. Low ileal atresia (small-bowel atresia), colon atresia, severe distal bowel stenoses
3. Hirschsprung's disease with aganglionosis of the entire colon

Anorectal Agenesis

Prevalence
The most common intestinal malformation, affecting 1:2500 to 1:3500 newborns

Diagnosis
Primary diagnosis is clinical; exploratory rectal catheterization is negative. Radiographs are useful for:
1. Evaluating an acute obstructive situation
2. Differentiating between a high-lying (supralevator) and low-lying (translevator) form
3. Demonstrating a fistula

Radiologic Signs
Plain radiographs should be taken at least 8-12 h after birth, since the terminal bowel needs to be adequately filled with air.
1. *Upside-down lateral abdominal film* on which the perineum and anal fossa are marked with barium past; the hips are held slightly flexed in a Babix sling (Fig. 241 a)

The air in the large bowel outlines the lower end of the blind pouch.

Caution: Escape of air through existing fistulae. Meconium in the blind pouch.

Reference lines to evaluate the form of the anorectal agenesis (Fig. 241 b)
Pubococcygeal (PC) line from the lower edge of the 5th sacral vertebra to the center of the pubis
I line (Kelly) through the lowest point of the ischium parallel to the PC line
M line (Cremin) midway between the PC line and I line, and parallel to them. The M line represents the boundary between the supra- and translevator forms.

2. With a visible and probable *fistula:* direct visualization of the blind pouch by injecting contrast medium through the catheterized fistula
3. *Visualization of the bladder and urethra (VCU):* The voiding cystourethrogram serves to demonstrate or exclude a retrovesical or retrourethral fistula and thus confirm or not a high or intermediate anomaly, for only these two categories are associated with retrouretheral or retrovesical fistulae.
4. *Visualization of the lower blind pouch* by percutaneous contrast injection from the perineum. Indication: high-lying form after the upside-down abdominal radiograph, no evidence of a fistula. The study is done supine

under sterile conditions. A spinal needle with stylet is inserted 1 cm anterior to the palpable tip of the coccyx, the stylet is withdrawn about 2 cm, and a syringe containing a nonionic contrast medium (e.g., metrizamide) is attached. The plunger is carefully raised and the needle advanced until meconium or air is aspirated. A small amount of contrast medium is injected, controlled by fluoroscopy, until the blind pouch is adequately visualized.
Spot films are taken in the strict lateral position with the perineum marked. The position of the blind pouch can vary considerably with the intra-abdominal pressure and contractile state of the levator sling; the lowest and highest positions of the pouch should be documented if possible (Fig. 241).

The various types of anorectal malformation are classified according to the Melbourne classification.

Note: Accurate classification is important, because the high-lying form of anorectal malformation requires an abdominal approach for surgical correction.

Atresia of the Colon

Prevalence
Very rare

Clinical Symptoms
Vomiting starting on the 2nd day of life, abdominal distension

Radiologic Signs
1. *Upright survey film of the chest and abdomen* in the sagittal projection shows abnormal air pattern with dilated bowel loops and multiple air-fluid levels in the upper and midabdomen.
2. *Contrast enema* (barium sulfate suspension or diluted water-soluble contrast). Isolated membranous atresia produces a "windsock sign" or windsocklike protrusion of the membrane, with microcolon distal to the membrane.

Congenital Megacolon, Hirschsprung's Disease

Prevalence
1:2000 to 1:5000 live births; males predominate by 4:1

Etiology
Aplasia of the intramural parasympathetic nerve ganglia in a segment of the colon. The narrow aganglionic segment may occur at a varying distance orad from the anus.

Clinical Symptoms
Drinking difficulties, bilious vomiting, abdominal distension, delay in passage of meconium, occasionally fulminating enterocolitis; in later cases, chronic constipation dating from birth.

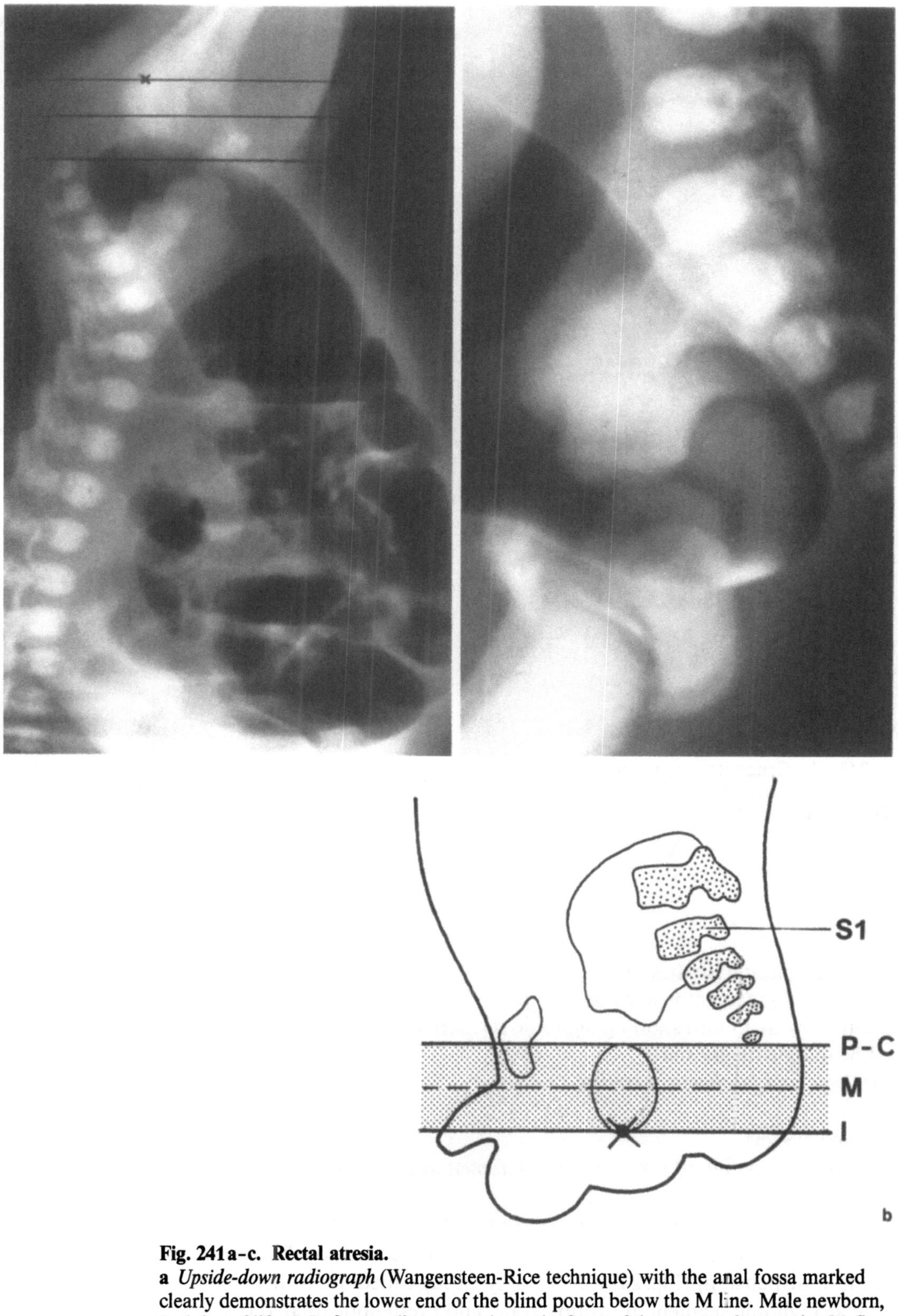

a c b

Fig. 241 a–c. Rectal atresia.
a *Upside-down radiograph* (Wangensteen-Rice technique) with the anal fossa marked clearly demonstrates the lower end of the blind pouch below the M line. Male newborn, 2nd day of life. **b** Reference lines to evaluate the form of the anorectal agenesis. *S1*, first sacral vertebra; *P-C*, pubococcygeal line between lower margin of S5 and center of pubic bone; *M*, line of Cremin halfway between P-C line and I line; *I*, line parallel to PC through the lowest point *(X)* of the ischium. **c** Visualization of the lower blind pouch by *percutaneous contrast injection* from the perineum: high form of rectal atresia (same child as in **a**)

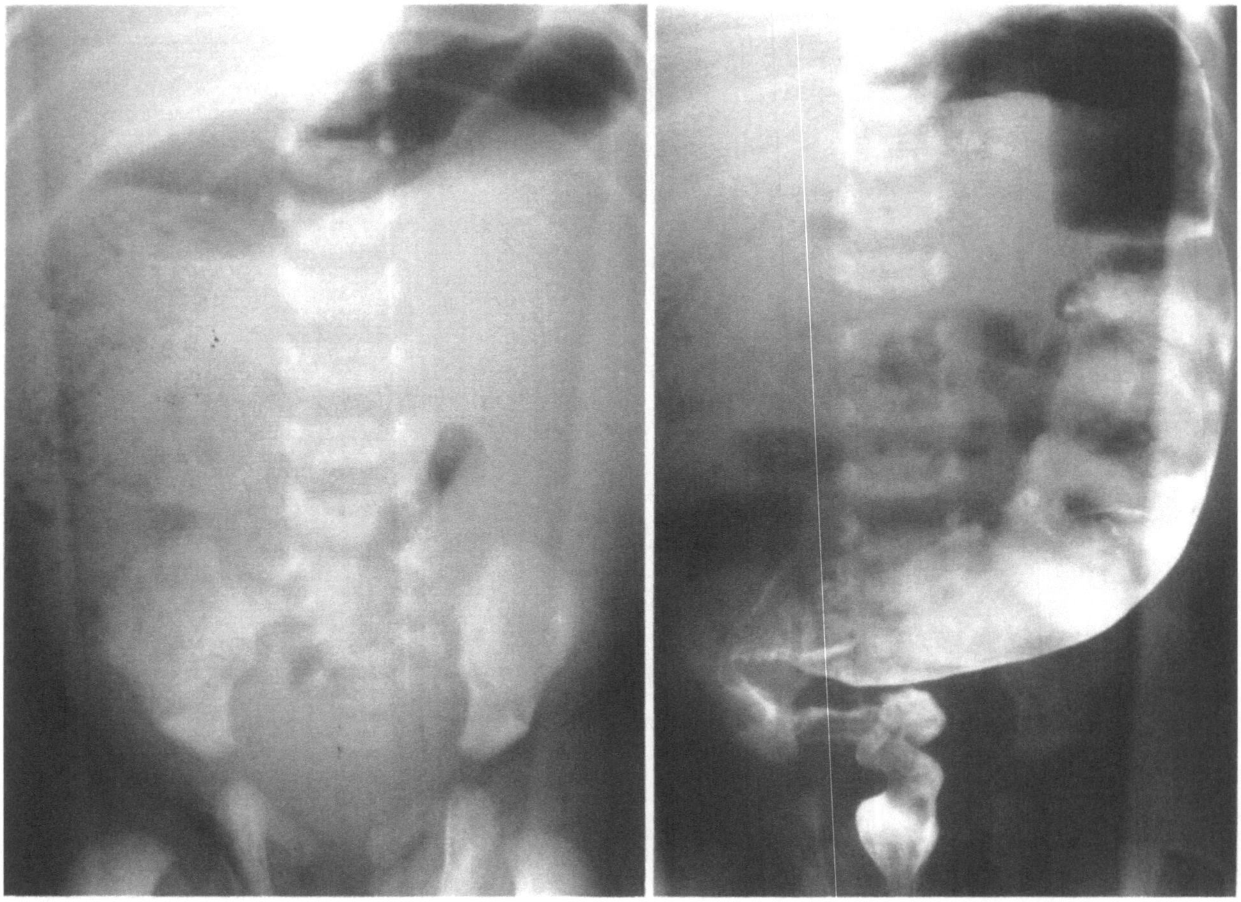

a b

Fig. 242 a, b. Congenital megacolon.
a *Upright abdominal film* in the sagittal projection shows a dilated colon containing a significant amount of stool.
b *Contrast enema* (dilute barium sulfate suspension/air) outlines the narrow segment in the region (newborn, 12th day of life)

Special Diagnostic Studies
Intraluminal manometry: accurate in up to 95% of cases; especially important with an ultrashort aganglionic segment (precluding radiographic and histologic diagnosis)
Histologic and biochemical studies

Radiologic Signs

1. *Upright survey film of the chest and abdomen* in the sagittal projection (Fig. 242 a)
2. *Lateral abdominal film* possibly with the Wangensteen-Rice technique
3. *Contrast enema* (diluted water-soluble contrast medium, or thin barium sulfate suspension) (Fig. 242 b). Use only enough medium to delineate the aganglionic segment, transition zone, and prestenotic dilated portion of the colon - normally about 10-30 ml! Double contrast as required. Short exposure times, small observation field (gonads!). Late films at 24 h and 48 h. Cleansing enema is contraindicated because it may distend the aganglionic segment and narrow the prestenotic dilatation of the sigmoid

Remarks on (1) and (2): Films show abnormal air pattern with distended bowel loops and fluid levels in the upper and midabdomen and also in the lower abdomen to a lesser degree; elevation of the diaphragm. Lateral view permits differentiation of colon and small-bowel loops (prevertebral descending colon), changes in the diameter of the affected colon, air in the rectum = incomplete obstruction.
Contrast enema produces transient improvement.

Caution: In newborns and infants, perforation of the colon and pneumoperitoneum can result from severe overdistension proximal to the narrowed segment, from ischemia and necrosis, or from manipulation with the rectal tube (damaged bowel wall).

Note: The aganglionic segment and prestenotic dilatation are not demonstrable during the first days of life, because both signs develop in mutual dependence on each other. Late films are necessary!

Generalized Aganglionosis of the Colon (very rare)

Clinical and Radiologic Signs

Intestinal obstruction. The caliber of the colon may be almost normal on contrast enema examination, but with significant microcolon, emptying will be impaired. Late films are necessary!

Meconium Ileus

Earliest manifestation of cystic fibrosis (mucoviscidosis). Most frequent cause of low intestinal obstruction in newborns.

Etiology

Prenatal obstruction of the terminal ileum by abnormal meconium. Danger of intrauterine perforation due to impaired intestinal blood flow

Clinical Symptoms

Bilious vomiting in the first days of life, abdominal distension, failure to pass meconium per rectum. Small-caliber rectum noted on rectal palpation

Radiologic Signs

1. *Upright survey film of the chest and abdomen* in the sagittal projection shows atypical air pattern: multiple dilated loops of small bowel *without* fluid levels. No air in the colon or rectum. Mottled "soap bubble pattern" within the bowel loops due to intermixture of gas with the viscid meconium
2. *Contrast enema* (diluted water-soluble contrast medium) shows microcolon. Study is both diagnostic and therapeutic, as the hyperosmotic contrast medium clears the obstruction and softens the inspissated meconium.

Caution: Meconium ileus may be complicated by a high localized atresia or volvulus.

Meconium Plug Syndrome

Etiology
Transitory functional obstruction of the distal large bowel by a viscous meconium plug

Clinical Symptoms
Vomiting, abdominal distension, visible peristalsis. Colonic emtying can occasionally be initiated by careful digital palpation of the rectum. Often the expelled meconium plug appears as a pencil-thin, greenish object several centimeters in length. If meconium passage fails to occur, X-ray examination is indicated.

Radiologic Signs
1. *Upright survey film of the chest and abdomen* in the sagittal projection shows abnormal air pattern with dilated loops of small bowel. Air-fluid levels with complete obstruction, foamy appearance of bowel contents due to intermixture of inspissated meconium with air bubbles
2. *Lateral film,* possibly with the Wangensteen-Rice technique: little or no air in the rectum
3. *Contrast enema* (diluted water-soluble contrast medium): both diagnostic and therapeutic. Demonstrates colon of normal caliber, expulsion of meconium plug

Note: Subsequent exclusion of congenital megacolon or mucoviscidosis is required.

Functional Transitory Intestinal Obstruction – Functional Neonatal Ileus

Etiology
Unknown

Clinical and Radiologic Signs
Features of low small-bowel obstruction without evidence of mechanical obstruction

5.1.3 Intestinal Pneumatosis

Causes
- Necrotizing enterocolitis (ischemic necrosis of the GI tract)
- Iatrogenic following umbilical catheterization } Rare
- Pneumomediastinum } Rare
- Enterocolitis with obstruction } Rare
- Hirschsprung's disease

Clinical Symptoms
Prematurity; abdominal distension; bilious vomiting; diarrhea; painful, bloody stools

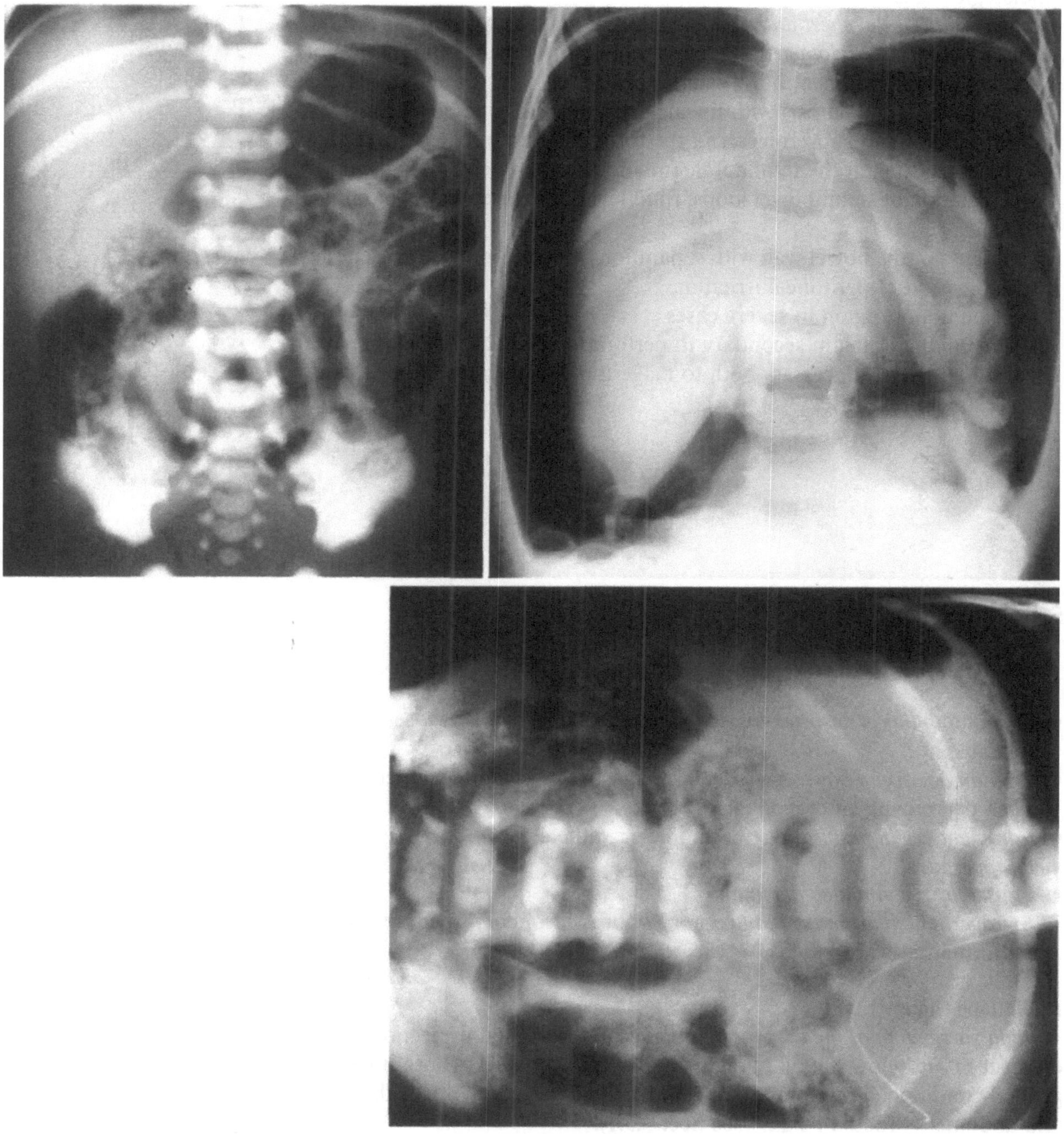

a c b

Fig. 243a–c. Pneumoperitoneum.
a *Supine abdominal film* in the sagittal projection shows intestinal pneumatosis. **b** *Left lateral film* in the horizontal projection shows pneumoperitoneum and intestinal pneumatosis. Multiple perforations of the small bowel (1-day-old newborn). **c** *Upright abdominal film* in the sagittal projection shows pneumoperitoneum after gastric ulcer perforation associated with a burn (infant)

Radiologic Signs

1. *Supine film of the chest and abdomen* in the sagittal projection
2. *L Lat film of the abdomen* in the cross-table projection, or upright film of the chest and abdomen in the sagittal projection
   - Intestinal pneumatosis with linear lucencies along the bowel wall, intramural and subserous air in the form of rings, bubbles, spots, or foam, starting at the terminal ileum and ascending colon (Fig. 243)
   - Dilatation of small-bowel loops, fluid levels as expression of paralytic ileus
   - Edema of the bowel wall with separation of bowel loops and ascites as expression of peritoneal irritation
   - Pneumoportogram in severe cases
   - Pneumoperitoneum secondary to perforation (Fig. 243). Abdominal radiography is necessary both to make the diagnosis and to evaluate treatment response.

Note: Intestinal pneumatosis is often already recognized in the portions of the upper abdomen that are depicted on the chest film.

5.1.4 Pneumoperitoneum

Perforation of the Gastrointestinal Tract

- *Proximal to bowel obstructions* (meconium ileus, atresias, stenoses, volvulus)
- *With an abnormal bowel wall* (defects in gastric muscular coat, neonatal ulcer, necrotizing enterocolitis)
- *Iatrogenic rectal perforation* (thermometer, catheter)
- *Postoperative*
- *Caused by pneumomediastinum*
- *Extraperitoneal air in the bladder* in newborns secondary to anorectal malformation with fistula

Radiologic Signs

Upright survey film of the chest and abdomen in the sagittal projection shows crescent of air below the diaphragm (Fig. 243 c). In babies whose poor general condition allows only supine and L Lat cross-table film of the chest and abdomen: "football sign" (see Sect. 3.5.1).

5.1.5 Intra-abdominal Calcifications

Sites of Occurrence

Abdominal wall: peritoneal calcifications after fetal meconium peritonitis from intrauterine bowel perforation (Fig. 244 b)
Liver: metastases, hepatoma
Retroperitoneum: tumor calcifications (neuroblastoma, Wilms' tumor)
Gastrointestinal tract
Peritoneal cavity: calcified mesenteric cyst (Fig. 244 b)
Meconium calcifications: possible in anal agenesis with cloaca due to intermixing of meconium and urine (fistula)

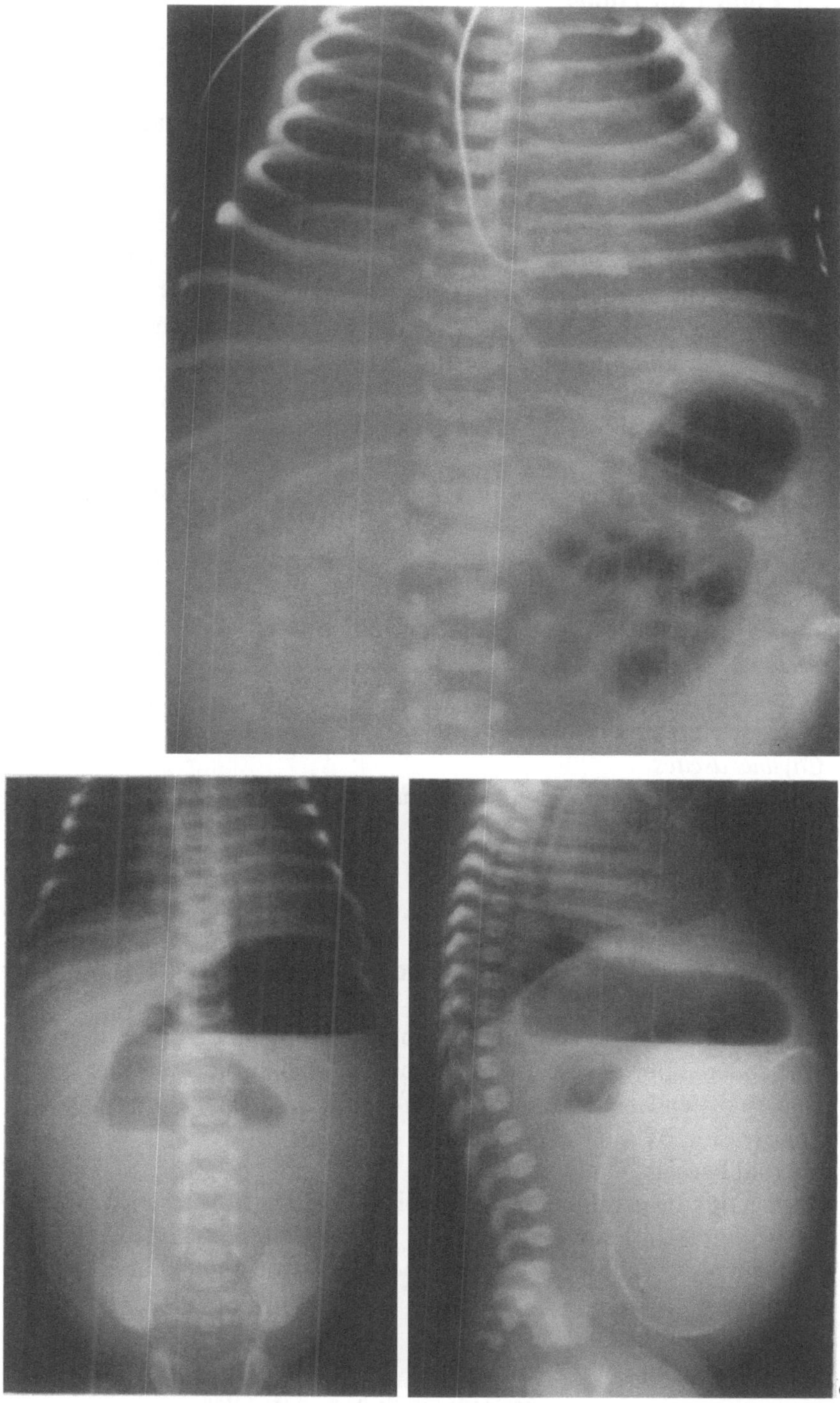

Fig. 244. a Peritoneal calcifications as a sequel to fetal meconium peritonitis from intrauterine bowel perforation, diagnosed prenatally by ultrasound. Male newborn, 1st day of life, mucoviscidosis.
b, c *Upright abdominal films* in anteroposterior and lateral projections show scaly calcifications in a mesenteric cyst (newborn) (Prof. H. J. von Lengerke, Department of Radiology, Westphalian Wilhelm University, Münster)

a

b

c

Note: Calcifications are uncommon after intrauterine bowel infarction. Contrast examination is occasionally necessary to pinpoint the calcifications.

5.1.6 Fluid Collections

Pyopneumoperitoneum

Caused by a postnatal perforation of the gastrointestinal tract

Radiologic Sings
1. *Sonography* demonstrates free intra-abdominal fluid.
2. *Upright survey film of the chest and abdomen* shows large air collection under the elevated diaphragm; caudal displacement of the liver and spleen; one or more fluid levels caused by exudation; uniform haziness of the lower abdomen due to effusion; paralytic ileus

Ascites

Causes are numerous; appropriate clinical-radiologic evaluation is necessary.
- *Urinary ascites:* due to perforation of the urinary tract (severe congenital obstruction)
- *Ascites:* due to perforation or anorectal malformation
- *Secondary to cardiac disease*
- *Secondary to hepatic disease*
- *Infectious* (especially syphilis)
- *Chylous ascites*
- *Rupture of large ovarian or mesenteric cyst*

5.1.7 Rare Causes of Acute Abdomen in Newborns

- Microgastria, gastric volvulus, lactobezoar, duplication of the stomach
- Preduodenal portal vein, duodenal hematomas (birth trauma), long duodenal stenosis due to absence of duodenal musculature or compression by a polycystic kidney
- Internal hernias, inguinal hernias
- Obstruction by clamping of the umbilical cord in the presence of an occult umbilical hernia
- Congenital short bowel syndrome (possible association with pyloric stenosis)
- Acute sigmoid volvulus
- Leiomyosarcoma of the colon
- Megacystis-microcolon syndrome with hypoperistalsis
- Torsion of an intra-abdominal testis
- Hepatic abscess caused by umbilical vein catheter
- Cholecystitis and hydrops of the gallbladder

5.2 Acute Abdomen in Infants

5.2.1 Paralytic Ileus

Intestinal Inflammations

Acute viral gastroenteritis is the most frequent cause of acute abdominal inflammatory diseases. An ominous complication in infants is dehydration with electrolyte disorders resulting from vomiting and diarrhea (toxicosis). Dehydration can be diagnosed from laboratory studies and also from the chest radiograph.

Radiologic Signs

1. *Sagittal chest film:* increased translucency of the lungs, decreased pulmonary vascular pattern, narrow cardiac silhouette
2. *Upright abdominal film,* or supine and L Lat film in infants whose general condition is poor: Features are variable. Often there are dilated bowel loops with air-fluid levels in both the small and large bowels.

Caution: If diarrhea is not (yet) present, these findings may be interpreted as mechanical bowel obstruction. Films are repeated as necessary.

Appendicitis (see Sects. 4.1.4 and 5.3.1)

Extraintestinal Inflammations

Pneumonia (especially pneumococcal and staphylococcal)

Note: A chest radiograph is always necessary in infants with acute abdomen!

Other inflammatory conditions: empyema, purulent meningitis, urinary tract infection, pertussis

5.2.2 Mechanical Bowel Obstruction

Hypertrophic Pyloric Stenosis

Prevalence

1:300 to 1:900 live births in Western countries. Males predominate by 5:1.

Clinical Symptoms

Symptoms appear at 2-10 weeks of age: forceful, copious vomiting after drinking; weight loss with dehydration; characteristic facies; palpable pyloric mass; peristaltic waves in the epigastrium and left upper quadrant shortly after feeding.

Laboratory tests show metabolic acidosis, hypochloremia, hypokalemia, hemoconcentration

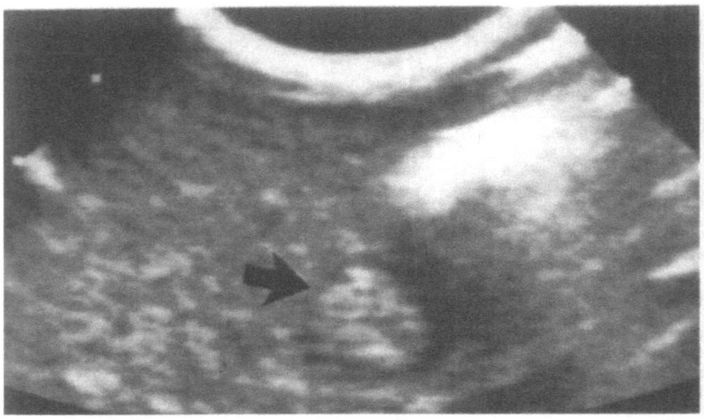
a

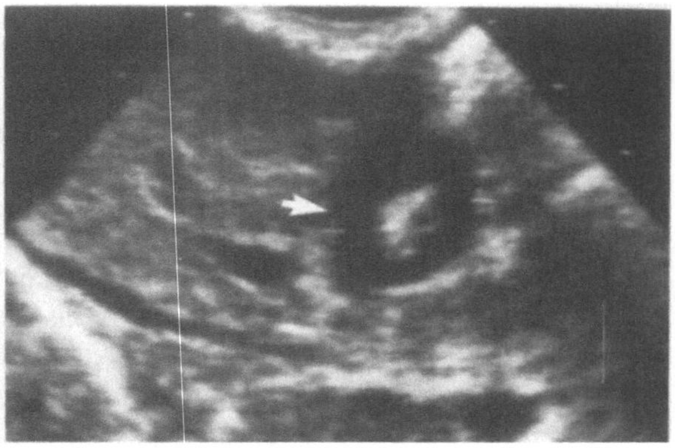
c

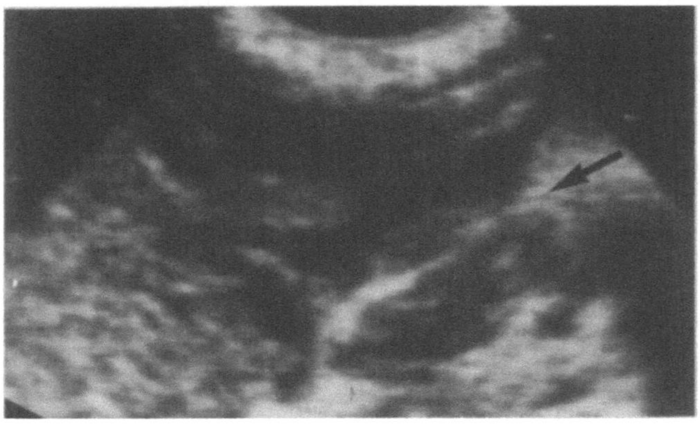
b

Fig. 245 a–e. Hypertrophic pyloric stenosis.
a *Sonographic appearance* of a normal pyloric canal (➧). Premature, newborn male, 3 weeks old. **b** *Sonographic appearance* of hypertrophic pyloric stenosis, longitudinal scan: thick pylorus muscle, narrow pyloric canal (→). **c** *Sonographic appearance* of hypertrophic pyloric stenosis (→), transverse scan 1.6 cm; 6-week-old male infant. **d** *Upright chest and abdomen film,* monozygotic twin, female, 3 weeks' old: marked gastric ectasia following aspiration of fluid and insufflation of about 30 ml of air by gastric tube. Abdomen distal to the stomach is almost gasless. **e** Sibling to patient in **d,** UGI series (dilute barium sulfate suspension): classic pattern with narrow and elongated pyloric canal and hoodlike duodenal bulb with marked delay of transit of contrast medium

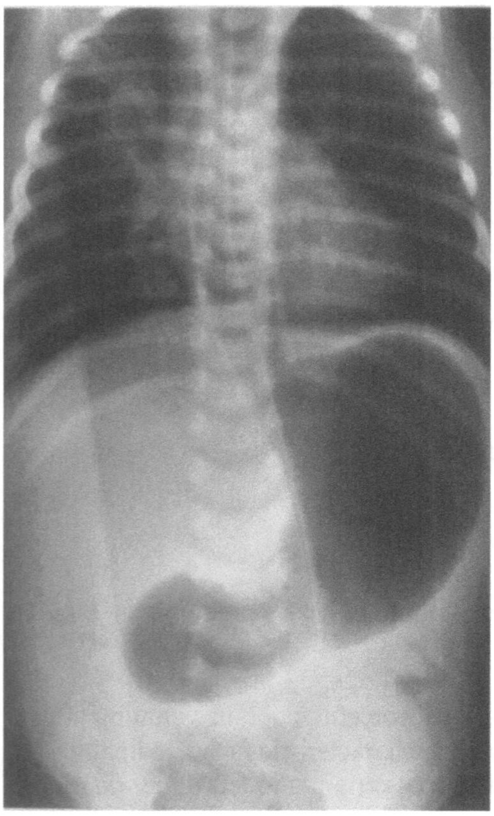
d

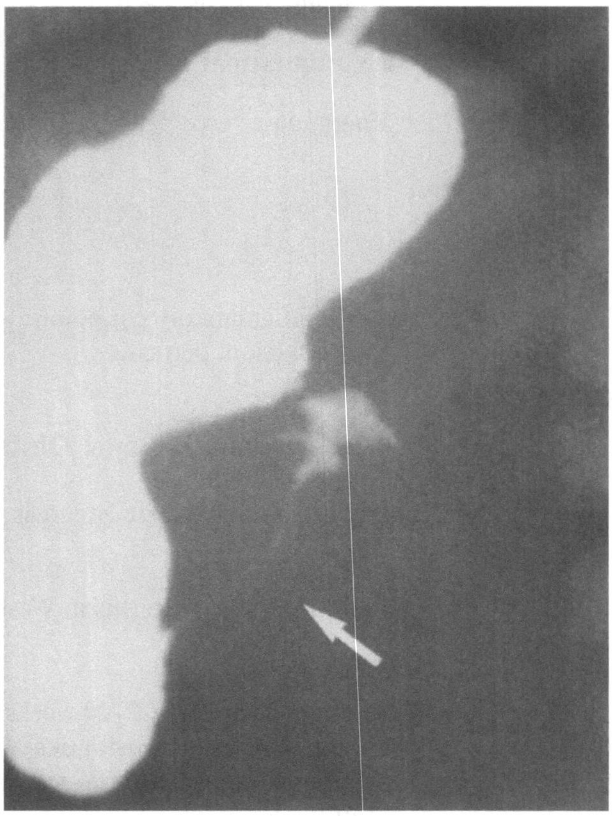
e

Radiologic Signs

Sonography
Examination is often hampered by a dilated, air-filled stomach, so air and residual stomach contents are aspirated by gastric tube, and approximately 20 ml of tea or 0.9% NaCl is instilled.
Examination in the R Lat position gives a good view of the pyloric region with a fluid-filled antrum. The pylorus appears directly adjacent to the gallbladder.
In hypertrophic pyloric stenosis the pylorus presents a target pattern in cross section with a markedly thickened, hypoechoic pylorus muscle and a hyperechoic central area representing the lumen (Fig. 245 c). In longitudinal section the thick pylorus muscle encloses the narrow, threadlike pyloric canal (Fig. 245 b).
The normal cross-sectional width of the pylorus in healthy children of this age is approximately 1.1 cm (Fig. 245 a). A width of 1.6–2.3 cm is considered an indication for surgery (Fig. 245 c). A pyloric width of 1.1–1.6 cm probably represents a spastic stenosis that can be treated nonoperatively.
The individual diameters of the muscular layer and canal are determined on the longitudinal scan.
Ratio of the muscular layer thickness to the central echo:
- less than 1 in healthy infants,
- usually greater than 2 in infants with hypertrophic pyloric stenosis (Fig. 245 b)

Plain Radiographs
Upright survey film of the chest and abdomen, or supine film for infants in poor general condition: large air- or food-filled stomach, caudal displacement of bowel loops containing little air. With equivocal findings, aspirate gastric contents and insufflate 20–30 ml of air (Fig. 245 d).
A post-aspiration condition is possible.

Contrast Examination
If evaluation of plain radiographs proves difficult, *upper GI series* (with barium sulfate suspension or nonionic contrast medium): Small amount of contrast medium administered in R Lat position using a special Förster bottle or nasogastric tube. Delayed gastric emptying, elongated pyloric canal, hoodlike duodenal bulb (Fig. 245 e).
After the pyloric canal has been opacified, the remaining contrast medium is aspirated.

Important:
Exclusion of Roviralta syndrome (combination of hiatal hernia and pyloric stenosis)

Incarcerated Inguinal Hernia (see Sect. 4.2.1)

Intussusception

Prevalence
The most frequent cause of acute abdomen in infants and small children: 70–80% of all intussusceptions occur in the first 2 years of life (75% in 1st year, 13% in 2nd year) with a peak between the 3rd and 9th months of life. Intussusception can also occur in utero. It is extremely rare in children of school age.
Males predominate by 3:2.

Pathogenesis
Usually occurs in the setting of enteritis as a result of increased intestinal mobility. Rarely it results from neoplastic changes in the bowel wall or mesentery (5%).
A segment of bowel with its mesentery invaginates into the lumen of the adjacent, aboral bowel segment. Peristalsis propels the invaginated bowel (the intussusceptum) farther analward (Fig. 246a).

Types of Intussusception
- Jejuno-jejunal intussusception (rare)
- Ileocolic intussusception with or without involvement of the cecum and appendix (80%)
- Colocolic intussusception
- Ileoileal intussusception

Results:
Venous congestion, edematous swelling, hyperemic bleeding and necrosis in the late stage due to mesenteric vascular constriction. Intestinal surfaces may become adherent to one another.

Clinical Symptoms
History of enteritis is common. Severe, recurring abdominal colic
Shock symptoms: pallor, sweating, vomiting
Symptom-free interval due to delayed onset of peritonitic irritation
The intussusceptum is palpable as a cylindrical abdominal mass.
Rectal examination: blood on the finger
Urgent late signs: heavier bloody discharge from the bowel, symptoms of intestinal obstruction
Exception: ileoileal intussusception (see below), intermittent jejuno-jejunal intussusception as a rare case with intermittent abdominal pain without ileus symptoms.

Note: A suspected intussusception demands swift action, because delays may necessitate bowel resection and increase the likelihood of a fatal outcome!

Fig. 246 a–h. Intussusception.
a Ileocolic intussusception. b *Upright film of chest and abdomen* shows little air in the abdomen. Terminal ileum is dilated and displaced laterally. Female infant, 5 months old, with 5 h history of ileocecal intussusception. Reduction. **c** *Upright film of chest and abdomen:* intestinal obstruction. Male infant, 3 months old. **Ileocecal intussusception** about 20 cm in length. Reduction was not possible, and 10 cm of bowel had to be resected.

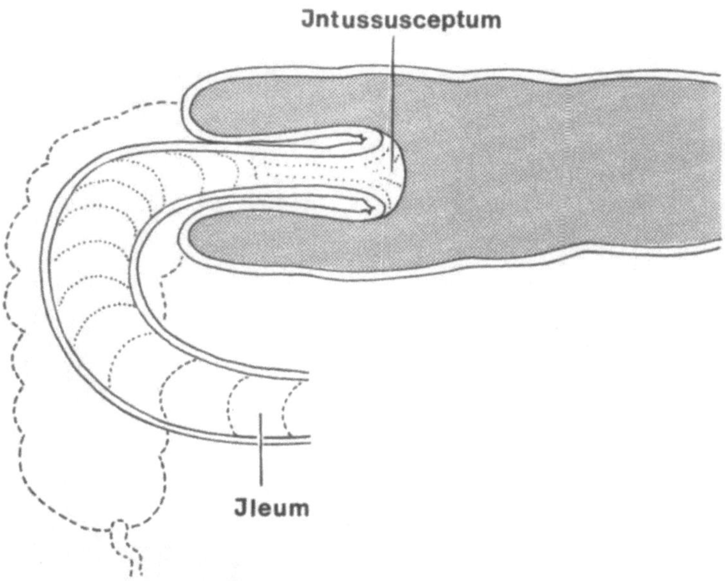

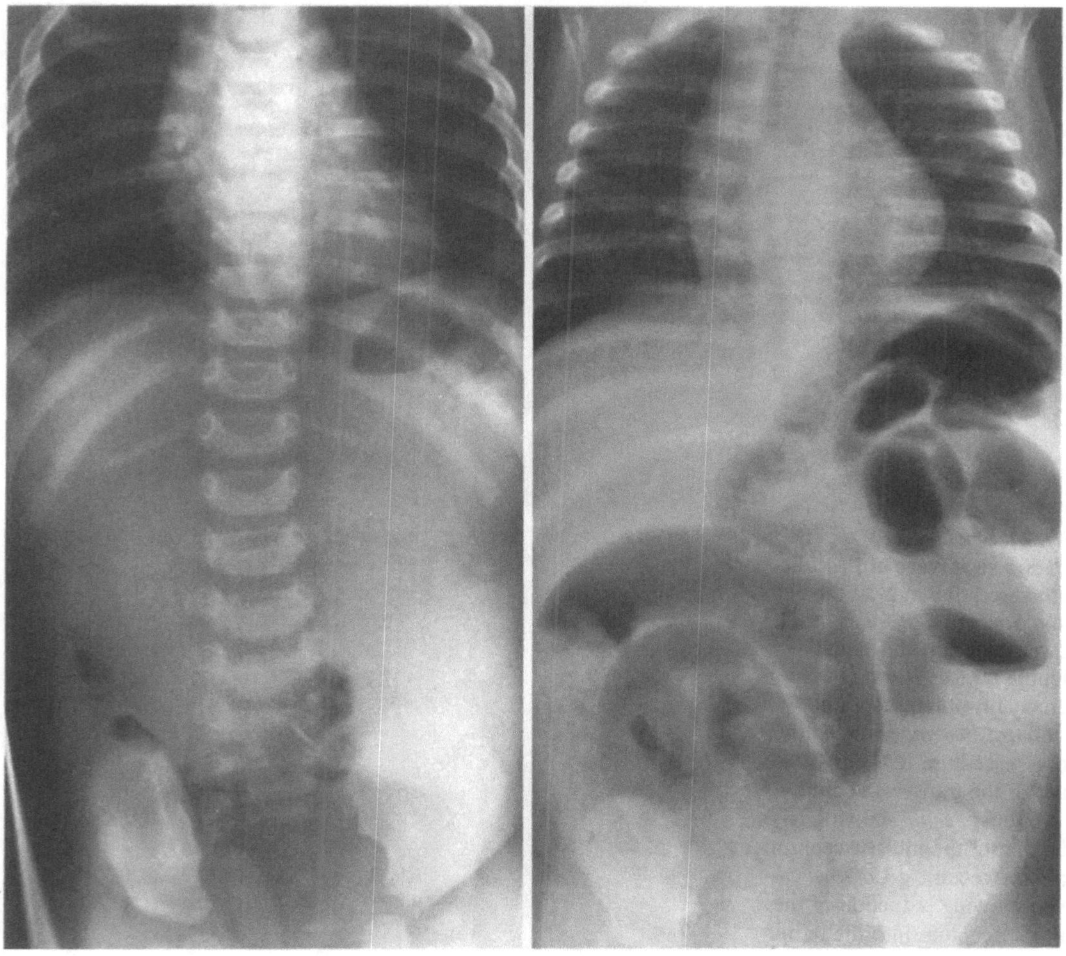

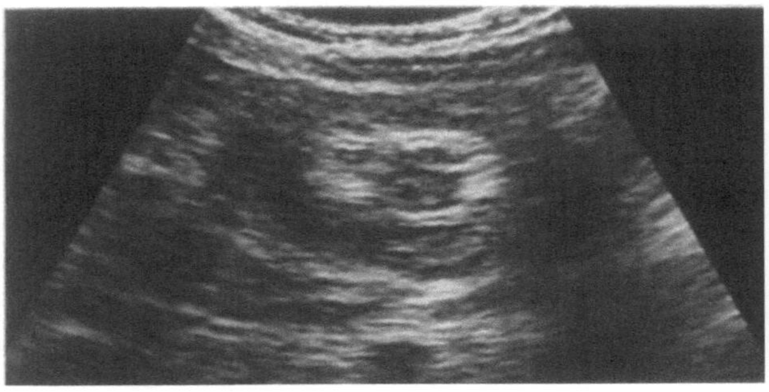
d

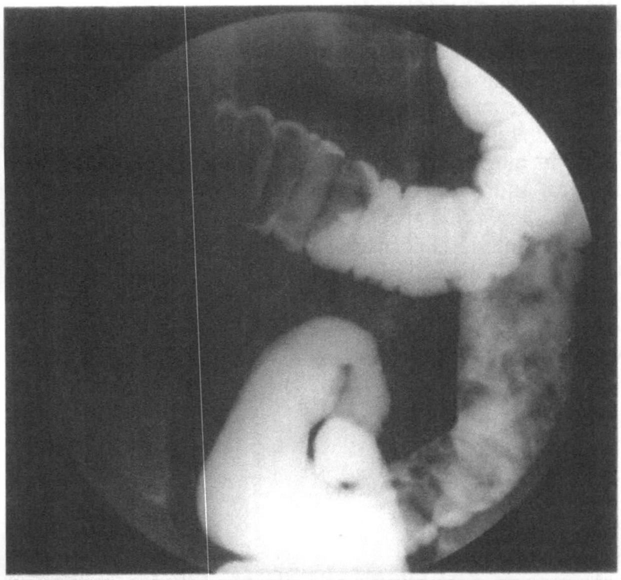
e

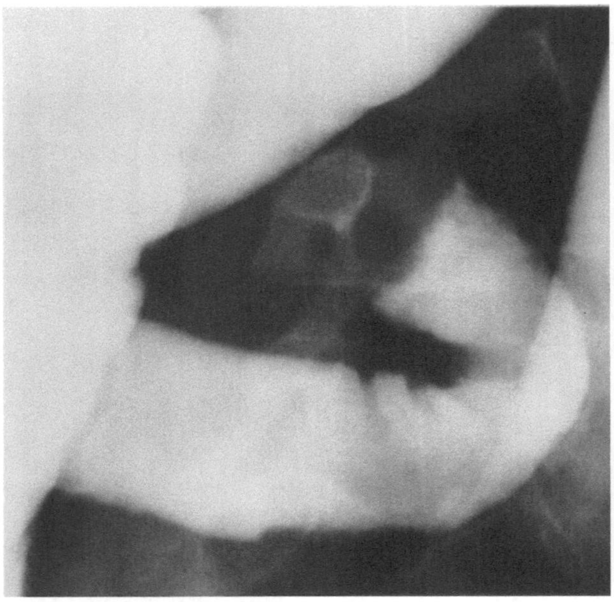
g

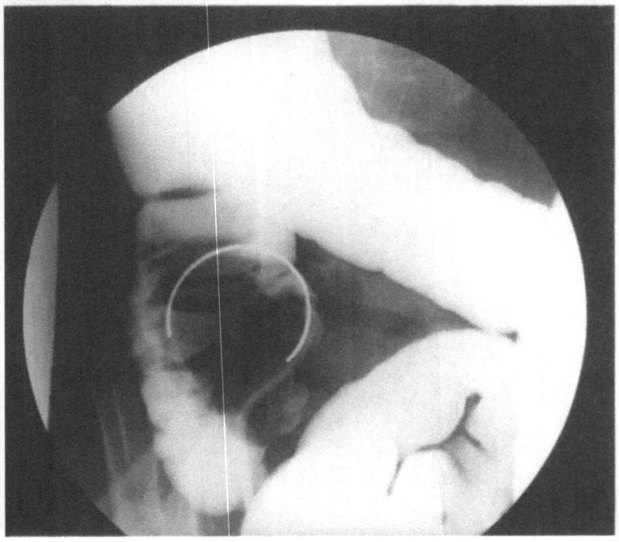
f

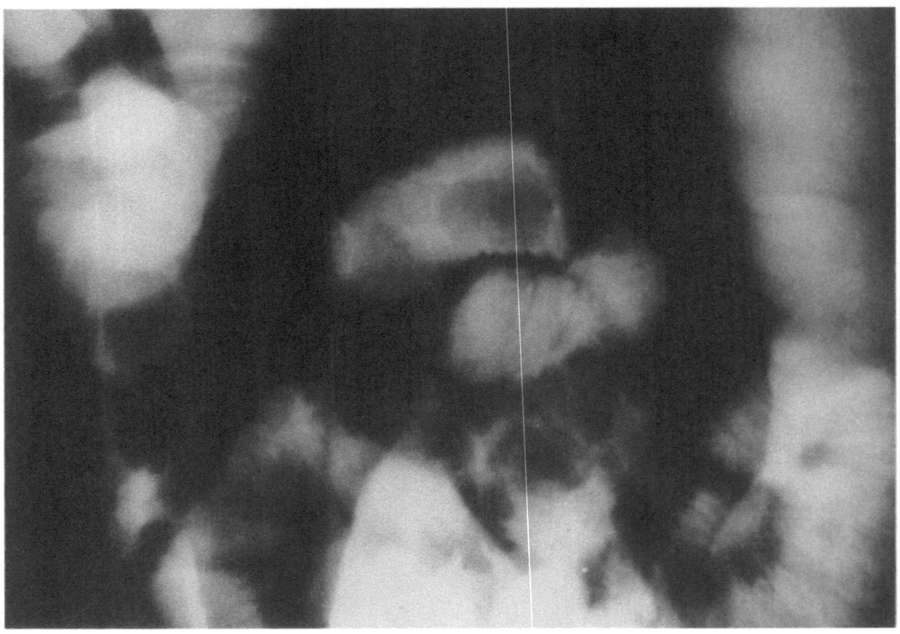
h

Fig. 246 (continued)
d Third recurrence of ileocolic intussusception in a 5-year-old boy. *Sonogram* of the right lower quadrant shows the double target pattern characteristic of intussusception. **e** *Contrast enema* showing the intussusceptum in the right half of the transverse colon. **f** *Contrast enema* showing reduction of the intussusceptum into the cecum. **g** *Contrast enema* showing reduction of the intussusceptum into the terminal ileum. **h** *Contrast enema* showing the intussusception completely reduced; there is normal reflux of contrast medium into the ileum. *Surgery* after fourth recurrence revealed a pedunculated leiomyoma of the ileum

Radiologic Signs

Plain Radiographs
Depending on the general condition of the child: *upright survey film of the chest and abdomen* or *supine and L Lat abdominal films*. Films show no abnormalities in the early stage.
In the advanced stage films show decreased air in the stomach and duodenum, dilatation and lateral displacement of the terminal ileum, and only little or no gas in the colon (Fig. 246b).
Occasionally the tip of the intussusception appears as a soft-tissue mass surrounded by air.
Signs and symptoms of intestinal obstruction do not appear until 12-24 h after the acute event (Fig. 246c).
Exception: ileoileal intussusception, which leads early to bowel obstruction with fluid levels, jejuno-jejunal intussusception without characteristic roentgen signs.

Sonography
Typical target lesion produced by edematous bowel wall, as in inflammatory bowel diseases. The thickened, hypoechoic margin represents the edematous intussuscipiens, which surrounds an echogenic center. The latter results from compression of the mucosal and serosal layers of the intussusceptum; however, the consistently thickened, hypoechoic wall of the intussuscipiens is an important differential diagnostic criterion and is specific for this condition (Fig. 246d).
A negative sonogram does not preclude intussusception and should be followed by a contrast enema. This study also possesses therapeutic value, although hydrostatic reduction under sonographic vision has been proposed as an alternative.

UGI series in cases with jejuno-jejunal intussusception (Fig. 247).

Contrast Enema
A water-soluble diluted contrast medium is safe in terms of perforation risk. Barium sulfate suspension is most commonly used in Scandinavia and the United States of America.
Following digital rectal examination, a balloon-tipped catheter of the largest possible caliber is introduced. The contrast medium is instilled under low pressure (90-100 cmH_2O) using the smallest possible fluoroscopic field (gonad protection!). Usually the head of the contrast column becomes concave on reaching the intussusception ("cup" form; Fig. 246). An onionskin pattern is produced when small amounts of contrast medium enter the space between the intussusceptum and bowel wall.
Other radiologic patterns of intussusception are shown in Fig. 248).

Fig. 247a–c. *UGI series* in an 8-year-old boy shows spontaneous resolution of **jejunojejunal intussusception**

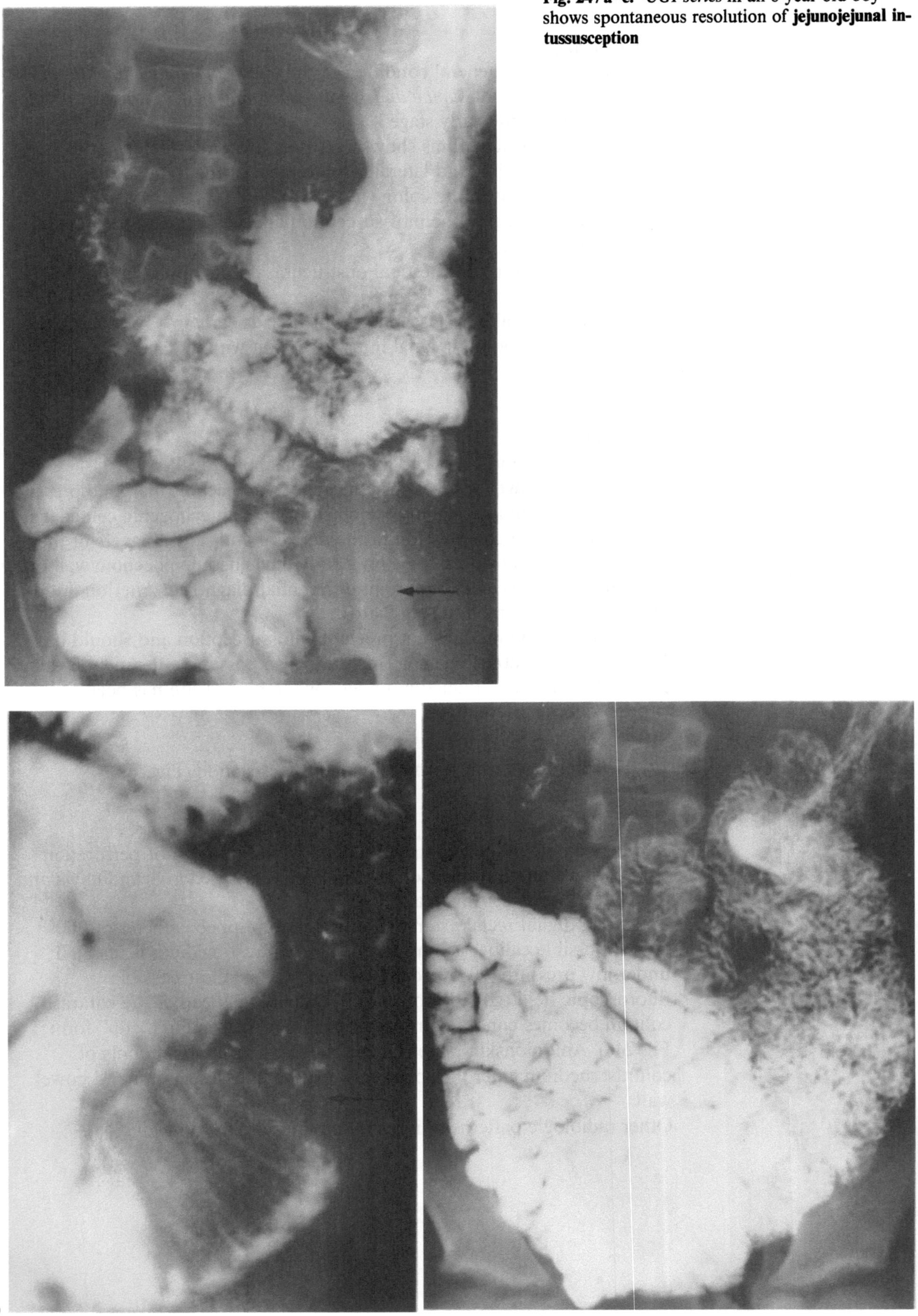

a

b

c

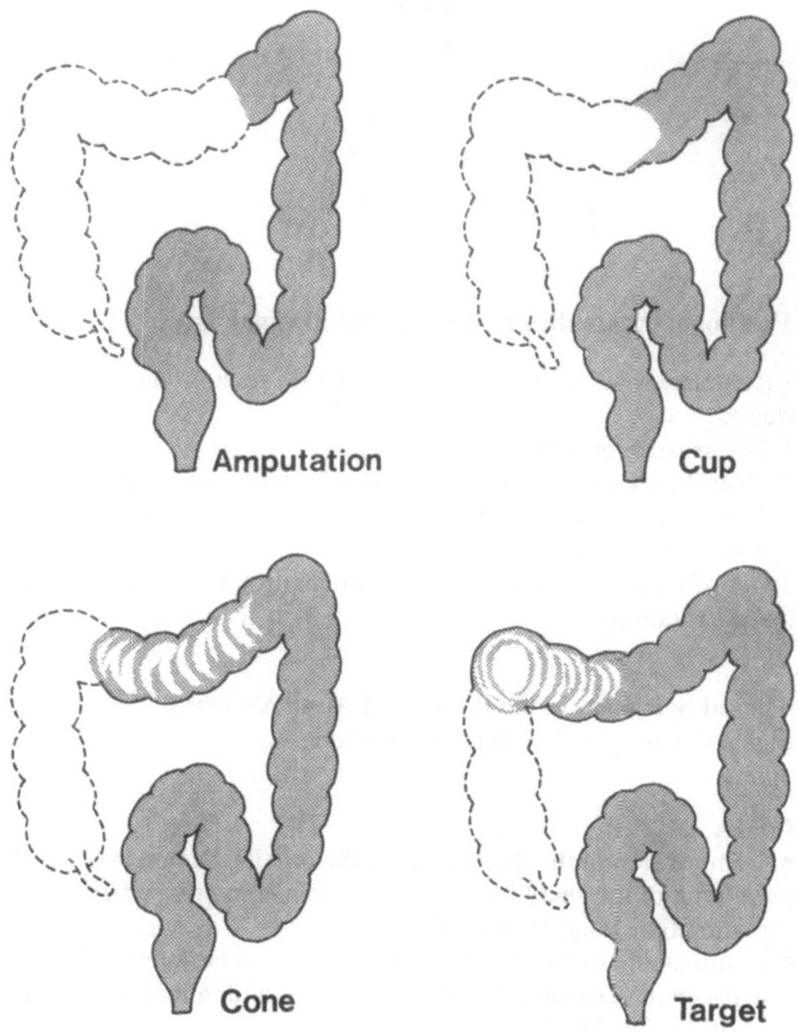

Fig. 248. Possible radiographic appearances of intussusception. (After Grob 1982)

Trial of Hydrostatic Pressure Reduction

Elected in consultation with the surgeon.

The immediate history may not exceed 12–24 h. There must be no evidence of peritonitis, minimal bloody discharge, and the child's general condition and electrolyte status must be satisfactory.

Contraindications: Suspicion of bowel damage with history longer than 24 h, shock, dehydration, peritonitis, complete intestinal obstruction, profuse bloody discharge

The intussusceptum having been demonstrated, diazepam is administered i.v., and additional contrast medium is carefully instilled under low pressure without palpating the bowel. The most difficult phase is getting past the ileocecal valve. Reduction has been successfully accomplished when the contrast column refluxes freely into the terminal ileum. Survey films are taken after the reduction to exclude reinvagination.

Note: If the contrast medium is discharged before reduction is accomplished, a second attempt may be made by the insufflation of air. A third attempt should *not* be made.
If reduction is not obtained or the immediate history is too long (more than 12–24 h), *laparotomy* is indicated.
Reduction of an ileoileal intussusception is *not* recommended!

Positional Anomalies of the Gastrointestinal Tract

Incomplete rotation (malrotation) of the GI tract in the early fetal period due to:
1. Disturbance of fetal bowel rotation
2. Disturbance in the intrinsic growth of certain bowel segments
3. Defect of mesenteric adhension that precludes normal fixation in the abdominal cavity

Types of fetal malrotation: nonrotation, malrotation I, malrotation II, inverse rotations

Clinical Symptoms in the Presence of Acute Abdomen

Signs of high-lying intestinal obstruction

Causes

- Compression of the duodenum by the proximal colon and possibly winding of the small bowel around the mesenteric pedicle (volvulus) in malrotation I and II (Fig. 249 a)
- Compression of the small bowel by fibrous adhesions (Ladd's bands) between the proximal colon and posterior abdominal wall in malrotation I and II (Fig. 249 a)

Note: Rapid diagnosis is imperative because of the potential for small-bowel infarction!

Radiologic Signs

1. *Upright film of chest and abdomen* or supine and L Lat abdominal film, depending on patient's condition: see Duodenal and Small-Bowel Obstruction (Fig. 249 b)
2. *Contrast enema* (barium sulfate suspension): Visualization of colon on the lower end of the cecum to establish the type of malrotation (Fig. 249 c)

Note: With signs of high intestinal obstruction of unknown cause, *contrast enema* is necessary to confirm or exclude a positional anomaly. *Gastric volvulus* produces a particularly acute surgical emergency with vomiting and severe abdominal pain.

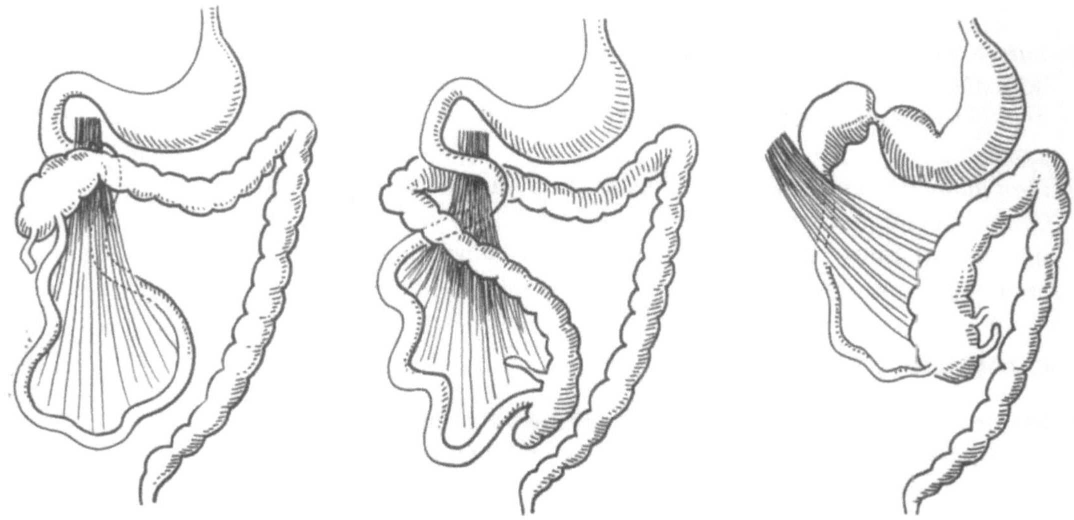

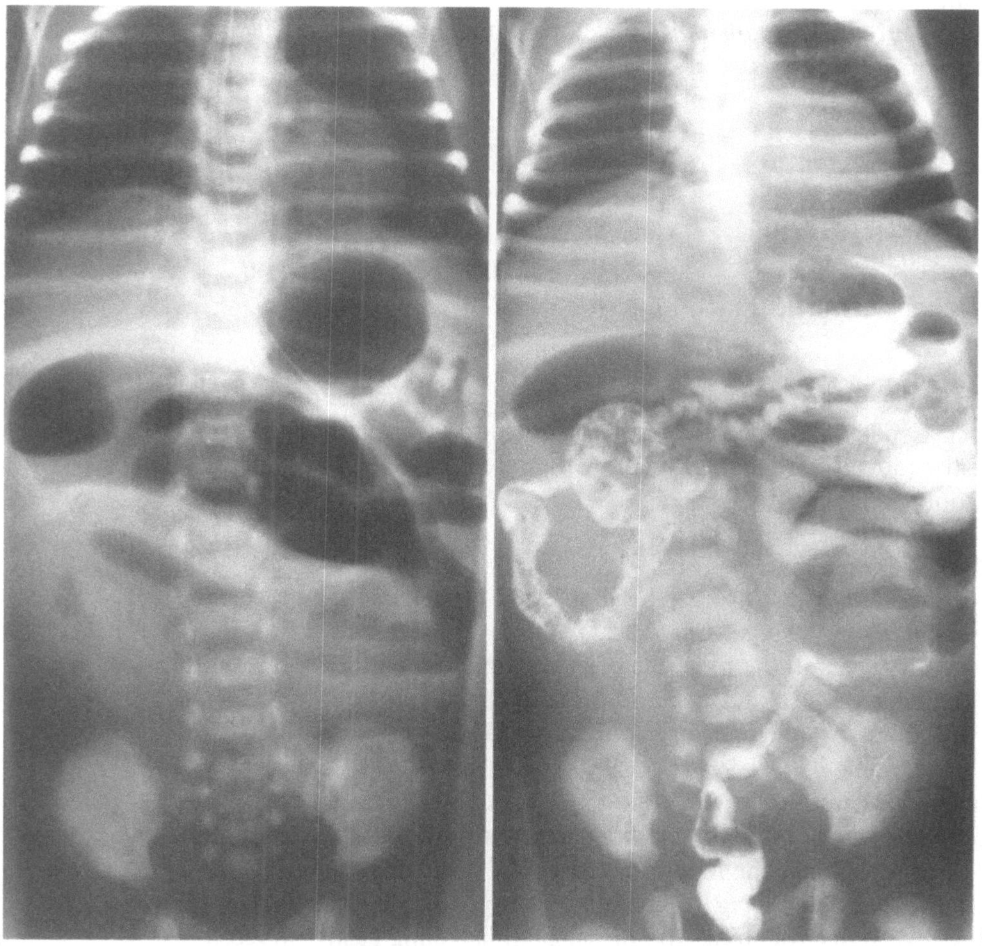

b c

Fig. 249 a–c. Positional anomalies of the gastrointestinal tract with compression of the small bowel.
a Scheme of Grob (1982). **b** *Upright film of chest and abdomen* after aspiration of stomach fluid and insufflation of air by gastric tube: bowel obstruction in **malrotation I due to volvulus.** Female newborn, 2nd day of life. **c** *Upright film of chest and abdomen* after contrast enema and oral contrast medium: **malrotation I with volvulus** (same child as in **b**)

Radiologic Signs in Gastric Volvulus

1. *Survey film of chest and abdomen* in supine and L Lat position in the horizontal projection: a large, wide stomach with elevation of the left hemidiaphragm; usually two fluid levels are observed in the volvulus stomach.
2. *Oral administration of contrast medium* (barium sulfate suspension): Contrast column terminates in the distal esophagus, indicating a high obstruction. Entry of the medium into the cardia will demonstrate the anomalous position of the stomach.

Internal Hernias (see Sect. 4.2.1)

1. Mesocolic hernia: In malrotation II and inverse rotation the entire small-intestinal mass can herniate into its mesentery, which envelops it like a sack.
2. Right mesocolic hernia: Envelopment of the small-bowel loops by the mesocolon in malrotation II

The picture of *acute abdomen* develops in the event of *strangulation of the mesenteric vessels.*

Meckel's Diverticulum

Causes

Persistence of the intra-abdominal portion of the omphalomesenteric duct. Usually the mucosa is orthotopic ileal mucosa, although ectopic gastric (50%), duodenal, and colonic mucosa may occur as well as ectopic pancreatic tissue.

Clinical Symptoms

Occasionally leads to recurrent abdominal complaints. The picture of *acute abdomen* results from:

- Peptic ulcers in the presence of gastric mucosa with penetration into the adjacent ileal mucosa and profuse intestinal bleeding
- Inflammatory changes in the mucosa (Meckel's diverticulitis)

Radiologic Signs

1. *Upright film of the chest and abdomen* or supine and L Lat abdominal films to disclose the nature of the bowel obstruction
2. *Radionuclide imaging* (^{99}Tc): only means available for demonstrating Meckel's diverticulum. The presence of secreting gastric mucosa causes accumulation of the radioisotope in the lesion.

Note: Meckel's diverticulum can lead to the following complications:
1. Intussusception
2. Ileal obstruction
3. Intestinal strangulation with volvulus due to congenital bands or antecedent inflammation
4. Necrosis of the diverticulum secondary to pedicular rotation and torsion
5. Contents of right-sided inguinal hernia

Congenital Megacolon (see Sect. 5.1.2)

5.3 Acute Abdomen in Small and School-Age Children

5.3.1 Acute Appendicitis (see Sect. 4.1.4)

Acute appendicitis is the most common surgical disorder of childhood. It is most prevalent between the 12th and 14th years of life, its icidence declining steadily before and after. Isolated cases have been described in newborns, but the disease is uncommon in children under 5 years of age. For this reason the possibility of acute appendicitis is *rarely* considered in *small children*. This fact, plus the difficulties of localizing pain in this age group and the variability in the position of the appendix, explain why in 90% of children who develop appendicitis before 5 years of age, a perforation already exists at the time of hospitalization, and the disease is taking a fulminant course.

Radiologic Signs

There is no standard diagnostic approach, because the picture of an acute abdomen is predominant:

1. *Upright film of the chest and abdomen* or supine and L Lat abdominal films. Features are highly variable; the following signs are present with greater consistency:
   - Dilatation of the cecum and terminal ileum with associated air-fluid levels (sentinal loops) (Fig. 250 b)
   - Pneumoperitoneum (Fig. 250 a)
   - Demonstration of a coprolith (fecolith) (Fig. 250 c)
2. *Sonography.* In many cases sonography provides additional evidence of appendicitis, a paratyphlitic abscess or a subhepatic abscess in Morison's pouch in cases of retrocecal appendicitis (Fig. 250 d) (see Sect. 4.1.4).

Fig. 250 a–e. Appendicitis.
a *Upright abdominal film* shows a perforated appendicitis, pneumoperitoneum. Female newborn, 15th day of life, Down's syndrome. **b** *Erect abdominal film* shows a low-sited, small-bowel obstruction (sentinel loops). Perforated appendicitis in a 7-year-old girl. **c** Small-bowel obstruction. Perforated appendicitis and coprolith in a 3.5-year-old boy.

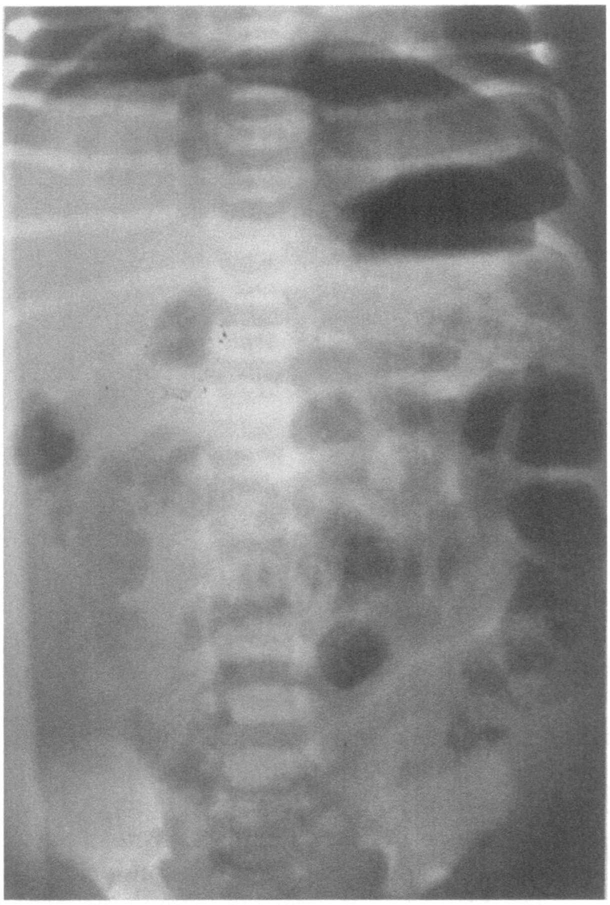

a

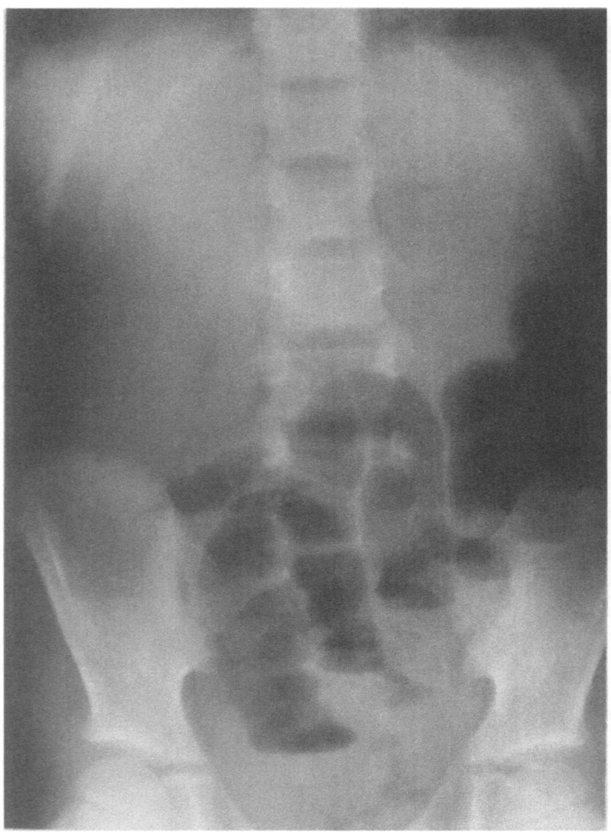

b

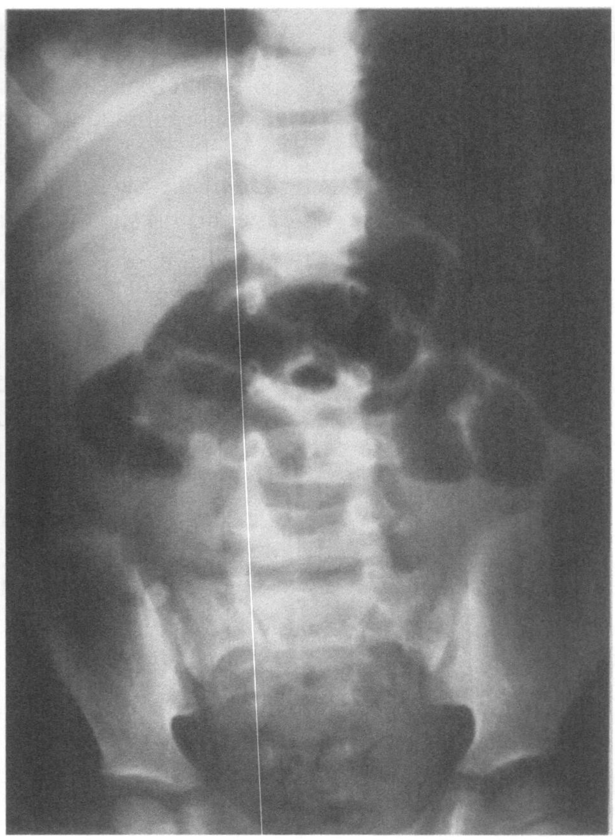

c

Fig. 250 (continued)
d *Sonogram*, right subcostal region: hepatorenal recess (Morison's pouch) caused by perforated appendicitis with abscess. *L*, liver; *A*, abscess; *K*, kidney. **e** *Upright film of abdomen* in the sagittal projection: air-fluid level in abscess in a 2.9-year-old girl. *Operation* revealed perforated retrocecal appendicitis with abscess

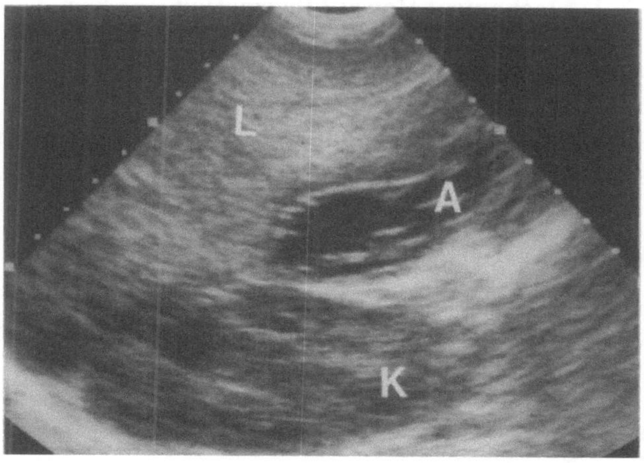

d

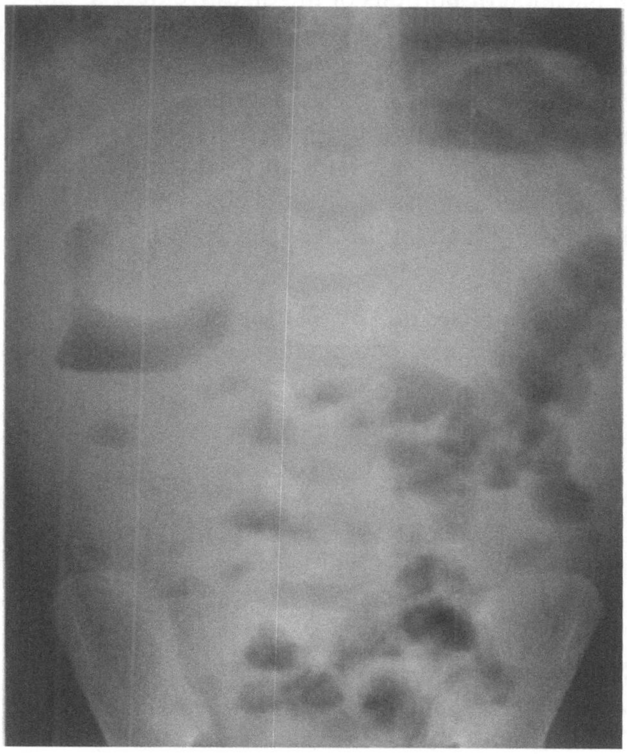

e

Purulent peritonitis in children is most commonly a seepage-type peritonitis following the perforation of an appendicitis.

Differential diagnosis of acute appendicitis in children:
Mesenteric lymphadenitis, Meckel's diverticulitis, urinary tract disease, adnexitis

5.3.2 Mechanical Bowel Obstruction (see Sect. 4.2.1)

Postoperative Adhesions

Volvulus due to Positional Anomalies of the Gastrointestinal Tract (see Sect. 5.2.2)

Meckel's Diverticulum (see Sect. 5.2.2)

Gastrointestinal Duplications (synonyms: enterogenic cyst, enterocystoma, giant diverticula)

Etiology
Duplication of portions of the digestive tract in the form of cystic or tubular cavities from the esophagus to the anus. The mesenteric side of the bowel is a site of predilection. Most of these lesions exhibit a typical bowel wall structure with the presence of mucosa and musculature. If the lesion lacks direct communication with the digestive tract, secretions may cause a rise of internal pressure with mucosal atrophy. Should a perforation occur, the signs and symptoms of acute abdomen will appear. Sane 40% become clinically apparent in the neonatal period.

Clinical Symptoms in Acute Abdomen
Vomiting, palpable abdominal mass, intestinal bleeding and/or obstruction

Note: There may be associated malformations of the intestine, urogenital tract, and vertebral column.
Duplications of the bowel can be tentatively diagnosed prenatally with ultrasound, and so overt disease in the form of an acute abdomen is becoming less frequent.

Radiologic Signs
1. *Sonography* demonstrates a cystic mass that usually cannot be assigned to a specific organ.
2. *Upright abdominal film* is useful for excluding bowel obstruction.

Note: The anatomic location of the duplication usually cannot be established from contrast studies!

Internal Hernias (see Sect. 2.2.4)

5.3.3 Other Causes of Abdominal Complaints

- *Diseases of the kidneys and urinary tract* such as urolithiasis, glomerulonephritis, urinary tract infection, hydronephrosis, and megaureter
- *Testicular torsion:*
  Sudden onset of rapidly increasing pain in the scrotum that radiates to the groin and lower abdomen.
  Shock symptoms. Erythema and swelling of the affected half of the scrotum indicates the acuteness of the condition → sonography!
  Incarcerated inguinal hernia must be considered in differential diagnosis.
- *Tumors*
  Tumors can produce the picture of an acute abdomen; the most common symptoms are abdominal pain and vomiting.
  - *Retroperitoneal tumors:*
    Neuroblastoma, nephroblastoma (Wilm's tumor)
  - *Intraperitoneal masses:*
    Duplications of the gastrointestinal tract (see Sect. 3.2.4)
    Non-Hodgkin's lymphoma of the bowel
    Posttraumatic pseudocysts of the pancreas
    Choledochal cysts
    Ovarian tumors
    Trichobezoar with gastric obstruction in neoropathic children

5.3.4 Recurring Abdominal Pain

- *Umbilical colic*
  Recurring bouts of colicky midabdominal pain for which a specific organic cause cannot be established. In rare cases an anomaly is discovered on radiographic contrast examination of the digestive tract.
- *Gastric or duodenal ulcer*
  Has assumed growing causal significance in patients with acute epigastric complaints.
- *Intermittent jejuno-jejunal intussusception* (see Sect. 5.2.2)
- *Catarrhal terminal ileitis* (hypertrophy and hyperplasia of Peyer's patches)
  Severe, colicky lower abdominal pain, at times accompanied by vomiting. Can be diagnosed radiologically by fractionated UGI series. Lesion is distinct from Croh's terminal ileitis.
- *Chilaiditi's syndrome* and *splenic flexure syndrome*
  Normal variant in which colon is interposed between the liver and diaphragm (Chilaiditi's syndrome). A corresponding condition may exist on the left side involving the higher-lying splenic flexure.

Radiologic Signs
Transient pathologic gas collection in the splenic flexure of the colon, possibly associated with temporary obstructive symptoms

Note: When serious abdominal distress is present, the finding of gaseous distension in the splenic or hepatic flexure should not be misinterpreted as free intraperitoneal air.

References

Bätz W, Hofmann-v. Kapherr S, Koltai JL, Pistor G (1985) Mesenterialzysten im Kindesalter. Monatsschr Kinderheilkd 133: 887

Berdon WE, Baker DH, Leonidas J (1968) Advantages of prone positioning in gastrointestinal and genitourinary roentgenologic studies in infants and children. AJR 103: 444

Blank E, Afshani E, Girdany BR, Pappas A (1974) "Windsock signs" of congenital membranous atresia of the colon. AJR 120: 330

Bowerman RA, Silver TM, Jaffe M (1982) Real-time ultrasound diagnosis of intussusception in children. Radiology 143: 527

Buffard P, Defrenne P (1961) Les possibilités de diagnostic des affections digestives du nouveau-né et du nourrisson. Par l'étude du simple contraste gazeux naturel. Arch Mal App Dig 50: 121

Caffey J (1985) Pediatric X-ray diagnosis, 8th edn. Year Book Medical Publishers, Chicago

Cipel L (1978) Radiology of the acute abdomen in the newborn. Grune and Stratton, New York

Ebel KD, Willich E (1979) Die Röntgenuntersuchung im Kindesalter, 2nd edn. Springer, Berlin Heidelberg New York

Griscom NT, Colodny AH, Rosenberg HK, Fliegel C, Hardy B (1979) Diagnostic aspects of neonatal ascites: report of 27 cases. AJR 128: 961

Grob M (1982) Kinderchirurgie, 2nd edn. Thieme, Stuttgart

Hatch EI Jr (1985) The acute abdomen in children. Pediatr Clin North Am 32: 1151

Lassrich MA, Prevôt R (1983) Röntgendiagnostik des Verdauungstraktes bei Kindern und Erwachsenen, 2nd edn. Thieme, Stuttgart

Leonidas JC, Harris DJ, Amoury RA (1975) How accurate is the roentgen diagnosis of acute appendicitis in children? Ann Radiol 4: 497

Meradji M, van Herreweghe M (1980) The plain film of the acute abdomen in the neonate and infant. J Belge Radiol 63: 42

Schumacher R (1982) Sonographische Diagnostik der hypertrophen Pylorusstenose. Kinderarzt 11: 1673

Swischuk LE (1979) Emergency radiology of the acutely ill or injured child. Williams and Wilkins, Baltimore

Wolf HG (1971) Das akute Abdomen in der Pädiatrie. Marseille, München

6 Evaluation of Imaging Procedures in the Diagnosis of Acute Abdomen

D. BEYER, U. MÖDDER, H. PICHLMAIER

We emphasize the fact that a thorough clinical examination with history taking is a necessary prelude to the selection of a diagnostic imaging procedure. This is the only way that we can "tailor" the diagnostic approach to the individual patient. The following evaluation and recommendation for a staged application of imaging procedures is marked by our personal experience with these modalities. To follow this scheme effectively, it is necessary to have a fully equipped radiology department with facilities for sonography, computed tomography, and angiography on a "round-the-clock" basis.

If two or more imaging procedures have an equivalent diagnostic value in a particular disorder, the physician should first use the method that is least invasive, least time-consuming, and most economical in order to confirm or refute the clinical impression.

The diagnostic workup *ends* when a diagnosis is made!

It is important that time-consuming and cost-intensive studies like CT and angiography be performed *completely* (e.g., CT with contrast opacification of the bowel and bolus injection) so that the necessity of surgery can be assessed and a plan of treatment devised without having to repeat or supplement the examination.

The main clinical diagnoses that are suggested by acute abdominal symptoms are listed in Table 2, which presents a rational approach to the use of diagnostic imaging procedures. The rating symbols (+ + +) reflect the anticipated diagnostic value of a given method for the presumed disease and generally do not correspond to the recommended sequence of the diagnostic procedures (①, ②, ③).

Thus, for example, it is appropriate to place CT with bolus injection only third in the sequence of investigations when pancreatitis is suspected, even though the table gives the procedure a + + + + rating in this setting. This is because sonography (1) can in many cases demonstrate or exclude acute pancreatitis, provided the pancreas is visible on the scans. The 2nd choice, plain radiography, evaluates for possible perforation or the gastrointestinal tract and the presence of fluid levels. CT (3) demonstrates the total extent of retroperitoneal exudation, enables a classification of grade 2 or 3 disease when a bolus injection is used, and therefore can direct the surgeon in selecting patients and planning the operation.

Although CT is frequently the best modality for demonstrating the pathoanatomic substrate of a disease, factors of time and cost *preclude* its use on a routine basis.

Clinical impression	Plain radio-graphy	Contrast examina-tion	Sono-graphy	CT **	Angio
Perforation of an intra-abdominal hollow viscus	① + + + + (no barium!)	+ Gastro-grafin	+	+	∅
Acute diseases of the gallbladder	②[a] +	(+) Cholecys-tography	① + + + +	+ +	∅
Acute pancreatitis	② +[a]	(+) Gastro-grafin	① + + +	③ + + + + (bolus injection)	∅
Diffuse peritonitis	① + + +	(+) Gastro-grafin	+	+ +	∅
Acute appendicitis	+[a]	∅	+ + + +	+ +	∅
Intraperitoneal abscess	②[a] + +	(+) Gastro-grafin	① + + +	③ + + + +	∅
Extraperitoneal abscess	② + +[a]	+ + Urogram	① + + +	③ + + + +	∅
Mechanical small-bowel obstruction	① + + + +	② + + + Gastro-grafin	③ + + +	(+)	∅
Mechanical colon obstruction	① + + + +	② + + + Contrast enema	+	(+)	∅
Intestinal pseudo-obstruction	① + +	② + + + + Gastro-grafin	∅	∅	∅
Acute intestinal ischemia	① + +	+ Gastro-grafin	② + +	+ +	③ + + + +
Toxic megacolon	① + + + +	∅	∅	∅	∅
Upper and lower gastrointestinal hemorrhage	+[a]	(+)	(+)	(+)	+ + +
Intramural bleeding	① + +	+ Gastro-grafin	② + + +	+ +	∅
Acute intraperitoneal hemorrhage	②[a] +	∅	① + + + +	Peritoneal lavage! + +	+
Renal colic	① + + + (plain film before ②)	② + + + Urogram	+ +	∅	∅

Clinical impression	Plain radio-graphy	Contrast examina-tion	Sono-graphy	CT **	Angio
Suspected penetration of abdominal aortic aneurysm	+[a]	∅	① ++	+++ (if time!)	∅
Blunt abdominal trauma	① +[a]	∅	② ++++	③ ++++	∅
Sharp, penetrating trauma	∅	∅	(+)	(+)	∅
Lesions of the abdominal wall and back with acute abdomen	(+)	∅	① +++	② ++++	∅
Acute diseases of the lesser pelvis	+[a]	++ Urogram	① ++++	② +++ (check for pregnancy!)	∅
Acute postoperative abdomen	① +++	++ Gastro-grafin	② ++	③ +++	∅
Foreign body	① ++ (if radio-paque!)	+ Gastro-grafin	+	++	∅
Acute abdomen in children	① +++	② ++	③ +++	(+) Trauma	∅

[a] To exclude perforation of an intra-abdominal hollow viscus
[b] To date (May 1988) there is no recognized indication for MRI in the acute abdomen!
[c] Gastrografin (Schering) water-soluble sodium amidotrizoate, meglumine amidotrizoate (370 mg iodine/ml)

7 Subject Index

MIX
Papier aus verantwortungsvollen Quellen
Paper from responsible sources
FSC® C105338

If you have any concerns about our products,
you can contact us on
ProductSafety@springernature.com

In case Publisher is established outside the EU,
the EU authorized representative is:
Springer Nature Customer Service Center GmbH
Europaplatz 3, 69115 Heidelberg, Germany

Printed by Libri Plureos GmbH
in Hamburg, Germany